Nonparametric Statistics for Health Care Research

Second Edition

SAGE was founded in 1965 by Sara Miller McCune to support the dissemination of usable knowledge by publishing innovative and high-quality research and teaching content. Today, we publish more than 850 journals, including those of more than 300 learned societies, more than 800 new books per year, and a growing range of library products including archives, data, case studies, reports, conference highlights, and video. SAGE remains majority-owned by our founder, and after Sara's lifetime will become owned by a charitable trust that secures our continued independence.

Los Angeles | London | New Delhi | Singapore | Washington DC

Nonparametric Statistics for Health Care Research

Statistics for Small Samples and Unusual Distributions

Second Edition

Marjorie A. Pett
University of Utah School of Medicine and School of Nursing

SAGE

Los Angeles | London | New Delhi
Singapore | Washington DC

SAGE

Los Angeles | London | New Delhi
Singapore | Washington DC

FOR INFORMATION:

SAGE Publications, Inc.
2455 Teller Road
Thousand Oaks, California 91320
E-mail: order@sagepub.com

SAGE Publications Ltd.
1 Oliver's Yard
55 City Road
London EC1Y 1SP
United Kingdom

SAGE Publications India Pvt. Ltd.
B 1/I 1 Mohan Cooperative Industrial Area
Mathura Road, New Delhi 110 044
India

SAGE Publications Asia-Pacific Pte. Ltd.
3 Church Street
#10-04 Samsung Hub
Singapore 049483

Acquisitions Editor: Vicki Knight
Editorial Assistant: Yvonne Mcduffee
eLearning Editor: Robert Higgins
Production Editor: Laura Barrett
Copy Editor: Gillian Dickens
Typesetter: C&M Digitals (P) Ltd.
Proofreader: Jen Grubba
Indexer: Jeanne Busemeyer
Cover Designer: Anupama Krishnan
Marketing Manager: Nicole Elliott

Printed in the United States of America

Library of Congress Cataloging-in-Publication Data

Pett, Marjorie A.

Nonparametric statistics for health care research: statistics for small samples and unusual distributions/Marjorie A. Pett, University of Utah College of Nursing. — Second edition.

pages cm
Includes bibliographical references and index.

ISBN 978-1-4522-8196-4 (pbk. : alk. paper)
1. Medicine—Statistical methods. 2. Nonparametric statistics. I. Title.

R853.S7P48 2016
610.72'7–dc23 2015022872

This book is printed on acid-free paper.

SFI Certified Sourcing
www.sfiprogram.org
SFI-00453

15 16 17 18 19 10 9 8 7 6 5 4 3 2 1

Brief Contents

Preface ix
Acknowledgments xiv
About the Author xv

1. Overview of Nonparametric Statistics 1
2. The Process of Statistical Hypothesis Testing 7
3. Evaluating the Characteristics of Data 17
4. "Goodness-of-Fit" Tests 47
5. Tests for Two Related Samples: Pretest-Posttest Measures for a Single Sample 91
6. Repeated Measures for More Than Two Time Periods or Matched Conditions 123
7. Tests for Two Independent Samples 152
8. Assessing Differences Among Several Independent Groups 201
9. Tests of Association Between Variables 269
10. Logistic Regression 323
11. Epilogue 397

Appendix: Statistical Tables 403
References 411
Author Index 428
Subject Index 437

Contents

Preface ix

Acknowledgments xiv

About the Author xv

1. Overview of Nonparametric Statistics 1

Common Characteristics of Parametric Tests 1
Development of Nonparametric Tests 2
Characteristics of Nonparametric Statistics 3
Use of Nonparametric Tests in Health Care Research 4
Some Common Misperceptions About Nonparametric Tests 5
Types of Nonparametric Tests 6

2. The Process of Statistical Hypothesis Testing 7

Choosing Between a Parametric and a Nonparametric Test 12

3. Evaluating the Characteristics of Data 17

Characteristics of Levels of Measurement 17
Assessing the Normality of a Distribution 21
Dealing With Outliers 35
Data Transformation Considerations 38
Examining Homogeneity of Variance 39
Evaluating Sample Sizes 42
Reporting Testing Assumptions and Violations in a Research Report 44
Summary 44

4. "Goodness-of-Fit" Tests 47

The Binomial Test 47
The Chi-Square Goodness-of-Fit Test 61
The Kolmogorov-Smirnov One-Sample Test 76

The Kolmogorov-Smirnov Two-Sample Test 83
Summary 89

5. Tests for Two Related Samples: Pretest-Posttest Measures for a Single Sample 91

The McNemar Test 92
The Sign Test 101
The Wilcoxon Signed-Ranks Test 111
Summary 120

6. Repeated Measures for More Than Two Time Periods or Matched Conditions 123

Cochran's *Q* Test 124
The Friedman Test 135
Summary 149

7. Tests for Two Independent Samples 152

Fisher's Exact Test 153
The Chi-Square Test for Two Independent Samples 164
The Wilcoxon-Mann-Whitney *U* Test 177
Summary 197

8. Assessing Differences Among Several Independent Groups 201

The Chi-Square Test for *k* Independent Samples 202
The Mantel-Haenszel Chi-Square Test for Trends 218
The Median Test 225
The Kruskal-Wallis One-Way ANOVA by Ranks 235
The Two-Way ANOVA by Ranks 251
Summary 265

9. Tests of Association Between Variables 269

The Phi Coefficient 269
Cramér's *V* Coefficient 276
The Kappa Coefficient 281
The Point Biserial Correlation 293
The Spearman Rank-Order Correlation Coefficient 301
Kendall's Tau Coefficient 311
Summary 319

10. Logistic Regression 323

The Logic of Logistic Regression 324
The Odds Ratio and Relative Risk 329
Simple Bivariate Logistic Regression 335
Multiple Logistic Regression 361

11. Epilogue 397

Nonparametric Statistical Procedures Identified in This Text 397
Some Promising Nonparametric Statistics 400

Appendix: Statistical Tables 403

References 411

Author Index 428

Subject Index 437

Preface

Consider this scenario: You have a wonderful idea for a health care intervention that you believe will have a strong positive impact on a particular client outcome. You work in a setting in which such an intervention can be undertaken feasibly. There is even an available comparison group that could receive usual patient care, *and* there is a pre- and posttreatment measure that is a reliable and valid assessment of the outcome in which you are interested. What more could a researcher in health care ask for? Your sample size is not so large as you would like—there are only 10 patients per group—but, realistically, given the setting, time constraints, and lack of funding, this is about as large as this sample is likely to be.

You undertake this study, collect the data, choose your statistical package, and are ready to determine the most appropriate statistics to use in this study. What statistics should you use? Not a problem, you think. Both your textbook on statistics and your software package indicate that there are plenty of tests to choose from. There are ANOVAs, ANCOVAs, and MANOVAs. There are also *t* tests, Pearson correlations, and multiple regression analyses. You recall that all these tests are labeled *parametric* and that they are based on some important assumptions, not the least of which is an adequate total sample size, a certain level of measurement, and a normal distribution of the dependent variable. Your study has violated a number of these assumptions.

Does this sound familiar? It should. This problem is relatively common in the health care research literature. That is, the research was undertaken on a limited budget, using a small sample of convenience, in a health care setting by a researcher whose primary interests are improving patient care and facilitating more satisfactory patient outcomes. Given these necessary limitations, it is inevitable that much of health care research is beset with potentially serious violations of the assumptions of parametric statistics. Unfortunately, most statistics textbooks at both the undergraduate and graduate levels tend to focus on parametric statistics, reserving only a few pages for their nonparametric counterparts. Most researchers in health care, therefore, have had limited exposure to alternatives to parametric tests. Yet it is the selection and interpretation of the most appropriate statistical tests which enable researchers to assess the effectiveness of a particular intervention. It is critical, therefore, that researchers be knowledgeable about the use and potential for misuse of parametric tests in health care research, know when to use such statistical techniques, and be aware of the availability of *nonparametric* alternatives when assumptions of parametric tests have been violated.

WHAT THIS TEXTBOOK IS

The purpose of this book is to present practical information concerning the most commonly used nonparametric statistical techniques that are available in user-friendly statistical computer packages and open-resource statistical websites via the Internet. The book's intention is to help the reader to understand when a particular nonparametric statistic would be used appropriately, to learn how to generate and interpret the computer printouts resulting from the application of this statistic, and to present the results of the analysis in table and text format.

For the sake of consistency, organization, and ease of use, two approaches to statistical analysis will be used throughout this textbook: IBM SPSS® Statistics[1] for Windows and the Mac (v. 22–23) and various free-access Internet resources. I realize that users of other equally suitable statistical computer packages (e.g., Excel, SAS, R, AMOS, Minitab, Stata, and SYSTAT) may initially view this conscious choice of a single environment to be disappointing and potentially restricting. They might even argue that the use of a single statistical package such as SPSS for Windows and the Mac severely limits the content area to that of the behavioral sciences.

During my more than 35 years' experience teaching and conducting research in the health care field, I have taught—and used—a variety of statistical computer packages (e.g., Excel, SPSS, SAS, LISREL, and AMOS) designed to answer different research questions. I have found that the statistical package of choice is often based more on the comfort level, knowledge, and statistical needs of the researcher than on the specific content area of his or her research interests. That is, SPSS is not just a tool for the behavioral sciences; it can also be used to help answer many key questions in such diverse areas as biology, economics, education, administration, geography, and zoology. Bottom line, despite our differences in choice of statistical package, the approach to examination and interpretation of the generated computer printouts will not change. I believe that you will find the information provided in the text will better enable you to select the most appropriate nonparametric test for your data in your particular research area of interest, whatever that may be. For those of you who prefer to use SAS, I have posted SAS syntax and output for all of the examples given in each chapter on the SAGE website (study.sagepub.com/pett2e).

It could also be argued that the free Internet resources that I am using today may be unavailable tomorrow. Despite that very real possibility, it is my opinion that we cannot ignore the many free Internet statistical analysis websites that were unavailable to us just a few short years ago. Certainly, a given site may fade from existence, but in its place will emerge other even more useful and free sites in the future.

1. SPSS is a registered trademark of International Business Machines Corporation.

WHAT THIS TEXTBOOK IS NOT

This textbook is *not* intended to be a replacement for the many invaluable quantitatively oriented textbooks on nonparametric statistics that offer more in-depth explanations and calculations of various nonparametric statistics. It was also not feasible to present in-depth discussions of some of the more challenging approaches to statistical analyses (e.g., kernel density estimation, expanded permutation tests, and time-to-event analyses). Rather, the intention is to provide the reader with a practical step-by-step approach to the application of the more readily available nonparametric statistics to clinically relevant research problems. Nevertheless, a brief discussion and references for these more challenging nonparametric approaches to statistical analyses are presented in Chapter 11. Additional resources can also be found throughout all chapters of this textbook.

While much of the focus of the textbook will be on statistics for "small" samples, the content presented in the text is *not* restricted to small sample applications. Much of what is discussed in the text applies to larger samples as well, particularly those with unusual distributions. A number of the presented examples will use larger data sets (e.g., $n > 30$). All data sets used in the examples are available to the reader on the SAGE website, study.sagepub.com/pett2e.

CHANGES/ADDITIONS TO THE FIRST EDITION

When I first embarked on a second edition to this textbook, I thought the revision would be a relatively easy task: I would update the chapters with the latest edition of the computer package, add a chapter on logistic regression, and be "home free." How naïve I was! So much has changed in both the statistical software and Internet environments since I completed the first edition back in 1997. To be responsible to you, the reader, it was imperative for me to undertake an extensive rewrite of the textbook. Hopefully, you will recognize that while the structure of the first edition has remained stable, additional content has been systematically added (e.g., confidence intervals, estimations/evaluations of effect sizes, and identification of useful Internet resources). In-depth material on other nonparametric multivariate statistics (e.g., two-way ANOVA by ranks and logistic regression) has also been added to this second edition.

In their reviews of the first edition of this textbook, several readers lamented the fact that tables of critical values for a given statistic had been omitted from the appendixes. These tables had been omitted deliberately in an attempt to avoid potentially overwhelming increases in page length. This omission has been corrected for the most commonly used nonparametric statistics and those for which a resource table was not available on the Internet. These tables can now be found in the Appendix. In addition, copies of the output and data sets for both SPSS and SAS are available for each chapter on the SAGE website (study.sagepub.com/pett2e). "Test Your Knowledge" and "Computer Exercises" have been added to the end of Chapters 1 to 10 to help reinforce the reader's understanding of the chapter material.

THOSE WHO MAY FIND THE TEXT USEFUL

This book is intended to be read by researchers, students, and professionals from a variety of settings and disciplines who do not necessarily have strong mathematics backgrounds but who are interested in finding reasonable and practical alternatives to parametric statistics when their data do not meet the assumptions of these tests. For that reason, presentation of mathematical formulas has been kept to a minimum.

This book is written at a level easily understood by people who have had at least a beginning course in statistics and therefore possess some familiarity with the concepts of levels of measurement, statistical hypothesis testing, shapes of distributions, outliers, various parametric statistics, and statistical power. For those readers who are unfamiliar with these topics, a close reading of Chapters 2 and 3 is strongly recommended. Additional resource references are provided in these chapters for further readings on these topics. Because nonparametric statistics have a particular usefulness in health care research, the examples given throughout the text have been directed to that area. Readers who have other research interests (e.g., studying kangaroo monkeys in the wild), however, should find that much of the information provided also applies to their areas of focus.

ORGANIZATION OF THE TEXT

This book consists of 11 chapters. Chapter 1 presents an overview of the development of nonparametric tests, a comparison of the characteristics of parametric and nonparametric tests, the use and common misperceptions of nonparametric statistics in health care research, and their current availability in statistical packages for personal computers. Chapter 2 examines the issues that are crucial in choosing the best statistical test given a particular data set. Included in the discussion is a brief review of the process of statistical hypothesis testing and an outline of criteria useful for choosing the most appropriate statistical test. Chapter 3 presents ways to evaluate the characteristics of data, such as level of measurement, normality of distributions, assessment of outliers, homogeneity of variance, and adequacy of sample size.

Chapters 4 through 10 each examine a particular set of nonparametric statistics using a common presentation format: the purpose of the particular statistic, a research question that could be answered using the statistic, an example of null and alternative hypotheses that would follow from the research question, an overview of the test procedure, a discussion of the test's underlying assumptions and limitations, the SPSS (and appropriate Internet website) commands used to generate the statistic, interpretations of the resulting computer printout, suggested ways to present the results in tabular and written formats, and examples from the published research literature from a variety of health care disciplines (e.g., exercise and sports science, health education, medicine, nursing, psychology, and social work) that have used the statistic in their analyses. Substantive references that provide further information about the statistic are located at the end of the textbook.

The reader will note that Chapter 10 consists of a presentation of logistic regression (LR) analysis. While some readers may question the presence of LR in a textbook on nonparametric statistical techniques ("How *is* logistic regression a nonparametric technique?"), it has been included in this textbook because it is an increasingly popular nonparametric alternative to ordinary least squares (OLS) linear regression when the outcome variable of interest is categorical, especially dichotomous. Chapter 11 presents a summary reference guide to the nonparametric statistics presented in the text, an identification of their parametric alternatives, and a discussion of promising nonparametric alternatives to parametric techniques that, hopefully, will soon find their way into more commonly used statistical computer packages. Although these chapters may appear to be a "cookbook" approach to the applications of nonparametric statistics, it is intended that the reader will become familiar with the use, logic, assumptions, and interpretations of these applications.

It should be noted that a critical assumption of *all* parametric and nonparametric tests is that the data be obtained from a random sample. Because of its universality, the assumption of random sampling will not be repeated for all the nonparametric tests discussed in this text. This is, however, an important assumption, especially when assessing generalizability of the obtained results. Without random selection, the ability of the researcher to assess the representativeness of his or her sample may be compromised.

So, sit back, open the book to Chapter 1, and let's begin our adventure into the exploration of nonparametric statistics for small samples *and* unusual distributions.

Acknowledgments

There are many people to whom I am very much indebted for helping to make this text a reality. First, I would like to thank the faculty in the College of Nursing at the University of Utah (Lauren Clark and Jia-Wen Guo in particular) for their patience and support not only for this text but also for our continued relationship. I am appreciative as well to the many graduate students in the health sciences and nursing, especially those who were willing to expand their creative thinking and skills to "embrace"—albeit at times reluctantly—the many challenges and potential rewards offered by statistics.

I am most indebted to Vicki Knight, SAGE Publications publisher for research methods, statistics, and evaluation, for her patience, determination, doggedness, and good humor. Without your perseverance, this second edition would have been just an afterthought. Thanks, too, to the staff at SAGE Publications and the reviewers for their helpful editing, suggestions, and critiques:

- Guogen Shan, University of Nevada Las Vegas
- Linda Highfield, PhD, MS, University of Texas School of Public Health Houston
- Jareen Meinzen-Derr, Cincinnati Children's Hospital Medical Center
- Justice Mbizo, The University of West Florida
- James H. Swan, University of North Texas

This book is dedicated to my husband Art—thanks for sharing both the dining room table and other parts of your busy life with the latest version of this manuscript.

About the Author

Marjorie A. Pett, MStat, DSW, is a Research Professor in the College of Nursing at the University of Utah, Salt Lake City, Utah, having been on the faculty since 1980. By her own admission, she is a "collector" of academic degrees: BA (Brown University), MS in sociology (University of Stockholm, Sweden), MSW (Smith College), DSW (University of Utah), and MStat (Biostatistics) (University of Utah).

Dr. Pett has a strong commitment to facilitating the practical application of statistics in the social, behavioral, and biological sciences, especially among practitioners in health care settings. She has designed and taught graduate courses to students from a variety of disciplines at the beginning and advanced levels, including research design and data management, parametric and nonparametric statistics, biostatistics, multivariate statistics, instrument development, and factor analysis. She has tried to approach the teaching of statistics with humor and from a clinician's perspective and has been the recipient of several distinguished teaching awards both at the college and university levels.

Her most recent research interests include the development of client-centered assessment tools and interventions to evaluate and enhance health-related quality of life (HRQoL) for persons with intellectual disabilities. She is the author of numerous research articles and chapters and is an author of *Making Sense of Factor Analysis: The Use of Factor Analysis for Instrument Development in Health Care Research*.

When not engaged in research, writing, or teaching, Marge is a (now retired) state soccer referee, devotee of tennis, an avid (high handicap) golfer, student of Italian and French, reader of mystery novels, grandmother to three, mother to two, and wife to (only) one.

CHAPTER 1

Overview of Nonparametric Statistics

Historically, the most popular statistical inferential techniques that have appeared in the research literature are those that make assumptions about the nature of the populations from which the data are drawn. These techniques are called *parametric* statistics because of their focus on specific parameters of the population, especially the population mean and variance.

COMMON CHARACTERISTICS OF PARAMETRIC TESTS

Parametric tests share a number of common characteristics (see Box 1.1). First, it is expected that there is independence of observations except when the data are paired. The data also are expected to be randomly drawn from a normally distributed, or bell-shaped, population of values. This condition is actually a proxy for the *real* assumption that the distributions of the parameters being tested (such as the mean) are normal. It is also expected that the dependent variable being analyzed is measured on at least an interval-level scale. That is, these data are rank ordered and have units or numbers that have equal intervals and whose values share similar meanings (e.g., a person's weight, a score on a depression scale that ranges from 1 to 100, or a preterm infant's heart rate).

Given that these data are assumed to be normally distributed, it is important to make some assessments of the normality assumption. Although not a requirement, to assess normality, a minimum sample size of approximately 30 subjects per group has been recommended. This traditional and somewhat arbitrary sample size recommendation is linked to the central limit theorem, which states that even when the population is non-normal, the sampling distribution of the mean (a critical parameter for parametric tests) becomes more like the normal distribution as the sample size increases (Field, 2009). Moreover, if comparing two or more groups, these sets of data should be drawn from populations having equal variances or spread of scores. The null and research hypotheses are formulated about numerical values, especially the means of a population. A typical null hypothesis is that the populations of interest share a common mean with regard to the dependent variable of interest (e.g., H_0: $\mu_1 = \mu_2$). The alternative or research hypothesis states that the population means are not the same (e.g., H_a: $\mu_1 \neq \mu_2$).

BOX 1.1 Common Characteristics of Parametric Tests

- Independence of observations, except when the data are paired
- The observations for the dependent variable have been randomly drawn from a normally distributed population
- The dependent variable is measured on at least an interval-level scale; that is, one that is rank ordered and has equidistant numbers, with the numbers sharing similar meaning
- A minimum sample size of approximately 30 subjects per group is recommended
- Data are drawn from populations having equal variances (rule of thumb: one variance cannot be twice as large as the other)
- Usually hypotheses are made about numerical values, especially the mean of a population (μ), for example:

$$H_0 : \mu_1 = \mu_2$$

$$H_a : \mu_1 \neq \mu_2$$

- Other possible requirements: nominal or interval-level independent variable, homoscedasticity, and equal cell sizes

Some parametric tests have additional requirements. These include assumptions regarding the level of measurement for the independent variables (nominal for analysis of variance [ANOVA], at least interval for Pearson product moment correlations), homoscedasticity, and equal cell sizes. *Homoscedasticity* implies that for every level of the independent variable, the dependent variable has a similar variance.

If a parametric test is the statistical technique of choice, the results should be, but unfortunately are not often, presented with this caveat:

> *If our assumptions concerning the shape of the population distributions are valid, we may conclude that. . .*

Because of this common set of assumptions, parametric tests are thought to be more clearly systematized, easier to apply, and supposedly easier to teach, although those of us who have taught or have taken classes in parametric statistics may think otherwise. Parametric tests, therefore, have been extremely popular in the research literature, almost to the point of excluding any other techniques.

DEVELOPMENT OF NONPARAMETRIC TESTS

Some alternative tests of statistical inference do not make numerous or stringent assumptions about the population from which the data have been sampled. These techniques have been called *distribution-free* or *nonparametric* tests. A substantial body of published information exists concerning these tests. A search of Google Scholar, for example, yielded 106,000 results related to nonparametric statistics, of which about 26,500 have been published since 2000.

A common misperception about nonparametric statistics is that they are relative newcomers to the statistics arena. This is not the case. Singer (1979) points out that, historically, parametric and nonparametric statistics appear to have been developed conjointly. In an entertaining overview of the historical development of nonparametric statistics, Singer indicates that the first attempt at hypothesis testing using a statistical test was undertaken by Artbuthnot in 1710. The procedure that was used was the nonparametric sign test. Singer also points out that Artbuthnot was friends with DeMoivre, the man who has been credited with first describing the normal distribution. It appears, therefore, that some of the best friends of statisticians of parametric persuasion are their nonparametric colleagues.

Despite having developed simultaneously, parametric and nonparametric tests have not shared the same popularity. Perhaps the term *nonparametric* implies that there is something lacking in nonparametric statistics, thus contributing to these statistics' second-class status among researchers. Even as early as the 1920s, however, there was concern expressed about the exclusive reliance on the normal distribution in the research literature. Singer (1979) reports that Karl Pearson, the man credited with naming the bell-shaped distribution as *normal*, warned that the normal distribution "has the disadvantage of leading people to believe that all other distributions of frequencies are in one sense or another 'abnormal' . . . that belief is, of course, not justifiable" (p. 289). It is interesting that Pearson made that comment more than 90 years ago, yet researchers still seem to hold that belief today.

BOX 1.2 Common Characteristics of Nonparametric Tests

- Independence of randomly selected observations, except paired
- Few assumptions of the population distribution
- The scale of measurement of the dependent variable may be categorical or ordinal
- The primary focus is on either the rank ordering or the frequencies of data
- Hypotheses are most often posed regarding ranks, medians, or frequencies of data
- Sample size requirements are less stringent than for parametric tests

CHARACTERISTICS OF NONPARAMETRIC STATISTICS

Just because these nonparametric or distribution-free tests do not have the strict assumptions of parametric tests does not mean that nonparametric tests are assumption free (see Box 1.2). Like parametric tests, nonparametric tests assume independence of randomly selected observations except when data are paired. Unlike parametric tests, however, there are limited assumptions required concerning the shape of the population's distribution. Because of the distribution *free-er* nature of the data, the distribution of values for the dependent variable may be very skewed, or nonnormal. That is, distributions can take on any shape and are not limited to the bell shape of the normal distribution. When comparing two or more groups using rank tests, however, the distributions of these values within each group must be similar in shape except for their locations (i.e., medians). The dependent variable may also be categorical or rank ordered (i.e., ordinal).

Examples of categorical data are a person's marital status (married, divorced, or single). Ordinal data could be a person's response on a 7-point Likert-type scale to a question concerning his or her current stress level (1 = *not at all stressed* to 7 = *extremely stressed*). Chapter 3 of this text reviews the levels of measurement of variables in greater detail.

In nonparametric tests, the primary focus is either on the *rank ordering* of scores, not their actual values, or on the *frequencies* or classification of data. The hypotheses that are posed, therefore, concern ranks, medians, or frequencies, not population means. Sample size requirements also are less stringent for nonparametric tests. It is not unusual for sample sizes of 20 or less to be reported.

A considerable body of research has indicated that parametric tests are more powerful than nonparametric tests only if the assumptions of the parametric test under consideration have been met. When choosing the most appropriate statistical test, therefore, it is important to examine carefully the extent to which the data to be analyzed adequately meet the test's assumptions. It is also necessary to evaluate the consequences of violating certain assumptions underlying the test that the researcher is considering.

No data will perfectly meet all of a test's assumptions. For example, the collected data may have a skewed or flat (i.e., nonnormal) distribution. Although some parametric tests are *robust* and can withstand certain violations of their assumptions, other tests are not so flexible. In the latter situation, the parametric test may be a poor choice in contrast to its nonparametric counterpart.

Statistics are tools designed to help the researcher in health care to make informed decisions about the outcomes of potentially important interventions. It is ultimately the client who pays the price for poorly planned and executed statistical analyses.

USE OF NONPARAMETRIC TESTS IN HEALTH CARE RESEARCH

Nonparametric statistics have a high potential for use in health care research. Their acceptance of small sample sizes, use of categorical- or ordinal-level data, and ability to accommodate unusual or irregular sampling distributions make them plausible alternatives to the more stringent parametric tests. Unfortunately, however, although most statisticians might agree on the need for both classes of tests in health care research, the reality is that nonparametric tests have been underused in research from a variety of disciplines.

Several years ago, for example, Gaither and Glorfeld (1985) reported that in an examination of 1,102 articles that appeared in the organizational behavior journals from 1976 to 1981, parametric tests dominated as the tests of choice. Only 169, or 9.3%, of the 1,824 statistical procedures used in these articles were nonparametric. The most common nonparametric procedures applied were the chi-square tests of independence and goodness of fit. These two tests accounted for 92 (54.4%) of the 169 nonparametric tests reported.

Horton and Switzer (2005) reported similar findings regarding chi-square tests in a more recent study of original research articles published in the *New England Journal of Medicine* for the years 2004–2005. Of the 311 articles that were reviewed, 265 articles reported having used at least one nonparametric statistical technique, 165 (53%) of which were contingency or chi-square analyses. Comparing the years 1978–1979, 1989, and 2004–2005, the authors reported an increase in the use of chi-square and Mann-Whitney tests but not nonparametric measures of association or other nonparametric tests. They also noted a dramatic increase in the use of more complex statistical techniques (e.g., survival analysis and advanced regression techniques). While the use of these more sophisticated techniques might be attributed to increased sample sizes reported in medical journals (Fagerland, 2012), the authors expressed concern that readers of such articles may lack the statistical skills to interpret and evaluate the appropriateness of such tests.

The scarcity of evidence to support the appropriateness of more sophisticated tests is not a new phenomenon. In an in-depth examination of 100 randomly selected articles identified in the Gaither and Glorfeld (1985) study, the authors concluded that, at best, there was insufficient evidence reported in the journal articles to indicate that the appropriate choice of parametric tests had been made. Conclusions similar to those of Gaither and Glorfeld were reached by D. G. Altman (1991, 2000) in medicine and Jenkins, Fuqua and Froehle (1984) in counseling psychology. As Altman (1994) has lamented,

> What should we think about a doctor who uses the wrong treatment, either willfully or through ignorance, or who uses the right treatment wrongly (such as by giving the wrong dose of a drug)? Most people would agree that such behaviour was unprofessional, arguably unethical, and certainly unacceptable. What, then, should we think about researchers who use the wrong techniques (either willfully or in ignorance), use the right techniques wrongly, misinterpret their results, report their results selectively, cite the literature selectively, and draw unjustified conclusions?
>
> We should be appalled. Yet numerous studies of the medical literature, in both general and specialist journals have shown that all of the above phenomena are common. This is surely a scandal. (p. 283)

These concerns are not at all uncommon and continue to be voiced in research journals from a variety of disciplines (Jin et al., 2010; Merrill, Lindsay, Shields, & Stoddard, 2007; Qualls, Pallin, & Schuur, 2010; Yim, Nahm, Han, & Park, 2010).

SOME COMMON MISPERCEPTIONS ABOUT NONPARAMETRIC TESTS

Why is it that, despite their promise and potential, nonparametric statistics tend to be underused in health care research? Common misperceptions related to nonparametric statistics on the part of readers, reviewers, and authors of research may contribute to the underuse of these statistics. These misperceptions include fears that readers of manuscripts might not understand the statistics and that the manuscripts might not be accepted by editors or reviewers. Some researchers also perceive that nonparametric statistics are inferior to parametric tests, that they are available only for the simplest of research designs, and that few statistical computer packages contain these statistics.

Such misperceptions appear to be related, in part, to a limited exposure to and training in the variety of uses to which nonparametric statistics can be applied. Unfortunately, nonparametric statistics often are relegated to the final pages of a chapter or textbook on statistics. In addition, the evaluation and reporting of the ability of research data to meet the assumptions of parametric tests has been underemphasized despite the availability of user-friendly computer packages that can be used to test underlying test assumptions.

TYPES OF NONPARAMETRIC TESTS

A wide variety of nonparametric tests are available for use in health care research. After reviewing how to decide when to use nonparametric tests in Chapter 2 and evaluating the characteristics of data in Chapter 3, Chapters 4 through 10 will examine specific nonparametric tests that are available for use in most statistical computer packages. These nonparametric tests include those that evaluate "goodness of fit" (Chapter 4), matched samples and repeated measures (Chapter 5), repeated observations across multiple time periods (Chapter 6), differences between two or more independent groups (Chapters 7 and 8), measures of association (Chapter 9), and logistic regression (Chapter 10). Chapter 11 will conclude with a summary table of the statistics reviewed in this text, along with a brief discussion of recent developments in nonparametric statistics.

TEST YOUR KNOWLEDGE

Here is a "test" of your knowledge on the main points of Chapter 1. You will want to review the chapter again should you find that you do not recall the answers to these questions.

1. What are the common characteristics of parametric tests?
2. What are the common characteristics of nonparametric tests?
3. How are the characteristics of a nonparametric test different from that of a parametric test?
4. What are three common misperceptions about nonparametric tests?

Visit **study.sagepub.com/pett2e** to access SAS output, SPSS datasets, SAS datasets, and SAS examples.

CHAPTER 2

The Process of Statistical Hypothesis Testing

A major function of both parametric and nonparametric statistics is statistical inference: We are interested in drawing conclusions about certain characteristics of a population of interest based on observations that we have obtained from a sample. To do this, we undertake the process of statistical hypothesis testing. To better understand this process, let us consider the hypothetical research example that was presented in the preface to this book and briefly examine the procedures that are common to most statistical hypothesis testing.

Recall from the Preface of this book that we are interested in the effects of a particular health care intervention on certain patient outcomes. To be more specific, suppose that we have formulated the following research hypothesis:

> Hospitalized pediatric cancer patients who receive a specially designed staff-initiated intervention to reduce the number of sleep environment interruptions by hospital staff will experience fewer nocturnal awakenings and lower levels of fatigue and distress compared to pediatric cancer patients who do not receive the intervention.

We propose to randomly assign a sample of 20 hospitalized pediatric cancer patients ages 6 to 10 years in equal numbers to one of two conditions (staff-initiated intervention vs. usual care); we will collect pre- and postintervention measures of the children's rate of nocturnal awakenings and their self-reported levels of fatigue and distress and then compare the changes in these outcome measures over time in the two groups. We will also document the efficacy of our intervention by recording the total number of sleep environment interruptions throughout the intervention in both groups.

After a careful review of the research literature, we have identified reportedly reliable and valid outcome measures to assess the number of sleep environment interruptions, the frequency of nocturnal sleep awakenings, and self-reported fatigue and distress in this sample of pediatric cancer patients. We were particularly interested in the measures used in a carefully designed study conducted by Hinds and colleagues (Hinds et al., 2007) to assess the relationships among nocturnal awakenings, sleep environment interruptions, sleep duration, and fatigue experienced by hospitalized pediatric cancer patients.

To undertake the test of this research hypothesis, we would follow a seven-step approach suggested in Box 2.1 (Siegel & Castellan, 1988). The reader will find variations in this process depending on the text chosen (Hinkle, Wiersma, & Jurs, 2003; Kellar & Kelvin, 2012; Warner, 2012), but basically the steps are similar. It should also be emphasized that, although they are presented separately, each of these steps is interdependent. For example, availability or unavailability of certain types of data may alter the hypotheses that have been formulated and the statistical tests that are subsequently run.

BOX 2.1 Steps in Statistical Hypothesis Testing

Step Procedure to Be Followed

1. State the null hypothesis (H_0) and its research alternative (H_a).
2. Decide what data to collect and the conditions under which the data will be collected.
3. Specify the significance level (alpha) and determine whether alpha is one- or two-tailed.
4. Identify those statistical tests that would most satisfactorily answer the research questions formulated for the study.
5. Determine the desired sample size (*n*).
6. Collect the data, evaluate their properties, and select (from among the statistical tests identified) those that most satisfactorily meet the requirements for the study and whose assumptions are best met by the collected data.
7. If the research data meet the test's assumptions, compute the value of the test statistic. If the computed value is in the rejection region, reject H_0. If the value falls outside the region of rejection, do not reject H_0.

1. *State the null hypothesis (H_0) and its research alternative (H_a).* The first step in any hypothesis testing procedure is that of stating the null and alternative hypotheses. These hypotheses are formulated and specifically stated for each dependent variable being examined. In our hypothetical example, one set of hypotheses could be stated as follows:

   H_0: There are no differences across time between the intervention and usual-care groups with regard to the children's self-reported levels of fatigue.

   H_a: The intervention group will report a significantly greater reduction in self-reported levels of fatigue across time compared to the usual-services group.

Note that the null hypothesis contains the statement of "no effect" and focuses on a single dependent variable. Since the alternative hypothesis is directional, we probably should also have stated in the null hypothesis that not only are there no differences between the groups but that potentially the usual-care group had a greater reduction in self-reported fatigue than the intervention group. It should also be noted that although the alternative or research hypothesis usually is the true focus of research interest, it is the null hypothesis that is tested in statistical analyses.

2. *Decide what data to collect and the conditions under which the data will be collected.* We propose to collect pre- and postintervention information on a small convenient sample of 20 pediatric cancer patients, ages 6 to 10 years, who have been admitted for treatment during a specified period of time to the children's hospital at which we are employed. The children will be randomly assigned in equal numbers to the intervention and usual-services groups.
3. *Specify the significance level (alpha) and determine whether alpha is one- or two-tailed.* The null hypothesis is the focus of statistical hypothesis testing. Based on the evidence that we have collected from our sample, we will decide to *reject* or *fail to reject* the null hypothesis. Because we are basing this decision on evidence obtained from a sample of observations and not an entire population, we can never be absolutely sure of the correctness of our decision. There is always room for error. Box 2.2 outlines the possible outcomes that can occur when undertaking statistical hypothesis testing.

BOX 2.2 Possible Outcomes Related to Decisions in Hypothesis Testing

	REALITY	
DECISION MADE	*Null hypothesis is really true*	*Null hypothesis is really false*
Fail to reject the null hypothesis	A. Correct decision!	B. Uh, oh . . .
		Type I error (α)
Reject the null hypothesis	C. Uh, oh . . .	D. Correct decision!
	Type II error (β)	

There are four possible outcomes when we decide to reject/fail to reject the null hypothesis (Box 2.2, A–D). Based on our sample evidence, we decide to

A. Fail to reject the null hypothesis when, if we knew "reality," the null hypothesis is really true; this is a correct decision.

B. Reject the null hypothesis when, in reality, the null hypothesis is really true; this is an error.

C. Fail to reject the null hypothesis when, in reality, the null hypothesis is really false; this, too, is an error.

D. Reject the null hypothesis when, in reality, the null hypothesis is really false; this is a correct decision and is known as "power."

There are, therefore, two possible types of decision-making error that could occur. These are called *Type I* and *Type II* errors. As Box 2.2 (cell B), indicates, Type I error occurs when, based on our sample evidence, we decide to reject the null hypothesis when, in fact, if we had evidence from the entire population, we would have ascertained that the null hypothesis was true. For example, we might conclude that, based on our sample evidence, there are differences between the intervention and usual-care groups with regard to changes in self-reported fatigue when in reality, the differences we observed were the result of error or random differences. Type II error (Box 2.2, cell C) occurs when, based on our sample evidence, we fail to reject the null hypothesis when, in fact, the null hypothesis is false. That is, we conclude that the evidence did not detect or demonstrate differences between the two groups with regard to changes in self-reported fatigue when, in fact, if we had evidence from the entire population, we would have found that differences existed.

The rates of occurrence of Type I and Type II errors are inversely related: Given the same sample size, decreasing the likelihood of one type of error will increase the likelihood of the other. In statistical hypothesis testing, the consequences of committing these errors need to be evaluated carefully given the context of the particular research. There are several excellent discussions presented in the statistics literature (Neter, Wasserman, & Whitmore, 1993; Warner, 2012) and on numerous websites (e.g., http://www.ncbi.nlm.nih.gov/pmc/articles/PMC2689604) concerning both the setting of Type I and Type II errors and the use of confidence intervals as an alternative to hypothesis testing in statistical inference.

In selecting the criteria for rejecting the null hypothesis, the researcher first needs to decide on the level of significance for his or her particular study. This level of significance, or alpha (α) level, represents the probability that the researcher will make a Type I error, the mistake of saying that differences exist between groups when in fact there are no differences.

Alpha must be set prior to conducting the study. Traditionally in health care research, alpha is set at .05, but as indicated, alpha could be set at any level depending on how serious it would be to make a Type I error. The statement "$\alpha = .05$" indicates that we are willing to make a Type I error 5 times out of 100.

Sometimes, because of the cost or potential negative side effects of the intervention, we might want to be more certain that the observed differences between the groups are not just random error. We might, therefore, set our level of alpha at a more stringent level, for example, $\alpha = .01$. On the other hand, if the study is exploratory and the sample size is small, we might want to identify differences that, although not statistically significant at $\alpha = .05$, might be of clinical interest. In such circumstances, we could set a more liberal alpha, for example, $\alpha = .10$. Remember, however, that if a more liberal alpha is set, the researcher increases the probability of committing a Type II error, or *beta error* (β).

Alpha provides us with guidance as to the conditions under which we will decide to reject or fail to reject the null hypothesis. The larger alpha is, the greater the rejection region of the null hypothesis for the statistic we are considering. Thus, all other things being equal, $\alpha = .05$ will give us greater opportunity to reject the null hypothesis than will $\alpha = .01$.

A second criterion for establishing the rejection region for the null hypothesis is whether our research hypothesis is directional or nondirectional. For example, if the research hypothesis predicts that there will be a difference between two groups but the direction of difference is not stated, the region of rejection, or alpha, is equally divided between two possibilities. Group 1 could do better or worse than Group 2. If, on the other hand, the research hypothesis not only states that there is a difference between the groups but also states the direction of difference (e.g., Group 1 will do better than Group 2), then there is only one region of rejection for the null hypothesis, making alpha one-tailed.

In our hypothetical example, we have decided that, for this study, we will set our alpha (α) at .05. It will be one-tailed because the research hypothesis states that the children in the intervention group will have more satisfactory outcomes than the children in the usual-care group. By stating a direction, we are putting all of our $\alpha = .05$ "in one basket," thus increasing the chances of rejecting the null hypothesis—provided that the differences that we observe between the two groups are in the direction that we have predicted.

4. *Identify those statistical tests that would most satisfactorily answer the research questions formulated for the study.* The identification of a proposed plan for statistical analysis needs to take place prior to any data collection. The identified statistical tests will then provide a basis for determining an appropriate sample size and conducting a power analysis. A full determination of the appropriateness of a particular statistic, however, will be undertaken after the data have been collected.

5. *Determine the desired sample size* (n). Determining the sample size that is appropriate to a particular study is also undertaken prior to conducting the study. This is not an easy task and requires careful consideration of each of the research hypotheses posed and the statistical tests that have been selected for the proposed data analysis. Several computer programs are available to help the researcher to undertake a statistical power analysis to determine the most appropriate sample size for most parametric and nonparametric statistical tests. These programs include G*Power 3 (Faul, Erdfelder, Lang, & Buchner, 2007), PASS 12 (Hintze, 2013), and IBM® SPSS® SamplePower3.0.1 (IBM® SPSS®, 2015). PASS 12 appears to be the most comprehensive in its ability to estimate sample size requirements for nonparametric tests.

In our hypothetical exploratory study, we have determined that, based on financial considerations and necessity, our sample will consist of 20 pediatric oncology patients. Moreover, our sample will not be randomly selected from all possible hospitals in our region but will be limited instead to all eligible pediatric oncology patients, ages 6 to 10 years, who are admitted to a specific hospital for treatment during a stated period of time. We will, however, randomly assign these 20 children in equal numbers to the intervention and usual-services groups, thus maintaining the integrity of our quasi-experimental design.

6. *Collect the data, evaluate their properties, and select from among the statistical tests identified those that most satisfactorily meet the requirements for the study and whose assumptions are best met by the collected data.* We have collected the data on our two groups of children and are set to analyze the results. Now we need to determine which of the statistical tests that we identified in our proposed plan for data analysis would be most appropriate to use given our specific hypotheses and the characteristics of the collected data. We have identified several alternative tests, both parametric and nonparametric, that might be appropriate for our needs. How do we determine which test would be most appropriate for our situation? To make this choice, it is necessary to arrive at some criteria for choosing between a parametric and a nonparametric test.

CHOOSING BETWEEN A PARAMETRIC AND A NONPARAMETRIC TEST

There are both statistical and substantive criteria to be applied when choosing between parametric and nonparametric tests (Harwell, 1988). *Statistical* criteria refer to the test's ability to control the Type I error rate at user-specified alpha levels (e.g., .05) and the power of a particular test. *Substantive* criteria refer to nonstatistical criteria, particularly the level of measurement of the variables under consideration.

Controlling Type I Error Rate

Recall that Type I error rate is the extent to which we incorrectly state that there is a difference between the two groups when in reality there is not a difference. We have set this error rate prior to our collection of data (e.g., $\alpha = .05$). A "good" statistical test will control this alpha at the level we have specified. The ability of a test to control this Type I error, however, depends on the extent to which the data being analyzed meet the underlying assumptions of the test being considered. Certainly no data are perfect (one would be suspicious of data that are!), and certain violations of a test's assumptions are to be expected.

A second consideration in choosing a test, therefore, is the extent to which the test being considered is "robust" with respect to departures from its assumptions. Harwell (1988) cautions that overconfident researchers have tended to rely too heavily on the robust properties of parametric tests and have continued to use them even in the face of serious assumption violations. Monte Carlo evaluation procedures have indicated that, with a sufficient sample size (e.g., $N > 30$ per group), some tests such as analysis of variance (ANOVA) are fairly robust even in the face of substantial departures from normality and other assumption violations. Other tests, however (e.g., analysis of covariance [ANCOVA], repeated-measures ANOVA, and multiple regression), are less able to withstand serious deviations from their assumptions.

Given the potential hazards of violating departures from normality, it is extremely important that the researcher consider the nature of the population from which the sample was drawn and whether it is realistic to expect that this population is, in truth, normally distributed. For example, would the preintervention self-reported fatigue scores for our target population of all 6- to 10-year-old hospitalized oncology patients undergoing radiation be normally distributed, or would it actually be negatively skewed, with a higher density of scores on the upper end of the fatigue scale?

We have already decided that, by necessity, our sample will be small. If we had, however, determined that we had sufficient funding to use a much larger sample, we would also need to consider the consequences of electing to use nonparametric rather than parametric tests. Fagerland (2012), for example, undertook a simulation study that compared the rejection rates for increasing sample sizes and skewed distributions of the Wilcoxon-Mann-Whitney (WMW) two-sample test and that of the independent *t* test. The findings indicated that the WMW test resulted on average in smaller *p* values than the *t* test. This discrepancy increased with larger sample sizes, severity of skewness, and differences in spread. Fagerland concluded that nonparametric tests are most useful for small studies and that *t* tests and their corresponding confidence intervals can and should be used with larger sample sizes, even when the data are heavily skewed.

Determining the Power of a Statistical Test

Given a parametric and a nonparametric test in competition, which test is more powerful? *Power* refers to the ability of a test to correctly reject the null hypothesis. A powerful test is also one whose assumptions have been sufficiently met. In comparing the power of two competing tests, therefore, the researcher needs to evaluate the ability of the data to meet the tests' assumptions.

Other things being equal, when data sufficiently meet the assumptions of a parametric test, the parametric test generally is more powerful. When there are serious departures from the parametric test's assumptions, however, Monte Carlo simulations have indicated that nonparametric tests tend to be more powerful than parametric tests when the distribution of the data being considered is unimodal but nonnormal in shape and the sample size is small (Harwell, 1988).

Because the power of a statistical test increases as the sample size increases, it is possible to accommodate a less powerful test by increasing the sample size. The *power efficiency* of a statistical test refers to the increase in sample size that would be necessary to make one test (e.g., a nonparametric test) as powerful as its rival (e.g., a parametric test) given that the assumptions of the rival test have been met, the alpha level is held constant, and the sample size of the rival test, N_1, is also held constant (Siegel & Castellan, 1988). In this situation, the power efficiency of a test is determined as follows:

$$\text{Power efficiency of Test 1} = (N_2/N_1)\ 100\%.$$

For example, if Test 1 requires a sample of 40 cases to have the same power as Test 2 with 30 cases, then Test 1 has a power efficiency of 75% ($[N_2/N_1]$ 100% = [30/40] 100% = 75%). A *power efficiency* of 75% implies that if the assumptions of both tests are met and Test 2 is more powerful than Test 1, then to achieve equality of power for the two tests, 10 cases would be required for Test 1 for every 7.5 cases used for Test 2 (Siegel & Castellan, 1988).

Level of Measurement of the Variables

There are nonstatistical criteria for selecting one test over another (Harwell, 1988). In particular, it is important to consider the level of measurement (i.e., nominal, ordinal, interval, or ratio) of the variables being considered for analysis. When two variables being considered are nominal or categorical in measurement, there is little choice of tests to be undertaken; the test of choice is typically nonparametric. The issue becomes less clear when the data are ordinal, interval, or ratio. For readers who are unfamiliar with the levels of measurement of variables, Chapter 3 provides a review.

Traditionally, nonparametric tests have been intended for use with nominal or ordinal data, whereas parametric tests were used with dependent variables that were interval or ratio in measurement. The issues, however, are not only the variables' level of measurement but also the size of the sample and the shape of the parent distribution behind the data. Some of the most powerful parametric statistical analyses can occur with large sets of observations of ordinal data with normally shaped distributions and equal variances. Some of the least powerful parametric statistical analyses occur when the interval or ratio data have distributions that are skewed, the variances are not equal, and the sample sizes are small.

The decision whether to use a parametric or nonparametric test, therefore, is not a simple one. The researcher needs to take into account not only the level of measurement of the variable(s) being considered but also the ability of the data being analyzed to meet the assumptions underlying the tests being considered. The most powerful test, parametric or nonparametric, is the one that best meets the underlying distribution of the data being considered in the hypotheses.

BOX 2.3 Situations That Suggest the Use of Nonparametric Tests

- The independent and/or dependent variables are nominal in measurement
- Ordered data with many ties
- Rank-ordered data specifying placement; no other metric assumed
- Unequal or small sample sizes
- Nonnormal distribution of the dependent variable
- Unequal variances across groups
- Unequal pairwise correlations across repeated measures
- Data with notable outliers

When to Consider a Nonparametric Test

Box 2.3 presents some situations that should suggest to the researcher that nonparametric tests are worthy of serious consideration. When both the dependent and independent variables consist of more than two unordered categories (e.g., religious preference and marital status), no parametric test can be used. The researcher may also find that although the data may be orderable (e.g., two variables that have five categories of pain and level of discomfort), there are many ties in the data. This also suggests that nonparametric tests may be preferable to parametric tests. The researcher may also have rank-ordered data in which no other metric is assumed. Examples of this situation might be a student's placement on a test or in a competition (e.g., first, second, third).

Unequal or small sample sizes (e.g., five subjects per group) may prevent our being able to determine the shape of the sample data's distribution even when the population distribution is normal. In our hypothetical example, a sample size of only 10 children in each group suggests that it may be difficult to ascertain the data's underlying distribution. Even with larger sample sizes, the distribution of observations may give evidence of gross nonnormality (e.g., a heavily skewed, peaked, or flat distribution). In that case, the researcher needs to carefully examine the consequences of choosing one test over another.

If several groups are being considered, there might also be unequal variances across groups, marked outliers, or unequal pairwise correlations across repeated measures. The bottom line is that the means may not be truly representative of the scores of the sample; therefore, other measures of central tendency (e.g., the median) might be better descriptors of the scores.

Researchers can use a number of readily available approaches to evaluate the extent to which their data meet the assumptions of a particular test. Because of the importance of this topic to statistical hypothesis testing, Chapter 3 focuses on this topic.

7. *If the research data meet the test's assumptions, compute the value of the test statistic. If the computed value is in the rejection region, reject H_0. If the value is outside the region of rejection, do not reject H_0.* The final task of hypothesis testing is to determine whether or not to reject the null hypothesis. That is, assuming that our data meet the assumptions of our chosen test (and that is a *big* assumption), we would use a statistical package to determine the value of the test statistic and whether this calculated value is in our identified region of rejection of the null hypothesis. If it is, we would reject the null hypothesis and conclude that our intervention group did have more positive postintervention outcomes than the usual-services group. If the calculated value of the test statistic is not in our identified region of rejection, we would fail to reject the null hypothesis and conclude that our evidence does not indicate any differences between the intervention and usual-services groups with regard to our postintervention outcomes.

Again, for each decision, we are faced with possible error: concluding that there is a difference between the intervention and usual-services groups with regard to postintervention outcomes when in reality there is no difference (Type I error) or failing to detect a difference between the two groups when in reality there is a difference (Type II error). A critical key to minimizing these error rates is our ability to choose the most appropriate test given the characteristics of our data. Chapter 3 presents some relatively easy approaches to the examination of these characteristics as a means of facilitating this choice.

TEST YOUR KNOWLEDGE

Here is a "test" of your knowledge on the main points regarding the process of hypothesis.

You will want to revisit the chapter should you find that you cannot recall the answers to the questions.

1. Outline the seven steps to statistical hypothesis testing.
2. Please define what is meant by the following:
    a. Type I error
    b. Type II error
    c. Alpha
    d. Beta
    e. Power
    f. Power efficiency of a test
3. In undertaking a statistical test, I decide that there is a difference between my intervention and usual-care group when in fact, the differences I found were merely the result of researcher error.
    a. What kind of error am I making?
    b. What is the alternative error that I could have made?
4. Under what conditions would you consider using a nonparametric test rather than a parametric one?
5. Is a parametric test always more "powerful" than a nonparametric test? Please explain.

Visit **study.sagepub.com/pett2e** to access SAS output, SPSS datasets, SAS datasets, and SAS examples.

CHAPTER 3

Evaluating the Characteristics of Data

Chapter 2 focused on the process of statistical hypothesis testing. Part of this process (Step 6) involves evaluating the extent to which the data being analyzed meet the assumptions of the tests being considered. Chapter 3 will outline available methods for evaluating the characteristics of data. First, the level of measurement of a variable needs to be identified to determine the most appropriate parametric or nonparametric statistical test. Next, it is important to evaluate the normality of the variable's distribution, the impact of outliers, the homogeneity of variance, and sample size adequacy.

CHARACTERISTICS OF LEVELS OF MEASUREMENT

Measurement is the process of assigning numbers or codes to observations according to certain prescribed rules. The way in which these values are assigned to the observations determines a variable's *level of measurement*. The most widely accepted set of rules for determining a variable's level of measurement is that developed by S. Stevens (1946). This typology consists of four levels of measurement whose order is based on how much information they carry. These levels are nominal, ordinal, interval, and ratio. Table 3.1 summarizes the characteristics of these four levels of measurement.

Nominal

The first level of measurement is nominal. A variable that is measured on a nominal scale is one that has distinct nonoverlapping categories. The numbers that are assigned to these categories have no intrinsic meaning, but all persons who share the same category are assigned a similar value.

There are three basic requirements for a "good" nominal-level variable: (1) all members of one level of the variable must be assigned the same number, (2) no two levels are assigned the same number, and (3) each observation can be assigned to one and only one of the available levels. Given that these three conditions have been fulfilled, the levels of the nominal-level variable are mutually exclusive and exhaustive.

Table 3.1 Overview of the Characteristics of the Levels of Measurement

Level of Measurement	*Mutually Exclusive Groups*	*Rank Ordering*	*Equidistant Values*	*Meaningful Zero Point*	*Example*
Nominal	•				Marital status
Ordinal	•	•			Stress level (1–7)
Interval	•	•	•		Depression scale (1–100)
Ratio	•	•	•	•	Weight (pounds)

The variable *gender* is a nominal-level measurement because it is composed of two independent, mutually exclusive (nonoverlapping), and exhaustive levels: male and female. In our hypothetical intervention study, each of the 20 participating children could be assigned a "0" or a "1" depending on whether the child is a male (0) or a female (1). The numbers 0 and 1 that have been assigned to these levels have no inherent order to them; these numbers could have been reversed. They merely indicate the gender group to which the child belongs. Additional variables in our hypothetical study that have a nominal level of measurement are the group to which the child was assigned (intervention = 0, usual care = 1), diagnosis (1 = solid tumor, 2 = acute myeloid leukemia, 3 = lymphoma, 4 = sarcoma), and race/ethnicity (1 = Caucasian, 2 = African American, 3 = Hispanic or Latino, and 4 = other).

Parametric statistics assume ordering and meaningful numerical distances between values; therefore, these statistics do not provide very useful information if the dependent or outcome variable has a nominal level of measurement. It does not make sense, for example, to report an average marital status. For nominal data, researchers rely instead on frequencies, percentages, and modes to describe their results. Nonparametric inferential statistics (e.g., the chi-square goodness-of-fit test or Fisher's exact test) may also be applied to these data.

Ordinal

The next level of measurement is ordinal. A variable that has an ordinal level of measurement is characterized by having mutually exclusive categories that are sorted and rank ordered on the basis of their standing relative to one another on a specific attribute according to some preset criteria. Although it may be possible to ascertain that one person has a higher rank relative to another person, it is not possible to determine exactly how much higher that person is than another.

Suppose the nurses in our hypothetical intervention study were asked to assess on a 7-point scale (1 = *not at all distressed* to 7 = *very distressed*) the extent to which a particular child appears to be distressed prior to our planned intervention. This variable, preintervention distress, is an ordinal-level variable. We know, for example, that Child A, who received a "6" on preintervention distress, was more distressed prior to the intervention than Child B, who received a "3" on this scale. Because there are not equidistant intervals on this 7-point scale, however, it is not possible to conclude that Child A is twice as distressed as Child B or that the difference between a "6" and a "7" is the same as the difference between a "3" and a "4." Moreover, not all values necessarily share the same intensity. For example, Nurse C's assignment of a "7" to a child may not have the same intensity level as Nurse D's "7." We only know that, for both nurses, a particular child was "very distressed" according to their criteria.

Because there is order to the values of an ordinal scale, descriptive statistics that rely on rank ordering (e.g., the median) can be used in addition to percentages, frequencies, and modes. Numerous nonparametric inferential statistics are available to test hypotheses about similarities of medians between groups and relationships among variables.

There has been much heated discussion in the research literature about the appropriateness of using parametric tests with ordinal-level data (Armstrong, 1981; Carifio & Perla, 2008; Jamieson, 2004; Knapp, 1990; Norman, 2010; Pell, 2005). Pedhazur and Schmelkin (1991) suggest that this controversy was sparked by early writings of S. Stevens (1951), who argued that means and standard deviations, the backbones of parametric statistics, were not appropriate measures of central tendency for ordinal data. Others have effectively argued (Knapp, 1990) that the critical issue is not so much that the data are ordinal but rather that the data have a sufficient sample size (e.g., $N > 30$) and a relatively normal distribution of the dependent variable to merit the use of parametric statistics. Norman (2010) presents a convincing argument that parametric statistics can be used with Likert data even with small sample sizes, unequal variances, and nonnormal distributions.

Interval

Interval-level scales are more refined than either nominal or ordinal scales. Like the ordinal scale, the interval-level scale has mutually exclusive groups and rank ordering. Unlike the ordinal scale, the interval-level scale has equidistant intervals. This means that we obtain information not only about the rank order of a particular score but also about how much greater or less a particular score is than another. That is, on an interval scale whose range is 1 to 100, the difference between 100 and 75 is, in some sense, the same as the difference between 75 and 50.

A classic example of an interval-level scale is temperature measured in degrees Fahrenheit. We know, for example, that a child whose body temperature is 102° has a temperature that is 2° higher than a child whose body temperature is 100°. Because an interval-level scale does not have an absolute zero point, however, the distances between values, although theoretically equidistant, do not carry exactly the same meaning. That is, the change in body temperature from 98° to 101° is not meaningfully the same as a change in body temperature from 102° to 105°. However, 100° is not twice as hot as 50° because 0° Fahrenheit is a numerical convenience, not an absolute.

A common practice among researchers is to use a multi-item scale to measure single or multiple constructs. The individual items tend to be either nominal (e.g., 0 = *agree* vs. 1 = *disagree*) or ordinal (e.g., 1 = *strongly agree* to 5 = *strongly disagree*) in nature, and the item responses are summed to produce a scale with interval-level properties and with a larger range of possible scores (e.g., 0–100). From these data, we can use all the measures of central tendency and variance. Parametric statistics such as the *t* test, analysis of variance (ANOVA), and Pearson product-moment correlation coefficient are all possible considerations.

In our intervention example, we might decide to use a 14-item self-reported fatigue assessment scale for children ages 7 to 12 years (Hinds et al., 2007; Hockenberry et al., 2003). This Childhood Fatigue Scale (CFS) is a 14-item instrument that first asks the child for a "yes" or "no" response regarding their experiences of 14 fatigue-related symptoms (e.g., *I have been tired*). If the child answers yes to the symptom, he or she is then asked to describe the intensity of the fatigue symptom on a scale of 1 (*not at all*) to 5 (*a lot*). From these 14 items, a total fatigue score can be generated with a range of scores from 0 (no fatigue) to 70 (high fatigue) along with three subscales: lack of energy, inability to function, and altered mood. (Hinds & Hockenberry-Eaton, 2001; Hockenberry et al., 2003).

Again, controversy exists as to the true nature of the level of measurement of such a multi-item scale (Knapp, 1990; Nunnally & Bernstein, 1994; Pedhazur & Schmelkin, 1991). That is, is an "interval" scale that has been generated from ordinal data truly interval? Should we even care? For statistical analysis, the concern is not so much the variable's "true" level of measurement as much as whether the information generated from the use of a particular statistic best represents the data. This conclusion can be reached only by examining the data thoroughly to determine the extent to which a particular test's assumptions have been violated. Pedhazur and Schmelkin (1991) indicate that, even in his later writings, S. Stevens (1968) argued, "The question is thereby made to turn, not on whether the measurement scale determines the choice of a statistical procedure, but on how and to what degree an inappropriate statistic may lead to a deviant conclusion" (p. 852).

Ratio

The highest level of measurement is ratio. In addition to maintaining the characteristics of the previous three levels of measurement (mutually exclusive and exhaustive categories, rank ordering, and equidistant intervals), a ratio-level variable also has a meaningful and absolute zero point that represents the complete absence of a given attribute. Because of its invariant zero point, the ratio of any two scores from a ratio scale is unchanged by transformations through multiplication and division.

Examples of ratio-level variables include weight, blood pressure, and temperature Kelvin. In our hypothetical study, a child's body weight and time to first voiding could be considered ratio-level variables. The age of the child might be more controversial. Our society has yet to agree on when an individual becomes a human being. At conception? At birth? Or at some other place along the way?

It does not matter much in statistics whether a variable is at the interval or ratio level of measurement. Both of these levels of measurement are appropriate for use with parametric statistics. To reiterate, equally important determinations regarding the use of parametric statistics are sample size and the shape of the distribution of the dependent variable.

Which Level of Measurement Is "Best"?

There is no clear answer as to which level of measurement is best for a particular research question. Clearly, the researcher wants to attain the very highest level of measurement possible given the time, financial, and design constraints of the research. The higher levels of measurement, interval and ratio, provide the researcher with the opportunity to use potentially more powerful statistical tests. Moreover, it is always possible to collapse data into lower levels of measurement. It is not possible, however, to resurrect interval-level data from precollapsed nominal data. The best approach is *not* to collapse data while entering them into the computer. Data can be collapsed, if necessary, later on during the statistical analyses.

ASSESSING THE NORMALITY OF A DISTRIBUTION

Returning to our hypothetical intervention study, suppose that we were interested in assessing the normality of the distribution of scores for children's self-reported fatigue during the 24 hours prior to the implementation of our intervention. As indicated above, this is a variable whose scores can range from 0 to 70, with higher scores suggesting greater intensity of fatigue. There are several ways that we could assess the normality of this variable. First, we could examine the distribution's skewness and kurtosis. Next, we could visually examine the distribution of the data to obtain a sense of its shape. Finally, we could statistically test the extent to which the data fit a theoretically normal distribution.

All three of these approaches are available in SPSS for Windows by choosing the following commands from the dropdown menu: (a) *Analyze . . . Descriptive Statistics . . . Frequencies . . .* (Figure 3.1) and (b) *Analyze . . . Descriptive Statistics . . . Explore . . .* (Figure 3.2). The *Frequencies* and *Explore* dialog boxes allow the researcher a number of options for evaluating data.

As indicated in Figure 3.1, by opening the *Frequencies . . . Charts* dialogue box and selecting *Histograms . . . with normal curve,* a normal distribution can be superimposed over the histogram of the variable of interest (1). This allows the researcher to visually inspect the data for violations of normality. The *Analyze . . . Descriptive Statistics . . . Explore* command may also be used to statistically test for normality (Figure 3.2, (1)). This procedure also produces information regarding descriptive statistics, stem-and-leaf plots, boxplots, outliers, normal probability plots, and statistical tests of normality. Separate analyses can be obtained for subgroups of data as well.

Figure 3.1 SPSS for Windows *Analyze . . . Descriptive Statistics . . . Frequencies . . .* commands for assessing normality of a distribution.

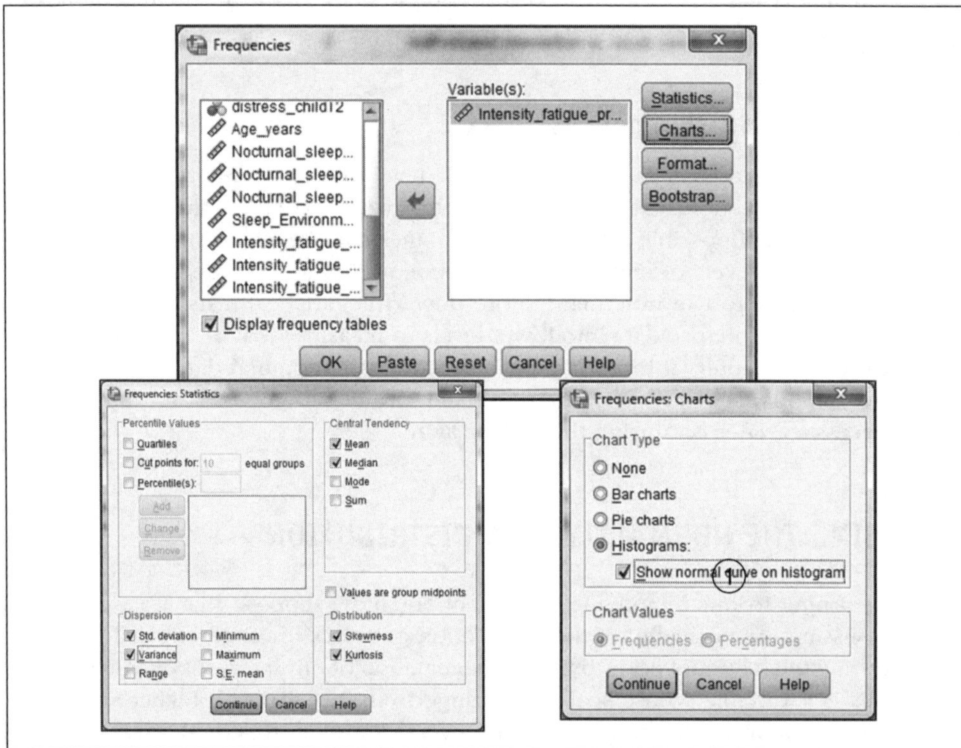

Skewness

Before we interpret the results of our SPSS output, let's review the meaning of skewness and kurtosis. You will recall that a normal distribution takes the form of a bell-shaped curve that is centered on the mean (Figure 3.3A). The normal distribution is symmetric, and all three measures of central tendency—the mean, median, and mode—share the same value. One simple way of assessing normality of a distribution, therefore, is to examine the measures of central tendency. If the mean, median, and mode are nearly equal in value, then there is evidence to suggest that the distribution is symmetric. If these three values are not at all similar, then the distribution is characterized as being asymmetric or *skewed;* that is, the distribution has one tail that is longer than the other.

There are two types of skewness: positive and negative skew. A distribution is *positively skewed* if the distribution's longer tail extends toward the right or toward the higher set

Figure 3.2 SPSS for Windows *Analyze . . . Descriptive Statistics . . . Explore . . .* commands for assessing normality of a distribution.

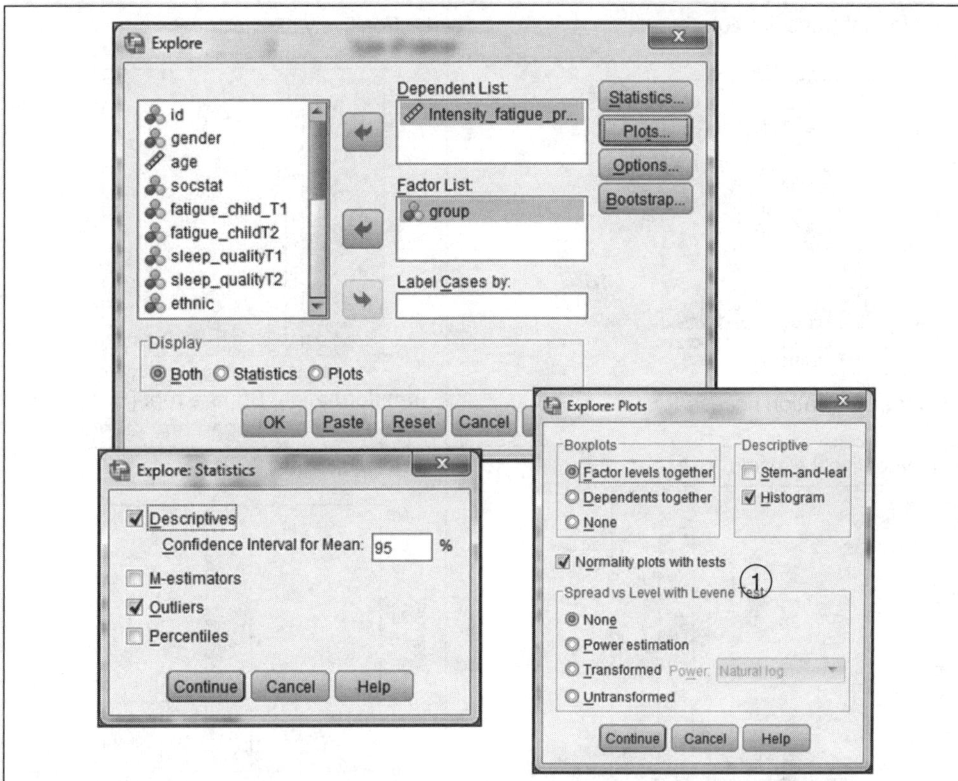

of values (Figure 3.3B). This results in the value of the mean being pulled to the right and being larger in value than the median or mode. A distribution that is *negatively skewed* has a longer tail that extends toward the left or toward the lower set of values (Figure 3.3C). This results in the mean being smaller in value than the median or mode.

The measure of skewness is referred to as the third moment about the mean, $\Sigma(X - \overline{X})^3/(n - 1)$ (Neter, Wasserman, & Whitmore, 1993; Park, 2008). Because this third moment is measured in cubed units (e.g., weight cubed), a standardized measure of skewness is considered more useful because its size does not depend on the units of measurement. This standardized measure is obtained by dividing the third moment by the cube of the standard deviation (s^3) of the variable being examined (Neter et al., 1993). This is the skewness value that is presented in the computer printout.

When a distribution is a symmetric bell-shaped curve, the value of this measure of skewness is 0. The measure has a negative value when the distribution is negatively

Figure 3.3 Comparison of the most common forms of distributions and suggested transformations.

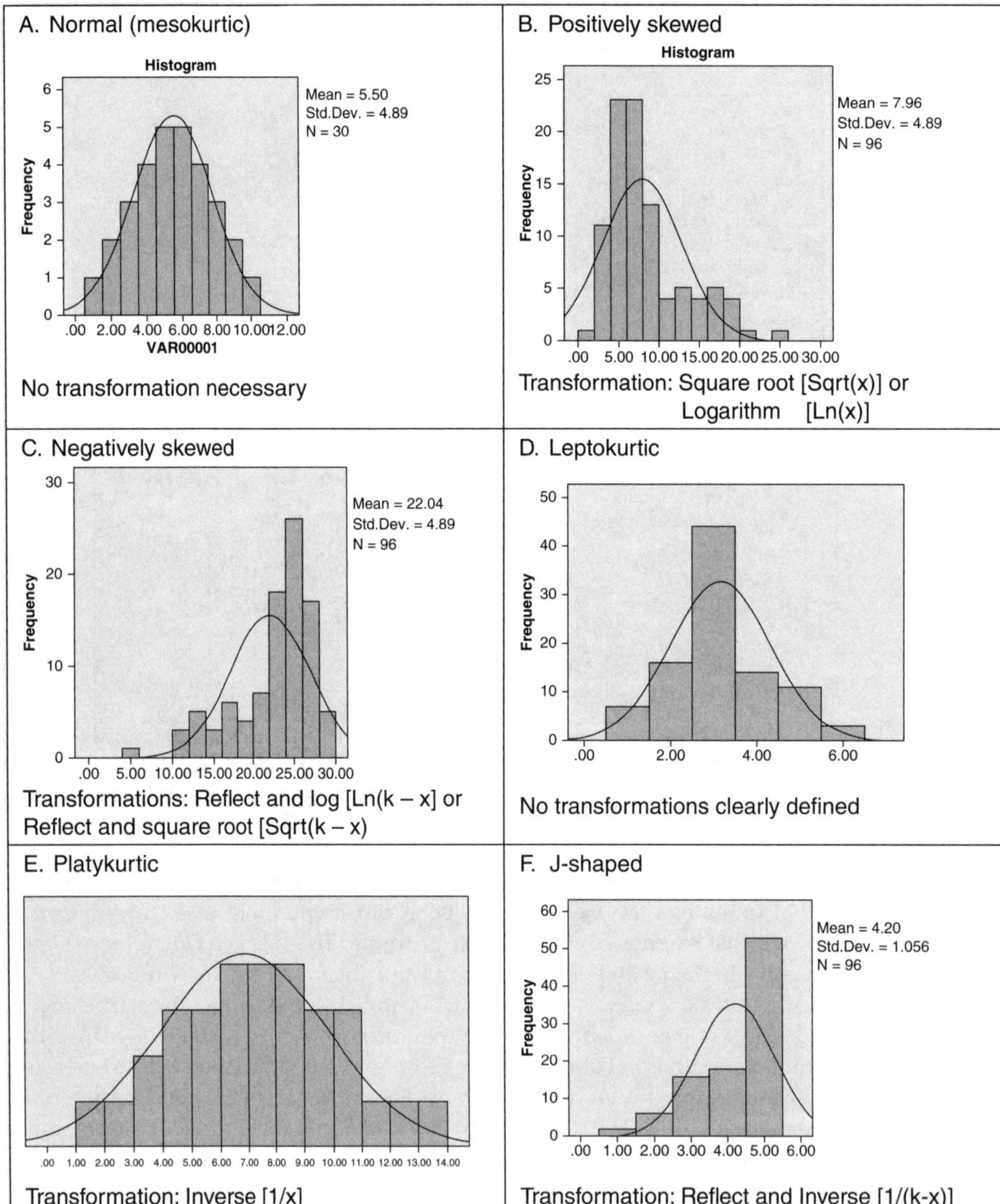

SOURCE: Transformation suggestions come from Hair, Anderson, Tatham, and Black (1995) and Tabachnick and Fidell (2013). In Panels C and F, *k* represents a constant, usually the largest score +1.

skewed and a positive value when the distribution is positively skewed. To determine the seriousness of the skewness of a distribution, one of two measures of skewness, Fisher's or Pearson's, can be used (Kellar & Kelvin, 2012; Lehman, 1991; Salkind, 2010). The Fisher's coefficient is as follows:

Fisher skewness coefficient = skewness / standard error skewness.

To calculate the Fisher skewness coefficient, the SPSS computer-generated value for skewness (Skewness) is divided by the standard error for skewness (SE Skew). If the resulting z statistic lies beyond the range of ±1.96 (the critical value for a two-tailed z statistic at $\alpha = .05$), the distribution is asymmetric and significantly skewed. Calculated values of this coefficient that fall between −1.96 and +1.96 suggest that the distribution is not significantly different from a normal distribution.

A second commonly used index for skewness is the Pearson skewness coefficient (Sk_p):

$$\text{Pearson skewness coefficient} = Sk_p = 3[(\overline{X} - Md) / s].$$

This statistic uses the difference between the mean ($\overline{X}$) and median (Md) of a distribution divided by the variable's standard deviation (s) to determine the level of skewness. If $Sk_p = 0$, the mean and median are equal and therefore the distribution is symmetric. A negative coefficient indicates a negative skew (i.e., the mean is smaller than the median), and a positive value represents positive skewness (i.e., the mean is larger than the median). Lehman (1991) suggests that values of Sk_p between −0.5 and +0.5 indicate generally acceptable levels of skewness.

Kurtosis

A second characteristic of a distribution is its *kurtosis,* or the fourth moment about the mean (Balanda & MacGillivray, 1988; DeCarlo, 1997; Neter et al., 1993; Park, 2008), calculated as $\Sigma(X - \overline{X})^4 / (n - 1)$. Because this fourth moment is measured in (units)^4, a standardized measurement of kurtosis is available in statistical packages that divides the fourth movement by s^4. Evaluation of a distribution's kurtosis is especially useful after it has been determined that the distribution is not unduly skewed. It is not very useful for asymmetric or skewed distributions.

Three terms are used to denote different levels of kurtosis: *mesokurtic, leptokurtic,* and *platykurtic*. A normal distribution has a standardized kurtosis value that is equal to zero and is referred to as being *mesokurtic* (Figure 3.3A). A positive value for the standardized kurtosis coefficient implies that the distribution is *leptokurtic,* or more peaked than a normal distribution (Figure 3.3D). (To remember what *leptokurtic* means, it might be helpful to recall Superman, *leaping* tall buildings in a single bound.) A negative value for the standardized kurtosis coefficient implies that the distribution is *platykurtic,* or flatter than a normal distribution (Figure 3.3E). (Remember that, like the platykurtic distribution, a platypus is an animal that stands low and close to the ground.) Kellar and Kelvin (2012) suggest using a Fisher coefficient to evaluate kurtosis:

Fisher coefficient of kurtosis = kurtosis / standard error of kurtosis.

That is, the standardized kurtosis value is divided by its standard error to determine the extent to which a bell-shaped symmetric curve deviates from a normal distribution. If this z statistic falls outside the range of ±1.96, then the bell-shaped distribution is significantly different from a standard normal distribution.

Computer Analysis of Skewness and Kurtosis

Assuming that the data for the 20 subjects in our hypothetical study have been entered into the computer data file (we are using "hospitalized children with cancer-20 cases.sav" located on the SAGE website, study.sagepub.com/pett2e), the syntax commands and computer-generated frequency output for the child's self-reported fatigue preintervention are presented in Figure 3.4. This output was obtained by running the commands presented in Figure 3.1 and selecting the preintervention fatigue variable for analysis.

We are first presented with the frequency distribution of the child's preintervention fatigue variable (Figure 3.4, (1)). Recall that the scores could range from 0 to 70, with higher scores indicating greater fatigue. Given that no child indicated that he or she was "very fatigued" during the preintervention phase, there are no values higher than 35. Notice that the mean (29.25), median (30.0), and mode (35.0) (2), although close, are not equal to one another, suggesting that the data may be skewed. Because the mean is smaller than either the median or the mode, the data are negatively skewed, with the longer tail in the direction of the smaller values, a condition that is verified by the skewness value of −1.103 (3). Dividing the measure of skewness by the standard error for skewness (−1.103/.512) results in a Fisher skewness coefficient of −2.15, which falls outside the acceptable limits of ±1.96, suggesting that the data may be seriously skewed. It is interesting that a different result is obtained for the Pearson Sk_p:

$$Sk_p = 3(\overline{X} - Md) / s = 3(29.25 - 30.0) / (6.54) = -.34.$$

The resulting value of −.34 is within the acceptable range of this coefficient (−.5 to + .5). This discrepancy may be explained by the extreme sensitivity of the Fisher measure of skewness to outliers (Kellar & Kelvin, 2012). Because the statistic is based on deviations from the mean raised to the third power, outliers have a very strong effect on this measure.

Ordinarily, when a distribution has serious skewness problems, indicating that it is not bell-shaped, it would not be necessary to examine its kurtosis. Given that we have conflicting information regarding this distribution's skewness, however, it would be useful to examine the distribution's kurtosis as well. The positive value (.380) for kurtosis (4) indicates that the distribution is leptokurtic, or more peaked than a normal distribution. Dividing the value for kurtosis by its standard error (.992), however, yields a Fisher coefficient of kurtosis of .383, which is well within the ±1.96 range for a normal distribution.

Visually Examining the Shape of the Distribution

Given these somewhat conflicting results, it is important that we examine the data visually to determine for ourselves the seriousness of the skewness. In fact, the

Figure 3.4 Computer-generated output obtained in SPSS for Windows (v. 22–23) for the frequencies and histogram of preintervention fatigue.

Frequencies (1)

Statistics

Child's self-reported fatigue-preintervention

N	Valid	20
	Missing	0
Mean		(2) 29.2500
Median		30.0000
Mode		35.00
Std. Deviation		6.54438
Variance		42.829
Skewness		-1.103
Std. Error of Skewness		(3) .512
Kurtosis		.380
Std. Error of Kurtosis		(4) .992

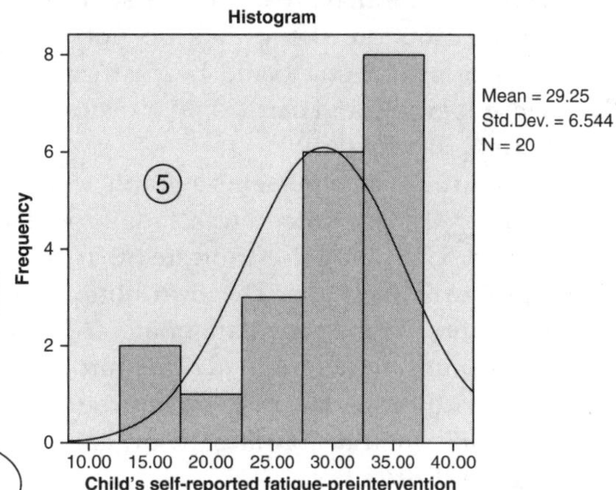

Child's self-reported fatigue-preintervention

		Frequency	Percent	Valid Percent	Cumulative Percent
Valid	15.00	2	10.0	10.0	10.0
	20.00	1	5.0	5.0	15.0
	25.00	3	15.0	15.0	30.0
	30.00	6	30.0	30.0	60.0
	35.00	8	40.0	40.0	100.0
	Total	20	100.0	100.0	

necessity of visually examining data for departures from normality cannot be overstressed. No statistical test of normality is superior to what my biostatistician friend, Dr. James Reading, refers to as the *eyeball test*.

The eyeball test consists of visually examining the data's distribution to determine if the distribution looks sufficiently comparable to a normal distribution for the researcher to feel comfortable using parametric tests. Is the mean an adequate representation of these data? Are there unusual "kinks" in the distribution? Is the distribution unimodal, or are there multiple modes? Are there outliers about which to be concerned? What effect does the sample size have on the potential shape of the distribution? Although the mean, median, and mode may be similar, a limited sample size may restrict one's ability to adequately distinguish the shape of the distribution. If the data do not have a normal distribution, is there a possible transformation that could be performed (e.g., log or square root) that would make sense logically and that would transform the nonnormal distribution into a more nearly normal distribution?

Figure 3.4 also presents a graph of the normal curve superimposed on the distribution for the preintervention fatigue variable for the 20 subjects in our hypothetical study (5). This figure indicates that the data are negatively skewed and somewhat leptokurtic in shape. The distribution also appears to have serious deviations from normality. With so few data points ($N = 20$), the shape of the distribution may also not be definitively determined. This information suggests that the use of nonparametric tests with these data may be in order. A second alternative would be to consider the possibility of transforming the preintervention fatigue variable to obtain a more nearly normal distribution.

Additional plots of normality may be generated in SPSS for Windows (v. 22–23) through the *Analyze . . . Descriptive Statistics . . . Explore . . . Plots . . . Normality plots with tests . . .* commands. These plots can be of help in visually examining data. They include normal probability plots and detrended normal plots. Figure 3.5 presents examples of normal and detrended normal probability plots for selected distributions.

Normal and Detrended Normal Probability Plots.

In the *normal probability plot,* each data point is paired with its expected value given a nearly normal distribution of similar range and sample size. If the sample is from a nearly normal distribution (Figure 3.5A), a normal probability plot of the observed and expected values would indicate that nearly all values lie along a 45° straight line running from the lower left corner to the upper right corner of the plot (6). Note that, except for a few minor deviations, the values fall along the 45° line.

A *detrended normal probability plot* is one in which the deviations from normal for each value in the sample are plotted against the observed values. If the sample is from a nearly normal distribution, these deviations will cluster evenly around zero along a horizontal band. This indicates that there is little difference between the observed values and expected values. The detrended normal probability plot for the nearly normal distribution in Figure 3.5A, third panel (7), illustrates this pattern. Note that the data do *not* need to fall *exactly* along a straight line but rather that the band of values is similar in width across all values of the data.

Distributions that are skewed or bimodal (e.g., Figures 3.5B–D) show markedly different patterns of deviations from normality. Curvilinear patterns often emerge, suggesting that the data are badly skewed (Figures 3.5B–C) (8) (9) or bimodal (Figure 3.5D) (10). Outliers can be identified on these plots because they occupy

Figure 3.5 Examples of normal probability, detrended normal probability, and boxplots for the normal and other selected distributions.

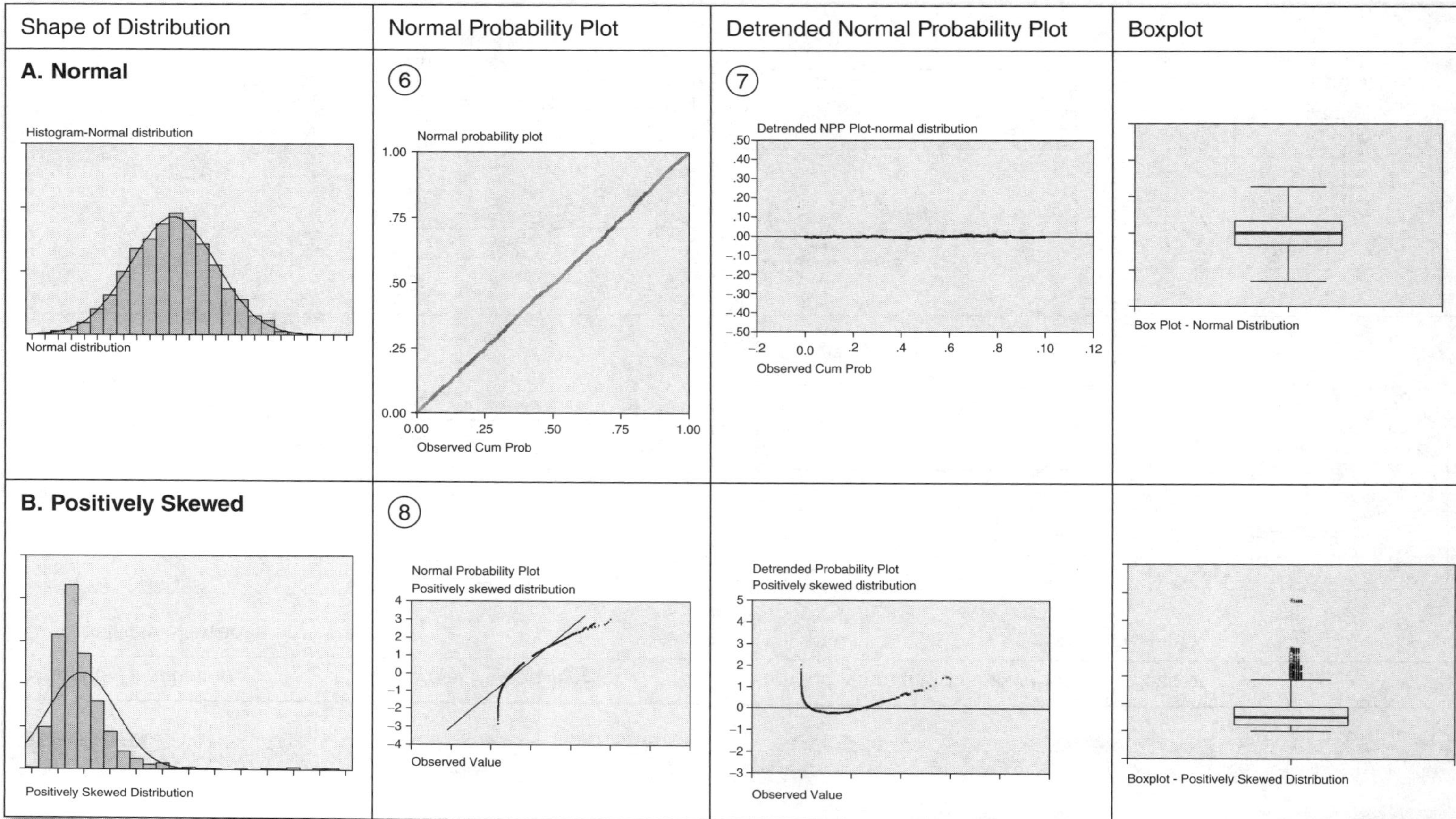

(Continued)

Figure 3.5 (Continued)

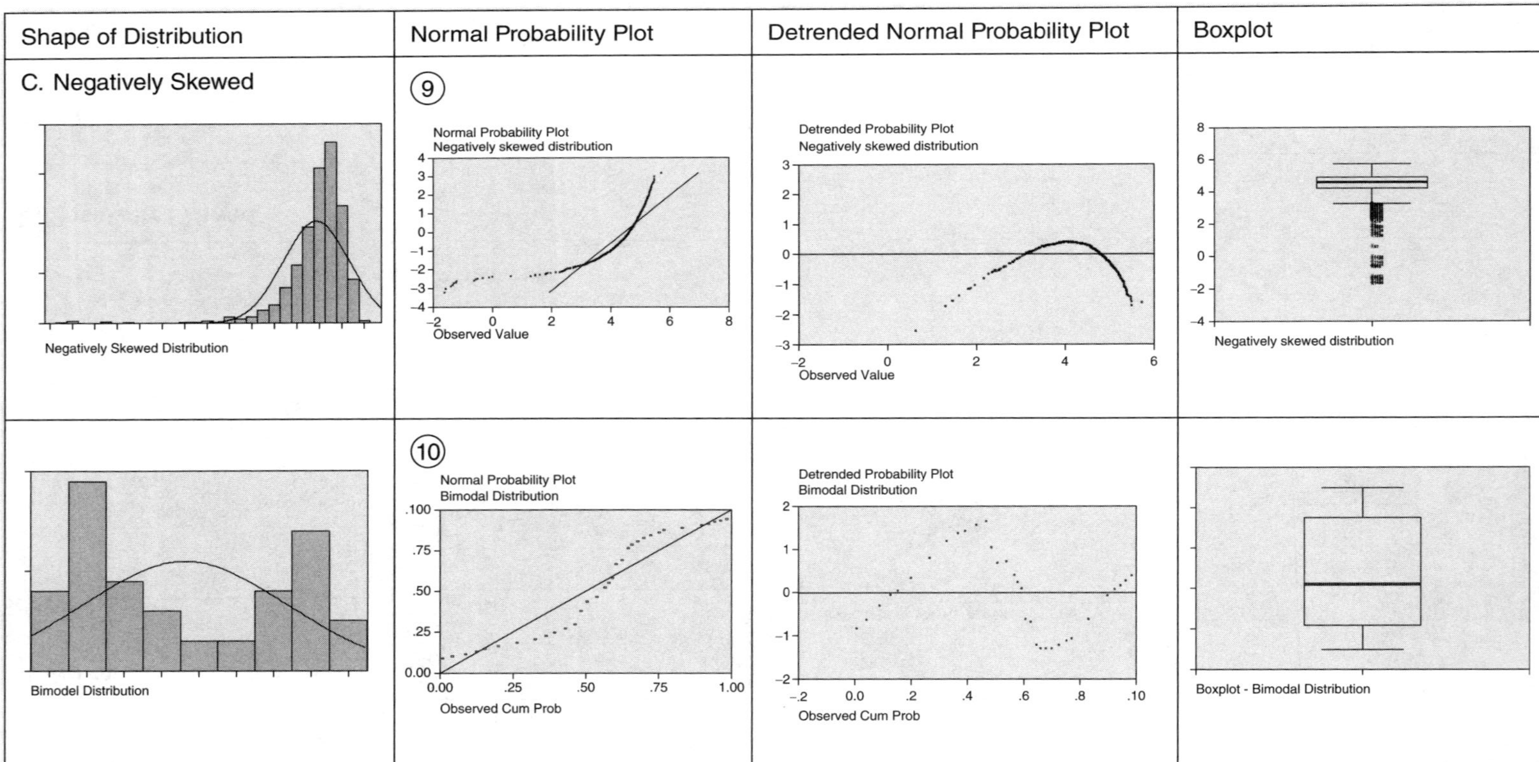

positions away from the other values and do not appear to be connected to them (Tabachnick & Fidell, 2013). For example, in Figure 3.5C (9), the values in the lower left-hand corner of the normal and detrended normal probability plots represent the outliers for this negatively skewed distribution.

Computer Examples of the Plots.

Figure 3.6 presents normal probability and detrended normal probability plots for the self-reported preintervention fatigue variable. The plots were generated from the SPSS for Windows (v. 22–23) commands *Analyze . . . Descriptive Statistics . . . Explore . . . Normality plots with tests . . .* illustrated in Figure 3.2. The data file that we are using is hospitalized children with cancer-20 cases.sav found on the SAGE website, study.sage pub.com/pett2e.

The two plots in Figure 3.6 confirm what we saw in Figure 3.4, that the preintervention fatigue data are not normally distributed. The values for this fatigue variable are not similar to the expected values and, therefore, are not situated on the 45° straight line of the normal probability plot (Figure 3.6A) (11). The detrended plot (Figure 3.6B) (12) indicates that the largest deviation from normality appears to be with the smaller values; they are farthest from the horizontal line that goes through 0.

Statistical Tests of Normality

The statistical tests for normality that are provided in SPSS for Windows (v. 22–23) are the Shapiro-Wilks and Kolmogorov-Smirnov (K-S) Lilliefors statistics. These can be obtained by selecting the *Analyze . . . Descriptive Statistics . . . Explore* commands from the menu, clicking on *Plots* and selecting *Normality plots with tests*. The objectives of these nonparametric goodness-of-fit tests are to compare the obtained distribution with a theoretically normal distribution of the same mean and standard deviation and to determine whether the deviations from normality are sufficiently large to conclude that the distribution under investigation is not normal. The null hypothesis is that the data are normally distributed; the alternative hypothesis is that the data are not normally distributed. The null hypothesis will be rejected if the obtained significance level is less than our stated level of alpha (e.g., $\alpha = .05$).

Both the Shapiro-Wilks and K-S Lilliefors statistics are extremely sensitive to departures from normality. It is strongly recommended, therefore, that the researcher supplement these statistical tests with the previously discussed methods for examining data for departures from normality (e.g., visually examining the data and assessing skewness and kurtosis).

The computer printout generated from SPSS for Windows for the Shapiro-Wilks and K-S Lilliefors statistics is presented in Table 3.2. For the preintervention fatigue variable, we have obtained similar results. Both tests indicate that the distribution is not normal (significance $< .001$ is less than $\alpha = .05$) (Table 3.2) (13). This is not always the case, however. Sometimes you will find that the two statistics disagree. Conover (1999) suggests that the Shapiro-Wilks test for normality may be more powerful than the K-S Lilliefors statistic in that it may be more likely to correctly reject the null hypothesis of normality.

Figure 3.6 Normal probability plots of preintervention fatigue scores (n = 20).

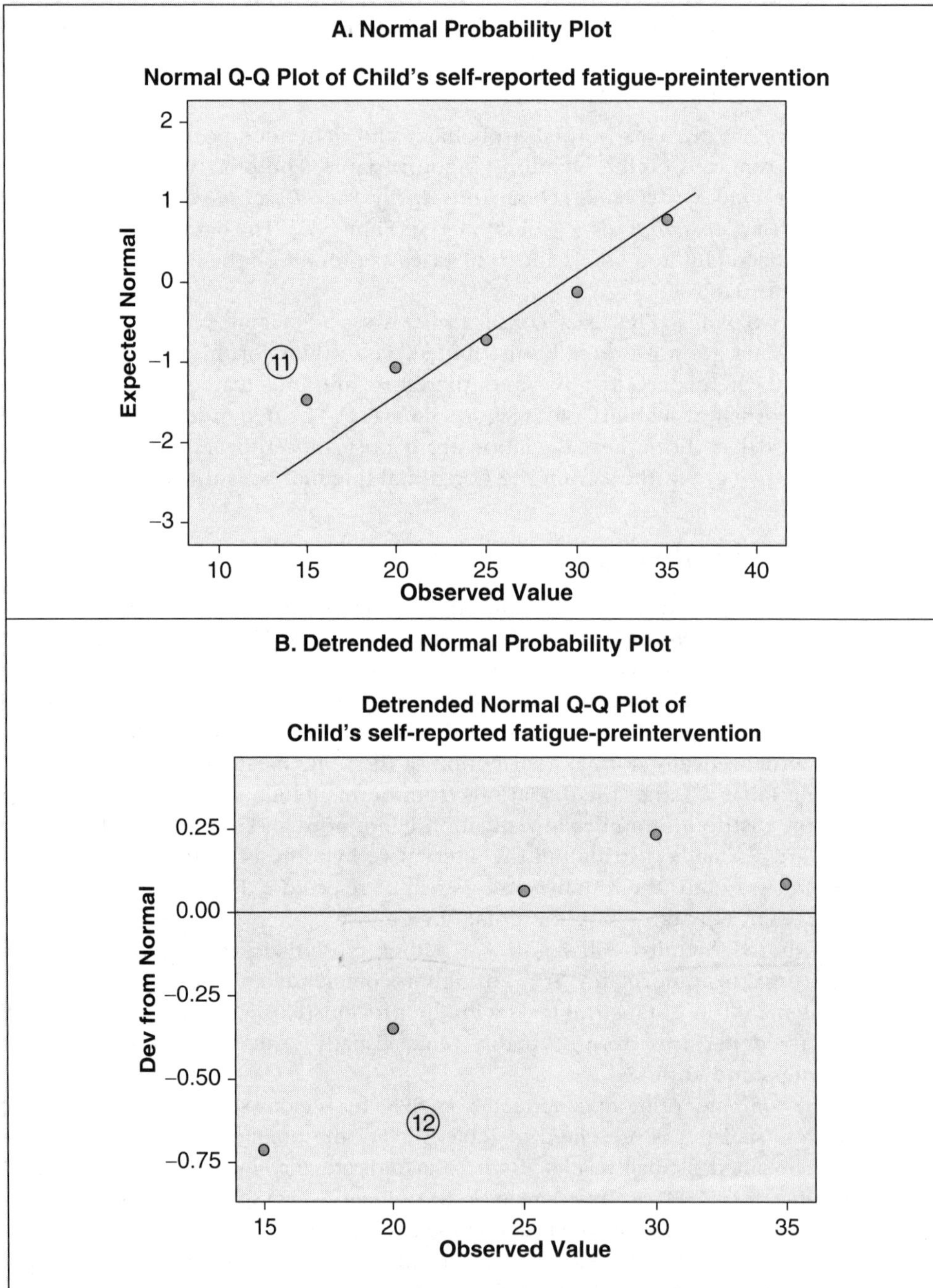

Table 3.2 Statistical Tests for Normality of the Preintervention Fatigue Variable

Tests of Normality

	Kolmogorov-Smirnov[a]			Shapiro-Wilk		
	Statistic	df	Sig.	Statistic	df	Sig.
Child's self-reported fatigue-preintervention	.2.46	20	(13) .003	.812	20	(13) .001

[a]Lilliefors significance correction.

Our determination of whether to accept or reject the preintervention fatigue distribution as normal should be based on all contributing factors: the level of measurement of the data, its visual representation, the similarity of the measures of central tendency, skewness and kurtosis, the statistics, and the sample size. Based on this evidence, we would most likely conclude that the data for preintervention fatigue are *not* normally distributed. This conclusion is based on the observation that although the data might be considered interval level of measurement, the visual representations suggest nonnormality; the mean, median, and mode are not similar; there is some skewness; the Shapiro-Wilks and K-S Lilliefors statistics support rejection of the null hypothesis of normality; and we had a sample size of only 20. This determination would suggest that we would seriously need to consider using nonparametric statistics when analyzing this variable.

Examining Distributions of the Dependent Variable by Subgroups

For many parametric tests, it is expected that the distribution of the dependent variable be normally distributed not only as a whole but also when broken down into subgroups of a particular independent variable of interest. Table 3.3 presents the syntax commands and a breakdown of the preintervention fatigue scores of the children by staff-initiated intervention and usual-care groups using the hospitalized children with cancer-20 cases.sav. These printouts were generated in SPSS for Windows by highlighting the *Analyze . . . Descriptive Statistics . . . Explore* commands (see Figure 3.2) and placing the dependent variable, *Intensity_Fatigue_preintervention,* in the *Dependent List* and the independent variable, *Group,* in the *Factor List.*

The resulting descriptive statistics (Table 3.3) and histograms (Figure 3.7) indicate that the staff-initiated intervention and usual-care groups have similar means and distributions. This suggests that we may have been successful in creating similar groups through random assignment—at least with regard to preintervention fatigue. The skewness statistics for the intervention group (skewness/standard error for skewness = −1.085/.687 = −1.579) and the usual-care group (−1.338/.687 = −1.95) also indicate that the variable's skewness for both groups is within an acceptable range (±1.96)

Table 3.3 Computer-Generated Printout of Pretreatment Fatigue by Group (Usual Care, Staff-Initiated Intervention) (SPSS for Windows, v.22–23)

```
EXAMINE VARIABLES=Intensity_fatigue_preintervention BY group
  /PLOT BOXPLOT HISTOGRAM NPPLOT
  /COMPARE GROUPS
  /STATISTICS DESCRIPTIVES
  /CINTERVAL 95
  /MISSING LISTWISE
  /NOTOTAL.
```

Descriptives

staff-initiated intervention vs. usual care				Statistic	Std. Error
Child's self-reported fatigue-preinteivention	usual care group	Mean		29.5000	2.03443
		95% Confidence Interval for Mean	Lower Bound	24.8978	
			Upper Bound	34.1022	
		5% Trimmed Mean		30.0000	
		Median		30.0000	
		Variance		41.389	
		Std. Deviation		6.43342	
		Minimum		15.00	
		Maximum		35.00	
		Range		20.00	
		Interquartile Range		10.00	
		Skewness		-1.338	.687
		Kurtosis		1.864	1.334
	staff-initiated intervention	Mean		29.0000	2.21108
		95% Confidence Interval for Mean	Lower Bound	23.9982	
			Upper Bound	34.0018	
		5% Trimmed Mean		29.4444	
		Median		30.0000	
		Variance		48.889	
		Std. Deviation		6.99206	
		Minimum		15.00	
		Maximum		35.00	
		Range		20.00	
		Interquartile Range		11.25	
		Skewness		-1.085	.687
		Kurtosis		.265	1.334

(14)
−1.338/0.687 = −1.95
−1.085/0.687 = −1.579

Tests Df Normality

	staff-initiated inteivention vs. usual care	Kolmogorov-Smirnov[a] Statistic	df	Sig.	Shapiro-Wilk Statistic	df	Sig.
Child's self-reported fatigue-preintervention	usual care group	.231	10	.139	.824	10	.028
	staff.initiated intervention	.257	10	.060	.835	10	.038

(16) (15)

a. Lilliefors Significance Correction

Figure 3.7 Boxplots of preintervention fatigue for the staff-initiated and usual-care group generated in SPSS for Windows (v. 22–23).

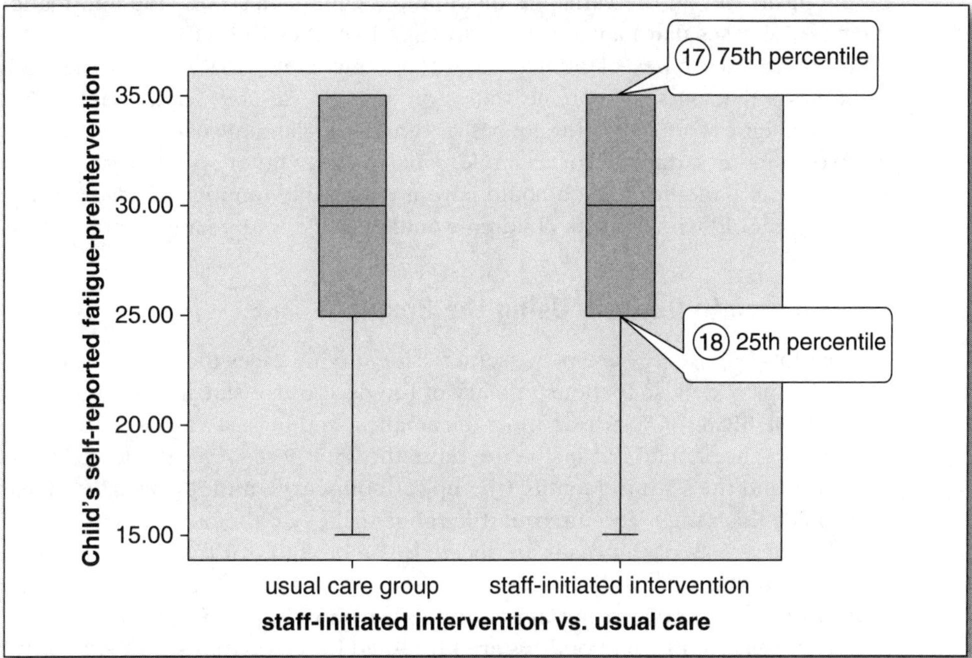

(Table 3.3, (14)). Given the small sample size for both groups (n = 10), however, as well as the shape of the histograms for both groups, nonparametric tests most likely would be used with these data. This conclusion is further supported by the significant Shapiro-Wilks tests for both groups, .028 and .038, which are less than α = .05 (15).

Notice, however that the Kolmogorov-Smirnov p values for the two groups are .139 and .06 (16), both of which are >.05. This test suggests that we should retain the null hypothesis, which states that the data are normally distributed. What should we do with this conflicting advice? Again, we need to return to the plots of the data (Figure 3.7) to determine for ourselves which of these two statistics we should believe. The results presented in Figure 3.7 suggest that both of the distributions for the usual-care and intervention groups appear to be negatively skewed. The conclusion, therefore, would be that, indeed, we do have skewed distributions for both groups.

DEALING WITH OUTLIERS

One of the disadvantages of the mean as a measure of central tendency is its sensitivity to outliers. Because outliers are extreme data points that are very much different from the rest of the data, they tend to pull the value of the mean in their direction. This can result in serious distortion of results. The median, on the other hand, is not at all influenced by atypical data points because the median assesses ranks, not actual values. The presence of outliers, therefore, requires a careful assessment of their influences both on the mean and on the variable's distribution. Outliers also provide information about the types of cases that may not fit a particular hypothesized model.

There are two types of outliers: univariate and multivariate. Univariate outliers are those cases that possess extreme values on a single variable (e.g., a child who has an extreme fatigue score). Multivariate outliers are cases with unusual combinations of scores on two or more variables. For example, a person may be of an acceptable age (e.g., 16 years old) and another person could have a reasonable number of children (e.g., four), but a 16-year-old who has four children would most likely appear as a multivariate outlier.

Assessing Univariate Outliers Using the Boxplot

Boxplots (Figure 3.7) are very useful for identifying cases that are univariate outliers. They also provide a snapshot summary of the descriptive statistics for the distribution. On request, SPSS for Windows plots the smallest and largest values of the data set, the median (the horizontal bar inside the box), the 25th percentile (the lower boundary of the box), and the 75th percentile (the upper boundary), and it presents values that lie far outside this range. The interquartile range makes up the box presented in this plot. This is where 50% of the cases are located. The boxplot for the normal distribution in Figure 3.5 A illustrates a distribution that is symmetrical, with equal tails, and a median that lies halfway between the upper and lower boundaries of the box.

Two types of univariate outliers are presented in the boxplots for SPSS for Windows. Any value that is more than three box-lengths (i.e., $3[P_{75} - P_{25}]$) from the upper or lower boundary of the box is designated on the plot with a "*" and is referred to as an *extreme value*. Each value that is between 1.5 (i.e., $1.5[P_{75} - P_{25}]$) and 3 box-lengths from the upper or lower boundary of the box is identified with an "O" and is called an *outlier*. The outliers and extreme values are also identified either by their case number (the default option) or by specifying a case label (e.g., the variable *id*). This information is useful for tracking down and correcting possible errors in data entry. The largest and smallest observed values that are not outliers are presented by lines drawn from the ends of the box to these values.

In general, boxplots are useful for comparing the distribution of a continuous variable for two or more subgroups in a sample. For example, Figure 3.5, in panels B to D, presents the boxplots for a positively skewed, a negatively skewed, and a bimodal distribution. The boxplots for the positively and negatively skewed distributions indicate that the distributions are asymmetrical, having a long tail in one direction. The median in each case is no longer in the middle of the box but rather lies closer to the bottom or top of the box, depending on the type of skew. Extreme values (*) and outliers (O) can also be found lying beyond the longer tail. It is interesting that the boxplot for a bimodal distribution (Figure 3.5D) is not very helpful in revealing the shape of the distribution. Although the box for this distribution is very large compared to the tails and there are no outliers, its bimodal shape has become hidden.

Boxplots are especially useful for comparing two distributions. For example, the boxplots for the preintervention fatigue scores for the staff-initiated intervention and usual-care groups are presented in Figure 3.7. These boxplots confirm our suspicion, based on visual inspection, that the preintervention fatigue data are negatively skewed for both groups: There is only one tail presented, directed toward the lower end of the values. Had the data been more normally distributed, two tails of equal length would have been presented, and the boxplots would have been similar to that in Figure 3.5A.

The lack of an upper tail for the preintervention anxiety scores in Figure 3.7 is understandable because there is a restricted range for this variable (14–35). For the staff-initiated intervention group, for example, the 75th percentile for this distribution is identified in the graph as the value of 35 (17) and the 25th percentile as the value 25 (18). Because 3 box-lengths is equal to 30 ($3[P_{75} - P_{25}] = 3\ [35 - 25] = 3\ [10] = 30$ and 1.5 box-lengths is equal to 15 ($1.5[P_{75} - P_{25}] = 1.5[35 - 25] = 1.5[10] = 15$), the extreme values (*) for this example would be those values that are either 65 or larger ($35 + 30=65$) or -5 or smaller ($25 - 30 = -5$). Outliers (O) would be 1.5 box-lengths above and below the upper and lower boundaries of the box, or the values of 50 ($35 + 15 = 50$) and 10 ($25 - 15 = 10$) respectively.

No children reported scores of less than 14 or higher than 35, so there were no outliers. Because there were no extreme values or minor outliers for this distribution, there are no "*" or "O" symbols in the computer printout. The conclusion to be drawn, therefore, is that the distribution of these data for both groups is relatively compact, of low range, and not normal.

Assessing Multivariate Outliers

Although the boxplot provides useful information about univariate outliers, it does not tell us anything about cases that have unusual patterns of scores with respect to two or more variables. These multivariate outliers can be screened by computer using techniques made available within SPSS using its regression analyses. Because the focus of this text is on nonparametric statistics, we will not examine these issues here. For the interested reader, these techniques (e.g., examining linear relationships, use of the Mahalanobis distance, and approaches to the analyses of residuals) are described in great detail and clarity by Hair, Black, Babin, Anderson, and Tatham (2010); J. Stevens (2009); and Tabachnick and Fidell (2013) in their excellent textbooks on multivariate statistical analysis.

What to Do About Outliers

Researchers appear to have mixed feelings about outliers and what to do about them. Some researchers view outliers as nuisance cases, ones that do not fit expectations. Others suggest that the outliers in a study are the cases that should be examined most closely. Kruskal (1988), for example, argues that "miracles are the extreme outliers of nonscientific life. . . . It is widely argued of outliers that investigation of the mechanism for outlying may be far more important than the original study that led to the outlier" (p. 929).

A critical task for the researcher is to determine why outliers exist in the first place. Are they a result of errors of coding or measurement, or are they legitimate cases that possess unique characteristics with respect to one or more variables? Different approaches to remedying problematic outliers and reducing their influence have been suggested, depending on the etiology of the outlier's presence (Hair et al., 2010; Johnson, 1985; Pedhazur & Schmelkin, 1991; Tabachnick & Fidell, 2013). Such techniques include eliminating the case altogether, reweighting or recoding the outlier to reduce its influence, and transforming the variable to create a more nearly normal distribution. It may also be useful to analyze the data both with and without the extreme data points to determine the extent of the outliers' influence.

An enormous advantage of nonparametric rank-order statistics is that the ranking of data that occur with these statistics serves to reduce the influence of outliers because the data being analyzed are ranks, not actual scores. There is no "quick fix" to the problem of outliers, and careful attention must be paid to the consequences of a particular remedy. These decisions must also be duly reported in the data analyses.

DATA TRANSFORMATION CONSIDERATIONS

When a particular distribution of a variable does not meet the normality assumption, it is possible to transform the values of that variable to create a new variable that has a more nearly normal distribution. Although this process appears easily accomplished, it does have serious problems, particularly with regard to both finding an adequate transformation index that will produce a more nearly normal distribution and interpreting the results of such a transformation. Figure 3.3 presents several common forms of nonnormal distributions and some suggested transformations that might help to create a more nearly normal distribution for the transformed variable. Hair et al. (2010) suggest that for flat (platykurtic) distributions (Figure 3.3E), the most common transformation is the inverse ($1/x$). A variable that is positively skewed (Figure 3.3B) might benefit from a log transformation ($\log(x)$), whereas one that is negatively skewed (Figure 3.3C) might be altered with a square root transformation. Leptokurtic distributions (Figure 3.3D) do not appear to have clearly defined transformations available in the research literature. Hair et al. (2010) also indicate that to achieve a noticeable effect from a transformation, the ratio of a variable's mean to its standard deviation should be less than 4.0 (i.e., mean/standard deviation < 4.0).

The goal of transforming data is to obtain a new distribution that is nearly normal in shape, with few outliers, and with skewness and kurtosis values near zero. It is important, therefore, that the researcher closely examine the distribution of the resulting transformation to ascertain if this goal has been achieved. Next, a careful interpretation of the resulting transformation needs to be made. Remember that a transformed variable no longer carries the original interpretation; the square root of preintervention fatigue is *not* the same as preintervention fatigue. Interpreting the meaning of a transformed variable is one of the most challenging tasks for the researcher.

In an attempt to obtain a more nearly normal distribution, the preintervention fatigue variable was transformed using two suggested transformations for negatively skewed distributions (Figure 3.3C). First we reflected the original variable such that the scores were reversed (i.e., *new score = (largest old score +1) – old score*), and then we took the square root and log of this newly created variable. We are using the "reflect" because our data are negatively skewed. The reflect allows us to reverse code the old variable and then take a square root or a log of the newly created variable. We need to be extremely careful, however, in our interpretation of this newly created variable since the interpretation of the direction of the scoring is now opposite of what it was before. If, for the untransformed variable, higher scores meant *greater* fatigue, then higher scores on this transformed variable will mean *lower* fatigue.

Transformations of variables can be undertaken easily in SPSS for Windows through its *Transform . . . Compute Variable* command (Figure 3.8). Using the data set, hospitalized children with cancer-20 cases.sav, two new target variables, *reflect_sqrt_fatigue_t1* and *reflect_log_fatigue_t1*, were obtained by indicating that they represent the reflect of the square root (and log) of the old variable, *Intensity_fatigue_preintervention*.

Figure 3.9 compares the newly formed reflect of the square root and log transformations with the original preintervention fatigue distribution. If the goal of data transformation is to obtain a nearly normal distribution with few outliers and with values of skewness and kurtosis near zero, it is apparent that while these transformations succeeded in lowering the skewness coefficients (Figure 3.9) to below the ±1.96 range, the shape of the resulting distributions is not normal. This failure to produce a more normal distribution may be a result of the small sample size (n = 20) and limited scale values (14–35). It also suggests that nonparametric statistics, which rely predominantly on the ranking of data, may be the approach of choice.

EXAMINING HOMOGENEITY OF VARIANCE

Another important assumption of parametric tests that compare differences between two or more groups is that the variances among the subgroups must be similar; that is, there is homogeneity of variance. A general rule of thumb is that the variance of one group should not be more than twice that of another. This assumption is especially important when groups of unequal size are being compared (Tabachnick & Fidell, 2013).

Several tests of homogeneity of variance are available in SPSS. These include Box's *M* and the Levene test. The null hypothesis for all tests of homogeneity is that the variances among the groups are equal, whereas the alternative hypothesis states that the variances are unequal. The null hypothesis will be rejected if the obtained level of significance is less than the preset level of alpha (e.g., α = .05).

The descriptive statistics presented for the preintervention fatigue variable in Table 3.3 indicate that the variance for the usual-care group was 41.39 compared to 48.89 for the intervention group. Because one variance is less than twice the other, it would appear that the homogeneity of variance assumption for preintervention fatigue has been met. The resulting Levene test generated from the *Analyze . . . Compare Means . . . Independent Samples T-test* command indicates that we would indeed fail to reject the null hypothesis

Figure 3.8 SPSS for Windows commands for transforming the negatively skewed fatigue variable.

A. Square Root of the Reflected Fatigue Variable

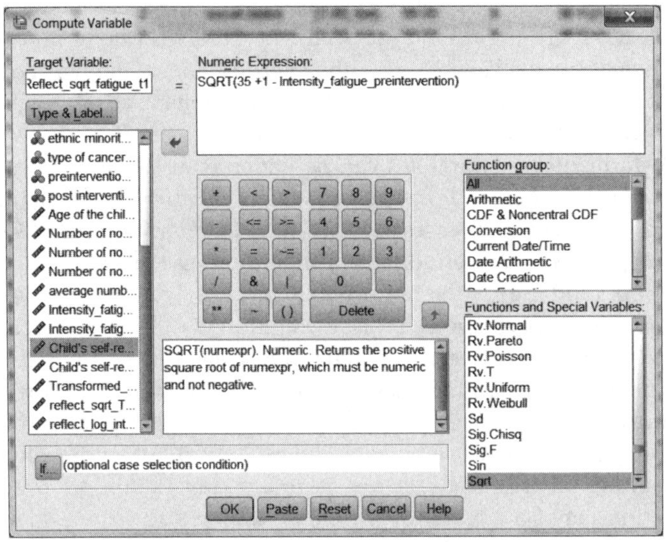

B. Log of the Reflected Fatigue Variable

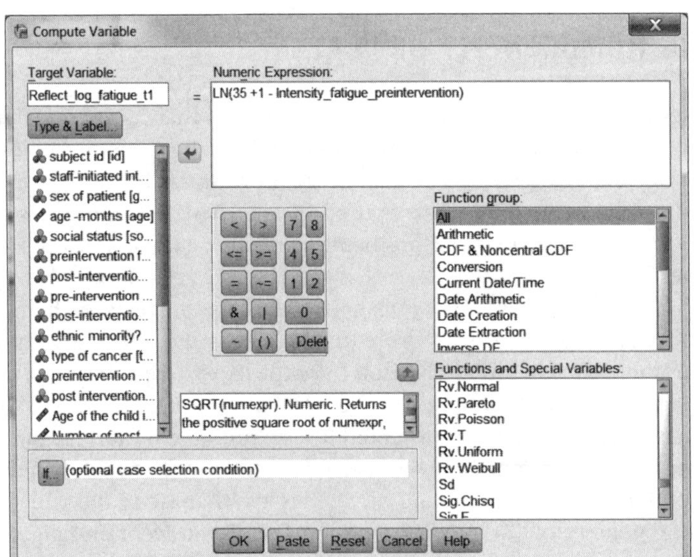

Figure 3.9 Results of reflect transformations of the preintervention fatigue variable.

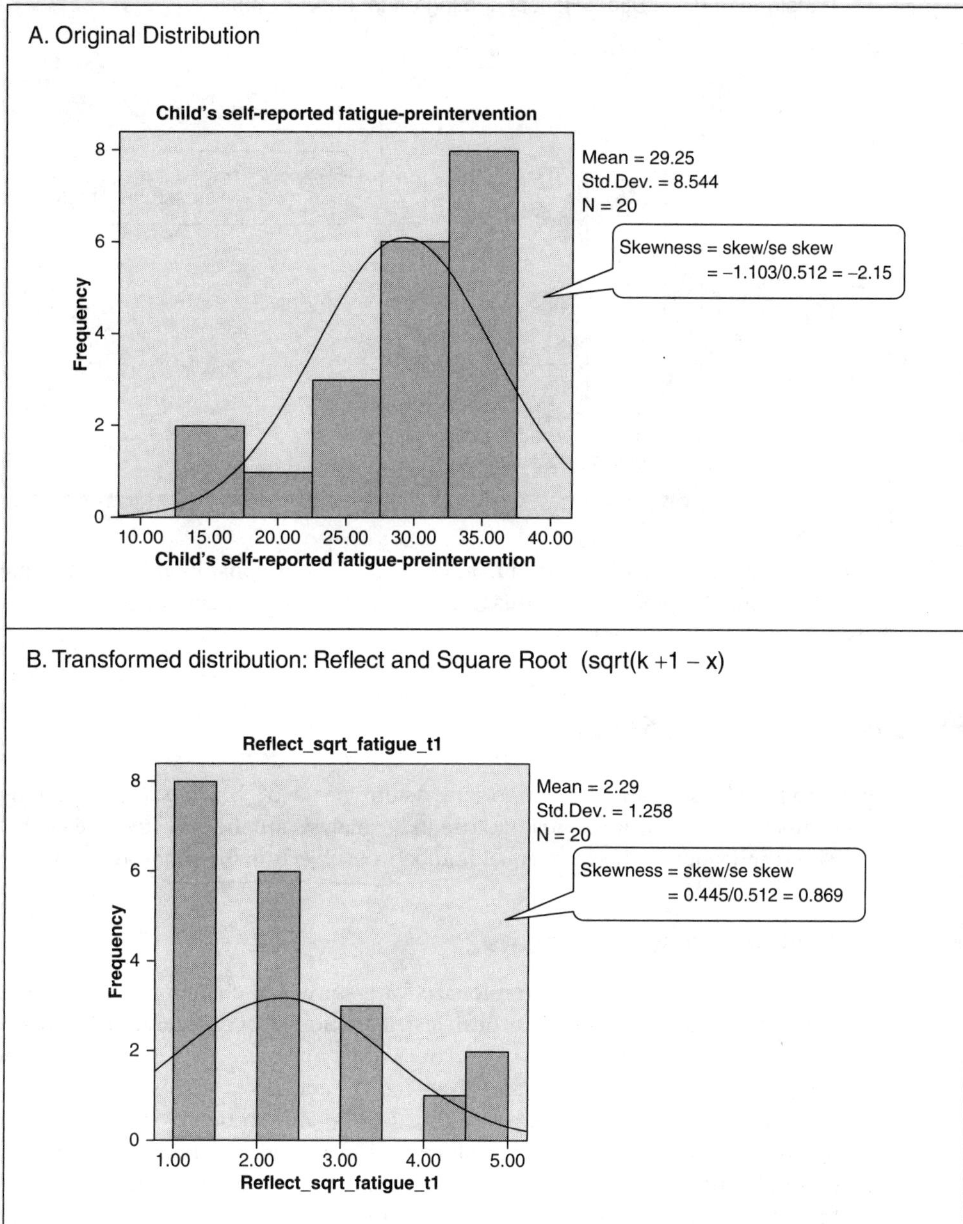

(Continued)

Figure 3.9 (Continued)

C. Transformed distribution: Reflect and logarithm (ln(k+1 – x)

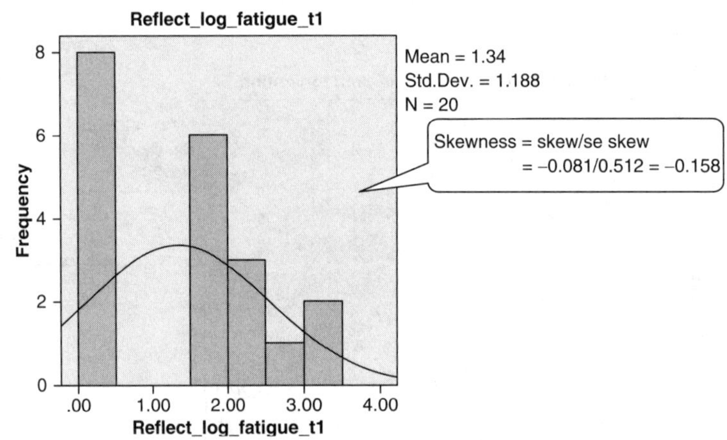

of equal variances because the significance level (.708) is considerably greater than our α = .05. We should be pleased with this "failure" because we can conclude that the variances between the groups are equal.

EVALUATING SAMPLE SIZES

Two additional issues that are important determinants of which statistic—parametric or nonparametric—is most appropriate to use in an analysis are the absolute size of the sample being used and whether there are equal numbers of subjects in the subgroups being analyzed.

Minimum Sample Size Requirements

Determining an appropriate sample size for a study is a challenging task and must be evaluated with each planned statistical test. Sample size consideration is also directly related to statistical power or the researcher's ability to correctly reject a null hypothesis. All other factors being equal (e.g., similar effect size and alpha level), the larger the sample size, the more likely it is that the researcher will be able to detect significant differences among groups. Smaller sample sizes reduce statistical power and increase the researcher's chance of making a Type II error or incorrectly concluding that the null hypothesis is true.

There is no definitive guideline as to how large a *large* sample is or what size sample is *too small* for use with a particular parametric test. The process of determining "how large is large enough?" is inextricably linked to issues of statistical power, the selected level of alpha, and the projected size of the expected differences among the groups (i.e., the "effect size").

Determining an adequate sample size also needs to be focused on the requirements of specific statistical tests (e.g., multiple regression, *t* tests, and ANOVA). An "adequate" sample size also depends in part on the normality of the distribution of the dependent variable of interest. It should be noted, though, that whatever the form of the original distribution, the central limit theorem has shown that as the sample size increases, the sampling distribution of the *mean* approaches normality. Because the mean plays a major role in most parametric statistics, this characteristic of the shape of the distribution of the mean is especially important.

In their classic text on nonparametric statistics, Siegel and Castellan (1988) argued that "if the sample size is very small, there may be no alternative to using a nonparametric statistical test unless the nature of the population distribution is known exactly" (p. 35). Unfortunately, the authors did not state specifically what they meant by a "very small" sample size. Other authors have discussed implications of using parametric statistical tests when sample sizes are *exceedingly* or *extremely* small (Neter et al., 1993) but, again, these limits are not specifically defined. Where does that leave us, as researchers, when we are faced with a total sample size of 20 and no likelihood of increasing the size? Do we use parametric or nonparametric tests to analyze our data?

The answer to this question is that "It depends." That is, the choice of a parametric or nonparametric test depends on the available sample, the variables' level of measurement, the shape of the distributions of the variables of interest, and the researcher's knowledge of the variables' distribution in the population. In addition, the researcher needs to consider the number of subgroups to be examined in the analyses. For example, dividing our sample of 20 hospitalized children into four subgroups depending on their type of cancer (e.g., solid tumor, acute myeloid leukemia, lymphoma, and sarcoma) will result in considerably smaller sample sizes (range: 2–8) to analyze than will merely breaking the group down by experimental and control groups (n = 10). Moreover, parametric analyses of the interaction of these two variables (group by type of minor surgery) would be rendered impossible given the resulting small and unequal sample sizes (n = 2 or 3 per group) within each subcategory of group by type of surgery interaction.

Assuming that we have sufficient funds to carry out this pilot study, should we consider increasing our sample size? Again, sample size determination is dependent on a number of factors (e.g., alpha, desired power, effect size, and planned statistical tests). Luckily, there are several computer programs available to help the researcher to undertake a statistical power analysis to determine the most appropriate sample size for most parametric and nonparametric statistical tests. These programs include G*Power 3 (Faul, Erdfelder, Lang, & Buchner, 2007), PASS 12 (Hintze, 2013), and IBM® SPSS® SamplePower (v. 3.0.1) (IBM® SPSS®, 2015).

Equal Numbers of Subjects Within Subgroups

As a general rule of thumb, it is highly desirable to have equal numbers of subjects within subgroups. Although this goal is attainable in experimental and quasi-experimental designs, it is often violated in descriptive studies because of natural selection. It is, therefore, a topic that cannot be avoided in health care research.

Unequal cell sizes have a differential impact on the results of a research study depending on the statistics selected. For example, the problems raised by unequal numbers of subjects are not disastrous when using *t* tests or simple one-way ANOVAs, particularly if the condition of homogeneity of variance is met (Tabachnick & Fidell, 2013). Serious problems regarding unequal cell sizes with or without homogeneity of variance arise, however, in factorial designs, such as two-way ANOVA, analysis of covariance (ANCOVA), multivariate analysis of variance (MANOVA), repeated-measures ANOVA, and multiple regression. These problems are generated because the hypotheses that test the main effects and interaction terms are no longer orthogonal (i.e., independent) when there are unequal cell sizes. Tabachnick and Fidell (2013) offer an in-depth discussion of both the problem of unequal cell sizes and possible solutions in their text on multivariate statistics. The problem of confounding of main effects for multiple factors when there are unequal cell sizes is present in some nonparametric analyses as well.

REPORTING TESTING ASSUMPTIONS AND VIOLATIONS IN A RESEARCH REPORT

The reporting of assessment of assumptions and their violations does not appear to be a common practice in health care research. Pett and Sehy (1996) found that less than 20% of the 238 randomly selected nursing research articles that they reviewed included even a brief discussion (i.e., a sentence or two) of the assumptions underlying the use of the statistical tests reported. Discussion of the formal testing of the assumptions underlying the statistical tests, management of violations of these assumptions, and handling of extreme data was also uncommon (15.5%, 14.7%, and 3.4%, respectively). Similar findings were reported by Gaither and Glorfeld (1983) in organizational behavior. These authors offer the hope that researchers do indeed consider the assumptions underlying their choice of statistical tests carefully but either choose not to report their findings or are discouraged to do so by reviewers or editors of journals.

The reporting of tests of assumptions and handling of violations does not have to be an arduous undertaking. A mere sentence or two would suffice. Robichaud-Ekstrand (1991), for example, did this very nicely in her report of responses to shower versus sink baths for 30 patients with myocardial infarction:

> Because the distribution of the overall subjective scores was skewed, a Friedman test ($p \leq .05$) and Wilcoxon post hoc pairwise tests ($p \leq .02$) were used. Pearson [product moment] correlations were used to compare the skewed scores of RPE [ratings of perceived exertion] and the overall subjective scores with the normally distributed HR [heart rate] and BP [blood pressure] scores. (p. 378)

Summary

This chapter has attempted to provide the reader with some guidelines for determining which statistics, parametric or nonparametric, are best suited for the data at hand. Box 3.1 presents a summary checklist of the procedures that the researcher can use to assess the characteristics of the data being analyzed. These steps include determining the level of measurement of the variables of interest, evaluating their distributions, assessing homogeneity of variances, considering sample sizes, determining the statistics that are best suited for these data, and duly reporting the results of this investigation. It is rare that data collected from the "real world" are perfectly suited to the requirements of a particular parametric or nonparametric test. Remember, however, that the bottom line to the choice of most parametric statistics is the important question: *Do the mean and standard deviation truly represent your data?*

BOX 3.1 Checklist for Assessing the Characteristics of Data

1. Determine the levels of measurement of the variables of interest.
2. Evaluate the distribution of these variables:
   - Compare the measures of central tendency for each variable
   - Determine skewness and kurtosis
   - Visually assess the distributions
   - Examine the probability plots
   - Transform the variables if necessary
   - Examine and interpret the results of the transformation
3. Check for homogeneity of variance.
4. Assess the total sample size and size of the subgroups.
5. Determine which statistic, parametric or nonparametric, is best suited for these data.
6. Report the process of evaluation and decisions in the data analysis section.

TEST YOUR KNOWLEDGE

Here are some questions that should help you recall the key points of this chapter. If you find that you cannot recall the answers, go back to the text and reread the appropriate sections.

1. What are the characteristics of the four levels of measurement?
2. What are the levels of measurement of the following variables?
   a. Time to wakefulness following anesthesia
   b. Weight of a child in pounds
   c. Scores on a single-item pain scale (0 = *little or no pain* to 10 = *severe pain*)
   d. IQ of your significant other
   e. Staging of breast cancer (Stages I through IV)
   f. A list of different specialties in your profession

(Continued)

(Continued)

g. Level of depression as measured by a 30-item (0 = no, 1 = yes) depression scale (total score: 0–30)
h. Ethnicity of the patient

3. What is the meaning of skewness and kurtosis, and how would you evaluate these conditions?
4. What is the difference between a univariate and multivariate outlier? How would you assess these conditions?
5. What kind(s) of transformations might I consider if I had the following distribution for a variable:
   a. Positively skewed distribution
   b. Negatively skewed distribution
   c. Mesokurtic distribution
   d. J-shaped distribution

COMPUTER EXERCISES

Here is a computer exercise that should help you to put into practice that which has been discussed in this chapter.

1. Using the data set provided to you at study.sagepub.com/pett2e (use hospitalized children with cancer-20 cases.sav or hospitalized children with cancer-20 cases.xlsx), please undertake the following assessments:
   a. Using SPSS for Windows (or another suitable statistical program), generate descriptive statistics including skewness and kurtosis coefficients, boxplots, and histograms for the following variables: age of the child in years, preintervention fatigue, and postintervention fatigue.
   b. In a sentence or two, describe the distributions of these three variables. Are there any outliers that you are concerned about?
   c. Which of these variables would you consider transforming? If so, what type of transformation would you choose?
   d. Undertake the transformation(s) of these variables. Rerun the descriptive statistics on these variables. How, if at all, did the transformation alter the shape, skewness, and kurtosis of your variables?

Visit **study.sagepub.com/pett2e** to access SAS output, SPSS datasets, SAS datasets, and SAS examples.

CHAPTER 4

"Goodness-of-Fit" Tests

- Binomial test
- Chi-square goodness-of-fit test
- Kolmogorov-Smirnov one-and two-sample tests

In this chapter, we will examine nonparametric "goodness-of-fit" tests. These types of tests are used when the researcher has obtained a sample of values and wants to know if this sample comes from a specified population distribution. For example, we might want to know whether the proportion of men and women obtained in a collected sample is similar to that in a target population. We might also like to test statistically whether a variable's distribution is similar to that of a normal or other distribution. These tests are described as *goodness-of-fit* tests because they compare the results obtained from a given sample to a prespecified distribution. The following tests that will be examined in this chapter are the binomial test, the chi-square goodness-of-fit test, and the Kolmogorov-Smirnov one- and two-sample tests for normal and other distributions.

THE BINOMIAL TEST

Many nominal-level variables are dichotomous. The variable "gender," for example, consists of two levels: male and female. In our hypothetical intervention study from Chapter 1, we created a grouping variable (*group*) that had two classes: a staff-initiated intervention and a usual-care group. A third type of dichotomous variable could be an outcome following an invasive intervention: cured or not cured.

Suppose we are interested in examining whether the proportion of 20 families in our hypothetical study who are ethnic minorities ($n = 5$) is different from that routinely seen in the hospital setting from which our sample has been drawn. The binomial test can provide us with this information. This test uses the binomial distribution to determine the likelihood of obtaining a number as extreme as or more extreme than that which we obtained in our sample (e.g., $n \leq 5$), given what we know about the numbers of ethnic minority families who routinely use the hospital facilities.

An Appropriate Research Question for the Binomial Test

The binomial test has been used in a number of different ways in the health care research literature. For example, Jagsi et al. (2009) used the binomial test to determine the underrepresentation of women in high-impact published clinical cancer research. Reed, Price, Grost, and Mantinan (2012) also used binomial tests to compare the proportions of male and female, White, and other park users in Michigan with similar cohorts in the general population. In our hypothetical intervention study, we are interested in comparing the ethnicity characteristics of our sample of convenience with those of the population of families who typically use the study hospital. The data set that we will be using for the binomial test is hospitalized children with cancer-20 cases.sav. It is located on the SAGE website, study.sagepub.com/pett2e. A research question that could be answered using the binomial test is as follows:

> Is the proportion of ethnic minority families who appear in the intervention study similar to the proportion of ethnic minority families who typically use the hospital facilities?

Null and Alternative Hypotheses

Table 4.1 presents the null and alternative hypotheses associated with this research question that are appropriate for the binomial test. Notice that these hypotheses focus on the proportions that would be expected under the null hypothesis that there is no difference between the proportions of ethnic minority families appearing in the sample and in the population. In statistical hypothesis testing, the alternative or research hypothesis can be directional or nondirectional. In our hypothetical intervention study, because our hypothesized proportion is less than .50 (it is .33) and we know our sample proportion is less than .33 (.25), we are going to use a directional alternative hypothesis (H_a: $p < p_0$); that is, the sample will be different from our hospital comparison population if too few of the families are in the "ethnic minority" group than would have been expected by chance. Since the hospital's proportion of ethnic minority families (.33) is definitely larger than that of our sample (.25), when stating the null hypothesis, we will not include the impossibility that our sample proportion is larger than that of the hospital (i.e., $p > p_0$).

Table 4.1 Example of Null and Alternative Hypotheses Appropriate for a Binomial Test

Null Hypothesis
H_0: There is no difference between the proportion of the ethnic minority families in our sample compared with that of the hospital in general; that is, $p = p_0$.
Alternative Hypothesis
H_a: The proportion of ethnic minority families in our sample is lower compared with that of the hospital in general; that is, $p < p_0$.

Overview of the Procedure

To use the binomial test, the data under examination must consist of a single nominal-level variable that is dichotomous. If the variable of interest is not dichotomous (e.g., an "ethnic status" variable that contains more than two classes), it needs to be collapsed carefully into two mutually exclusive categories (e.g., minority and nonminority). Defining the criteria used to define these two distinct classes, however, is the task for the researcher, not the computer. Values of "1" are assigned to those individuals who make up the category of interest (e.g., 1 = ethnic minority), and values of "0" are assigned to those individuals who belong to all other categories (e.g., 0 = ethnic nonminority).

Next, the proportion (p) of subjects who reside in the population of interest who would have been assigned a value of 1 for the target variable had they taken part in the study needs to be determined. Because it is a proportion, this value can take on values only between 0 and 1. Finally, the proportion of subjects in the target population (1 − p = q) who would have been assigned a value of 0 for the target variable is identified. Values for p and q could be obtained from a variety of sources, such as official records, census data, and prior research. In our hypothetical example, we might have patient census information available for the previous 12 months that indicates that the proportion of ethnic minority families who have used the hospital facilities is one third. Our p, therefore, would equal .33, and 1 − p = q = .67.

The binomial test is based on the binomial distribution. This distribution enables the researcher to determine the probability that the given sample of subjects (e.g., 20 families, of whom 5 are ethnic minorities and 15 are nonminorities) could have come from a binomial population whose values of p and q are similar to those of the target population (e.g., .33 and .67). The formula for a binomial distribution is:

$$\mathrm{P}[Y = k] = \binom{N}{k} \mathrm{p}^{k}\mathrm{q}^{N-k}$$

where

$\mathrm{P}[Y = k]$ = the probability of obtaining exactly k observations in one class and $N - k$ observations in the other;

Y = a random variable that can take on any number of values that are greater than 0 but no larger than the sample size, N;

k = the number of subjects in the sample who were assigned the value of 1 on the target variable;

$\binom{N}{k}$ = N *choose* $k = \dfrac{N!}{(k!)(N-k)!}$; and

N = the total sample size.

The exclamation point (!) indicates a factorial; for example, $N! = (N)(N-1)(N-2)\ldots(2)(1)$. Suppose that we want to know the probability of obtaining exactly five minority families in our study given p = .33. This random variable, Y, would take on the value of

5, and the probability that a random sample of size 20 will contain exactly 5 minority families would be calculated as follows:

$$P[Y = k] = \binom{N}{k} p^k q^{N-k} = P[Y = 5] = \binom{20}{5} .33^5 \ .67^{15}$$

$$= \frac{20!}{5!15!} (.0039)(.0025) = .1493.$$

The probability, therefore, that we would obtain exactly 5 ethnic minority families in a sample of 20 is .1493.

In hypothesis testing, we are not usually interested in the probability of obtaining *exact* values; instead, we often want to know the probability of obtaining values *as extreme as or more extreme than* our obtained value. In our intervention study, for example, we might want to know the probability of obtaining 5 or fewer ethnic minority families in a sample of size 20 given the proportion of such families in the target population (i.e., p = .33). In this case, we would want to calculate $P[Y \le k]$, which would be the sum of the probabilities that Y = 0, 1, 2, 3, 4, and 5, or $P[Y=0]+P[Y=1]+P[Y=2]+P[Y=3]+P[Y=4]+P[Y=5]$.

Performing such calculations by hand quickly involves a lot of pencil pushing. There are binomial distribution tables for small sample sizes ($n \le 25$) in many statistics textbooks, but these tables are large and cumbersome, difficult to interpret, and often do not offer exact comparisons (e.g., we might be given a p = .30 or p = .35 instead of p = .33 as in our example). Fortunately, we can access via the Internet free cumulative distribution function (CDF) calculators.

For the binomial calculator, we could go to a site such as DanielSoper.com and click on *Statistics Calculators . . . Cumulative Binomial Probability Calculator.* We would enter the "probability of success" (p = .33) (the proportion of ethnic minorities typically seen in this hospital setting), the number of successes (5) (the number of ethnic minorities in our sample), and the number of trials (20) (our sample size). Having input that information, we are quickly given the output presented in Figure 4.1. From this output, we can see that the probability of having up to 5 ethnic minorities in a sample of 20, given that the proportion of ethnic minorities in the hospital population is .33, is .3082 (1).

We could have obtained this same information had we painstakingly calculated the probabilities by hand using the formula given above. That is,

$$P[Y \le 5] = P[Y = 0] + P[Y = 1] + P[Y = 2] + P[Y = 3] + P[Y = 4] + P[Y = 5]$$

$$= .0003 + .0033 + .0153 + .0453 + .0947 + .1493 = .3082$$

What does that mean to us? It means that the probability of having up to five minorities in our sample, given the hospital rate of .33, is .3082. Comparing that *p* value (.3082) to α = .05, we would fail to reject the null hypothesis of no differences between the proportion of minorities in our group and the hospital population.

Figure 4.1 Results obtained using an Internet-accessed cumulative binomial probability calculator.

This calculator will compute cumulative probabilities for a binomial outcome, given the number of successes, the number of trials, and the probability of a successful outcome occurring. For the number of successes x, the calculator will return P(X < x), P(X ≤ x), P(X > x), and P(X ≥ x).

Please supply the necessary parameter values, and then click 'Calculate'.

Probability of success: 0.33 — Proportion in population of interest

Successes: 5 — # Persons of interest in sample

Trials: 20 — Sample size

Calculate!

P(X < 5): 0.15892403

P(X ≤ 5): 0.30825006 (1)

P(X > 5): 0.69174994

P(X ≥ 5): 0.84107597

SOURCE: Copyright © 2006–2015 by Dr. Daniel Soper. All rights reserved. Retrieved from http://www.danielsoper.com/statcalc

Using the *z* Approximation to the Binomial Distribution

The binomial distribution also approximates a normal z distribution as N becomes large and p is not too close to the extreme values of 0 or 1. This z distribution can be used when Np and Nq (where q = 1 – p) are both greater than 5 (Daniel, 2000). If this approximation is used in place of the binomial distribution, $P(Y \leq k)$ is obtained by examining the probability of obtaining a z statistic as extreme as or more extreme than the following:

$$z = \frac{(Y \pm .5) - N\text{p}}{\sqrt{N\text{p}q}}$$

Note that $(Y + .5)$ is used when $Y < N\text{p}$, and $(Y - .5)$ is used when $Y > N\text{p}$.

In our hypothetical study, we could use this approximation because we meet Daniel's (2000) criteria (Np = (20)(.33) = 6.7 and Nq = (20)(.67) = 13.3). We would also use the value $(Y + .5)$ to calculate the z statistic because Np = 6.7 is greater than 5. Our z statistic, therefore, would be calculated as follows:

$$z = \frac{(Y+.5)-Np}{\sqrt{Npq}} = \frac{(5+.5)-20(.33)}{\sqrt{(20)(.33)(.67)}} = -.52$$

Using the table of values for the cumulative distribution function for the standard normal curve that is available in Appendix A (Table A.1a–b) in the back of this textbook, we can calculate the area under the curve that lies to the left of $z = -.52$. Since, by definition the z distribution is symmetric about its mean (0), the area under the curve that lies to the left of $-.52$ is the same as that which lies to the right of $+.52$. Since Table A.1a represents the cumulative distribution function for the standard normal curve (from $-\infty$ to z), we would go to the first column, identify the first decimal for z (+.5), and move across to the third column (.02) to arrive at +.52. The area under the curve that lies to the left of +.52 is .6985.

Since the whole area under the curve from $-\infty$ to $+\infty = 1.0$, then $1 - .6985$ or .3015 represents the area that lies to the right of both $z = +.52$ and $z = -.52$. Except for approximation error, this area is similar to that which we obtained from the exact values of the binomial distribution (.3082). Because this p value is considerably larger than $\alpha = .05$, we will fail to reject the null hypothesis and conclude that our sample is not significantly different from the target population. The meaning of these results will be discussed in greater detail when we examine the computer printout generated in SPSS for Windows.

Confidence Intervals for the Binomial Test

Sometimes we are less interested in hypothesis testing but rather would like to determine the range of possible values of our statistic in our population of interest. This range is called the *confidence interval* (*CI*). A CI represents the confidence that we have that the true population value for a given statistic lies within a given range. Typically, the CI is set at the $100(1 - \alpha)\%$ level, where α represents the level of Type I error we are willing to set (e.g., .05). In our example, we would be interested in the 95% CI for the proportion of minority families in the population. That is, we could say that there is a 95% probability that the true value for the proportion of minority families in our population of interest ranges between the two calculated values.

As we discussed above, as N becomes larger, the probabilities of the binomial distribution can be approximated by the standard normal distribution, where the mean of this distribution = p and the standard deviation = $\sqrt{\frac{PQ}{N}}$. When the sample size is small, the 95% CI for a proportion can be estimated by the following approximation (Hays, 1994):

$$\frac{N}{N+z^2}\left[P + \frac{z^2}{2N} \pm z\sqrt{\frac{PQ}{N} + \frac{z^2}{4N^2}}\right]$$

where

N = the sample size (e.g., 20);

Z = a two-tailed Z score for our chosen alpha (e.g., 1.96 for $\alpha = .05$);

P = the proportion of "successes" (i.e., minorities) in our sample (e.g., 5/20 or .25); and

$Q = 1 - P$ (e.g., 1 − .25 or .75).

For our example, we would obtain the following 95% CI:

$$\frac{20}{20+1.96^2}\left[.25+\frac{1.96^2}{2(20)}\pm 1.96\sqrt{\frac{(.25)(.75)}{20}+\frac{1.96^2}{4(20)^2}}\right]$$

$$.8389\left[.3460 \pm 1.96(.1085)\right]$$

$$.8389\left[.1333, .5587\right]$$

$$\left[.112, .469\right]$$

According to our calculations, there is a 95% probability that the true proportion of minority families in our population of interest ranges between .112 and .469. Given that the comparison proportion that we had for ethnic minority families in the hospital population was .33, we could not reject the null hypothesis of similar proportions since .33 falls within the range for our potential population proportion.

For larger sample sizes (e.g., $N \geq 100$), Hays (1994) indicates that this confidence interval can be reduced to the following formula:

$$(1-\alpha)\%\ \text{CI} = P \pm Z_{\alpha/2}\sqrt{\frac{PQ}{N-1}}$$

This standard interval is similar to the Wald interval for the binomial case (Brown, Cai, & DasGupta, 2001).

If we were to use this formula for our data ($P = .25$, $Q = .75$, $N = 20$, and $Z = 1.96$), we would arrive at yet another range of values for the 95% CI:

$$95\%\ \text{CI} = .25 \pm 1.96\sqrt{\frac{(.25)(.75)}{19}}$$

$$= .25 \pm .1947$$

$$= \left[.055, .445\right]$$

That is quite a different confidence interval from that which we obtained above! Which one should we believe?

Brown et al. (2001) indicate that there are problems with using this Wald interval formula to accurately estimate confidence intervals for binomial proportions, particularly with small sample sizes and with P near 0 or 1. Both Brown and colleagues and Agresti and Coull (1998) argue that this Wald interval is a poor estimator even when p is not at the extremes, given that it is subject to erratic and unpredictable behavior. Agresti and Coull (1998) provide an adjustment to the Wald interval formula, which Brown et al. (2001) suggest is a good alternative to use when $n > 40$. That is, when $\alpha = .05$, the value of "2" is used instead of 1.96, and 2 "successes" and 2 "failures" are added to the formula:

$$Adj(1-\alpha)100\%\text{CI} \cong \tilde{P} \pm 2.00\sqrt{\frac{\tilde{P}\tilde{Q}}{\tilde{N}}}$$

where

$\tilde{P} = (X + 2)/(N + 4)$,

$\tilde{Q} = 1 - \tilde{P}$, and

$\tilde{N} = N + 4$.

If we were to use this adjusted Agresti-Coull interval with our data, we would arrive at the following confidence interval:

$$Adj(95)\%\text{CI} = \frac{(5+2)}{(20+4)} \pm 2.00\sqrt{\frac{\left(\frac{7}{24}\right)\left(\frac{17}{24}\right)}{24}}$$

$$= .2917 \pm 2.00(.0928)$$

$$= .2917 \pm .1856$$

$$= .106, .477$$

This is much closer to our Hays (1994) estimate. Given the varied results obtained in estimating confidence intervals for proportions, Brown et al. (2001) suggest using the equal-tailed Jeffrey prior interval for small sample sizes ($n \leq 40$) (Brown et al., 2001) and the Agresti-Coull interval (Agresti & Coull, 1998) for $n \geq 40$. We will go over some of these approaches to estimation when generating the SPSS output.

Undertaking the Binomial Test in SPSS for Windows

Given that we have access to SPSS for Windows, it will be quite easy to run this example using that program with our data set, hospitalized children with cancer-20 cases.sav. We could obtain the output for the binomial test in two ways. First, we would click on *Analyze . . . Nonparametric tests . . .* and then choose either the *One Sample tests . . .* or *Legacy Dialogues*. While the *Legacy Dialogues . . .* approach generates output similar to earlier versions of SPSS, the *One Sample test* approach has the advantage of also estimating confidence intervals for the binomial test.

Figure 4.2 SPSS for Windows commands for generating the binomial test.

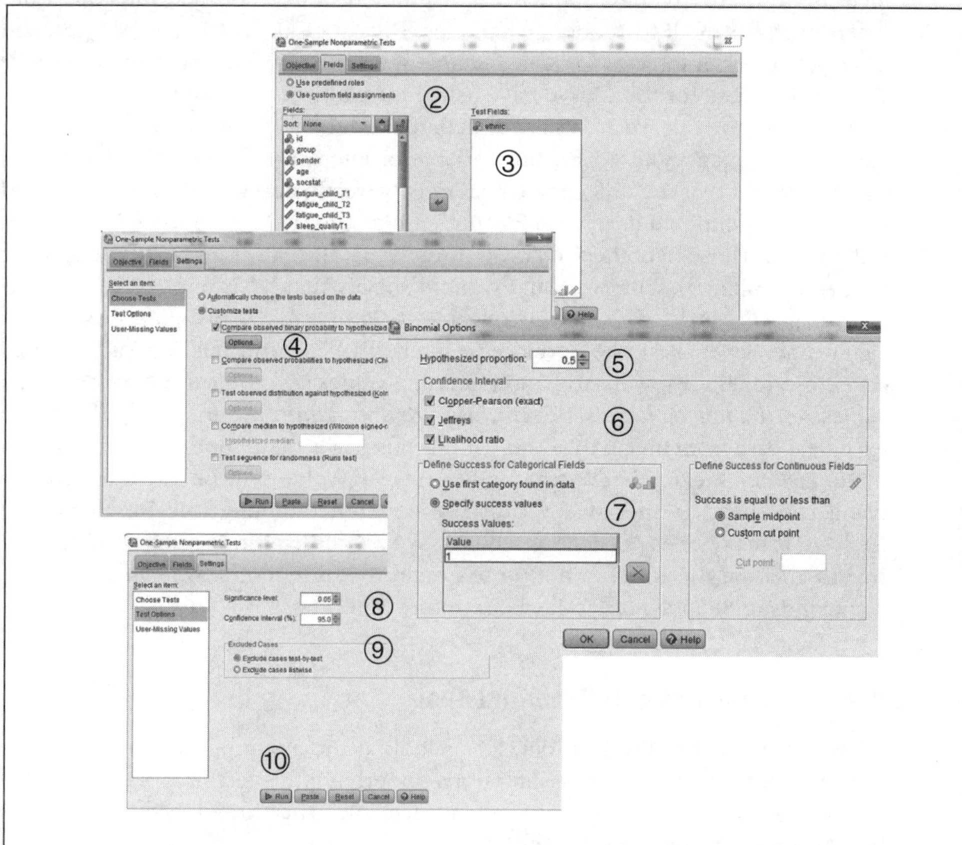

Clicking on the *One-sample nonparametric tests* . . . command will open the *One Sample Nonparametric Tests* Dialog Box (Figure 4.2). Our first task is to identify the variable(s) that we will be using in our analysis (2). We can do that by clicking on the *Fields* . . . and *Use custom field assignments* . . . buttons. The variables to be tested (e.g., *ethnic*) should be moved over to the *Test Fields* . . . box (3). The variables that we will not be examining will remain in the *Fields* box.

Clicking on *Settings* . . . will open the dialog box, which enables you to *Customize* and select the *Binomial test*. Clicking on the *Options* . . . button directly underneath this choice (4) will allow us to change the *Hypothesized proportion* from the default (.50) to our hypothesized proportion of interest (.33) (5).

We can also obtain a 95% confidence interval (CI) for our proportion (6). There are three methods available for computing CIs for binary data: the *Clopper-Pearson* CI, which is an exact interval based on the cumulative binomial distribution; the *Jeffreys,* which is a Bayesian interval; and the *likelihood ratio,* an interval based on the likelihood function for p. Agresti (2013) suggests that the likelihood ratio test-based interval is preferable when we have small to moderate samples. Brown et al. (2001) also suggest the equal-tailed Jeffrey prior interval for small sample sizes ($n \leq 40$). For the sake of comparing the three estimations for the CI, we have asked for all three estimates.

Just below the CIs, we are asked to define "Success" for categorical fields. We can either use the first category listed for our variable of interest or specify the "Success" value(s) (7). Be careful that the "Success" category is correctly defined. Since we have coded ethnicity as 1 = ethnic minority and 2 = not ethnic minority, our "Success" value = 1, which is the group whose hypothesized proportion is .33. Had we coded *ethnic* as 0 = nonminority and 1 = minority, then we could want to specify that "1" is our "Success" value.

Under *Settings . . .* we can also select *Test Options . . . .* This allows us to choose the significance level (.05), the confidence interval (95%), and missing values (8). We can also indicate how we want to handle missing values (9). We can either exclude missing values *test by test* or *listwise. Excluding missing values test by test* means that we will exclude a case from the analysis only if it is missing a value for the variable we are examining. *Listwise* means that a case with a missing value will be excluded from all tests being conducted in the run. Because we are only running one binomial test in this analysis, it really does not matter which way we will handle missing values. Now we are free to click on the *Run . . .* button to obtain the output (10). We can also *Paste . . .* the commands to SPSS Syntax to facilitate future SPSS runs.

Critical Assumptions of the Binomial Test

Before we review the printout, let us look at the assumptions for the binomial test. Because there are not many assumptions underlying this test, it is a valuable test to use when other, more powerful tests are not feasible. The three basic assumptions of the binomial test are described below.

1. *The randomly selected observations are independent and obtained from a single sample.* This assumption means that there are no duplicate observations in which a respondent's answers are counted twice, and no respondent has exerted an undue influence on the other responses. In addition, there is a single sample that consists of all the respondents who are taking part in the study. The binomial test is not appropriate for repeated observations obtained from the same sample or when two or more groups are being compared.

2. *The data must be in two discrete categories to which the values of 0 and 1 have been assigned.* It may be that the variable of interest is at the nominal level of measurement but not dichotomous. If that is the case, the multiple levels of the variable need to be collapsed into two mutually exclusive categories. Better yet, a new variable could be created from the old one, thus retaining the old variable's values for future reference. In our hypothetical example, we may have had several

types of ethnic minority families, requiring collapsing of the data into a single category for minorities. In SPSS for Windows, a new dichotomous variable containing two levels can be created easily from a multilevel variable by highlighting the commands *Transform . . . Recode . . . Into a Different Variable* in the menu.

3. *The probability of an event occurring in a given population can be specified (e.g., p = .5).* To use the binomial test, the value of p, or the proportion of events in the population that is likely to take on the value of 1 for the variable of interest, must be specified or estimated. As indicated, these theoretical proportions can come from a variety of sources, such as public records, census data, or prior research.

Computer-Generated Output

Figure 4.3 presents the syntax commands (11) and computer-generated printout obtained from SPSS for Windows. The data set that was used was hospitalized children with cancer-20 cases.sav. In the future, the syntax commands could be used in lieu of using the menu by replacing *ethnic* with the variable of interest.

When examining the Hypothesis Test Summary, you need to be careful when making a decision whether to reject or fail to reject the null hypothesis. Do not rely totally on the posted decision listed in the output (e.g., *Retain the null hypothesis . . .*) (12). Review your stated null and alternative hypotheses. Was your alternative hypothesis a one- or a two-tailed test, and do these results (e.g., two-tailed $p = .308$) (13) fit with your predicted alternative hypothesis, or do you need to divide this value in half to obtain a one-tailed p value (e.g., if two-tailed p=.308, then one-tailed p=.308/2=.154).

Double-clicking on the *Hypothesis Test Summary* will open up the *Model Viewer*. At the bottom of the *Model Viewer,* we can toggle between the *Hypothesis* and *Confidence Interval Summary* views. Looking at the *Hypothesis Test Summary* (Figure 4.3), we are first presented with a set of plots that compare the *observed* proportion of ethnic minorities in our sample (.25) with that of the *hypothesized* proportion obtained from the hospital proportion (.33) (14). To determine whether the difference between these proportions, .33 and .25, is large enough to reject the null hypothesis of no difference in proportions, we need to turn to the one-tailed asymptotic (.300) and exact (.308) significance or p values (15) and compare them to our stated alpha level (.05). The decision rule is that we would reject the null hypothesis of similarity of proportions if the obtained one-tailed significance level is less than .05.

Since both of these p values are greater than our alpha, we fail to reject the null hypothesis of no difference in proportions. They are also similar to what we obtained when using a table of probabilities for the binomial distribution. Our conclusion is, therefore, that there is no significant difference between the proportion of ethnic minority families in our sample and that in the hospital in general.

Should we be pleased with or concerned about this decision not to reject the null hypothesis? In this particular situation, we might be pleased to note that our sample is not unlike the hospital population, at least with regard to the proportion of ethnic minority families participating in our study. This finding increases the potential generalizability of our findings.

Figure 4.3 SPSS output for the binomial test.

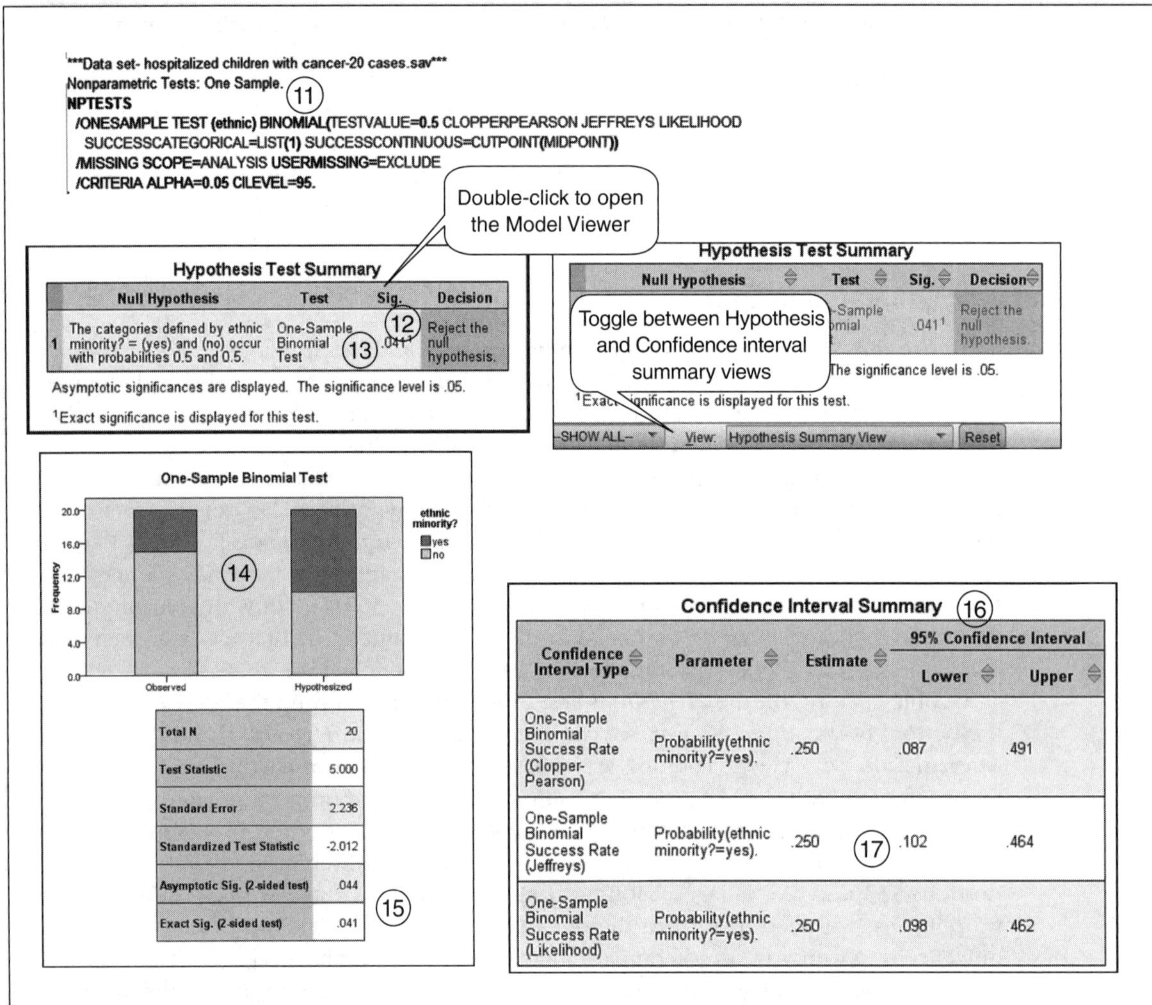

Figure 4.3 also presents a summary of the three confidence intervals (CIs) that we requested (16). It appears that both these CIs and those that we calculated earlier are somewhat different from one another:

Estimates obtained from our earlier calculations:

Hays estimate	.112, .469
Wald estimate	.055, .445
Agresti-Coull	.106, .477

From the computer printout

Clopper-Pearson	.087, .491
Jeffreys	.102, .464
Likelihood	.098, .462

We have six estimates, five of which are within reasonable range of each other. Which one should we report? As indicated earlier, for small samples, it has been recommended that either the Jeffreys (Brown et al., 2001) or the likelihood (Agresti, 2003, 2013) confidence intervals be used. Since they are approximately the same, we will report the Jeffreys estimate (17). That is, there is a 95% probability that the true proportion of minorities in our population of interest ranges between .10 and .46. Since our hypothesized proportion, .33, falls in that interval, we cannot reject the null hypothesis that the proportion of minorities in our sample is similar to that of the hospital proportion.

There are a number of resources that the reader might find useful concerning the choice of exact confidence intervals for discrete data. These include the works by Agresti (2003, 2013); Kabaila and Lloyd (2000); Lloyd (2007, 2013); Shan, Ma, Hutson, and Wilding (2012); and Wang (2006, 2010). Shan and Wang (2013) have presented an R package for computing exact confidence intervals for the difference of two proportions. Hopefully, additional contributions will also find their way into the repertoire of the commonly used statistical computer packages.

Presentation of Results

Several approaches could be taken to present the data obtained from a binomial test. A very simple but effective approach would be to present the results in text form as follows:

> No statistically significant differences were found between the proportion of ethnic minority families who participated in this study (.25) and that which would have been expected (.33) given the numbers of minority families who utilize the hospital's services (p = .30) (95% CI: .10, .46).

A second approach might be to present these results in tabular form similar to Table 4.2.

Advantages, Limitations, and Alternatives to the Binomial Test

The binomial test is extremely useful in many different types of situations because all that is required is a dichotomous variable and knowledge about the expected

Table 4.2 Comparison of the Numbers and Proportions of Ethnic Minority Families in the Study and in the Hospital Population

	Observed		Expected			
Ethnic Minority?	N	*Proportion*	N	*Proportion*	*95% CI*[a]	p
Yes	5	.25	6.3	.33	.10, .46	.30
No	15	.75	13.7	.67		
Total	20	1.00	20.0	1.00		

[a]Jeffreys 95% CI interval estimate.

proportions in the population. Data also could be collapsed to obtain these dichotomous categories. Conover (1999) indicates that with a bit of ingenuity, the binomial test can be adapted to nearly any data set. Siegel and Castellan (1988) caution, however, that when a continuous variable is dichotomized (e.g., collapsing a person's age into two categories such as younger than 30 and 30 and older), the choice of the binomial test may result in a waste of rich information contained in the data.

Because the binomial test uses only categorical data, there is no parametric counterpart to this nonparametric test. A nonparametric alternative is the chi-square goodness-of-fit test.

Sample Size Determination for the Binomial Test

Because ours was a pilot study undertaken by clinical researchers with little or no funding, we were restricted in the number of hospitalized children that we could include in our sample ($n = 20$). Suppose we wanted to know how big of a sample size would we have needed to detect a statistically significant greater difference between our group and that of the hospital population with regard to ethnicity with 80% power, $\alpha = .05$, and contrasting proportions of .25 (for our sample) versus .33 (our hospital population). To determine how large our sample for this one-tailed test would have needed to be, we could use a number of different sample size determination packages, for example, Sample Power (IBM, 2012) and PASS12 (Hintze, 2013). Using PASS12, we arrived at the following sample size determination:

> A sample size of 171 from a population of 1,000 achieves 81% power to detect a superiority proportion (P0) of .2500 using a one-sided binomial test for superiority. The target significance level is .0500. The actual significance level achieved by this test is .0465. These results assume that the actual proportion (P1) is .3300.

Examples From Published Research

Harsham, J., Keller, J. H., & Disbrow, D. (1994). Growth pattern of infants exposed to cocaine and other drugs in utero. *Journal of the American Diet Association, 94*, 999–1007.

Jagsi, R., Motomura, A. R., Amarnath, S., Jankovic, A., Sheets, N., & Ubel, P. A. (2009). Underrepresentation of women in high-impact published clinical cancer research. *Cancer, 115*(14), 3293–3301. doi: 10.1002/cncr.24366

Reed, J. A., Price, A. E., Grost, L., & Mantinan, K. (2012). Demographic characteristics and physical activity behaviors in sixteen Michigan parks. *Journal of Community Health: The Publication for Health Promotion and Disease Prevention, 37*(2), 507–512. doi: 10.1007/s10900-011-9471-6

THE CHI-SQUARE GOODNESS-OF-FIT TEST

Nominal-level variables often are not dichotomous but rather have multiple levels. For example, we may want to be more specific regarding a family's ethnic origins rather than simply distinguishing between ethnic minority and nonminority families. We may also be interested in comparing the types of cancers experienced by the children in our sample with what we would have expected given what we know about the hospital population of children in general.

The chi-square goodness-of-fit test (Cochran, 1952) is a useful tool to analyze such data. This chi-square test compares the frequencies for a categorical variable actually obtained from a sample with what would have been expected given what we know or hypothesize about the target population.

An Appropriate Research Question for the Chi-Square Goodness-of-Fit Test

The chi-square goodness-of-fit test is particularly appropriate when researchers want to compare their sample of categorical values to what is known or hypothesized about a target population. For example, in addition to their use of the binomial test, Reed et al. (2012) used the chi-square goodness-of-fit test to examine whether the observed proportions for age groups observed using the park differed from the actual proportions for age groups in Michigan. This goodness-of-fit test also has been used in combination with logistic regression to evaluate rates of exposure to abuse, disease, or mortality in various populations (Ratner, 1995; Ruttimann & Pollack, 1991; Zahniser, Gupta, Kendrick, Lee, & Spirtas, 1994). In occupational therapy, Huebner, Johnson, Bennett, and Schneck (2003) used this test to compare their sample of brain-injured adults with that of a national sample. In an interesting study that underscores the need for greater use of nonparametric tests in health care research, Gaddis and Gaddis (1994) used the chi-square goodness-of-fit test to evaluate the shape of the distributions of the Glasgow Coma Score (GCS) and Revised Trauma Score (RTS) in a Level I trauma center. The authors concluded that the GCS and RTS distributions were not normally distributed for all data sets that they examined.

In our hypothetical intervention study, we were interested in comparing the types of cancer experienced by our sample of convenience with those of the hospital population in general. The data set we will be using is hospitalized children with cancer-20 cases.sav which can be found on the SAGE website, study.sagepub.com/pett2e. A research question that could be answered using the chi-square goodness-of-fit test is as follows:

> To what extent are the types of cancer experienced by the 20 children in the sample representative of the target population of children who are hospitalized with cancer?

Null and Alternative Hypotheses

Table 4.3 presents the null and alternative hypotheses for this research question that can be used with the chi-square goodness-of-fit test. The null hypothesis will be rejected if the probability associated with the computed value of the chi-square statistic with $df = k - 1$ (where k = number of categories for the variable of interest) is less than the stated level of alpha (e.g., $\alpha = .05$). Note that the hypotheses reflect *frequencies* of observed and expected data and that the alternative hypothesis is nondirectional, or two-tailed.

Table 4.3 Example of Null and Alternative Hypotheses for the Chi-Square Goodness-of-Fit Test

Null Hypothesis
H_0: There is no difference between the obtained frequencies of types of cancer experienced by the children in our sample and the expected frequencies obtained from the hospital in general.
Alternative Hypothesis
H_a: There *is* a difference between the obtained frequencies of types of cancer experienced by the children in our sample and the expected frequencies obtained from the hospital in general.

Overview of the Procedure

The chi-square (χ^2) goodness-of-fit test requires that the data being analyzed be at a nominal level of measurement, with two or more levels. These data must also be presented in the form of frequencies, not scores. The researcher also needs to have available information concerning what frequencies would have been expected given what is known about a particular population.

A chi-square statistic is used to examine differences between observed and expected frequencies generated for each category or cell. That is,

$$\chi^2 = \sum_{1}^{k} \left(\frac{(O_i - E_i)^2}{E_i} \right)$$

where

O_i = observed frequencies in the ith cell,

E_i = expected frequencies in the ith cell,

k = the number of levels of the categorical variable, and

$df = k - 1$.

If the sum of the differences between the observed and expected values across all the cells of the variable is sufficiently large, the resulting chi-square value with $k - 1$ degrees of freedom (*df*) will also be large, increasing the likelihood that the null hypothesis will be rejected. Our decision rule is that we will reject the null hypothesis if and only if the actual chi-square value that we obtain is larger than our critical value, which has $df = k - 1$ at the alpha level that we have chosen.

Let us suppose that our $\alpha = .05$ and that, for whatever reason, we need to undertake our analysis without the aid of a statistical computer package. In our hypothetical example, the categorical variable of types of cancer scheduled for the children has four levels with the following corresponding values and sample sizes: 1 = solid tumor (seven children), 2 = acute myeloid leukemia (two children), 3 = lymphoma (eight children), and 4 = sarcoma (three children). Each child was assigned to one and only one of the four categories, and the data are expressed in frequencies, not scores on a particular test. That means, then, that the degrees of freedom $(df) = k - 1 = 4 - 1 = 3$.

Suppose that we also knew from past records that the expected percentages for the types of cancer for the children were as follows: solid tumors = 50%, acute myeloid leukemia = 20%, lymphoma = 25%, and sarcoma = 5%. The expected values for each of the four categories, therefore, would be 20 * .50 = 10, 20 * .20 = 4, 20 * .25 = 5, and 20 * .05 = 1. These values (10, 4, 5, and 1) would represent our expected values. Note that the expected values add up to 20, our sample size. With this information, we can calculate the chi-square goodness-of-fit test using the formula given above:

$$\chi^2 = \sum_{1}^{k} \left(\frac{(O_i - E_i)^2}{E_i} \right)$$

$$\chi^2 = \frac{(7-10)^2}{10} + \frac{(2-4)^2}{4} + \frac{(8-5)^2}{5} + \frac{(3-1)^2}{1}$$

$$\chi^2 = .90 + 1.0 + 1.8 + 4.0 = 7.70$$

To determine whether or not to reject our null hypothesis of no difference in the proportion of types of cancer in our sample compared to our hypothesized distribution, we would compare our calculated χ^2 value (7.70) to a critical value of the χ^2 statistic when $\alpha = .05$ and $df = 3$. We would reject our null hypothesis if and only if our calculated value for the χ^2 (7.70) exceeds the critical value. Critical values of the χ^2 statistic are presented in the χ^2 table (Table A.2) in Appendix A of this textbook.

Interpreting a Chi-Square Table

The χ^2 is both a statistic and a family of distributions. The shape of each χ^2 distribution varies depending on its degrees of freedom (*df*) (Figure 4.4). Because it is generated from squared standardized scores, χ^2 values are restricted in range from 0 to $+\infty$. While the χ^2 shape is positively skewed, the amount of skewness decreases as the *df*s increase (Figure 4.4) and, eventually, its shape approximates a normal distribution.

Figure 4.4 Three examples of chi-square distributions with varying degrees of freedom.

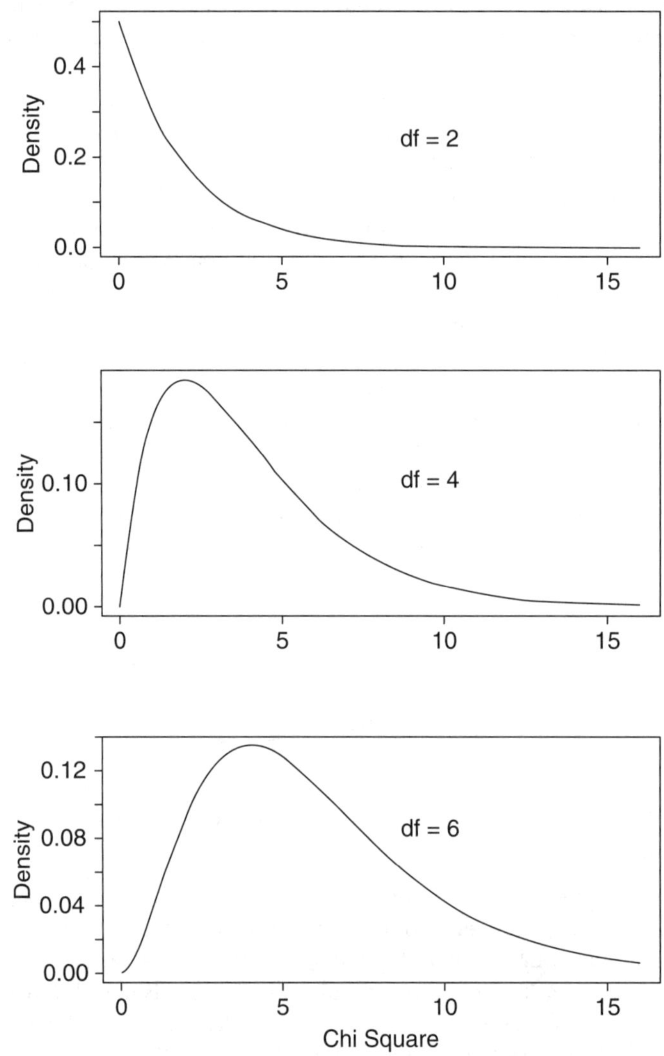

SOURCE: Online Statistics Education: A Multimedia Course of Study (http://onlinestatbook.com/). Project Leader: David M. Lane, Rice University, an online course in the public domain.

Table 4.4 presents a portion of Table A.2 (Appendix) in order to facilitate your understanding of how to determine the critical value of a χ^2 for a given α level and specified *df*s. Please note that, as illustrated in Table 4.4, the shaded area represents the cumulative probability distribution function for a typical χ^2. The area under this curve can range from

0 to 1.0, with higher values meaning that the shaded area is covering more of the distribution. Where the shaded area stops is where the critical value of the χ^2 (χ^2_{cv}) is located (1). Thus, the area under the curve that lies to the right of this value represents α. If, in our example, α = .05, then we are looking for a χ^2_{cv} such that the area under the curve that lies to the right of that value is .05. That would be the same value that has an area of .95 lying to the left of it (1 – .95 = .05) (2).

Now we need to determine which row we should be looking at. Since our *dfs* = 3, we will be looking on row 3 of the first column of *dfs* (3). If we move across to the column for .95, we find that the χ^2 = 7.81. Our rule of thumb will be that we will reject the null hypothesis of similar proportions if and only if our actual χ^2 is greater than χ^2_{cv} .

Was it? Looking at our calculations above, we see that our actual χ^2 (7.70) is less than our χ^2_{cv} (7.81). What is our conclusion? We fail to reject the null hypothesis and conclude that the distribution of types of cancer in our sample of hospitalized children is similar to that of our hospital population. Are we happy with this conclusion? Yes . . . it means that our sample may be representative of our target population.

Determining the Value of a Chi-Square Statistic Using an Internet Website

We can also easily obtain the same chi-square value by using a website interactive calculator (e.g., http://www.quantpsy.org/chisq/chisq.htm) (Figure 4.5). To use this calculator, we would enter both the actual (7, 2, 8, 3) and hypothesized (10, 4, 5, 1) values for the four types of cancer the children experienced. We have already calculated those values in our example above.

Table 4.4 Determining the Critical Value of the Chi-Square Distribution Using Table A.2 in Appendix

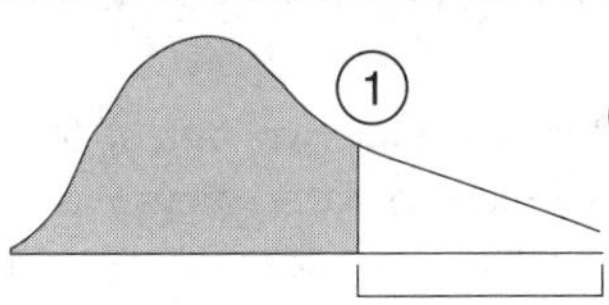

Critical Points of the Chi Square Distribution

(2) ↓

Cumulative probability

	D. F.	0.005	0.010	0.025	0.05	0.10	0.25	0.50	0.75	0.90	0.95	0.975	0.99	0.995
	1	0.39E-4	0.00016	0.00098	0.0039	0.0158	0.102	0.455	1.32	2.71	3.84	5.02	6.63	7.88
	2	0.0100	0.0201	0.0506	0.103	0.211	0.575	1.39	2.77	4.61	5.99	7.38	9.21	10.6
(3) →	3	0.0717	0.115	0.216	0.352	0.584	1.21	2.37	4.11	6.25	7.81	9.35	11.3	12.8
	4	0.207	0.297	0.484	0.711	1.06	1.92	3.36	5.39	7.78	9.49	11.1	13.3	14.9

SOURCE: This public table is in the public domain. It was produced using APL programs written by the author, William Knight/ Univ. of New Brunswick/Canada

Figure 4.5 Example of chi-square goodness-of-fit output generated by an interactive Internet site.

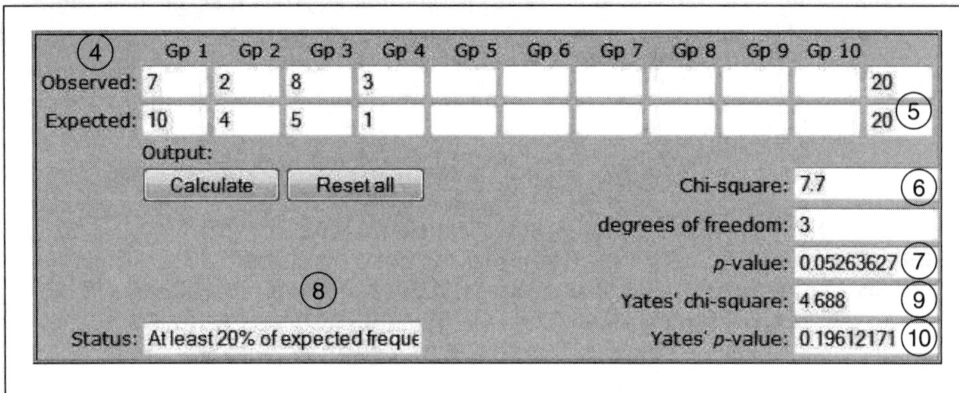

SOURCE: © 2010-2015, Kristopher J. Preacher Calculation for the chi-square test: An interactive calculation tool for chi-square tests of goodness of fit and independence [Computer software]. (2001). Available from http://quantpsy.org.

Using the quantpsy.org website (http://quantpsy.org), we can enter the values for our χ^2 goodness-of-fit statistic (Figure 4.5). Given that we have both the actual and hypothesized values for our types of cancer, we can enter them directly into the cells (4). Be sure that both sets of values equal the sample size (e.g., $n = 20$) (5). Click on the *Calculate . . .* button, and the result appears almost immediately. The actual value of our χ^2 is similar to our hand-calculated value (7.70) (6). This time, however, we are presented with the exact *p* value (.0526) (7). In this case, we can compare this *p* value to our $\alpha = .05$. We will reject the null hypothesis if and only if our $p < \alpha$. Since .0526 is close but still greater than .05, we cannot reject the null hypothesis and conclude that the distribution of types of cancer in our sample is similar to our comparison group.

But wait! We are given a message that more than 20% (in fact two out of four) cells have *expected* frequencies less than 5 (8). As a result, we have violated a critical assumption of this test (see discussion below). We will examine this issue more closely when we address the assumptions of this test.

Note, too, that we are given a second χ^2 value: a *Yate's* χ^2 and a *Yate's p value* (9). What do these values mean? Yates (1934) pointed out that there is an error when using a continuous chi-square distribution to approximate the probabilities of categorical data, especially when the sample size is small (e.g., $n < 20$). As a result, statistical significance tends to be overestimated for small sample sizes, especially when the expected frequencies for at least one cell of the table is < 5. To correct for this error, Yates proposed a continuity correction to the chi-square statistic by subtracting .5 from the difference between the observed and expected values in each cell:

$$\chi^2_{\text{Yates}} = \sum_{i=1}^{N} \frac{\left(|O_i - E_i| - 0.5\right)^2}{E_i}$$

The result is that the χ^2 value is reduced and the p value is increased. We can see this result in Figure 4.5, where the Yates $\chi^2 = 4.688$ and $p = .1961$ (10). With this Yates correction, we now have a very conservative estimate of both the χ^2 and p value, a result that can also increase the likelihood of a Type II error (failing to reject the null hypothesis of no differences when we should have). When should we consider using the Yates correction? Howell (2011) suggests that there are both supporters and naysayers and that it is an extremely conservative approach even when the sample size is less than 20. It is also more likely to be reported with goodness-of-fit tests and 2 × 2 contingency tables (Preacher, 2001). A greater concern is that we have violated a critical assumption of the χ^2 statistic, as we will see below.

Critical Assumptions of the Chi-Square Goodness-of-Fit Test

1. *The variable of interest must be categorical with two or more mutually exclusive and exhaustive levels.* Like the binomial test, the chi-square goodness-of-fit test requires nominal-level data for a single variable that are reflected in frequencies of data, not scores. Unlike the binomial test, this test can be used with data that have more than two levels of mutually exclusive categories.

In our hypothetical example, the categorical variable of types of cancer scheduled for the children has four levels that have the following corresponding values: 1 = solid tumor, 2 = acute myeloid leukemia, 3 = lymphoma, and 4 = sarcoma. Each child was assigned to one and only one of the four categories, and the data are expressed in frequencies, not scores on a particular test.

Thus, we have met this assumption.

2. *The randomly selected observations are independent.* Like the binomial test, the chi-square goodness-of-fit test assumes that the randomly selected observations are independent; that is, there cannot be duplicate observations from the same respondent, and one set of observations should not unduly influence another set. Regarding our data, we do not have randomly selected observations (this was a sample of convenience). We do know, however, that we do not have duplicate observations. However, we do not know if the sample of hospitalized children had undue influence on one another. For example, they could have shared a room and therefore might have influenced one another's responses.

3. *The expected frequencies for the variable in the target population must be specified.* As with the binomial test, it is necessary to specify the expected frequencies for the chi-square goodness-of-fit test. Expected values for a particular variable are obtained from the knowledge the researcher has regarding the population of interest.

In our hypothetical example, we are comparing the obtained frequencies of types of cancer for our sample of children with those of the hospital population of children who were hospitalized with cancer during a particular time period to determine whether our sample could possibly have been obtained from such a population. Since we have obtained the expected percentages for the types of cancer for this population of children (i.e., solid tumors = 50%, acute myeloid leukemia = 20%, lymphoma = 25%, and sarcoma = 5%), we have our expected values. They could be expressed in numbers that sum to 20 (e.g., 10, 4, 5, and 1), percentages (e.g., 50, 20, 25, and 5), or proportions (e.g., .50, .20, .25, and .05).

4. *If the categorical variable is dichotomous, the expected frequencies for each cell should be at least 5. If there are more than two levels for the categorical variable, no more than 20% of the cells should have expected frequencies of less than 5, and no cell should have an expected frequency of less than 1.* If the variable of interest is dichotomous, the degrees of freedom associated with it is 1 ($df = k - 1 = 2 - 1 = 1$). For dichotomous variables, the expected value for each of the two cells must be at least 5. This requirement suggests that a minimum sample size for a dichotomous variable needs to be 10 if the expected proportion is equal to .50 for each cell and greater than 10 if the proportions are unequal.

If the nominal-level variable of interest has more than two levels, such as our variable "type of cancer," no more than 20% of the cells should have expected frequencies of less than 5, and no cell should have an expected frequency of less than 1. This rule of thumb suggests that a minimum sample size for a categorical variable with four levels when equal proportions are expected is 20; the minimum sample size would increase as the proportions become more disparate.

The reason for this requirement is that the chi-square goodness-of-fit test is only asymptotically chi-square; that is, it approaches a chi-square distribution as the expected frequencies become larger. Monte Carlo simulation studies have indicated that the approximation is sufficient when the expected values are greater than 5 (Gibbons, 1985). Hays (1994) suggests that the expected frequency for each cell should be 10 or more when the degrees of freedom are equal to 1 (i.e., the variable is dichotomous) and should be equal to 5 or more if the degrees of freedom are greater than 1 (i.e., the variable has more than two levels). Note that it is the *expected values,* not actual values, that need to meet this requirement.

Should the results of the statistical analysis indicate that the data fail to meet this requirement, it is possible to collapse the data to create a smaller number of cells. Such collapsing of cells, however, needs to be undertaken carefully so that the combined cells make intuitive sense. For example, if the categories were ordered (e.g., level of income), it would be preferable to collapse adjacent cells rather than those at the extremes. Care should also be taken when collapsing data, because the procedure may reduce information available and obscure potentially important findings.

In our example, we have violated this assumption when we use our "type of cancer" variable with four levels. Since we are in the data analysis phase, it is a bit late to increase our sample size. That should have occurred at the beginning of the study. Alternatively, we could collapse the original variable into a new one that has two or three levels. The problem would be in deciding how to collapse such a variable. For example, where would one place those children with a sarcoma? Would they best fit with those children with solid tumors, or would it be better to place them with those children with lymphoma or leukemia?

Computer Commands

The chi-square goodness-of-fit test can be generated in SPSS for Windows (v. 22–23) by highlighting the *Statistics . . . Nonparametric Tests . . . One Sample . . .* commands in the menu (Figure 4.6). By clicking on *Choose Tests . . .* we can indicate that we wish to *Customize tests . . .* (11).

We can then check the box next to the chi-square test. By selecting *Test Options . . .* (12) we can customize the expected probability values (13). The default option is that the expected frequencies are equal. Unequal expected frequencies can be listed as proportions (e.g. .50, .20, .25, .05), percentages (e.g., 50, 20, 25, and 5), or actual values (e.g., 10, 4, 5, 1) in ascending order of the values of the categorical variable (e.g., 1, 2, 3, and 4). Actual values will be reinterpreted as expected proportions. These proportions (e.g., .50) are then multiplied by the total number of cases, *N,* to arrive at the expected number of cases in each corresponding category.

Selecting the *Fields* icon, we can click on *Custom Field Assignments . . .* to choose the variable (*Type of cancer*) that we wish to evaluate (14). Under *Test Options . . .* we are given a choice of *Significance level* (e.g., $\alpha = .05$) and *Confidence Interval . . .* (15) although the output does not produce confidence intervals for the chi-square goodness-of-fit statistic.

Computer-Generated Output

Figure 4.7 presents the syntax commands and computer-generated printout obtained from SPSS for Windows. As with the binomial test, the syntax commands (16) can be used in lieu of using the menu by replacing *type_of_cancer* with the variable of interest.

When examining the Hypothesis Test Summary, be careful when making a decision whether to reject or fail to reject the null hypothesis. Do not rely totally on the posted decision listed in the output (e.g., ***Retain the null hypothesis . . . .***) (17). Review your stated null and alternative hypotheses to confirm whether you have a one- or two-tailed alternative hypothesis. Given that our goodness-of-fit test is two-tailed, our result (asymptotic significance [two-sided test] = .053) (18) fits with our nondirectional null and alternative hypotheses.

Double-clicking on the *Hypothesis Test Summary* will open up the *Model Viewer* (Figure 4.7). We are first presented with a set of plots that compare the *observed* proportion of types of cancer in our sample with those of the *hypothesized* proportions obtained from the hospital population (19). To determine whether the differences in proportions are large enough to reject the null hypothesis of comparable proportions, we need to compare the two-tailed asymptotic (.053) significance (20), or *p* value, to our stated alpha level (.05). The decision rule is that we will reject the null hypothesis of similarity of proportions if the obtained two-tailed significance level is less than .05.

Figure 4.6 SPSS commands for the chi-square goodness-of-fit test.

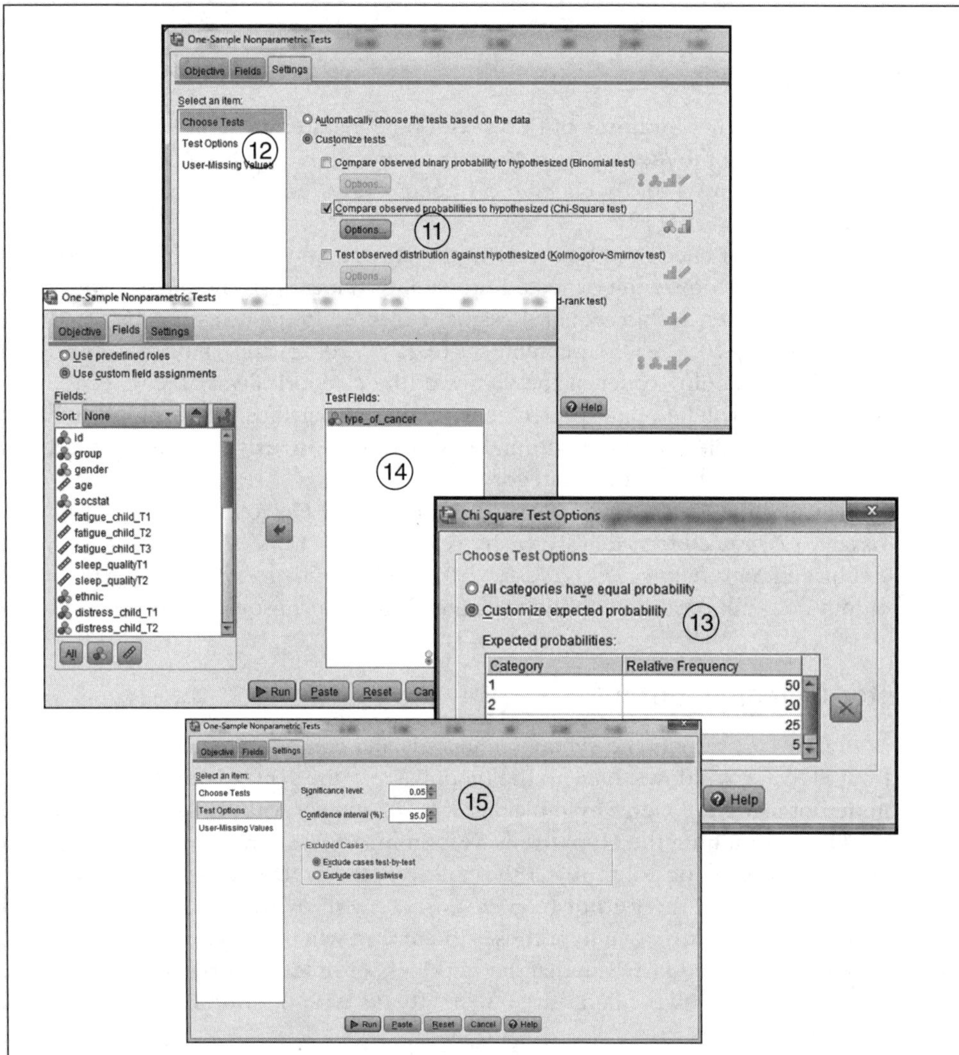

Since this *p* value (.053) is somewhat greater than our alpha (.05), we fail to reject the null hypothesis of no difference in proportions. Note, too, that the *Test Statistic* (7.70) (21) is similar to what we obtained when we hand-calculated the chi-square statistic. Our conclusion is, therefore, that there is no significant difference between the proportions of types of cancer in our sample and that in the hospital in general.

Figure 4.7 SPSS syntax and computer-generated output for chi-square goodness-of-fit test.

```
***Data set: Hospitalized children with cancer-20 cases.sav***
NPTESTS
  /ONESAMPLE TEST (type_of_cancer) CHISQUARE(EXPECTED=CUSTOM(CATEGORIES=1 2 3 4
   FREQUENCIES=50.0 20.0 25.0 5.0 ))
  /MISSING SCOPE=ANALYSIS USERMISSING=EXCLUDE
  /CRITERIA ALPHA=0.05 CILEVEL=95.
```

(16)

Hypothesis Test Summary

	Null Hypothesis	Test	Sig.	Decision
1	The categories of type of cancer occur with the specified probabilities.	One-Sample Chi-Square Test	(18) .053	Retain the null hypothesis. (17)

Asymptotic significances are displayed. The significance level is .05.

One-Sample Chi-Square Test

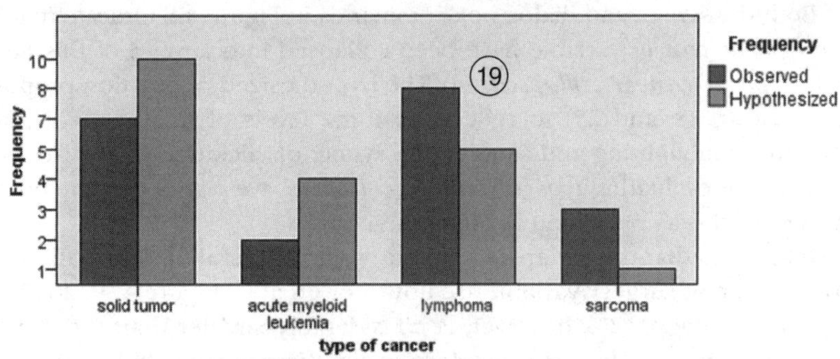

Total N	20
Test Statistic	7.700 (21)
Degrees of Freedom	3
Asymptotic Sig. (2-sided test)	.053 (20)

1. There are 2 cells (50%) with expected values less than 5. The minimum expected value is 1. (22)

There continues to be the problem that there are two cells, or 50%, with expected values less than 5 (22). This warning suggests that the results from this particular chi-square test may be questionable and that we need to consider collapsing a few cells. We can find out which cells have violated this assumption by hovering the cursor over the cells presented for the one-sample chi-square test. This will open a set of boxes that indicate that *acute myeloid leukemia* (hypothesized = 4) and *sarcoma* (hypothesized = 1) both have expected values of less than 5. As discussed earlier, combining these two cells would reduce the number of cells to three and eliminate the expected frequency violation. The question to be answered by the researcher, however, is whether it makes intuitive sense to combine these two cells, leukemia and sarcoma, leaving three cells: lymphoma, solid tumors, and "other cancers."

Collapsing Cells to Eliminate Minimum Size Violations

Figure 4.8 presents the syntax and dialog box commands for collapsing the variable, *type_of_cancer*, into a different variable with three levels (*type_of_cancer_collapsed*). First, we would recode the old variable into a new one using the commands *Transform . . . Recode . . . Into a Different Variable,* identifying the variable to be collapsed and the new variable to be created, clicking on the *Old and New Values* button, and indicating which of the levels we intend to collapse (23).

Both the syntax and dialog box commands in Figure 4.8 indicate that Levels 2 and 4 of the *type_of_cancer* variable have been collapsed into Level 3 of this newly created variable, *type_of_cancer_collapsed* (24). The hypothesized population proportions have been altered (50, 25, and 25) to reflect the three levels of this newly created variable (25). By either highlighting and running the syntax or clicking on *OK* after we have indicated that we are evaluating *type_of_cancer_collapsed,* we can obtain the output for the goodness-of-fit test as presented in Figure 4.9.

It appears that the collapsing of data was successful, because all the expected values for the type of surgery variable are now 5 or greater (Figure 4.9) (26). The generated chi-square statistic of (27), however, is considerably smaller than the statistic presented in Table 4.5 and is no longer even close to significance ($p = .259$) (28). Our decision, therefore, would be to fail to reject the null hypothesis. There are no statistically significant differences between the obtained and expected frequencies with regard to types of cancer experienced by the children in our sample and that of the target population.

Presentation of Results

The results of this analysis could be presented in either text or tabular form. For example, the following could be stated in the text:

> No statistically significant differences ($p = .26$) were found between the types of cancer experienced by the children in this sample and what would have been expected given the types of cancer ordinarily experienced by the children in this hospital.

The data also could be presented in tabular form similar to that in Table 4.5.

Figure 4.8 SPSS syntax and commands for generating output for collapsed type of cancer variable.

```
***Data set: hospitalized children with cancer-20 cases.sav***

RECODE type_of_cancer (1=1) (3=2) (2=3) (4=3) (MISSING=SYSMIS) INTO
    type_of_cancer_collapsed.
VARIABLE LABELS  type_of_cancer_collapsed 'Collapsed types of cancer-3 levels'.
VALUE LABELS type_of_cancer_collapsed 1 'solid tumor' 2 'lymphoma' 3 'other cancers-
    leukemia and sarcoma'.

NPTESTS
/ONESAMPLE TEST (type_of_cancer_collapsed) CHISQUARE(EXPECTED=CUSTOM(CATEGORIES=1 2 3
FREQUENCIES=50.0 25.0 25.0 ))
/MISSING SCOPE=ANALYSIS USERMISSING=EXCLUDE
/CRITERIA ALPHA=0.05 CILEVEL=95.
```

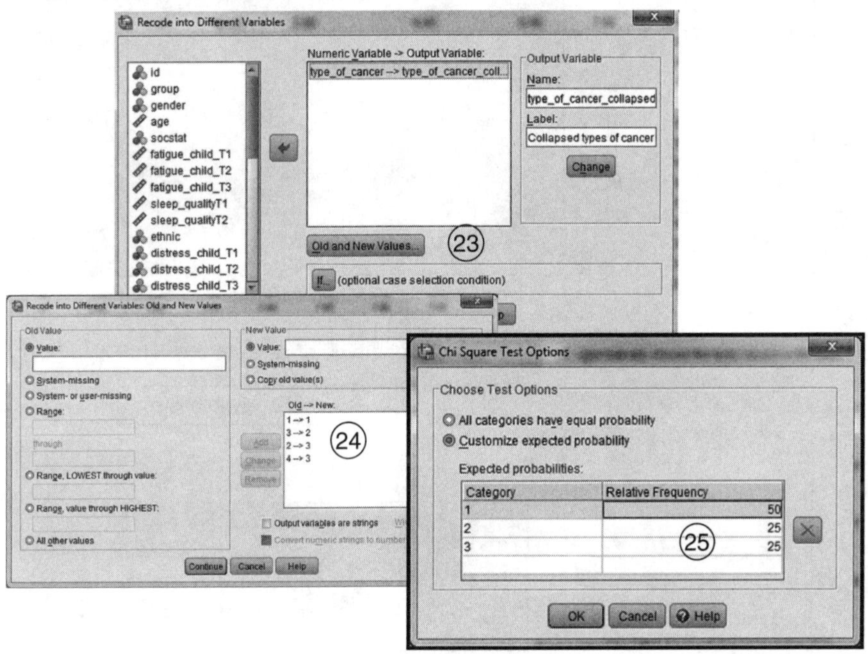

Advantages, Limitations, and Alternatives to the Chi-Square Goodness-of-Fit Test

The chi-square goodness-of-fit test can be used to test a variety of problems concerning whether the obtained frequency distribution for a given categorical variable fits a hypothetical theoretical distribution. These theoretical distributions could take on

Figure 4.9 SPSS-generated output for collapsed type of cancer variable.

Hypothesis Test Summary

	Null Hypothesis	Test	Sig.	Decision
1	The categories of Collapsed types of cancer-3 levels occur with the specified probabilities.	One-Sample Chi-Square Test	.259	Retain the null hypothesis.

Asymptotic significances are displayed. The significance level is .05.

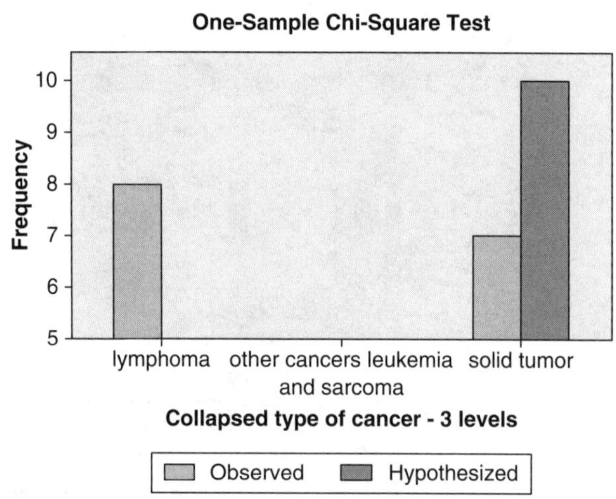

Total N	20	
Test Statistic	2.700	(27)
Degrees of Freedom	2	
Asymptotic Sig. (2-sided test)	.259	(28)

1. There are 0 cells (0%) with expected values less than 5. The minimum expected value is 5. (26)

Table 4.5 Types of Cancer Experienced by the Children Compared to Hospital Population

		Percent (%)			
Type of Cancer	N	*Actual*	*Expected*	χ^2	p
Solid tumor	7	35.0	50.0		
Acute myeloid leukemia	2	10.0	20.0	2.70[a]	.26
Lymphoma	8	40.0	25.0		
Sarcoma	3	15.0	5.0		
Total	20	100.0	100.0		

[a] $df = 2$; two cells, acute myeloid leukemia and sarcoma, were collapsed because these two cells had expected frequencies < 5.

several different forms. Neter and colleagues (1993) outline an approach using the chi-square statistic to test the null hypothesis that the obtained distribution is Poisson. Hays (1994) and Daniel (2000) provide information concerning the approach to testing whether the distribution is normal. In both instances, it is required that the researcher estimate the expected values for such distributions given the number of levels of the discrete (categorical) variable.

In SPSS for Windows, testing of specific distributions using the chi-square goodness-of-fit test is limited to either its default, the uniform distribution (i.e., equal frequencies expected in each category), or specified values for the unequal frequencies. An additional disadvantage of this test is that although, technically, numerous theoretical distributions could be tested using this test, it is necessary to have at hand the actual values of the expected frequencies, and these are not always readily available. Moreover, this test does not arrive at unique results because the value of the statistic depends, to some extent, on the number of levels of the categorical variable being examined (Daniel, 2000; Kallenberg, Oosterhoff, & Schriever, 1985). Other, more suitable, nonparametric statistics could be used when a comparison of obtained and theoretical distributions is desired. One such test is the Kolmogorov-Smirnov test for one and two samples. We will examine these statistics later in this chapter.

Given that the chi-square goodness-of-fit test is intended for use with categorical data, there is not a suitable parametric counterpart to this test. Alternative nonparametric tests include the binomial test and the Kolmogorov-Smirnov one-sample test.

Examples From Published Research

Gaddis, G. M., & Gaddis, M. L. (1994). Non-normality of distribution of Glasgow Coma Scores and Revised Trauma Scores. *Annals of Emergency Medicine, 23,* 75–80.

Kelly-Hayes, M., Wolf, P. A., Kase, C. S., Brand, F. N., McGuirk, J. M., & D'Agostino, R. B. (1995). Temporal patterns of stroke onset: The Framingham Study. *Stroke, 26,* 1343–1347.

Reed, J. A., Price, A. E., Grost, L., & Mantinan, K. (2012). Demographic characteristics and physical activity behaviors in sixteen Michigan parks. *Journal of Community Health: The Publication for Health Promotion and Disease Prevention, 37*(2), 507–512.

Salls, J. S., Silverman, L. N., & Gatty, C. M. (2002). The relationship of infant sleep and play positioning to motor milestone achievement. *American Journal of Occupational Therapy, 56,* 577–580.

Zahniser, S. C., Gupta, S. C., Kendrick, J. S., Lee, N. C., & Spirtas, R. (1994). Tubal pregnancy and cigarette smoking: Is there an association? *Journal of Women's Health, 3,* 329–336.

THE KOLMOGOROV-SMIRNOV ONE-SAMPLE TEST

The chi-square goodness-of-fit test is useful when the researcher has nominal-level data that she or he wants to compare to a theoretical distribution. Sometimes, the variable we wish to compare is a continuous one. The Kolmogorov-Smirnov (K-S) one-sample test is useful for this type of comparison. In SPSS for Windows (v. 22–23), it is possible to evaluate whether the distribution of the sample variable is similar to a hypothesized normal, Poisson, exponential, or uniform distribution.

At this point, the reader should be familiar with the shape of a normal distribution. Like the normal distribution, the Poisson distribution (Neter et al., 1993) is a family of distributions. Its shapes are determined by a single rate parameter represented by the Greek symbol λ. The Poisson distribution is often used to compare the likelihood that a number of events (x) (e.g., 25 calls to a community crisis hotline) could occur during a fixed time interval (e.g., in a 24-hour period) given a theoretically known Poisson distribution of events (e.g., $\lambda = .3$).

The probability function for a Poisson distribution is as follows:

$$P(x) = \frac{\lambda^{x} e^{-\lambda}}{x!}$$

where

$P(x)$ = the probability that x events will occur during the time interval in question given a theoretical Poisson distribution with rate parameter λ,

λ = the rate parameter of the hypothetical Poisson distribution, and

e = the base of the natural logarithm, which is equal to 2.71828.

λ can assume any positive value between 0 and ∞. Poisson distributions are skewed to the right, but as λ becomes larger, the shape of the distribution becomes more symmetric and eventually approximates a normal distribution.

Like the Poisson and normal distributions, the exponential distribution is a family of continuous probability distributions. It describes the time between consecutive events in a Poisson process—that is, a process in which events occur continuously and independently at a constant average rate (Conover, 1999). It is often used as a test for randomness or the time to wait before a given event occurs, such as the next phone call or the next patient request for help.

The uniform distribution, on the other hand, is rectangular and has a uniform or constant probability across each of its values (Neter et al., 1993). This means that the frequencies associated with each value of the variable being examined are equal. The upper (*b*) and lower (*a*) endpoint values of the variable determine the probability function for the uniform distribution:

$$f(x) = 1/(b - a)$$

The uniform distribution has been used in simulation studies and to generate random numbers. It also has been used to evaluate whether the distribution of a phenomenon in a sample is similar across all categories. In our hypothetical example, we might want to know whether a distribution that looks uniform does, indeed, take on that shape.

An Appropriate Research Question for the Kolmogorov-Smirnov (K-S) One-Sample Test

The K-S one-sample test is especially useful for assessing the normality of a distribution. As we saw in Chapter 3, this is especially important when we wish to determine whether a parametric statistic is appropriate for a particular analysis. Rosen, Debanne, Thompson, and Dickinson (1992) used this approach in their study to examine distributions of the relationship between abnormal labor and infant brain damage. The K-S one-sample test also has been used to evaluate circadian rhythms in the request for helicopter transport of cardiac patients (Fromm, Levine, & Pepe, 1992), to assess the properties of the Timed 'Up-and-Go' Scale (Herman, Giladi, & Hausdorff, 2011), for sequential detection of influenza epidemics using exponential distributions (Closas, Coma, & Méndez, 2012), and to evaluate the similarity between panic symptom sequence distributions and hypothesized pathophysiologic models (Katerndahl, 1990).

In our hypothetical intervention study, suppose that we wish to determine whether the average number of sleep environmental interruptions per night during the intervention for the children in the sample was normally distributed. Our research question for this example would be the following:

> To what extent does the average number of sleep environmental interruptions per night during the intervention for the children in our sample resemble a normal distribution?

Null and Alternative Hypotheses

The null hypothesis for the K-S one-sample test is that the cumulative distribution for the sample variable, $F(x)$, is similar to the theoretical cumulative distribution, $F_0(x)$. The alternative, or research, hypothesis may be directional or nondirectional, although it is probably rare that a directional hypothesis would be used. A nondirectional alternative hypothesis merely states that the theoretical and obtained cumulative distributions are disparate, $F(x) \neq F_0(x)$. Table 4.6 presents the null and nondirectional alternative hypotheses that would follow from the research question that we have generated.

Table 4.6 Example of Null and Alternative Hypotheses Appropriate for the Kolmogorov-Smirnov One-Sample Test

Null Hypothesis
H_0: The cumulative distribution of the average number of sleep environmental interruptions per night during the intervention for the children in our sample is similar to that of a normal distribution.
Alternative Hypothesis
H_a: The cumulative distribution of the average number of sleep environmental interruptions per night during the intervention for the children in our sample is not similar to that of a normal distribution.

Overview of the Procedure

To determine whether the sample distribution could conceivably have come from a given theoretical distribution, the K-S one-sample test compares the cumulative distribution of the sample variable with what would have been expected to occur had the sample been obtained from the theoretical parent distribution. In our example, the K-S test compares the cumulative distribution of average number of sleep environmental interruptions per night during the intervention of the children in our sample with what would have been expected had the distribution been a perfectly bell-shaped normal distribution. If the point of greatest divergence between the obtained and expected cumulative distributions is sufficiently large, the null hypothesis of normality will be rejected.

The exact methods used to determine the value of the test statistic for the K-S test are more mathematically cumbersome than is desired for presentation in this text. The interested reader is referred to Conover (1999), Daniel (2000), and Sprent and Smeeton (2001) for excellent descriptions of the mathematical approach to calculating this statistic.

Critical Assumptions of the Kolmogorov-Smirnov One-Sample Test

1. *The sample variable should consist of a randomly selected set of observations that are at least on an ordinal scale of measurement.* As with all nonparametric statistics, the K-S one-sample test assumes that the data have been generated from a sample that has been randomly selected. As is often the case in health care research, our hypothetical data were collected from a sample of convenience; therefore, we have violated this assumption. It is important, therefore, to assess the extent to which our nonrandom sample is representative of the general population of hospitalized children with cancer. This becomes an issue not only for choice of statistic but also for generalizability.

The K-S one-sample test uses the cumulative distribution function to compare the obtained and theoretical distributions. It is assumed that the variable being examined is at least ordinal level of measurement. Our variable, average number of sleep environmental interruptions per night during the intervention, consists of an average count of the number of interruptions per night, indicating that we have met this assumption.

2. *The theoretical distribution to which the sample variable is being compared must be completely specified*. This assumption requires that for every value of the study variable, the value of the cumulative distribution function can be determined (Siegel & Castellan, 1988). Sometimes, values for a theoretical distribution do not exist (e.g., negative or zero values for a logarithm scale), and therefore the cumulative distribution function for those values cannot be defined. The K-S test could not be used to compare the distribution of a study variable that has negative or zero values to that of a log distribution without first shifting the range of the scale values to exclude the negative and zero values. For example, we could add the value of +4 to every observation in a scale that ranges from −3 to +3 to create an adjusted scale that ranges from +1 to +7.

SPSS for Windows is limited in the number of distributions to which the researcher can compare her or his obtained cumulative distribution: the normal, Poisson, exponential, and uniform distributions. The limited availability of comparison distributions may be a result, in part, of the fact that, for distributions that are not determined by the population mean and variance, it is sometimes difficult to estimate, from sample data, the parameters that are critical to defining the distribution.

Computer Commands

There are two ways that the K-S one-sample test can be generated in SPSS for Windows. In Chapter 3, we saw that this test is used in the *Analyze . . . Descriptive Statistics . . . Explore . . .* dialog box to assess whether a continuous variable is normally distributed. In addition to the K-S one-sample test, the Shapiro-Wilks test and the Lilliefors significance level for the K-S test are presented in this dialog box. The Shapiro-Wilks test is similar to the K-S test in that it also tests for normality of distributions. The Lilliefors significance level for the K-S test is used because it provides a better approximation to the normal distribution than does the K-S statistic alone (Conover, 1999). Chapter 3 addressed the interpretation of the computer-generated printout obtained from these commands.

A second way to obtain the K-S one-sample statistic in SPSS for Windows is by highlighting the *Analyze . . . Nonparametric test . . . One-Sample . . . Customize analysis . . .* commands in the drop-down menu (Figure 4.10). The *Settings . . . Choose tests . . .* command (1) enables the researcher to choose the K-S statistic to test the hypotheses that the sample distribution is not only normal but also uniform, exponential, or Poisson. Clicking on the *Test Distribution . . . Normal* box will generate a normal distribution for comparison (2). Clicking on the *Fields . . .* button will allow us to use *Custom Field Assignments* to choose our variable of interest (*average number of sleep environment interruptions during the intervention*) (3).

Figure 4.10 Menu options for generating the Kolmogorov-Smirnov (K-S) statistic.

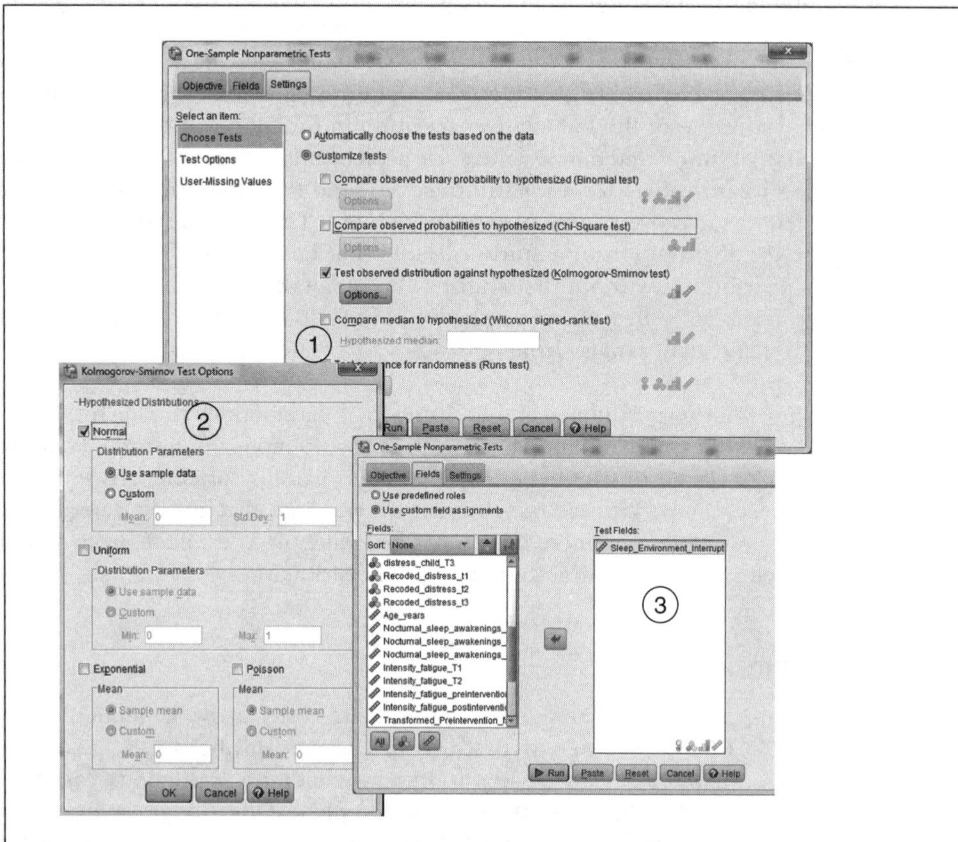

Computer-Generated Output

Figure 4.11 presents the syntax commands and computer-generated output obtained for the K-S statistic from SPSS for Windows. The data set that we are using is hospitalized children with cancer-20 cases.sav which is found on the SAGE website, study.sagepub.com/pett2e. The syntax commands indicate that the normal distribution has been specified (4). Next, the computer-generated printout presents the *Hypothesis Test Summary,* which spells out the null hypothesis for our K-S statistic for our variable of interest, *average number of sleep environmental interruptions per night during the intervention* (5). Where does the mean (9.95) and standard deviation (4.63) come from? These values were generated from our sample data. Had we wanted to, we could have hypothesized a different mean and standard deviation. The p value (*Sig*) is .998 (6), which is larger than our α = .05. Therefore, we would fail to reject (i.e., *Retain*) the null hypothesis and

Figure 4.11 SPSS syntax and computer-generated output for the Kolmogorov-Smirnov statistic.

```
***Data set: Hospitalized children with cancer-20 cases.sav***

NPTESTS
 /ONESAMPLE TEST (Sleep_Environment_Interruptions) KOLMOGOROV_SMIRNOV(NORMAL=SAMPLE ) (4)
 /MISSING SCOPE=ANALYSIS USERMISSING=EXCLUDE
 /CRITERIA ALPHA=0.05 CILEVEL=95.
```

Hypothesis Test Summary

	Null Hypothesis	Test	Sig.	Decision
1	The distribution of average number of sleep environmental interruptions per night during intervention is normal with mean 9.95 and standard deviation 4.63. (5)	One-Sample Kolmogorov-Smirnov Test	.998 (6)	Retain the null hypothesis.

Asymptotic significances are displayed. The significance level is .05.

One-Sample Kolmogorov-Smirnov Test

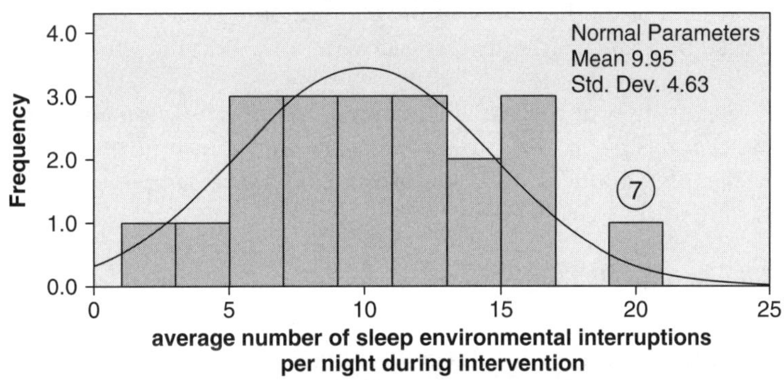

Total N		20	
Most Extreme Differences	Absolute	.088	(8)
	Positive	.088	
	Negative	-.062	
Test Statistic		.394	(9)
Asymptotic Sig. (2-sided test)		.998	(10)

conclude that this variable, *average number of sleep environmental interruptions per night,* is normally distributed.

By double-clicking on the *Hypothesis Test Summary,* we are given additional information about our variable. We are first presented with the plot of our data with a normal curve superimposed on it. This hypothesized normal curve is what we would have expected the curve to look like given that same mean and standard deviation (7). Visually, the curve does have some deviations from normality but not enough to reject the null hypothesis.

In the next box, we are given the most extreme absolute (.088), positive (.088), and negative (–.062) differences between the actual and theoretical (normal) distributions. The most extreme absolute difference (.088) (8) is used to obtain a z statistic (.394) (9). If the significance level (p value) of this test statistic is smaller than our stated level of alpha (e.g., $\alpha = .05$), we will reject the null hypothesis that states that the actual and theoretical distributions are similar. Our generated two-tailed p value, .998 (10), is larger than our stated level of alpha (.05), indicating that we must fail to reject the null hypothesis that our distribution is similar to a normal distribution.

Presentation of Results

The results of the K-S one-sample test are best presented in text form. For example, they could be stated in the text as follows:

> An examination of the variable, *average number of sleep environmental interruptions per night during the intervention*, using the Kolmogorov-Smirnov one-sample goodness-of-fit test indicates that the sample data were normally distributed (K-S $z = .394$, $p = .99$).

It would be difficult and confusing to present this information in table format.

Advantages, Limitations, and Alternatives to the Kolmogorov-Smirnov One-Sample Test

The K-S one-sample test is especially useful when evaluating the underlying structure of a variable's distribution. It is more powerful than its alternative, the chi-square goodness-of-fit test, especially when sample sizes are small and the level of measurement is ordinal (Goodman, 1954; Lilliefors, 1967; Siegel & Castellan, 1988; Slakter, 1965).

SPSS for Windows has four available distributions that can be tested using this statistic: the normal, uniform, exponential, and Poisson. Although the normal distribution is the one most commonly compared, the K-S test has been found to be extremely sensitive to even slight deviations from normality, particularly with larger sample sizes. This makes it more likely that the null hypothesis of normality of distributions will be rejected even when, visually, the data distribution appears to be nearly normal. It is recommended, therefore, that the researcher use this statistic only as a beginning assessment of normality. Chapter 3 outlined additional methods for assessing normality.

There is no parametric counterpart to the K-S test. A nonparametric alternative is the chi-square goodness-of-fit test.

Examples From Published Research

Closas, P., Coma, E., & Méndez, L. (2012). Sequential detection of influenza epidemics by the Kolmogorov-Smirnov test. *BMC Medical Informatics and Decision Making, 12,* 112.

Fromm, R. E., Levine, R. L., & Pepe, P. E. (1992). Circadian variation in the time of request for helicopter transport of cardiac patients. *Annals of Emergency Medicine, 21,* 1196–1199.

Herman, T., Giladi, N., & Hausdorff, J. M. (2011). Properties of the 'timed up and go' test: More than meets the eye. *Gerontology, 57*(3), 203–210.

Katerndahl, D. A. (1990). Comparison of panic symptom sequences and pathophysiologic models. *Journal of Behavior Therapy and Experimental Psychiatry, 21,* 101–111.

Rosen, M. G., Debanne, S. M., Thompson, K., & Dickinson, J. C. (1992). Abnormal labor and infant brain damage. *Obstetrics and Gynecology, 80*(6), 961–965.

THE KOLMOGOROV-SMIRNOV TWO-SAMPLE TEST

A second type of K-S goodness-of-fit test is the two-sample alternative. This test was originally developed by Smirnov (1939) but subsequently was named the Kolmogorov-Smirnov two-sample test because both Kolmogorov and Smirnov developed similar types of tests (Kolmogorov for the single sample, Smirnov for two samples) (Daniel, 2000).

In this test, the distribution of a continuous variable for two independent samples is compared. The goal of this test is to determine whether the two samples that represent two levels of a categorical variable have been drawn from populations sharing the same distribution (e.g., self-reported preintervention level of fatigue for our intervention and control groups). This K-S two-sample test compares the cumulative distributions of the dependent variable within the two categories. If the two cumulative distributions diverge too greatly at any particular point, there may be reason to believe that these distributions do not share the same parent distribution, whatever that distribution might be. Note that, unlike the K-S one-sample test, the two-sample test does not specify the exact form of the two distributions.

Examining the similarity of distributions of a variable within different groups provides the researcher with valuable information. It could be, for example, that although two samples share similar measures of central tendency, the shapes of their distributions are disparate. The K-S two-sample test will examine these discrepancies to determine whether the divergence between the two distributions is sufficiently large to reject the null hypothesis of similarity of distributions. In many ways, the K-S two-sample test is similar to the median, Mann-Whitney, and *t* tests in that it compares distributions of two independent samples. A huge advantage of the K-S test over these others is its more complete examination of the similarity of cumulative distributions, not merely the measures of central tendency.

An Appropriate Research Question for the Kolmogorov-Smirnov Two-Sample Test

The K-S two-sample test has been used in numerous ways to compare distributions of two populations. Cao, Lake, Griffin, and Moorman (2004) used the K-S two-sample test to evaluate increased nonstationarity of neonatal heart rate before the clinical diagnosis of sepsis. King, Gotch, and Larsson-Sciard (2001) used the same K-S statistic to evaluate T-cell repopulation in HIV-infected children on highly active antiretroviral therapy, while Thornbury (1992) used the same statistic to compare cognitive performance on Piagetian tasks by 30 Alzheimer disease patients and their controls.

In our hypothetical intervention study, we might be interested in comparing the similarity of the preintervention fatigue score distributions for the intervention and control groups. A research question that could be answered using the K-S two-sample test would be as follows:

> To what extent are the distributions of preintervention fatigue scores for the staff-initiated intervention and usual-care groups similar?

Null and Alternative Hypotheses

Table 4.7 presents the null and alternative hypotheses for the K-S two-sample test that follow from the research question posed. Note that the hypotheses do not state the form of the distributions. Unlike the K-S one-sample test, the two-sample test does not evaluate this issue.

Table 4.7 Example of Null and Alternative Hypotheses Appropriate for the Kolmogorov-Smirnov Two-Sample Test

Null Hypothesis
H_0: The cumulative distributions of the self-reported preintervention fatigue scores for the children assigned to the staff-initiated intervention and usual-care groups in our sample are similar.
Alternative Hypothesis
H_a: The cumulative distributions of the self-reported preintervention fatigue scores for the children assigned to the staff-initiated intervention and usual-care groups in our sample are not similar.

Overview of the Procedure

To use the K-S two-sample test, the cumulative frequency distribution for each sample of observations is determined, using similar intervals for both distributions. Next, for each interval, the difference between the two cumulative distribution functions is obtained. The K-S two-sample test then determines the largest discrepancy between the two functions. This discrepancy forms the basis for determining the test statistic.

The K-S two-sample test can be one- or two-tailed, depending on the stated hypotheses; that is, one distribution can be predicted to be different from the other in a particular direction. In our hypothetical example, the alternative hypothesis is nondirectional, indicating that the test is two-tailed.

The mathematical method for determining the significance for this two-sample test depends on the sample size and is offered in Conover (1999). SPSS for Windows provides this test among its series of nonparametric statistics.

Critical Assumptions of the Kolmogorov-Smirnov Two-Sample Test

1. *The randomly selected dependent variable must be at least ordinal in its level of measurement.* Like the one-sample test, the K-S two-sample test derives a statistic that is based on a cumulative distribution. For that reason, the randomly selected dependent variable must be at least ordinal in its level of measurement. The scores for our variable, self-reported preintervention fatigue, are derived from a 7-point ordinal scale (1 = *not at all fatigued* to 7 = *extremely fatigued*), suggesting that we have met the assumption of ordinal-level measurement. Our data, however, are from a sample of convenience and are not a random sample.

2. *The independent or grouping variable must have two mutually exclusive levels.* To determine differences between two groups, it is necessary to have a grouping variable with two mutually exclusive levels. This means that a subject may be assigned to one and only one level of the independent variable. Should this categorical variable have several levels to it (e.g., ethnic status), the multiple levels may be collapsed to two mutually exclusive categories, or the levels may be compared two at a time. Our variable of interest, type of intervention, has only two levels to it (staff-initiated intervention vs. usual care); therefore, we have met this assumption.

Computer Commands

Figure 4.12 presents the dialog boxes used to generate the K-S two-sample test in SPSS for Windows. We will continue to use the data set, hospitalized children with cancer-20 cases.sav found on the SAGE website, study.sagepub.com/pett2e. These dialog boxes were opened by highlighting *Analyze . . . Nonparametric Tests . . . Independent-Samples . . . Customize Analysis . . .* and selecting the *Kolmogorov-Smirnov (two-sample)* test in the *Settings* menu ①. In the *Fields* dialog box, we will select the variable *preintervention fatigue* for our Test Field ② and *group (staff-initiated intervention vs. usual care)* in the Groups box ③. Since we set our α at .05, our significance level will be set at .05 ④. Despite a listing for a confidence interval, this is not offered for the K-S statistic.

As indicated, this K-S statistic cannot determine the shape of the distributions. To determine whether the two-sample distributions came from a specified normal distribution, it would be necessary to use the *Analyze . . . Descriptive statistics . . . Explore . . .* dialog box. A grouping variable is then selected (e.g., Group) for evaluations of the subgroups. To obtain assessments of other distributions (e.g., the uniform, exponential, or Poisson), it would be necessary to first separate out the levels of the independent variable through the *Data . . . Split File . . . Organize Output by Groups . . .* dialog box. It is also possible to use conditional expressions to select cases through the *If Condition Is Satisfied* command in SPSS for Windows to isolate the groups (e.g., if Group = 0). Either way, a one-sample K-S test for each level of the independent variable could then be undertaken.

Figure 4.12 SPSS commands for generating the Kolmogorov-Smirnov two-sample test.

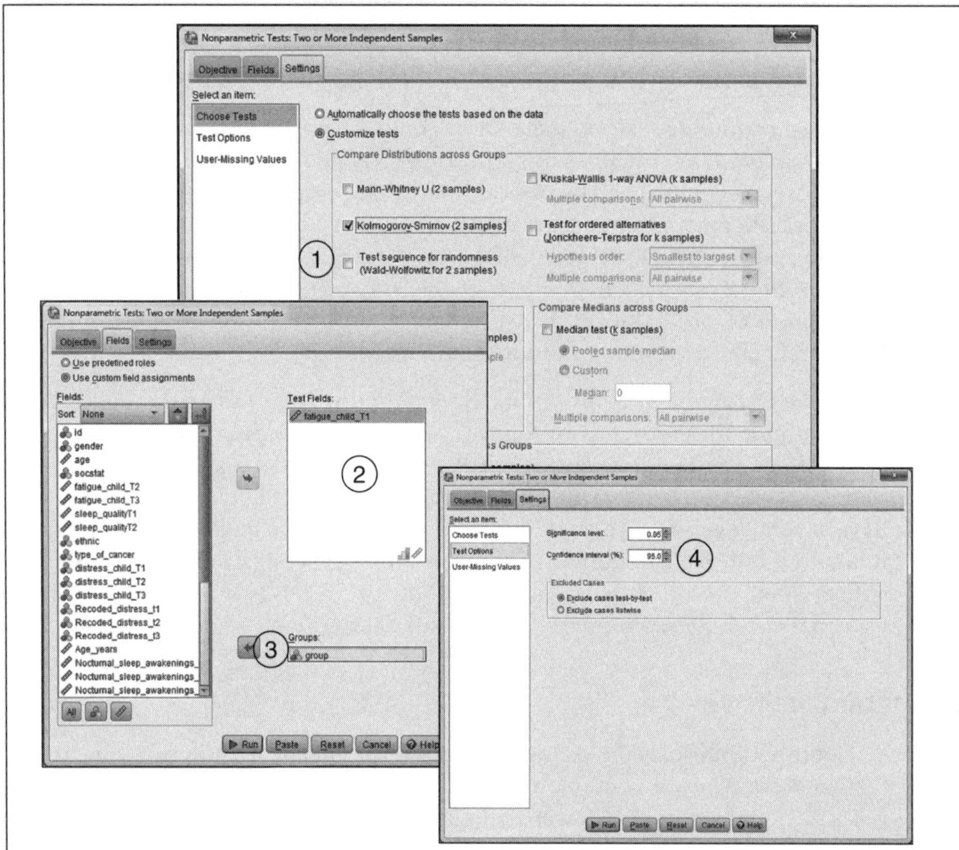

Reprints Courtesy of International Business Machines Corporation, © International Business Machines Corporation

Computer-Generated Output

Figure 4.13 presents the syntax commands and computer-generated printout obtained for the K-S two-sample test obtained in SPSS for Windows. The syntax commands (5) can be saved and used in later analyses. The first line (***Data set: hospitalized children with cancer-20 cases.sav***) is merely a note to you indicating the data set that will be used in this analysis. Because the message lies between the ***'s, the SPSS program will ignore the message.

As with the K-S one-sample test, we are presented with the most extreme differences between the two distributions, but this time we are comparing the intervention and control groups (6). The most extreme absolute difference between the two distributions, .100, will be used to generate a K-S z statistic (7). If the two-tailed p value (8) is smaller than our prestated alpha (e.g., $\alpha = .05$), we will reject the null hypothesis that states that the distributions of the intervention and control groups are similar.

Figure 4.13 SPSS syntax and computer-generated printout for the Kolmogorov-Smirnov two-sample test.

```
***Data set: hospitalized children with cancer-20 cases.sav***

NPTESTS
 /INDEPENDENT TEST (fatigue_child_T1) GROUP (group) KOLMOGOROV_SMIRNOV
 /MISSING SCOPE=ANALYSIS USERMISSING=EXCLUDE
 /CRITERIA ALPHA=0.05 CILEVEL=95.
```

(5)

Hypothesis Test Summary

	Null Hypothesis	Test	Sig.	Decision
1	The distribution of preintervention fatigue is the same across categories of staff-initiated intervention vs. usual care.	Independent-Samples Kolmogorov-Smirnov Test	1.000	Retain the null hypothesis.

(9)

Asymptotic significances are displayed. The significance level is .05.

Independent-Samples Kolmogorov-Smirnov Test

staff-initiated intervention vs. usual care

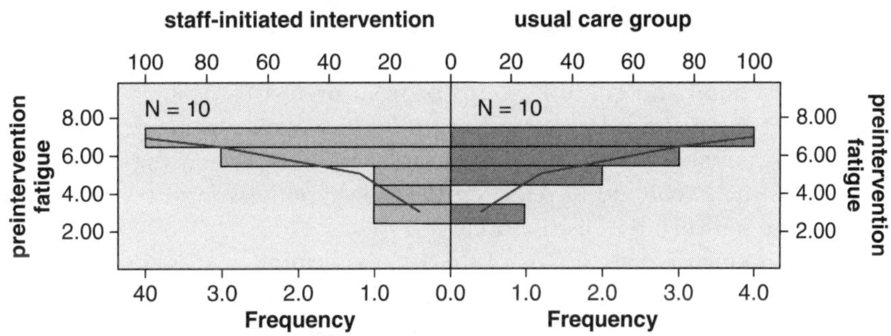

(6)

Total N		20
Most Extreme Differences	**Absolute**	.100
	Positive	.000
	Negative	-.100
Test Statistic		.224
Asymptotic Sig. (2-sided test)		1.000

(7) (8)

Our obtained two-tailed p value, 1.000, is considerably larger than our $\alpha = .05$. In fact, it could not get any larger! Our decision, therefore, is that we must fail to reject the null hypothesis and conclude that the distributions for the preintervention fatigue variable for both groups are similar. That is also the message that we receive in the Hypothesis Test Summary (*Retain the null hypothesis*) (9).

Presentation of Results

As with the K-S one-sample test, the results of the K-S two-sample test are best presented in text form:

> The results of the Kolmogorov-Smirnov two-sample test indicate that the distributions of preintervention fatigue for the staff-initiated intervention and usual-care groups were similar (K-S $z = .22$, $p = 1.00$).

Advantages, Limitations, and Alternatives to the Kolmogorov-Smirnov Two-Sample Test

The K-S two-sample test is useful for comparing similarity of two distributions. It has the unique advantage over its parametric counterpart, the t test, of comparing the entire distribution, not just measures of central tendency. This would be a useful test, therefore, if the researcher did not find any differences in the measures of central tendency between the intervention and control groups or from pretest to posttest but suspected that the shapes of the distributions were very different. A disadvantage of this test is that it is extremely sensitive to unusually large deviations between the two distributions. This increases the likelihood of rejecting the null hypothesis and concluding that there is a difference between the distributions.

The parametric counterpart of the K-S two-sample test is the t test for independent samples. Alternative nonparametric tests include the chi-square goodness-of-fit test, the median test, and the Mann-Whitney U test. Siegel and Castellan (1988) report that, for small samples, the K-S two-sample test is nearly as powerful as the parametric t test (95% efficiency) but declines somewhat in power as n becomes larger. It is more powerful, however, than either the chi-square test or the median test and is slightly less powerful than the Mann-Whitney U test (see Chapter 6) when samples are large.

Examples From Published Research

Campbell, J. P., Gratton, M. C., Salomone, J. A., & Watson, W. A. (1993). Ambulance arrival to patient contact: The hidden component of prehospital response time intervals. *Annals of Emergency Medicine, 22,* 1254–1257.

Cao, H., Lake, D. E., Griffin, M. P., & Moorman, J. R. (2004). Increased nonstationarity of neonatal heart rate before the clinical diagnosis of sepsis. *Annals of Biomedical Engineering, 32*(2), 233–244.

King, D. J., Gotch, F. M., & Larsson-Sciard, E. L. (2001). T-cell re-population in HIV-infected children on highly active anti-retroviral therapy (HAART). *Clinical and Experimental Immunology, 125*(3), 447–454.

Thornbury, J. M. (1992). Cognitive performance on Piagetian tasks by Alzheimer's disease patients. *Research in Nursing and Health, 15,* 11–18.

Summary

In this chapter, we have examined four goodness-of-fit tests that are useful for one- and two-sample designs: the binomial test, the chi-square goodness-of-fit test, and the K-S one- and two-sample tests. These goodness-of-fit tests are useful for testing whether the data being examined fit a prespecified distribution or model. The binomial test is used when the categorical variable being examined is dichotomous. It is especially useful for small sample sizes and when the assumptions of the chi-square goodness-of-fit test are not met. The chi-square goodness-of-fit test is used when the sample size is sufficiently large to meet the expected frequency requirements (e.g., expected $n \geq 5$ when $df = 1$). It also can be used when there are multiple levels to the categorical variable.

The chi-square goodness-of-fit test was designed for use with frequency data. When data are continuous (i.e., measurement on at least an ordinal scale), the more powerful K-S one- and two-sample tests can be used. The K-S one-sample test compares the cumulative distribution of the target variable to that of a theoretical distribution (e.g., normal, uniform, or Poisson). The K-S two-sample test, on the other hand, examines the goodness of fit of a cumulative distribution of the dependent variable for two levels of a dichotomous categorical variable. The K-S one- and two-sample tests are considered more powerful than either the binomial or the chi-square goodness-of-fit test but do require that the dependent variable be continuous.

TEST YOUR KNOWLEDGE

This section is designed to test your knowledge regarding the nonparametric statistical procedures that have been discussed in this chapter. If you find yourself struggling to answer the questions, please review, once again, that part of the chapter that addresses this material.

1. List an appropriate research question (in addition to that which was discussed in the chapter) that could be addressed by the following nonparametric statistical tests:
   a. The binomial test
   b. The chi-square goodness-of-fit test
   c. The Kolmogorov-Smirnov one-sample test
   d. The Kolmogorov-Smirnov two-sample test
2. Under what conditions would you use a Kolmogorov-Smirnov one-sample test compared to the chi-square goodness-of-fit test?
3. When might you elect to use a Kolmogorov-Smirnov two-sample test instead of the parametric independent *t* test?

COMPUTER EXERCISES

Using the data set provided to you on the SAGE website (study.sagepub.com/pett2e) hospitalized children with cancer-20 cases.sav or hospitalized children with-cancer-20 cases.xlsx, please undertake the following analyses:

1. The researcher wanted to determine whether her nonrandom sample of 20 hospitalized children with cancer were similar to the hospital population with regard to their social status: upper, middle, and working class. From the hospital records, she determined that, for the previous year, the hospital had the following social status distribution: high (10%), middle (65%), and low (25%). Her research hypothesis was that there was no difference between her sample and that of the hospital population with regard to the children's social status.
    a. Using either SPSS for Windows or an Internet website (e.g., http://www.quantpsy.org/chisq/chisq.htm), prepare to undertake a chi-square goodness-of-fit test for these data.
    b. Why would you use a chi-square (χ^2) goodness-of-fit test instead of a binomial test?
    c. What are the null and alternative hypotheses for this test? Assuming that $\alpha = .05$, what will be your rule of thumb regarding rejecting or failing to reject the null hypothesis?
    d. Using either SPSS for Windows or an Internet website, undertake this χ^2 test.
    e. What are your conclusions regarding the null hypothesis?
    f. Briefly interpret your findings.

Visit **study.sagepub.com/pett2e** to access SAS output, SPSS datasets, SAS datasets, and SAS examples.

CHAPTER 5

Tests for Two Related Samples: Pretest-Posttest Measures for a Single Sample

- McNemar test
- Sign test
- Wilcoxon signed-ranks test

In Chapter 4, we examined nonparametric tests that could be used to determine the extent to which a single sample is similar to a hypothesized theoretical sample. In health care research, we frequently try to assess whether a particular intervention is effective with a certain population. In our hypothetical example from Chapters 1 and 3, we were interested in evaluating the effects of a staff-initiated intervention to reduce the number of sleep environment interruptions for hospitalized pediatric cancer patients on the frequency of their nocturnal awakenings, levels of fatigue, and distress compared to a usual-care group. In this study, there may be certain characteristics of the sample, such as type of cancer, age, or gender of the child, that are known from prior research to confound and potentially misrepresent the outcomes of the intervention.

Two approaches that can be used to address this problem prior to the intervention are the following: (1) matching the subjects with regard to these extraneous confounding variables and then randomly assigning one of the pairs to the control and the other to the intervention group and (2) using each subject as his or her own control. Data being analyzed then become paired, either through the use of related samples or through repeated observations on a single sample. A third occurrence of matched pairs can occur when the researcher has sampled observations in pairs (e.g., husband and wife). Although each member of the pair may have separate scores on a dependent variable (e.g., marital satisfaction), there is reason to believe that knowing the scores of one member of the pair (e.g., wife's marital satisfaction) will give information about the scores of the other member (husband's marital satisfaction).

There are many types of naturally occurring situations in which respondents are paired, such as mothers and fathers, husbands and wives, twins, and parents and children. A research design could also be longitudinal, with multiple observations of a single sample but lacking a control group. In these situations, a statistical test for independent groups is inappropriate because the data are paired. We are restricted instead to paired tests that acknowledge the dependence of the observations in the samples.

If we were using parametric statistics, the paired *t* test typically would be used to analyze paired samples. This type of *t* test is very useful and robust to violations of its assumptions. Sometimes, however, it is not possible to use the paired *t* test because the data do not sufficiently meet the test's assumptions. Perhaps the sample size is too small, the continuous dependent variable is severely skewed, or the data are categorical. In these situations, the statistical test of choice would be nonparametric.

Several nonparametric statistical procedures are suitable for use with paired observations or repeated measures using a single sample across two time periods. Three tests will be examined in this chapter: the McNemar test, the sign test, and the Wilcoxon signed-ranks test. Two additional tests for repeated measures across more than two time periods (Cochran's *Q* and the Friedman test) will be examined in Chapter 6. The McNemar test and Cochran's *Q* test are used when the measurement of the dependent variable is dichotomous, whereas the remaining tests are used when the dependent variable is at least ordinal in its level of measurement.

THE MCNEMAR TEST

The McNemar test is especially useful when the researcher has a pretest-posttest design in which the subjects serve as their own controls and the dependent variable is dichotomous (Bennett & Underwood, 1970; Feuer & Kessler, 1989; Siegel & Castellan, 1988). In health care research, for example, we might be interested in comparing the performance of two procedures, comparing the opinions of two experts, or determining whether an educational program altered people's preferences for a particular type of health provider (e.g., nurse practitioner vs. physician). The McNemar test examines the extent of change in the dichotomous variable from pretest to posttest. If the proportion of changed responses in one direction is sufficiently greater than what would be expected by chance, the null hypothesis of no disproportionate change is rejected.

An Appropriate Research Question for the McNemar Test

Numerous examples from the research literature illustrate the versatility of the McNemar test. Demir and Erdil (2013) used both the McNemar and other nonparametric tests to evaluate the effectiveness of home monitoring in hip replacement surgery patients. Price (2013) used the same test to assess creatinine normalization of workplace urine drug tests, and Elizondo-Montemayor et al. (2013) used the test to evaluate a school-based individualized lifestyle intervention to decrease obesity and the metabolic syndrome in Mexican children. Using this same test, Snoey and colleagues (1994) compared error rates of physicians and cardiologists regarding their interpretations of emergency department electrocardiograms (ECGs). In all these examples, the data that were analyzed using the McNemar test were dichotomous variables that were paired either through matched samples or through a design in which the subjects served as their own controls.

In our hypothetical intervention study, the children in both the staff-initiated intervention and usual-care groups were asked before and after the intervention whether they were distressed about their current hospitalization. Because the pretest-posttest measure is dichotomous (the children answered "yes" or "no" to the question concerning distress) and the data are paired, the use of the McNemar test is appropriate. An example of a research question that could be answered using this test would be as follows:

> Is the staff-initiated intervention effective in reducing children's distress concerning their current hospitalization?

Note that we are examining the pretest and posttest responses of one sample of children who have served as their own controls. We are not comparing the two groups.

Null and Alternative Hypotheses

Table 5.1 presents the null and alternative hypothesis for the McNemar test that would follow from the research question. Although nondirectional tests are possible, our alternative hypothesis predicts a direction for the probability statement; therefore, the test is directional, and we will be using a one-tailed alpha level (e.g., $\alpha = .05$).

Table 5.1 Example of Null and Alternative Hypotheses Appropriate for the McNemar Test

Null Hypothesis
H_0: Among those children who took part in the intervention and who change their reported distress concerning their current hospitalization, the probability that a child's distress is reduced is the same as the probability that the child's distress is increased. $P_{reduced} = P_{increased}$
Alternative Hypothesis
H_a: Among those children who took part in the intervention and who change their reported distress concerning their current hospitalization, the probability that a child's distress is reduced is greater than the probability that the child's distress is increased. $P_{reduced} > P_{increased}$.

Notice that the McNemar test focuses only on those children in the sample who change their opinions regarding their distress and does not include those children whose reported distress does not change. The test also does not compare intervention and usual-care groups, because this is a test of change in a single group.

Overview of the Procedure

To undertake a McNemar test, the data first need to be cast into a 2 × 2 table that represents the change in an individual's response from before to after the intervention. If the original response data are not nominal, they need to be reduced to a form such that the coding scheme (e.g., 0s and 1s) represents identical values for the paired variables being examined. Table 5.2 presents the form that such a table typically takes.

Table 5.2 2 × 2 Tables for the McNemar Test for Children's Expressed Distress Concerning Hospitalization

			After Intervention	
Expressed Distress			*Yes* *(1)*[a]	*No* *(0)*
Before Intervention				
	No	(0)[a]	A ①	B
	Yes	(1)	C	D ②

[a]The inconsistent ordering of the categories was deliberate, as a means of duplicating the pattern presented on the computer printout.

In our hypothetical example, "A" represents the number of children in the intervention group who reported not being distressed regarding their hospitalization prior to the intervention but reported being distressed following the intervention ①. "D" represents the number of children in the experimental group whose distress regarding their hospitalization decreased following the intervention ②. "A + D" therefore is the total number of subjects who changed their responses from before to after the intervention.

When sample sizes are reasonably large (i.e., when the total frequency of changes is greater than 10 (Siegel & Castellan, 1988)), the McNemar test uses a chi-square test to compare the number of subjects who changed in a specific direction (i.e., A – D) with the frequency of change that would be expected under the null hypothesis of a change being equally likely in both directions ([A + D]/2). This chi-square statistic is similar to the goodness-of-fit statistic that was presented in Chapter 4:

$$\chi^2 = \sum_1^k \frac{(O_i - E_i)^2}{E_i}$$

where

O_i = the observed number of cases in cell *i*,

E_i = the expected number of cases in cell *i*,

k = the number of cells that represent change.

For the McNemar test, we are interested only in the *observed* and *expected* values of two cells, A and D, because these are the only cells that represent change. The *expected* values for each of these cells are (A + D)/2. The chi-square statistic for the McNemar test is given by

$$\chi^2 = \sum_1^k \frac{(O_i - E_i)^2}{E_i} = \frac{[A - (A + D)/2]^2}{(A + D)/2} + \frac{[D - (A + D)/2]^2}{(A + D)/2}$$

If the sum of the differences between the observed and expected values across the change cells is sufficiently large, the resulting chi-square value with 1 degree of freedom ($df = k - 1 = 2 - 1$) will also be large, increasing the likelihood that the null hypothesis will be rejected. When the sample size is smaller (e.g., when the expected change frequency, (A+D/2) is less than 10), a binomial test is used instead (see Chapter 4) (Siegel & Castellan, 1988). In our case, (A + D)/2 = (0 + 6)/2 = 3, which is smaller than the criterion. The printout in SPSS for Windows, therefore, represents the binomial test instead.

Critical Assumptions of the McNemar Test

There are four major assumptions of the McNemar test.

1. *The dichotomous variable being assessed has assigned values for each level (e.g., 0 and 1), the meaning of which is similar across both time periods.* This assumption implies that the dichotomous variable for the pretest and posttest is coded similarly. In our hypothetical study, for example, children who expressed no distress concerning their hospitalization were assigned the value of 0, whereas children who did express distress were assigned the value of 1 for both the pretest and the postintervention measure.

2. *The data being examined represent frequencies, not scores.* As with all chi-square statistics, the assumption is made that the data being examined are frequency data, not scores. In our hypothetical study, the children answered "yes" (1) or "no" (0) to the question of whether they were distressed about their hospitalization. These data represent frequencies or counts and, therefore, meet this assumption.

3. *The dichotomous measures are paired observations of the same randomly selected subjects or matched pairs.* It is expected that the data consist of paired responses from a set of randomly selected subjects or matched samples of subjects. In our hypothetical study, the children were not randomly selected because this was a sample of convenience. The observations were paired, however, because the children served as their own controls by responding to the question concerning their distress at two different points in time.

4. *The levels of the dichotomous variable are mutually exclusive; that is, a subject can be assigned to only one level of the dichotomous variable that is being examined over time.* This assumption implies that a subject cannot be assigned to both a 0 and a 1 on the dichotomous variable at pretest and posttest. In our hypothetical intervention study, a child could not report *both* a *"yes" and* a "no" on the pre- or postintervention distress variables.

Computer Commands

The data set that we will be using for this example is "hospitalized children with cancer-20 cases.sav." This file can be found on the SAGE website (study.sagepub.com/pett2e). Figure 5.1 presents the SPSS for Windows dialog boxes that are used to generate the McNemar test. This dialog box was opened by choosing the following items from the menu: *Analyze . . . Nonparametric Tests . . . Related Samples.* Because we were interested in restricting the analysis to only those children who received the intervention ($n = 10$), the sample was restricted by first using the *Select Cases* command (*Data . . . Select Cases . . . If the Condition is Satisfied . . .*) and instructing the computer to select only those cases that met the condition that they had been assigned to the intervention group (i.e., Group = 1).

Selecting *Customize Analysis . . .* will allow us to choose the McNemar test ③. Next, the pair of dichotomous variables to be examined is selected from the menu. These variables can be either repeated measures from subjects who are being used as their own controls (e.g., *Distress_Child_T1* = preintervention distress and Distress_Child_T2 = postintervention distress) ④ or dichotomous variables obtained from matched samples (e.g., husbands' and wives' marital satisfaction). Be sure that both variables have been labeled "nominal" in the data set ⑤. We will also instruct the computer that the value of "1" for pre- and postintervention distress is the "success" value. If desired, values could also be combined into the success category ⑥.

Computer-Generated Output

Figure 5.2 presents the SPSS for Windows syntax commands and computer-generated output for the McNemar test. The syntax commands can be saved for future analyses. They indicate that the sample selection has been restricted to only those children from the staff-initiated intervention group (Group = 1) because a filter has been placed on the data set (filter_$) ⑦ and that a McNemar test has been run on the restricted sample ⑧. The subcommand, */missing scope = analysis,* indicates that we

Figure 5.1 SPSS for Windows commands for generating the McNemar test (study.sagepub.com/pett2e).

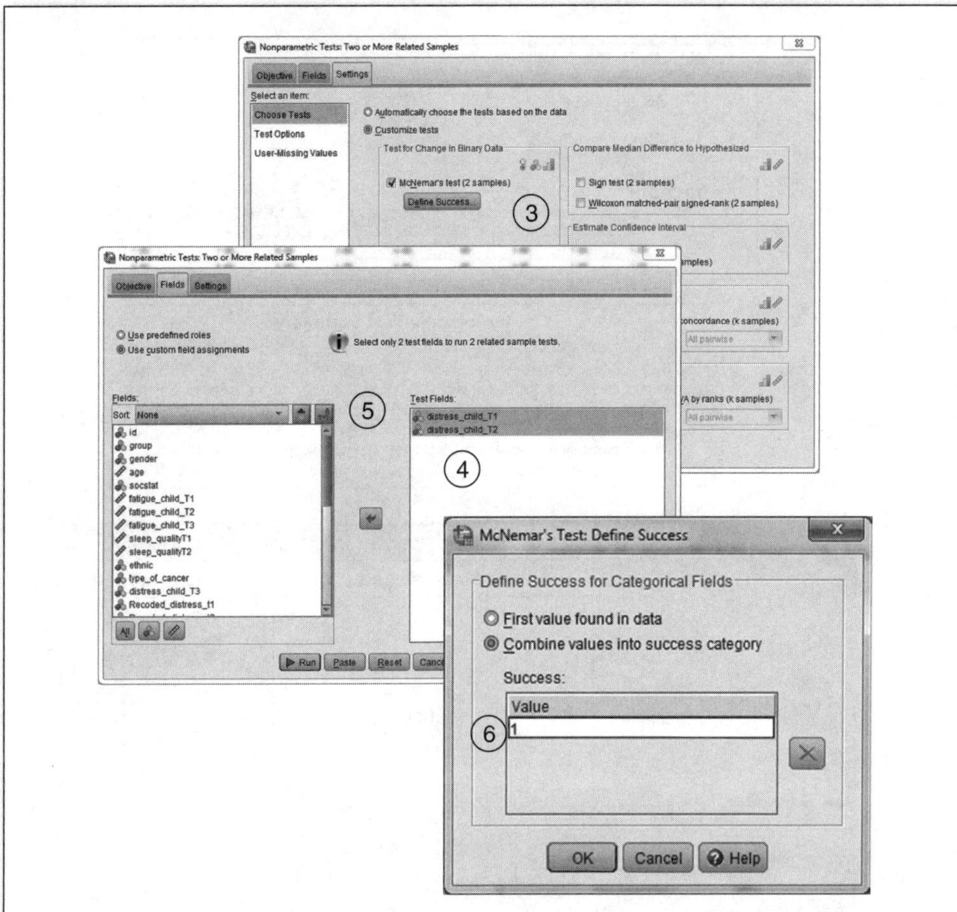

have selected the default option for the handling of missing values: Cases will be omitted on a test-by-test basis.

In the printout, we are presented with the Hypothesis Test Summary. The significance level is .031, and the "decision" is to reject the null hypothesis (9). Before we accept what the output suggests, we should first reexamine our null and alternative hypotheses. Were they directional or nondirectional? Since our alternative hypothesis was directional, we have a directional test. Since the p value (.031) in the SPSS output is two-tailed, we need to divide that value in half (.031/2 = .016) and compare the resulting value to $\alpha = .05$. The null hypothesis will be rejected if our generated p value (.016) is less than our alpha (.05), which indeed it is.

Figure 5.2 Syntax and computer-generated output obtained for the McNemar test in SPSS for Windows (v. 22–23). Data file: hospitalized children with cancer-20 cases.sav (study.sagepub.com/pett2e).

```
COMPUTE filter_$=(group = 1).
VARIABLE LABELS filter_$ 'group = 1 (FILTER)'.
      VALUE LABELS filter_$ 0 'Not Selected' 1 'Selected'.
FORMATS filter_$ (f1.0).
      FILTER BY filter_$.
EXECUTE.
NPTESTS
 /RELATED TEST(distress_child_T1 distress_child_T2) MCNEMAR(SUCCESS=LIST(1))
      /MISSING SCOPE=ANALYSIS USERMISSING=EXCLUDE
      /CRITERIA ALPHA=0.05 CILEVEL=95.
```

(7) (8)

Hypothesis Test Summary

Null Hypothesis	Test	Sig.	Decision
The distributions of different values across preintervention distress and post intervention distress are equally likely for the specified categories.	Related-Samples McNemar Test	.031[1] (9)	Reject the null hypothesis.

Asymptotic significances are displayed. The significance level is .05.

[1]Exact significance is displayed for this test.

Preintervention distress	post intervention distress: yes, distressed	post intervention distress: no, not distressed
yes, distressed	Observed Frequency = 3	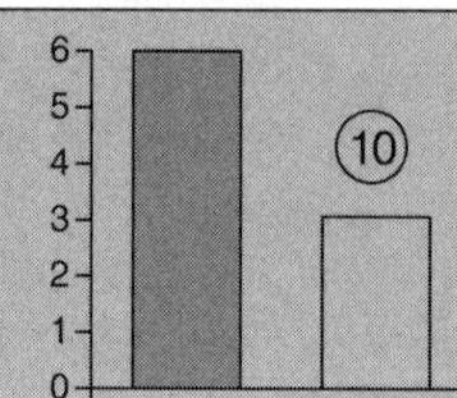 (10)
no, not distressed	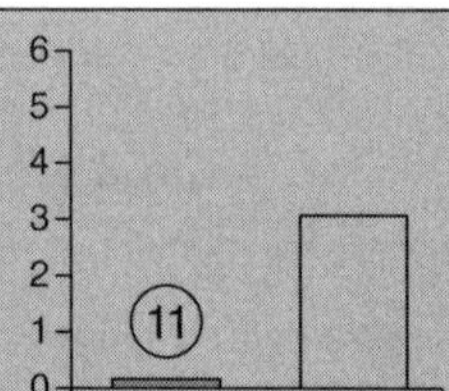 (11)	Observed Frequency = 1

Total N	10
Test Statistics	4.167
Degrees of freedom	1
Asymptoic Sig. (2 sided test)	0.41
Exact Sig. (2 sided test)	.031

1. The exact p-value is computed based on the binomial distribution because there are 25 or fewer records.

How will we interpret these results? To examine whether our decision to reject the null hypothesis is in our hypothesized direction, we need to examine the results presented for the change test. The results from this printout indicate that six children from our staff-initiated intervention group who reported preintervention distress no longer reported distress following the intervention (10). No children reported increased distress following the intervention (11). Our conclusion, therefore, is that, among the 10 children in the staff-initiated intervention group, the change in distress levels was in the direction of lowering distress.

Determining the Outcome of a McNemar Test Using a Website

Several useful websites provide interactive calculators that enable the researcher to calculate a McNemar test without the need for a statistical computer package. Because some of these websites have publishing restrictions, we will illustrate how to use this type of calculator using www.vassarstats.net, a website that is in the public domain.

In the vassarstats website, click on *Proportions . . . McNemar's test for correlated proportions.* Once there, we can input our summary data for the distress levels of the children in the staff-initiated intervention group (1). By clicking on the *Calculate* button (2), we are given the one- and two-tailed McNemar test result (3). Because our research

Figure 5.3 Internet-generated output for the McNemar test.

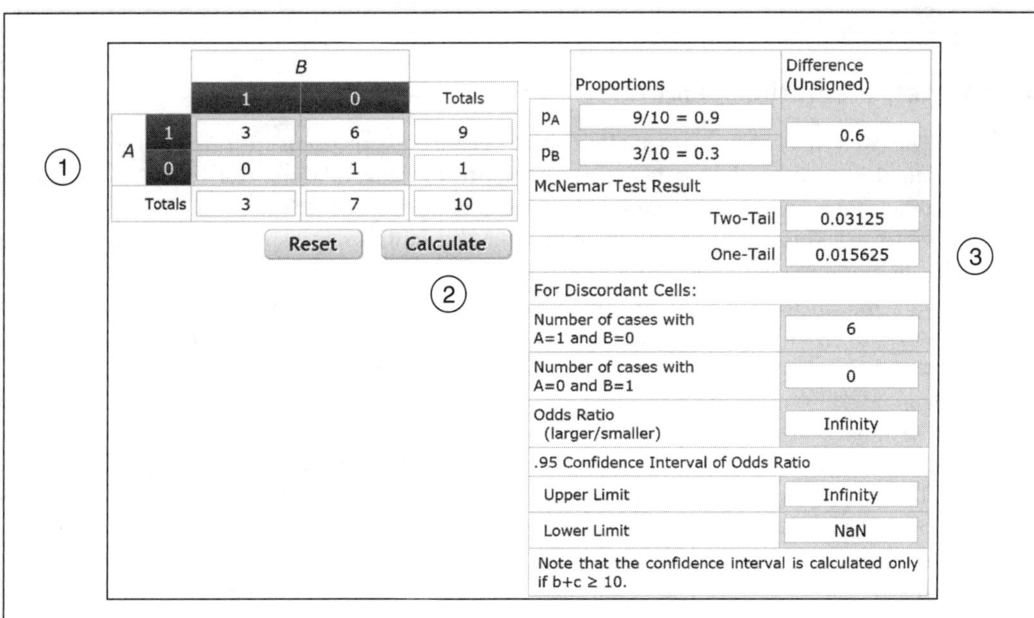

SOURCE: www.vassarstats.net.

hypothesis was directional, we will focus on the one-tailed result (p = .0156). This is the same result we obtained from the output generated in SPSS for Windows. Again, we can conclude that the staff-initiated intervention was effective in lowering the children's distress levels from pre- to postintervention.

Presentation of Results

Table 5.3 presents a suggested approach to presenting the results of the McNemar test. Percentages are omitted from the table to prevent confusion resulting from such a small sample. An alternative method would be to present the results in written format:

> The results of the McNemar test indicate that the staff-initiated intervention was effective in changing distress levels in the direction of reduced distress from pre- to postintervention (one-tailed p = .016).

Table 5.3 Suggested Presentation of McNemar Test Results

	Distress Following Intervention?			
	Yes	*No*	*Total*	*p (1-tailed)*
Distress prior to intervention?				
Yes	3	6	9	.016
No	0	1	1	
Total	3	7	10	

Advantages, Limitations, and Alternatives to the McNemar Test

The McNemar test is especially useful because it can be used to examine change in nominal-level data. A disadvantage of this test is that it does not examine extent of change, only whether change has occurred. In the hypothetical example, it is not possible to ascertain the extent of change in the children's distress, only whether they changed and, if so, in what direction.

The McNemar test also does not allow for a comparison group (e.g., the control group) because this is a test using dependent observations. Feuer and Kessler (1989) have presented a two-sample situation for the McNemar test in which the marginal changes in a nominal-level variable for two independent cohorts (a control and an intervention cohort) are examined across two time periods. If the researcher wanted to compare two groups, two additional nonparametric approaches are possible. McNemar tests could be run on each of the independent groups independently and their results compared. Alternatively, a 2 × 2 contingency table representing group membership (intervention, control) by change classification (change in a positive direction, change in a negative direction) could be created. The Fisher's exact test (Chapter 7) could then be used to examine group-by-time interaction between the two dichotomous variables, group and direction of change.

Because the McNemar test is used primarily with nominal-level data, there is no parametric counterpart to this test. If there are more than two periods of data collection (e.g., pretest, posttest, and follow-up), Cochran's *Q* test is recommended (see Chapter 6). If the data are continuous and meaningfully ranked, it would be advisable to use more sensitive nonparametric tests that use paired data, such as the sign test and the Wilcoxon test.

Examples From Published Research

Demir, S. G., & Erdil, F. (2013). Effectiveness of home monitoring according to the Model of Living in hip replacement surgery patients. *Journal of Clinical Nursing, 22*(9/10), 1226–1241.

Elizondo-Montemayor, L., Gutierrez, N. G., Moreno, D. M., Martínez, U., Tamargo, D., & Treviño, M. (2013). School-based individualised lifestyle intervention decreases obesity and the metabolic syndrome in Mexican children. *Journal of Human Nutrition & Dietetics, 26,* 82–89.

Price, J. W. (2013). Creatinine normalization of workplace urine drug tests: Does it make a difference? *Journal of Addiction Medicine,* 7(2), 129–132.

Snoey, E., Housset, B., Guyon, P., ElHaddad, S., Valty, J., & Hericord, P. (1994). Analysis of emergency department interpretation of electrocardiograms. *Journal of Accident & Emergency Medicine, 11*(3), 149–153.

THE SIGN TEST

The sign test is one of the oldest of all nonparametric tests, dating back to 1710 (Conover, 1999). It is called the sign test because the statistic is generated from data that have been reduced to +'s or −'s. The test can be used with paired data that are either dichotomous, ordinal, or continuous and that have been collected across a single sample or matched pairs. If the data are dichotomous, the two categories making up the variable need to have some rank order to their measurement (e.g., "success" vs. "failure" or "yes" vs. "no"), and the test reduces to the McNemar situation.

The sign test can be used in any situation in which the researcher can determine whether one of two paired or matched observations is "greater" or "less" than the other with regard to some identified attribute. The exact quantitative amount of the difference does not need to be determined for this test because the focus of the analysis is on the signs of the differences between each pair of variables.

An Appropriate Research Question for the Sign Test

The sign test has not been very popular in the research literature, possibly because it has been overshadowed by the more powerful Wilcoxon signed-ranks test. Several examples from the literature, however, demonstrate the potential usefulness of the sign test. Graves, Carter, Anderson, and Winett (2003) used the sign test to evaluate an 8-week pilot intervention based on social cognitive theory to improve quality of life for women with breast cancer. A similar sign test was used by Miletic, Sekulic, and Ostojic (2007) to examine body physique and prior training experience as determinants of Self-Estimated Functional Inability Because of Pain (SEFIP) scores for university dancers, and Whellan et al. (2012) used the same test to determine time from admission to 50% improvement in impedance and to when a heart patient was medically ready for discharge.

In our hypothetical health care intervention study, suppose we were interested in examining the reduction in self-reported levels of fatigue from pretest to posttest within the group of 10 children who received the staff-initiated intervention. An example of a research question for which a sign test would be appropriate would be as follows:

> Do the children in the staff-initiated intervention group reduce their self-reported fatigue from pretest to posttest?

Note that because the pretest and posttest fatigue measures that we are using are scales of ordinal level of measurement that range from 1 to 7, we cannot use the McNemar test.

Null and Alternative Hypotheses

Table 5.4 presents the null and alternative hypotheses for which a sign test would be appropriate given the research question outlined above. Note that the alternative hypothesis is directional; therefore, the test will be one-tailed. Because the fatigue variable consists of a 7-point Likert scale (range: 1 = *not at all fatigued* to 7 = *very fatigued*), we are predicting that the number of negative differences formed by Fatigue_T2 – Fatigue_T1 will be greater than the number of positive differences. That is, self-reported fatigue was greater at pretest than at posttest.

Table 5.4 Example of Null and Alternative Hypotheses Appropriate for the Sign Test

Null Hypothesis
H_0: The self-reported level of fatigue for the children who took part in the staff-initiated intervention will not change from pretest to posttest; that is, the number of children whose fatigue is reduced from pretest to posttest is the same as the number of children whose fatigue is increased.
Alternative Hypothesis
H_a: The self-reported level of fatigue for the children who took part in the staff-initiated intervention will decrease from pretest to posttest; that is, the number of children whose fatigue is reduced from pretest to posttest is greater than the number of children whose fatigue is increased.

Overview of the Procedure

To compute the sign test, the differences in the paired data are obtained and the direction of the differences ("+" or "–") recorded and summed. The test then takes the form of a binomial test (see Chapter 4 for calculations) in which the sum of the negative signs is compared to the sum of the positive signs, ignoring the instances of no differences. Depending on the direction stated in the alternative hypothesis, the null hypothesis of no difference between the number of positive and negative signs will be rejected if the probability of obtaining as extreme an occurrence of the obtained values is less than the prestated alpha level.

Either a one- or a two-tailed test may be used, depending on the wording of the alternative hypothesis. In a one-tailed test, the alternative hypothesis states which sign, positive or negative, will occur more frequently. A two-tailed alternative test merely states that there will be a difference in the number of positive and negative signs.

When the sample size is relatively large ($N > 25$ in SPSS for Windows), the normal approximation to the binomial distribution is used for the sign test. This distribution has a mean, μ_x, that is equal to np and a variance, σ_x^2, equal to $n$pq. The value of the z statistic with a continuity correction for categorical data and p = q = .5 is given as follows:

$$\mathrm{z} = \frac{x - \mu_x}{\sigma_x} = \frac{(x \pm 0.5) - n\mathrm{p}}{\sqrt{n\mathrm{pq}}} = \frac{(x \pm 0.5) - 0.5n}{0.5\sqrt{n}}$$

where

x = the number of +'s or –'s, depending on the stated direction of the alternative hypothesis, and

n = the number of paired observations that have been assigned a "+" or "–" value.

When calculating the z statistic, (x + .5) is used when $x < .5n$ and (x – .5) is used when $x > .5n$. The calculated value of this z statistic is then compared to the critical value of the standard normal distribution at the prestated one- or two-tailed alpha level.

Hand-Calculating the Value of the Sign Test

We could hand-calculate the value of this sign test by using the formula given above. The difference in fatigue scores (postintervention fatigue minus preintervention fatigue) is presented in Table 5.5. The data set we are using is hospitalized children with cancer-20 cases.sav (study.sagepub.com/pett2e). These difference scores were obtained in SPSS for Windows (v. 22–23) by using the SPSS commands *Transform . . . Compute Variable . . .* and creating a difference variable by subtracting the preintervention fatigue variable (*Fatigue_T1*) from the postintervention fatigue variable (*Fatigue_T2*) for the staff-initiated intervention group (Group = 1).

Table 5.5 indicates that there were one positive and eight negative changes in the children's fatigue levels. Since our research hypothesis indicated that there would be a reduction in the children's fatigue levels from pre- to postintervention, we are interested in the negative values (see discussion below). Our "x," therefore, is 8, and $n = 9$ since there was one tie. We will also use (x – .5) since 8 > (.5) (9) > 4.5. We will reject the null hypothesis of no change in fatigue levels if and only if our generated z value is less than our one-tailed critical value ($z = 1.64$) at $\alpha = .05$.

Using the formula above, we obtain the following actual value of z:

$$z = \frac{(x - 0.5) - (0.5)n}{0.5\sqrt{n}} = \frac{(9 - 0.5) - (0.5)9}{0.5\sqrt{9}} = \frac{(8.5) - 4.5}{1.5} = 2.67$$

Table 5.5 Difference in Fatigue Scores (Postintervention Minus Preintervention Generated in SPSS for Windows [v. 22–23])

Difference scores: Postintervention Minus Preintervention					
		Frequency	*Percent*	*Valid Percent*	*Cumulative Percent*
Valid	−4.00	1	10.0	10.0	10.0
	−3.00	2	20.0	20.0	30.0
	−2.00	2	20.0	20.0	50.0
	−1.00	3	30.0	30.0	80.0
	.00	1	10.0	10.0	90.0
	3.00	1	10.0	10.0	100.0
	Total	10	100.0	100.0	

Since our actual z (2.67) is greater than our critical value of z (1.64), we will reject the null hypothesis and conclude that the children in the staff-initiated intervention group reduced their self-reported fatigue levels from pre- to postintervention.

Critical Assumptions of the Sign Test

One of the advantages of the sign test is that there are not many assumptions attached to it. Unlike the paired t test, the sign test makes no assumptions regarding the form of the distribution of differences between the two variables being examined. The assumptions for this test are as follows.

1. *The data to be analyzed may be dichotomous or continuous. For dichotomous data, there must be some order implied in the coding system (e.g., "0" and "1").* The data that we are examining, pre- and postintervention fatigue, have been measured on a 7-point Likert-type scale and are, therefore, at the ordinal level of measurement.

2. *The randomly selected data are paired observations from a single sample, constructed either through matched pairs or through using subjects as their own controls.* The data from our hypothetical intervention study consist of a pre- and postintervention measure that has been conducted on the same sample of children and are, therefore, paired observations. The data are not, however, randomly selected.

Computer Commands

Figure 5.4 presents the SPSS for Windows dialog boxes used to generate the sign test for pre- and postintervention fatigue levels for the 10 children who received the staff-initiated intervention. The data set that we are using is hospitalized children with cancer-20 cases.sav that is found on the SAGE website (study.sagepub.com/pett2e).

As with the McNemar test (Figure 5.2), only those children who were in the staff-initiated intervention were selected (*Data . . . Select Cases . . . If the Condition is Satisfied . . . If Group = 1*). Next, the following items were selected from the drop-down menu: *Analyze . . . Nonparametric tests . . . Related samples.* Note that the Wilcoxon signed-ranks test also can be generated for the fatigue data from the same dialog box by clicking on the appropriate test box (1). A confidence interval for the difference in the pre- and postintervention fatigue medians using the Hodges-Lehmann confidence interval estimation procedure (Hodges & Lehmann, 1963) could also be selected (2). Since the sign test is not concerned with medians but rather with the number of positive versus negative changes, estimating a confidence interval for the medians will be addressed when discussing the Wilcoxon signed-ranks test.

Figure 5.4 SPSS for Windows (v. 22–23) dialog boxes used to generate the sign test. Data set: hospitalized children with cancer-20 cases (study.sagepub.com/pett2e).

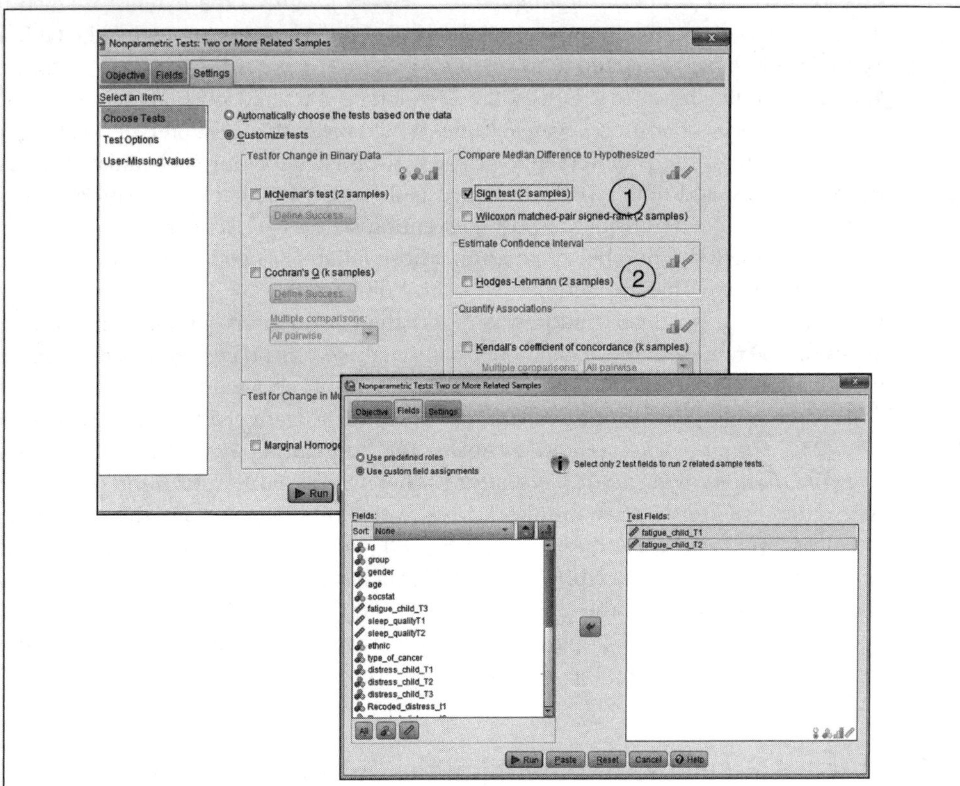

Computer-Generated Output

Figure 5.5 presents the syntax commands and computer-generated output for the sign test obtained in SPSS for Windows (v. 22–23). As indicated, the sample has been filtered to include only the 10 children in the staff-initiated intervention group (3). The syntax commands for the sign test are then presented (4).

Recall from Table 5.4 that the alternative hypothesis is directional. We are hypothesizing that the children in the staff-initiated intervention group will report lower levels of fatigue from pre- to postintervention. The test, therefore, is one-tailed. We will reject the null hypothesis if and only if our one-tailed p value is less than the stated alpha (e.g., .05) and if the results are in the predicted direction.

According to the output presented in Figure 5.5, the two-tailed p value is .0391 (5), which means that the one-tailed p value is .0391/2 or .0195, which is less than $\alpha = .05$. Note that the output suggests that the null hypothesis should be rejected (6). Should we then reject the null? Before that decision is made, it is imperative that we first determine whether the results are in the predicted direction. To do that, those "positive" ($n = 1$) and "negative" ($n = 8$) differences that are presented in the output need to be interpreted (7).

It is important to review the scoring of the fatigue variables. The children indicated on a scale of 1 to 7 (1 = *not at all fatigued* to 7 = *very fatigued*) the extent to which they felt "fatigued." Lower scores, therefore, indicated lower fatigue. Please note that the table element for the results table presented to us on the X-axis (*preintervention fatigue – postintervention fatigue*) is confusing (8). If indeed the computer subtracted postintervention scores from preintervention scores, then negative values would mean that postintervention fatigue scores were *higher* than the preintervention scores, a disaster for our staff-initiated intervention. However, the stated null hypothesis suggests the opposite, that the preintervention fatigue scores were subtracted from the postintervention scores (9). If so, the negative differences ($n = 8$) represent the number of children whose fatigue at postintervention was *lower* than at preintervention, that the number of positive differences ($n = 1$) represents those children whose fatigue at postintervention was *higher* than at preintervention, and that the number of ties ($n = 1$) represent those children for whom there was no change in fatigue scores. Note, too, that because the sample size was small ($n < 25$), a binomial test was undertaken (10).

To determine the meaning of the positive and negative differences, a new variable (*Post_Pre_Fatigue*) was created by using the commands *Transform . . . Compute . . . . Post_Pre_Fatigue = fatigueT2 - fatigueT1*. This new variable represented the differences when the preintervention fatigue scores were subtracted from the postintervention fatigue scores. These results (Figure 5.5 (9)) indicate that indeed the negative values represent those children who reported higher fatigue scores at preintervention. Given that these results are in the predicted direction, we will reject the null hypothesis and conclude that there was a significant reduction in self-reported levels of fatigue from pretest to posttest among the children who took part in the intervention.

Using Internet Resources to Determine the Outcome of a Sign Test

As with the McNemar test, several useful websites provide interactive statistical resources that enable the researcher to generate findings from a sign test without the

Figure 5.5 SPSS for Windows (v. 22–23) syntax and computer-generated output for the sign test.

```
***DATA SET: hospitalized children with cancer-20 cases.sav (www.Sagepub.com)***
COMPUTE filter_$=(group = 1).
VARIABLE LABELS filter_$ 'group = 1 (FILTER)'.
VALUE LABELS filter_$ 0 'Not Selected' 1 'Selected'.
FORMATS filter_$ (f1.0).
FILTER BY filter_$.
EXECUTE.
.
NPTESTS
 /RELATED TEST(fatigue_child_T1 fatigue_child_T2) SIGN
 /MISSING SCOPE=ANALYSIS USERMISSING=EXCLUDE
 /CRITERIA ALPHA=0.05 CILEVEL=95.
```

Hypothesis Test Summary

	Null Hypothesis	Test	Sig.	Decision
1	The median of differences between post-intervention fatigue and pre-intervention fatigue equals 0.	Related-Samples Sign Test	.0391[1]	Reject the null hypothesis.

[1]Exact significance is displayed for this test.

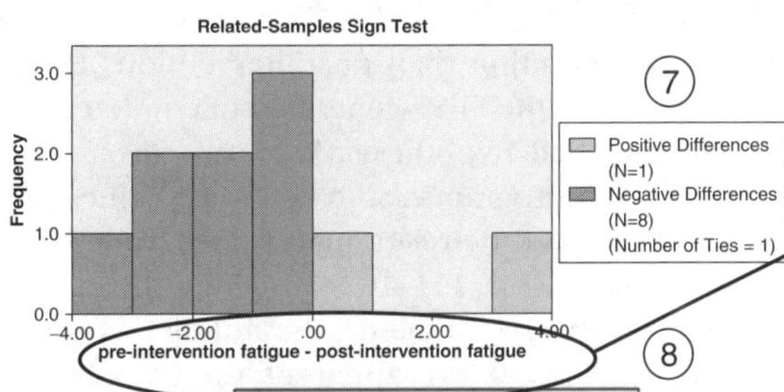

Difference scores: Post-intervention minus Pre-intervention

		Frequency	Percent	Valid Percent	Cumulative Percent
Valid	-4.00	1	10.0	10.0	10.0
	-3.00	2	20.0	20.0	30.0
	-2.00	2	20.0	20.0	50.0
	-1.00	3	30.0	30.0	80.0
	.00	1	10.0	10.0	90.0
	3.00	1	10.0	10.0	100.0
	Total	10	100.0	100.0	

Total N	10
Test Statistic	1.000
Standard Error	1.500
Standardized Test Statistic	-2.000
Asymptotic Sig. (2-sided test)	.046
Exact Sig. (2-sided test)	.039

1. The exact p-value is computed based on the binomial distribution because there are 25 or fewer cases.

need for a stand-alone statistical computer package. One such website that is in the public domain is http://www.socr.ucla.edu. While this is not the only free site available, it should illustrate how one might use such a website to generate the sign test. We will also use the same site to generate other nonparametric statistics such as the Wilcoxon signed-ranks test.

Given that the data for pre- and postintervention fatigue are ordinal level of measurement, we can no longer simply enter the numbers into a 2 × 2 table as we did for the McNemar test. Instead, the data need to be downloaded into the site via a spreadsheet program such as Excel. This example is available to you in Excel format (hospitalized children with cancer-20 cases.xlsx) at study.sagepub.com/pett2e. You may also need to upgrade your Java script.

After accessing the website and the spreadsheet (Figure 5.6), you will need to first click on the *Analyses* button (11) and then indicate which test you wish to undertake (e.g., *two paired samples sign test*) (12). Next, return to your own spreadsheet containing the data of interest, copy, and, using the *Paste* button, (13) paste the values that will be used for the sign test into the SOCR spreadsheet presented on the website (Figure 5.6 (14)). Note that the data of interest in this example are those children who were in the staff-initiated intervention. If desired, you can also change the variable names from C1 and C2 to Fatigue_t1 and Fatigue_t2 (15).

By clicking on the *Calculate* button (16), the output for the sign test is generated (Figure 5.6). Notice that the difference between the two variables is *Fatigue_T1 – Fatigue_T2* (17). That means that the number of cases with differences >0 are those whose fatigue scores were higher at preintervention than postintervention (18). Our one-tailed p value is .01 (19), which is lower than the SPSS-generated one-tailed p value (.0195) but still small enough to reject the null hypothesis. Why this discrepancy? Because the sample size was less than 25, both programs estimated the p values based on the binomial distribution, so one would expect the resulting p values to be similar. In fact, Conover (1999) gives a similar example (pp. 161–162) in which the resulting one-tailed p value is .0195 when $n = 9$ (ties are not counted), the number of positive (as opposed to negative) differences = 8, and $p = .50$. It is apparent, therefore, that the discrepancy seems to be with the p value generated from the SOCR website.

Presentation of Results

Table 5.6 presents an example of how the results for the sign test might be reported. The information for this type of table can be obtained in SPSS for Windows (v. 22–23) by clicking on *Analyze . . . Tables . . . Custom Tables . . .* bringing the variables of interest (e.g., *Fatigue_T1* and *Fatigue_T2*) into the drawing frame and choosing the summary statistics that are desired. Be sure that the appropriate cases have been selected for presentation (e.g., *Data . . . Select Cases . . . If the condition is satisfied (Group = 1)*).

Notice that the median is presented along with the mean and standard deviation. Given that the sign test is nonparametric, some authors might prefer to limit the presentation to only the medians. Because the sample size was small, the binomial distribution was used to evaluate the sign test. For that test, only the p value can be presented in the

Figure 5.6 Spreadsheet format and output generated for the sign test from the website http://www.socr.ucla.edu.

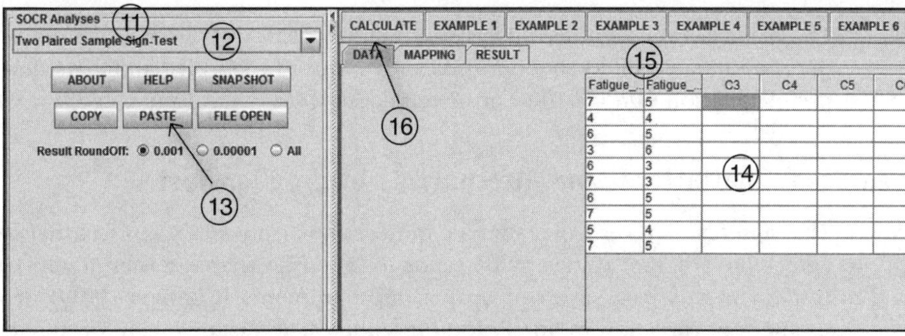

Variable 1 =Fatigue_T1 (17)

Variable 2 =Fatigue_T2

Let Difference = Fatigue_T1 - Fatigue_T2

Result of Two Paired Sample Sign Test: (18)

Number of Cases with Difference > 0: 8 case(s).
Number of Cases with Difference < 0: 1 case(s).
Number of Cases with Difference = 0: 1 case(s).

Sign-Test Statistic = 8 ~ B(n=9, p=0.5)

One-Sided P-Value = .010 (19)

Two-Sided P-Value = .020

Table 5.6 Suggested Presentation of Sign Test Results

Fatigue Scores	N	*Mean*	*Median*	*Standard Deviation*	p[a]
Preintervention	10	5.8	6.0	1.4	.019
Postintervention	10	4.4	4.5	1.0	

[a]The calculated one-tailed *p* value is for the sign test.

table. For larger sample sizes, the normal approximation to the binomial distribution is used. For that reason, the generated z statistic also could be presented.

The results from statistical analysis using the sign test could also be more easily presented in the text as follows:

> The results of the sign test analysis indicated that the 10 children who took part in the staff-initiated intervention significantly reduced their median fatigue levels from preintervention ($Md = 6.0$) to postintervention ($Md = 4.5$) (one-tailed $p = .019$).

Advantages, Limitations, and Alternatives to the Sign Test

The sign test is a versatile, simple, and easy-to-apply statistical test that can be used to determine whether one variable tends to be larger than another. It also can be used to test for trends in a series of ordinal measurements (Conover, 1999) or as a quick assessment of direction in an exploratory study. The disadvantage of this test is that it does not take into account the order of magnitude of the differences between two paired variables. When data are at least ordinal in level of measurement, the Wilcoxon signed-ranks test is preferred.

The parametric alternative to the sign test is the paired t test. Both Siegel and Castellan (1988) and Walsh (1946) report that the sign test is about 95% as efficient as the paired t test. Recall from Chapter 3 that *power efficiency* refers to the sample size that is required for one test (e.g., the sign test) to be as powerful as its rival (e.g., the paired t test) given the same alpha level and that the assumptions of both tests have been met. A 95% efficiency rating implies that, for small samples, only 20 cases are needed for the sign test to achieve the same power as the paired t test with 19 cases (i.e., N_2/N_1 [100%] = 19/20 [100%] = 95%). This suggests that the sign test is especially useful for small sample sizes and in situations in which meeting the assumptions of the robust paired t test either is not possible (e.g., the data are nominal) or is questionable (e.g., a severely skewed distribution with small sample sizes). A more powerful nonparametric alternative to the sign test when the data are at least ordinal in level of measurement is the Wilcoxon signed-ranks test, which makes better use of the quantitative differences between the paired observations.

Examples From Published Research

Graves, K. D., Carter, C. L., Anderson, E. S., & Winett, R. A. (2003). Quality of life pilot intervention for breast cancer patients: Use of social cognitive theory. *Palliative & Supportive Care, 1*(2), 121–134.

Miletic, D., Sekulic, D., & Ostojic, L. (2007). Body physique and prior training experience as determinants of SEFIP score for university dancers. *Medical Problems of Performing Artists, 22*(3), 110–115.

Whellan, D. J., Droogan, C. J., Fitzpatrick, J., Adams, S., McCarey, M. M., Andrel, J., . . . Keith, S. (2012). Change in intrathoracic impedance measures during acute decompensated heart failure admission: Results from the Diagnostic Data for Discharge in Heart Failure Patients (3D-HF) pilot study. *Journal of Cardiac Failure, 18*(2), 107–112.

THE WILCOXON SIGNED-RANKS TEST

The reduction of data in the sign test to +'s or –'s results in the loss of potentially important quantitative information: the *size* of the differences between two paired variables. In our fatigue data, for example, no use is made by the sign test of the information that 5 of the 10 children reduced their fatigue by more than 2 points and that one child increased his fatigue by 3 points (Table 5.5). By taking into account the magnitude and the direction of changes, the Wilcoxon signed-ranks test, which was developed by Wilcoxon (1945), produces a more sensitive statistical test. It is used with paired data that are measured on at least the ordinal scale and is especially effective when the sample size is small and the distribution of the data to be examined does not meet the assumptions of normality, as is required in the paired *t* test.

An Appropriate Research Question for the Wilcoxon Signed-Ranks Test

The Wilcoxon signed-ranks test has been used widely in the health care research literature. It is a very flexible test that can be used in a variety of situations with different sample sizes and few restrictions. The only requirements are that the data be at least ordinal level of measurement and be paired observations; that is, there are either pretest-posttest measures for a single sample or subjects who have been matched on certain criteria.

This test has been used frequently in the research literature to evaluate changes in attitudes on a variety of topics, such as changes over time in satisfaction with health care and medical mistrust among Native American cancer patients (Guadagnolo, Cina, Koop, Brunette, & Petereit, 2011) and nursing students' attitudes toward Australian Aborigines (Hayes, Quine, & Bush, 1994). It has been particularly useful in evaluating the effectiveness of interventions, such as the effects of a cardiac rehabilitation paradigm for non-acute ischemic stroke patients (Lennon, Carey, Gaffney, Stephenson, & Blake, 2008), a pilot walking program for Mexican American women living in colonias at the border (Mier et al., 2011), magnetic resonance imaging in patients with low-tension glaucoma (Stroman, Stewart, Golnik, Curé, & Olinger, 1995), and the effects of a mindfulness stress reduction program on distress in a community-based sample (Evans, Ferrando, Carr, & Haglin, 2011).

Numerous assessments have also been made between two alternative approaches to data collection methods. For example, Vereecken, Covents, and Maes (2010) compared a food frequency questionnaire with an online dietary assessment tool for assessing preschool children's dietary intake. Waninge and colleagues (Waninge, Evenhuis, van Wijck, & van der Schans, 2011; Waninge, van der Weide, Evenhuis, van Wijck, & van der Schans, 2009) used the Wilcoxon to evaluate the feasibility and reliability of body composition measurements and two different walking tests in adults with severe intellectual and sensory disabilities. The Wilcoxon signed-ranks test was also used by Bowring et al. (2012) to measure the accuracy of self-reported height and weight in a community-based sample of young people. Bottom line, there are limitless possibilities for the application of the Wilcoxon signed-ranks test.

In our hypothetical intervention study, we will continue to use the fatigue data that were collected on the children at preintervention and then immediately following the staff-initiated intervention. This will enable us to compare the results that we obtain from the Wilcoxon signed-ranks test with those from the sign test. A research question similar to that of the sign test could, therefore, be asked:

> Do the children in the staff-initiated intervention group reduce their fatigue from pretest to posttest?

As with the sign test, the Wilcoxon signed-ranks test can only examine changes in one group over time.

Null and Alternative Hypotheses

Table 5.7 presents an example of null and alternative hypotheses that would be appropriate for the Wilcoxon signed-ranks test. Note that this nonparametric test examines the differences between medians, not means. Because our alternative hypothesis is directional (i.e., we are predicting a drop in fatigue level following our intervention), the test that will be undertaken is one-tailed. Our level of alpha for this test will remain the same as before ($\alpha = .05$).

Table 5.7 Example of Null and Alternative Hypotheses Appropriate for the Wilcoxon Signed-Ranks Test

Null Hypothesis
H_0: The median fatigue scores of the children who took part in the staff-initiated intervention will not change from pretest to posttest (i.e., $Md_{pretest} = Md_{posttest}$).
Alternative Hypothesis
H_a: The median posttest fatigue scores of the children who took part in the staff-initiated intervention will be lower than at pretest (i.e., $Md_{pretest} > Md_{posttest}$).

Overview of the Procedure

To conduct the Wilcoxon signed-ranks test, the differences between the paired data are calculated and the absolute values of these differences are recorded. Next, the absolute values of the differences between the two variables are ranked from lowest to highest. Finally, each rank is given a positive or negative sign depending on the sign of the original difference. The positive and negative ranks are then summed and averaged. Pairs that indicate no change are dropped from the analysis.

A z statistic is used to test the null hypothesis of no differences in the matched pairs. This z statistic takes the following form:

$$z = \frac{\text{x} - \mu}{\sigma} = \frac{T - [n\,(n+1)\,/\,4]}{\sqrt{n(n+1)\,(2n+1)\,/\,24}}$$

where

T = the absolute value of the sum of the positive or negative ranks, depending on the proposed alternative hypothesis, and

n = the number of positive and negative ranks, excluding ties.

If the null hypothesis is true, the absolute value of the sum of the positive ranks should be nearly equal to the absolute value of the sum of the negative ranks. If the differences in positive and negative ranks are sufficiently large, the null hypothesis is rejected. Either a one- or a two-tailed test is undertaken, depending on the wording of the alternative hypothesis.

Hand-Calculating the Value of the Wilcoxon Signed-Ranks Test

We could arrive at a hand-calculated value for the Wilcoxon signed-ranks test using the test statistic outlined above. We have eight negative ranks whose sum (T), according to Table 5.5, is the absolute value of (–4)1 + (–3)2 + (–2)2 + (–1)3 = $|-38| = 38$. Since $n = 9$ (1 positive + 8 negative ranks = 9), the actual value of our z, therefore, would be as follows:

$$\text{z} = \frac{T - \left[n(n+1)/4\right]}{\sqrt{\dfrac{n(n+1)(2n+1)}{24}}} = \frac{38 - \left[9(9+1)/4\right]}{\sqrt{\dfrac{9(9+1)((2)9+1)}{24}}} = \frac{38 - 22.5}{8.44} = 1.84$$

Since the research hypothesis in Table 5.7 is directional and our one-tailed $\alpha = .05$, the critical value of our z statistic will be +1.64. We will reject the null hypothesis if and only if the actual value of our z statistic is greater than our critical value. Since 1.84 is greater than 1.64, we will reject the null hypothesis and conclude that, according to the Wilcoxon signed-ranks test, the children in the staff-initiated intervention reported statistically significantly lower levels of fatigue following the intervention.

Critical Assumptions of the Wilcoxon Signed-Ranks Test

The assumptions of the Wilcoxon signed-ranks test are fairly liberal.

1. *The data are paired observations from a single randomly selected sample, constructed either through matched pairs or through using subjects as their own controls.* It is assumed either that the data being analyzed are test-retest measures of the same

group of randomly selected subjects or that the data have been collected from subjects who have been paired on one or more variables. The data for our hypothetical study only partially meet this assumption. Although the fatigue data consist of Time 1 and Time 2 measures for the same sample of 10 children who took part in the staff-initiated intervention, our sample is a nonrandom sample of convenience.

2. *The data to be analyzed must be at least ordinal in level of measurement, both within and between pairs of observations.* This assumption means that not only must the variables themselves be at least ordinal in level of measurement, but the generated values of the difference scores must also be at least ordinal level of measurement. In fact, Daniel (2000) indicates that these differences should be measured on at least an interval scale.

The fatigue data from our hypothetical intervention study consist of two pretest and posttest Likert-type scale measurements (1 = *not at all fatigued* to 7 = *extremely fatigued*). Both of these scales and their difference scores are at least ordinal in level of measurement.

3. *There is symmetry of the difference scores about the true median for the population.* This assumption implies that, if it were possible to view the distribution of the difference scores in the population, the distribution of these difference scores would be symmetric (though not necessarily normal) about the population median (Daniel, 2000). One approach to assessing this third assumption might be to plot the difference scores for the sample to assess their symmetry. Figure 5.7 presents the plot that was generated for the DIFF12 variable that was created by subtracting the children's Fatigue_T1 scores from their Fatigue_T2 scores using the *Transform . . . Compute* commands. This histogram was obtained by opening the *Statistics . . . Summarize . . . Frequencies* dialog box and selecting histograms from the *Charts* option. The histogram indicates that although the data for the 20 children are not completely symmetric, they are not badly skewed. We could conclude, therefore, that we approach meeting this assumption.

Computer Commands

The SPSS for Windows (v. 22–23) dialog box that was used to generate the sign test (Figure 5.4) also produces the Wilcoxon signed-ranks test. The data set used was hospitalized children with cancer-20 cases.sav (study.sagepub.com/pett2e). The Wilcoxon signed-ranks test was obtained by clicking on the *Wilcoxon* box under *Compare median differences to hypothesized.* Note, too, that we are also asking for the Hodges-Lehmann 95% confidence interval for the difference in the medians as well.

Computer-Generated Output

Figure 5.8 presents the syntax commands and computer-generated output from SPSS for Windows (v. 22–23) for both the Wilcoxon signed-ranks test and the Hodges-Lehmann 95% confidence interval. As with the sign test, we are interested only in the results for the 10 children in the intervention group since the Wilcoxon can examine

Figure 5.7 Histogram of difference scores: Fatigue2 – Fatigue1 generated in SPSS for Windows (v. 22-23). Data set: Hospitalized children with cancer-20 cases. sav (study.sagepub.com/pett2e).

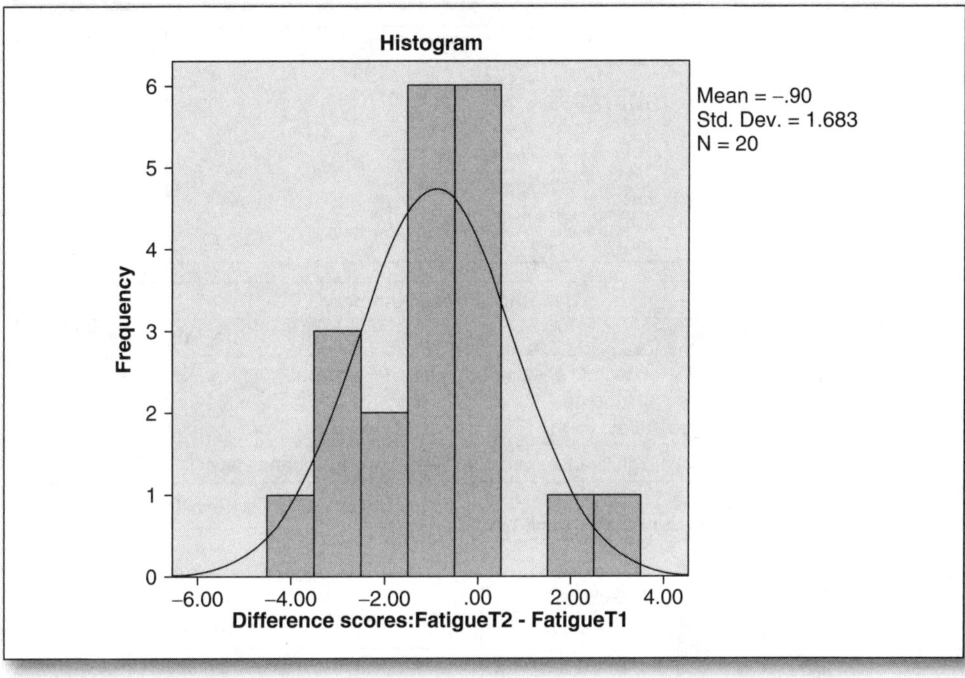

only one group at a time. Therefore, the *Select Cases* . . . command obtained from the *Data* menu is operative (1). The SPSS for Windows syntax commands for the Wilcoxon signed-ranks test are then presented along with the request for the Hodges-Lehmann confidence interval (2).

The computer-generated printout for the Wilcoxon signed-ranks test indicates that eight children had a negative rank (their scores postintervention were lower than preintervention), one child's fatigue level increased from pre- to postintervention, and one child did not alter his or her fatigue level (3). This is the same information that we obtained for the sign test.

Notice that the z statistic generated in SPSS for Windows (–1.851) (4) is a negative value. The T value used by SPSS for Windows was the *sum* of the positive differences ([7][1] = 7) instead of the sum of the negative values (38) (5). It is also not exactly clear why the absolute value of the z statistic (1.851) should be slightly larger than our hand-calculated value (1.84).

The two-tailed p value for this z statistic is .064 (6). If our alternative hypothesis test had been nondirectional, we would not have been able to reject the null hypothesis

Figure 5.8 Syntax and SPSS output for the Wilcoxon signed-ranks test, the Hodges-Lehmann 95% confidence interval, and the descriptive statistics for pre- and postintervention fatigue.

```
***Data set: Hospitalized children with cancer-20 cases***
COMPUTE filter_$=(group = 1).                                   (1)
VARIABLE LABELS filter_$ 'group = 1 (FILTER)'.
VALUE LABELS filter_$ 0 'Not Selected' 1 'Selected'.
FORMATS filter_$ (f1.0).
FILTER BY filter_$.
EXECUTE.
*Nonparametric Tests: Related Samples.
NPTESTS
  /RELATED TEST(fatigue_child_T1 fatigue_child_T2)
  WILCOXON
  HODGES_LEHMAN                                    (2)
  /MISSING SCOPE=ANALYSIS USERMISSING=EXCLUDE
  /CRITERIA ALPHA=0.05 CILEVEL=95.
```

Hypothesis Test Summary

Null Hypothesis	Test	Sig.	Decision
The median of differences between pre-intervention fatigue and post-intervention fatigue equals 0.	Related-Samples Wilcoxon Signed Rank Test	.064 (6)	Retain the null hypothesis. (7)

Asymptotic significances are displayed. The significance level is .05.

Related-Samples Wilcoxon Signed Rank Test

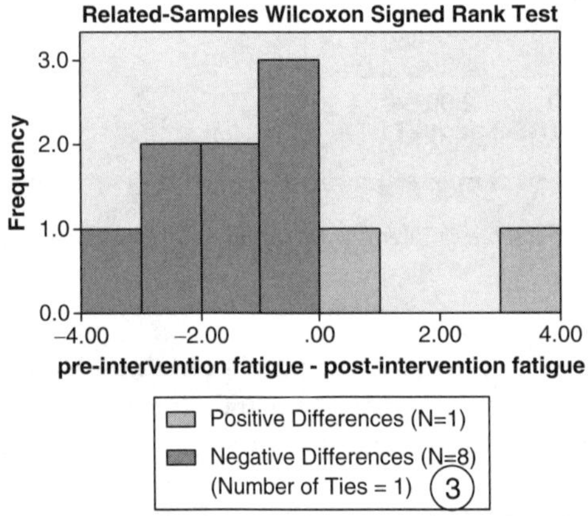

Statistics

		pre-intervention fatigue	post-intervention fatigue
N	Valid	10	10
	Missing	0	0
Mean		5.8000	4.4000
Median		(8) 6.0000	4.5000
Std. Deviation		1.39841	96609

Total N	10	
Test Statistic	7.000	(5)
Standard Error	8.374	
Standardized Test Statistic	−1.851	(4)
Asymptotic Sig. (2-sided test)	.064	

Confidence Interval Summary

Confidence Interval Type	Parameter	Estimate	95% Confidence Interval Lower	95% Confidence Interval Upper
Related-Samples Hodges-Lehman Median Difference	Median of the difference between pre-intervention fatigue and post-intervention fatigue.	-1.500	-2.500	.000 (9)

because this two-tailed p value (.064) is greater than a two tailed $\alpha = .05$. Note that the decision suggested by the output is to retain the null hypothesis (7). Our alternative hypothesis, however, was directional, in that we stated that the children would have lower median fatigue scores at postintervention than at preintervention (Table 5.7). The output that we have obtained from running the frequency statistics for the two variables (*Analyze . . . Frequencies . . .*) (Figure 5.8) supports our predicted direction in that the median postintervention fatigue score (4.5) *is* lower than the median pretest value (6.0) (8).

To determine whether this difference in medians is large enough to reject the null hypothesis, we need to compare our one-tailed $\alpha = .05$ to half the presented two-tailed p value (.064/2 = .032). Because this one-tailed p value, .032, is less than our $\alpha = .05$ and our medians are in the direction predicted, we can reject the null hypothesis of equal medians. Our conclusion, therefore, is that the intervention group significantly reduced its self-reported fatigue from pre- to postintervention.

Note that this generated one-tailed p value for the Wilcoxon test, .032, is greater than the p value that was generated for the sign test, .019 (Table 5.6). The reason for this discrepancy is that the Wilcoxon signed-ranks test is picking up the *size* of the negative and positive ranks, not just noting the direction of differences. The significance of the Wilcoxon statistic has been influenced by the fact that the one child who did increase his or her fatigue from pretest to posttest did so substantially.

Hodges-Lehmann Confidence Interval for the Wilcoxon Signed-Ranks Test

The $(1 - \alpha)100\%$ confidence interval for median differences for both paired and independent samples was developed by Hodges and Lehmann (1963) and is described in detail in Lehmann's (2006) textbook on nonparametric statistics. Using the normal approximation to the Wilcoxon signed-ranks distribution, an asymptotic confidence interval can be obtained as illustrated in Han (2009) and Newson (2006, 2007).

For our data set, the interpretation for such a confidence interval would be as follows: *We can be $(1 - \alpha)100\%$ confident that the true median difference in the children's pre- and postintervention fatigue scores for the population lies between ____ and ____.* If "0" falls in that confidence interval, we cannot reject the null hypothesis because it could conceivably be the true median difference.

The Hodges-Lehmann 95% confidence interval (CI) for the median differences is presented in Figure 5.8 (9). This 95% CI has a lower limit of –2.500 and an upper limit of .000. Note that because this CI contains "0," we should not reject the null hypothesis. Yet our one-tailed p value (.032) indicated that we should reject the null since $.032 < .05$. What is going on here?

The answer is rather straightforward. The 95% CI is two-tailed. Therefore, using a 95% CI, we could not reject the null as indicated in the printout in Figure 5.8 (7). To build a more appropriate CI when we have a one-tailed test (and $\alpha = .05$), we should use a 90% CI instead. This 90% CI would result in a range of values between –2.500 and –.500. Since this range does not contain "0," we can reject the null hypothesis of no difference in medians.

Using Internet Resources to Determine the Outcome of the Wilcoxon Signed-Ranks Test

As we did with the sign test, we will generate the results of the Wilcoxon signed-ranks test using the website http://www.socr.ucla.edu (Figure 5.9). Again, this is not the only site that is available to calculate the Wilcoxon but is illustrative of what is possible using free websites available in the public domain.

After accessing the website and the spreadsheet (Figure 5.9), we will first click on the *Analyses* button (10) and then indicate that we would like to undertake the Wilcoxon signed-ranks test (e.g., *two paired sample signed rank test[Wilcoxon])* (11). Next, using the Excel workbook (Hospitalized Children with Cancer-20 cases.xlsx) that is available on the website, study.sagepub.com/pett2e, highlight and copy the Fatigue_T1 and Fatigue_T2 data for the group that we are interested in evaluating (e.g., the staff-initiated

Figure 5.9 Internet-generated output for the Wilcoxon signed-ranks test (http://www.socr.ucla.edu).

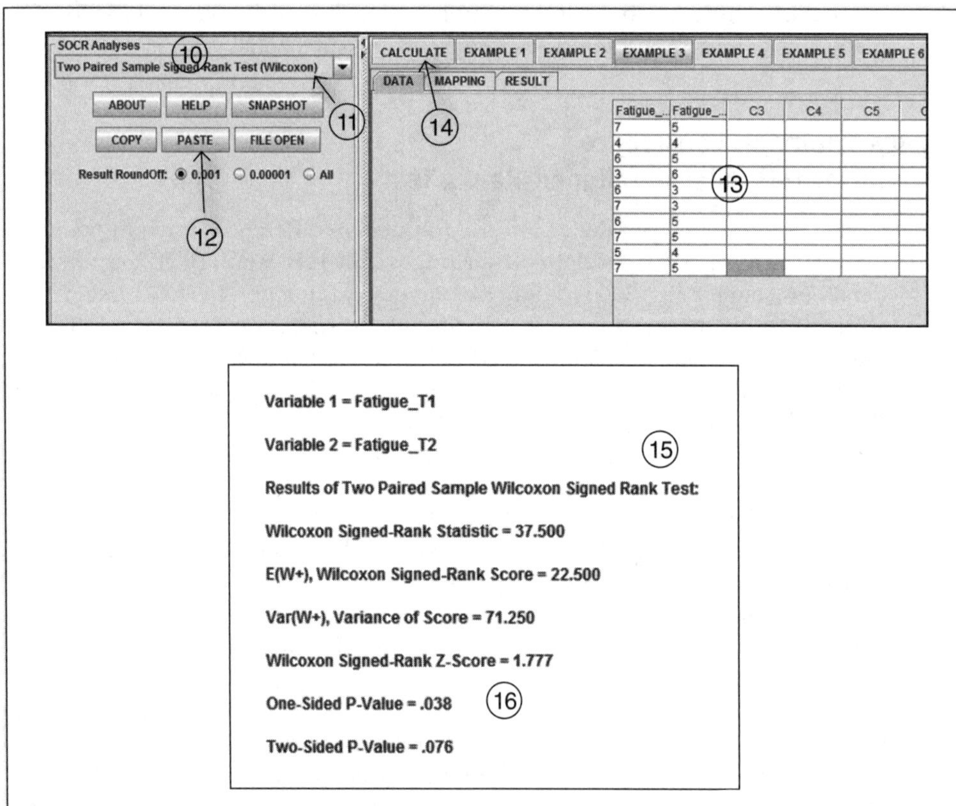

intervention or Group = 1). Bring the data over into the www.socr.ucla.edu spreadsheet and, using the *Paste* button (12), paste the values that will be used for the Wilcoxon signed-ranks test into the SOCR spreadsheet presented on the website (Figure 5.9). Note that the data of interest in this example are those children who were in the staff-initiated intervention. If desired, you can also change the variable names from C1 and C2 to Fatigue_t1 and Fatigue_t2 (13).

By clicking on the *Calculate* button (14), the output for the Wilcoxon signed-ranks test is generated (Figure 5.9) (15). While the resulting one-tailed *p* value (.033) (16) is negligibly higher than the SPSS-generated one-tailed *p* value (.032) (Figure 5.8), it is still low enough to reject the null hypothesis. It does not appear that this website provides us with the Hodges-Lehmann confidence interval for the median difference.

Presentation of Results

The Wilcoxon signed-ranks test can be presented in tabular form in much the same way as the sign test (Table 5.6). The only change that would be required would be the size of the *p* value (.03) and the type of test reported (Wilcoxon signed-ranks test). The results could also be presented in the text as follows:

> The results of the Wilcoxon signed-ranks test indicated that the 10 children who took part in the staff-initiated intervention significantly reduced their self-reported fatigue levels from preintervention (*Md* = 6.0) to postintervention (*Md* = 4.5) ($p = .03$). The Hodges-Lehmann 90% confidence interval for the median difference ranged from –2.500 to –.500.

Advantages, Limitations, and Alternatives to the Wilcoxon Signed-Ranks Test

The Wilcoxon signed-ranks test is very easy to apply and has an advantage over the sign test in that it uses more of the information provided by the data. There are no specific limitations that have been identified for this test.

The parametric alternative to the Wilcoxon signed-ranks test is the *t* test for related samples or paired *t* test. This is the statistical test of choice if the data are found to be normally distributed. The paired *t* test, however, has been found to be unsatisfactory when the distributions of the variables being considered have heavy tails (Wilcox, 1992). Blair and Higgins (1985) used Monte Carlo methods to assess the relative power of the paired *t* test and the Wilcoxon signed-ranks test under 10 different distributional shapes. They report that, when the data were not normally distributed, the Wilcoxon was more often the more powerful test and that the magnitude of the Wilcoxon's power advantage over the paired *t* test often increased with the sample size. Lehmann (2006) also compared the Wilcoxon to the *t* test and reported that, when the distribution is normal, the *t* test is more powerful but that the efficiency loss of the Wilcoxon is slight (about 5%). When the shape of the distribution is unknown, however, the Wilcoxon may be considerably more efficient than the *t* test.

The nonparametric alternatives to this test are the sign and binomial tests. As indicated above, these tests are not as sensitive as the Wilcoxon signed-ranks test but could be used if that test's assumptions are not sufficiently met.

Examples From Published Research

Chaplin, D., Deitz, J., & Jaffe, K. M. (1993). Motor performance in children after traumatic brain injury. *Archives of Physical Medicine and Rehabilitation, 74,* 161–164.

Guadagnolo, B. A., Cina, K., Koop, D., Brunette, D., & Petereit, D. G. (2011). A pre-post survey analysis of satisfaction with health care and medical mistrust after patient navigation for American Indian cancer patients. *Journal of Health Care for the Poor and Underserved, 22*(4), 1331–1343. doi: 10.1353/hpu.2011.0115

Hayes, L., Quine, S., & Bush, J. (1994). Attitude change amongst nursing students towards Australian Aborigines. *International Journal of Nursing Studies, 31*(1), 67–76.

Lennon, O., Carey, A., Gaffney, N., Stephenson, J., & Blake, C. (2008). A pilot randomized controlled trial to evaluate the benefit of the cardiac rehabilitation paradigm for the non-acute ischaemic stroke population. *Clinical Rehabilitation, 22*(2), 125–133. doi: 10.1177/0269215507081580

Mier, N., Tanguma, J., Millard, A. V., Villarreal, E. K., Alen, M., & Ory, M. G. (2011). A pilot walking program for Mexican-American women living in colonias at the border. *American Journal of Health Promotion, 25*(3), 172–175. doi: 10.4278/ajhp.090325-ARB-115

Novack, C. M., Waffarn, F, Sills, J. H., Pousti, T. J., Warden, M. J., & Cunningham, M. D. (1994). Focal intestinal perforation in the extremely-low-birth-weight infant. *Journal of Perinatology, 14,* 450–453.

Summary

In this chapter, we have examined three nonparametric statistical techniques that could be used when data collected from a single sample are paired through using subjects either as their own controls (e.g., pretest and posttest measures) or as matched pairs (e.g., husband-wife pairs). The McNemar test is used when the pretest-posttest data being examined are dichotomous. The sign and Wilcoxon tests require that the distribution of the variable being considered be continuous. Although the sign test can be used with ordered dichotomous data, the Wilcoxon signed-ranks test assumes at least an ordinal level of measurement.

In Chapter 6, several nonparametric tests that can be used when data have been collected over more than two time periods will be presented. These tests include Cochran's *Q* test, which is used with dichotomous data, and the Friedman test, which is used with continuous data.

TEST YOUR KNOWLEDGE

Here is a "test" of your knowledge on the main points regarding the various nonparametric statistics that have been discussed in this chapter. You will want to reread the chapter should you find that you cannot recall their content.

1. What are the main differences between the McNemar, sign, and Wilcoxon signed-rank tests, and when would you consider using each of these nonparametric tests?
2. What are the critical assumptions of each of these three nonparametric tests? Did the distress and fatigue data that were used in this chapter meet those assumptions?
3. Why was it necessary to separate out the staff-initiated intervention group from the usual-care group when running the three nonparametric tests discussed in this chapter?
4. Why was it preferable to change from a 95% to a 90% confidence interval when reporting the median difference for our one-tailed test at $\alpha = .05$?

COMPUTER EXERCISES

The following computer exercises should enable you to build on your skills in using SPSS for Windows, Excel, and/or Internet-based programs.

1. Using either the SPSS for Windows data set (hospitalized children with cancer -20 cases.sav) or Excel spreadsheet (hospitalized children with cancer -20 cases.xlsx) made available to you at study.sagepub.com/pett2e, undertake the sign and Wilcoxon signed-ranks test for the pre- and postintervention fatigue data (*fatigue_T1, fatigue_t2*) for the usual-care group (Hint: be sure to select only those cases for whom *Group* = *2*). Set a two-tailed alpha at .05 and request a Hodges-Lehmann 95% confidence interval (CI) for the median difference.
   a. Looking at your results in Question 1, what was your decision with regard to the null hypotheses for these two tests? Does the Hodges-Lehmann 95% CI support your decision? Why or why not?
   b. Compare the results that you have obtained for the usual-care group with that of the staff-initiated intervention as detailed in this chapter. Were the results for the two groups different or similar? What conclusions would you draw from your results?
2. Eighty participants, ages 48 to 49 years, who were enrolled in a workplace health maintenance plan attended a 3-hour educational workshop addressing the need for routine colorectal cancer screening after age 50. Prior to the workshop, the participants were asked whether they would be likely to obtain a routine colonoscopy once they reached age 50. This same question was asked again immediately following the workshop. The research hypothesis for this study was that the educational workshop would increase the likelihood that the participants would undergo a colonoscopy screening once they reached age 50.

(Continued)

(Continued)

a. What nonparametric statistical test would you use to analyze these data?
b. State the null and alternative hypotheses for this analysis.
c. Is this a one- or a two-tailed test? Please justify your answer.
d. Using the SPSS for Windows data set provided to you at study.sagepub.com/pett2e (colorectal cancer screening data.sav), undertake your analysis of these data using $\alpha = .05$. Alternatively, use an available website (e.g., www.vassarstats.net) to undertake your analyses using the data outlined in the table below.
e. Based on the results you have obtained, were the participants more likely to seek an immediate colonoscopy once they reached age 50? Justify your answer.
f. Create a table and written paragraph that would reflect your results.

		Following Workshop		
Recommend Colonoscopy Screening?		*Likely*	*Not Likely*	*Total*
Prior to workshop	Likely	25	10	35
	Not likely	22	23	45
	Total	47	33	80

Visit **study.sagepub.com/pett2e** to access SAS output, SPSS datasets, SAS datasets, and SAS examples.

CHAPTER 6

Repeated Measures for More Than Two Time Periods or Matched Conditions

- Cochran's *Q* test
- Friedman test

In Chapter 5, we examined tests that are useful for examining data for matched pairs or a single sample with "before-and-after" observations. In clinical research, we are often interested in extending our data collection to include repeated observations across more than two time periods, such as preintervention, postintervention, and 6 months follow-up. Because these data are collected for more than two time periods, the McNemar, sign, and Wilcoxon signed-ranks tests are no longer suitable choices for statistical analysis.

It may also be that we have blocks of subjects who have been matched on a *nuisance* factor that is thought to have an unwanted effect on the dependent variable of interest. This type of design is called a *randomized block design* (Hinkelman & Kempthorne, 2007), in that blocks of matched subjects are formed such that the number of matched subjects in each block is equal to the number of levels of the independent variable. For example, subjects might be matched or *blocked* according to diagnosis. A subject from each diagnosis block is then randomly assigned to each level of the independent variable. The intent of this matching is to obtain an equal number of patients with given diagnoses in each group, thus reducing the amount of error variance that could be attributed to this factor. For this method to be effective, it is important that the researcher be certain that this blocking factor (e.g., children's type of cancer) does indeed have a statistically significant effect on the dependent variable (e.g., reported level of fatigue).

In this chapter, we will examine two nonparametric tests that can be used for multiple or repeated observations on single or matched samples: Cochran's *Q* test and the Friedman test. Cochran's *Q* test is used with dichotomous data, whereas the Friedman test is used with multiple observations of data that are at least at the ordinal level of measurement. It should be noted that our decision to examine a single group across time is not an endorsement for running separate analyses for the treatment and control groups. It is done here to illustrate the repeated measures analyses that can be undertaken using Cochran's *Q* test and the Friedman test.

Why would a researcher want to undertake a repeated measurement study with more than two time points? A major reason is that a study with only two data collection points does not give us sufficient information about the paths that the individuals or groups took to arrive at point 2 from point 1. Given below are three hypothetical paths that could have been taken to arrive at one point from another. In each instance, if we had only examined the differences in numerical values between points 1 and 2, we would have concluded that the three groups (or individuals) were similar to one another when in fact their trajectories were vastly dissimilar.

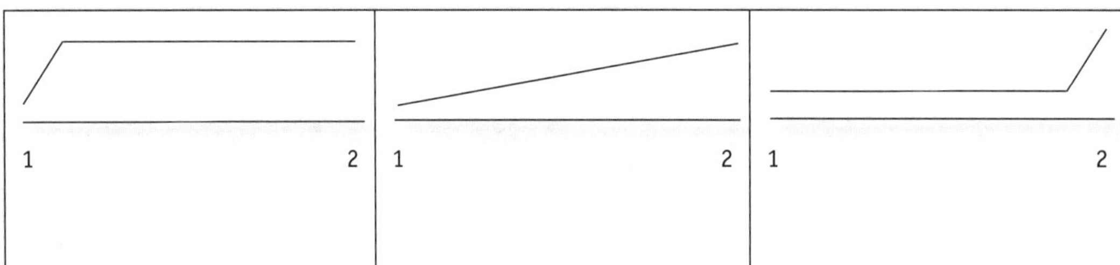

COCHRAN'S *Q* TEST

As indicated in Chapter 5, the McNemar test is used to evaluate change in a dichotomous variable across two time periods. Cochran's *Q* test extends this test to examine change in a dichotomous variable across more than two observations. It is a particularly appropriate test when subjects are used as their own controls and the dichotomous outcome variable is measured across multiple time periods or under several types of conditions. For example, using a randomized block design, subjects may be exposed to more than one intervention. If the treatment outcome can be classified into one of two categories (e.g., success or failure), Cochran's *Q* test would be appropriate for examining whether the proportion of cases in a particular category is the same across all conditions or time periods.

An Appropriate Research Question for Cochran's *Q* Test

Cochran's *Q* test has been used in a wide variety of statistical analyses in health care research. For example, Schrager, Wong, Weiss, and Kipke (2011), in a study of human immunodeficiency virus (HIV) testing and risk behaviors among homosexual men, used Cochran's *Q* test to evaluate the presence or absence of quantifiable changes in their binary risk measures over time. Rentinck, Gorter, Ketelaar, Lindeman, and Jongmans

(2009) used this same statistic to evaluate changes across time in perceptions of family participation among parents of children with cerebral palsy.

A variation of Cochran's *Q* test , I^2, has been used extensively in systematic reviews and meta-analysis studies to evaluate whether there are systematic differences underlying the results of studies (heterogeneity) or whether variation in findings across studies can be attributed to chance alone (homogeneity) (Higgins & Green, 2011; Higgins, Thompson, Deeks, & Altman, 2003). Examples of meta-analysis studies that have used these statistics include a meta-analysis of the relationship between non–high-density lipoprotein cholesterol reduction and risk for coronary heart disease (Robinson, Wang, Smith, & Jacobson, 2009) and an evaluation of obstetric outcomes after conservative treatment for intraepithelial or early invasive cervical lesions (Kyrgiou et al., 2006).

Siegel and Castellan (1988) have also illustrated the use of Cochran's *Q* to evaluate which items of a test are more difficult to answer correctly than others for a given group of respondents. In this example, the samples of dichotomous responses are the correct or incorrect answers to each item. These are related samples to the extent that a set of items is internally consistent. That is, all of the items in the set test the same content. The analysis will also only use data from subjects who have completed all of the items of that set.

In our hypothetical intervention example, the children who were hospitalized with cancer were asked prior to and immediately following the staff-initiated intervention to identify whether they were distressed about their current hospitalization. The McNemar test from Chapter 5 evaluated the direction of change in children's fears from pretest to posttest. Suppose a third point of data collection took place 3 days after the staff-initiated intervention. Because there are now three points of data collection, the McNemar test can no longer be used. Cochran's *Q* test, however, would be appropriate. The following research question could then be posed:

> Is the proportion of children in the staff-initiated intervention who indicate distress (yes, no) regarding their current hospitalization the same across all three data collection periods?

Note that we are only examining the pretest, immediate posttest, and 3-day follow-up responses of the children who were assigned to the staff-initiated intervention. We cannot compare the intervention and usual-care groups simultaneously.

Null and Alternative Hypotheses

Table 6.1 presents an example of null and alternative hypotheses for which a Cochran's *Q* test would be appropriate. Note that the alternative hypothesis is not directional. Like the *F* test in analysis of variance (ANOVA), Cochran's *Q* test determines whether or not there is a significant difference in the proportion of specific responses across the three conditions. Post hoc tests using the McNemar test with a Bonferroni correction for increased Type I error are used to determine where the differences lie.

Table 6.1 Example of Null and Alternative Hypotheses Appropriate for Cochran's *Q* Test

Null Hypothesis
H_0: The proportion of "yes" responses with regard to the children's distress concerning their current hospitalization will be the same across all three time periods for those children who took part in the staff-initiated intervention.
Alternative Hypothesis
H_a: For those children who took part in the staff-initiated intervention, the proportion of "yes" responses with regard to the children's distress concerning their current hospitalization will differ depending on which of the three time periods is being considered.

Overview of the Procedure

To undertake a Cochran's *Q* test, the data are first cast into a two-way table consisting of *N* rows and *k* columns, where *N* represents the number of subjects and *k* represents the number of conditions or time periods (Siegel & Castellan, 1988). Table 6.2 presents the frequency data generated for the 10 children in our hypothetical intervention study.

Table 6.2 Frequencies of Staff-Initiated Intervention Group Children's Responses to Distress (1 = Yes, 0 = No)

	Children's Distress ($k = 3$)			
Subject	*Preintervention*	*Immediately Postintervention*	*3 Days Postintervention*	*L_i (Row 1s)*
1	1	0	1	2
2	1	0	0	1
3	1	1	1	3
4	0	0	0	0
5	1	0	1	2
6	1	0	1	2
7	1	1	1	3
8	1	0	0	1
9	1	1	1	3
10	1	0	0	1
Gj	9	3	6	18

The data set that we will be using is hospitalized children with cancer-20 cases.sav (study.sagepub.com/pett2e). We will only be using the data for those 10 children who were in the staff-initiated intervention.

Next, the data are evaluated to determine whether the proportion of subjects who indicate a preference for a particular dichotomous response (e.g., "yes" = 1) is similar across all *k* conditions. The statistic that is used to evaluate these proportions is as follows (Cochran, 1954):

$$Q = \frac{(k-1)\left[k\sum_{j=1}^{k} G_j^2 - \left(\sum_{j=1}^{k} G_j\right)^2\right]}{k\sum_{i=1}^{N} L_i - \sum_{i=1}^{N} L_i^2}$$

where

k = the number of conditions or time periods,

N = the number of subjects,

G_j = the total number of 1s in the *j*th column, and

L_i = the total number of 1s in the *i*th row.

This Q statistic is distributed approximately as a chi-square (χ^2) with $df = k - 1$ if the size of the sample is greater than 4 and the calculated value, $(N)(k)$, is greater than 24. For smaller sample sizes, Patil (1975) offers exact distributions of Q, but as Siegel and Castellan (1988) point out, Cochran's Q quickly approximates the χ^2 distribution. The null hypothesis of equality of proportions of 1s across all levels of k will be rejected if the calculated value of Q exceeds the critical value of the χ^2 with $df = k - 1$ at the prespecified level of alpha (e.g., $\alpha = .05$). If there are only two time periods, Cochran's Q is nothing more than the McNemar test.

The Q statistic for the data from our hypothetical study will be distributed approximately as a χ^2 with $df = 2$ because our sample size is greater than 4 ($N = 10$), and $(N)(k) > 24$, that is, $(10)(3) > 24$. Calculating Cochran's Q from the data presented in Table 6.2, we obtain the following value:

$$Q = \frac{(k-1)[k\sum_{j=1}^{k} G_j^2 - (\sum_{j=1}^{k} G_j)^2]}{k\sum_{i=1}^{N} L_i - \sum_{i=1}^{N} L_i^2}$$

$$= \frac{(3-1)[3(9^2+3^2+6^2)-(18^2)]}{3(2+1+3+2+2+3+1+3+1)-(2^2+1^2+3^2+2^2+2^2+3^2+1^2+3^2+1^2)}$$

$$= \frac{2(378-324)}{3(18)-42} = \frac{108}{12} = 9.0$$

As indicated above, this Q statistic is distributed approximately as a χ^2 with $df = 2$. Therefore, to determine the critical value of the χ^2, we would turn to the χ^2 table in Appendix A (Table A.2). With $df = 2$ and $\alpha = .05$, the critical value of the $\chi^2 = 5.99$. The rule of thumb is to reject the null hypothesis if and only if (iff) the Q statistic is greater than the critical value of the χ^2 or if $p < \alpha$. Since our generated Q value, 9, is greater than the critical value of the χ^2 at $df = 2$ (5.99), the null hypothesis of equality of proportions of "yes" responses across all three time periods therefore will be rejected. The implications of this finding and its significance level will be addressed when we examine the computer printout.

Critical Assumptions of the Cochran's *Q* Test

Cochran's Q test shares many of the assumptions of the McNemar test but extends these assumptions to more than two conditions or time periods.

1. *The variables being assessed across all time periods are dichotomous with levels that have been assigned similar values (e.g., 0s and 1s).* This assumption means that the same dichotomous variables have been measured across multiple conditions or time periods. The researcher also needs to make certain that the levels that are coded with 0s and 1s share the same meaning across all time periods. In our hypothetical intervention example, the children were asked to assess their distress (yes, no) concerning their hospitalization across three time periods—preintervention, immediately postintervention, and 3 days postintervention. Their "yes" or "no" answers were coded similarly each time (1 = yes, 0 = no); therefore, these data meet this assumption.

2. *The data being examined represent frequencies, not scores.* The data being examined are the frequencies of occurrence of a particular event (e.g., the number of times in a particular time period that a "yes" or a "1" occurred). These data do not represent scores on a particular test. Our hypothetical data, children's responses to a question concerning their distress (yes, no), meet this assumption.

3. *The dichotomous measures are multiple observations of the same subjects or matched samples.* This assumption implies that (1) the dichotomous data have been collected on the same subjects across more than two time periods, (2) the same group of subjects have been exposed to multiple conditions, or (3) N sets of three or more subjects have been matched on certain characteristics and that, within each set, each matched subject has been randomly assigned to one of the designated conditions. In our hypothetical intervention study, the children who took part in the intervention were asked the same question at three different points in time: prior to the intervention (*distress_child_T1*), immediately following the intervention (*distress_child_T2*), and 3 days postintervention (*distress_child_T3*). Our data, therefore, meet this assumption.

4. *The levels of the categorical variables are mutually exclusive.* This assumption means that a subject can be assigned to only one level (0 or 1) of the dichotomous variable at each of the time periods or conditions. The children in the intervention group could be assigned only a "1" or a "0," depending on whether or not they

expressed distress concerning their hospitalization. The levels of these dichotomous variables (*distress_child_T1, distress_child_T2,* and *distress_child_T3*) therefore are mutually exclusive.

Computer Commands

Figure 6.1 presents the SPSS for Windows (v. 22–23) commands used to generate Cochran's *Q* test. This dialog box was opened by selecting the following items from the menu: *Analyze . . . Nonparametric Tests . . . Related Samples . . . Objective: Custom Analysis.* After choosing the Cochran's *Q* test (Figure 6.1) (1), we are then directed to "define success." Since our "success" value = 1 (i.e., answering yes to the question related to distress) is the second value found in the data, we need to indicate that it is not the first value found in the data (0 = no) but rather "success" equals another value (1) (2).

Next we indicate the three time periods we are interested in (3). Make sure that any time period variable that is analyzed with this statistic has been labeled as a nominal level measure in the SPSS database. Finally, under *Settings . . . Test Options . . .* we will indicate that α = .05 and that we will exclude cases test by test (4). Since we have only one "test" that we are examining (and we do not have any missing values), it does not matter which

Figure 6.1 SPSS for Windows (v. 22–23) commands for generating Cochran's *Q* test.

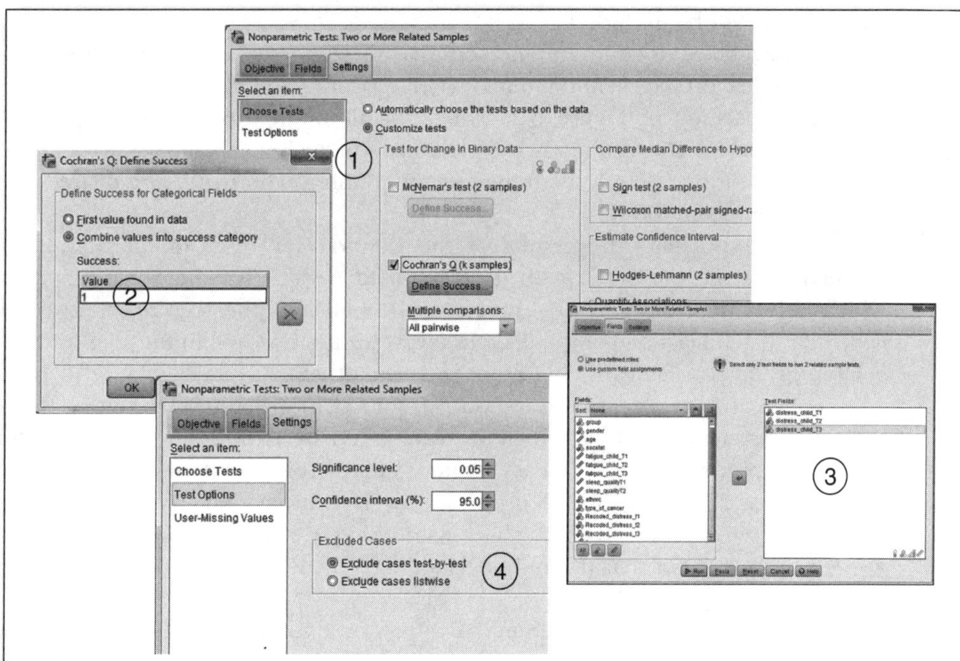

"excluded cases" option we choose. Note, too, that as with the McNemar test from Chapter 5, the data set that we will be using is hospitalized children with cancer-20 cases. sav (study.sagepub.com/pett2e) and the analysis will be restricted to only those 10 children who took part in the intervention. This restriction is obtained by opening the *Data . . . Select Cases . . .* dialog box and selecting only those children who were in the staff-initiated intervention (i.e., *Group = 1*).

Computer-Generated Output

To begin this analysis, we will run the frequencies for our three distress variables using the SPSS pull down menu, *Analyze . . . Descriptive statistics . . . Frequencies . . .* and bringing our three distress variables over into the variables box. That will give us a sense of what our data look like. The SPSS for Windows syntax and computer-generated output for these analyses are presented in Figure 6.2. Note that a filter variable (*filter_$*) has been created as a result of the *Select Cases* command that excludes the children from the control group from the analysis (5). The syntax commands therefore indicate that only the data for the 10 children who took part in the staff-initiated intervention (Group = 1) will be examined.

Next the syntax command for generating frequencies for our three distress variables is presented (6). Also included are the syntax commands for the Cochran's Q test (7). Note that we have also asked for pairwise comparisons of the three time periods (8). The command *Usermissing=Exclude* (9) means that cases that have missing values for this analysis will be excluded.

The frequencies of children who reported distress (1's) and no distress (0's) for the three variables, preintervention, immediately postintervention, and 3 days postintervention, are presented in Figure 6.2. Note that although the number of children who expressed distress concerning their hospitalization declined from preintervention ($n = 9$) to postintervention ($n = 3$), the frequency of children who expressed distress increased 3 days postintervention ($n = 6$).

Figure 6.3 presents the results of the Cochran's Q test. In the Hypothesis Test Summary, we are presented with the generated p value for the Q statistic (.011) (10), which is less than our $\alpha = .05$; therefore, the null hypothesis is rejected, and we can conclude that at least one of the distress levels for the children in the staff-initiated intervention group is significantly different from the others.

Next, we are presented with the output for Cochran's Q test. Note that the test statistic, 9.0, is similar to that which we calculated by hand (11). Be careful, however, when interpreting the bar charts. Earlier versions of SPSS (versions < 22 and some editions of v. 22) had mislabeled the output. If you have such versions, be sure that the upper "blue" part of the bar chart is coded as 1, not 0 (12). Check the frequencies as well to be certain that the output is similar to the frequencies (e.g., that which is presented in Figure 6.2).

To determine where the differences lie, we would look first at the plot of the pairwise comparisons that are presented to us (13). These are pairwise comparisons using McNemar tests. Unfortunately, this plot is confusing to interpret (at least in SPSS for Windows) and needs to be examined carefully. Typically, a plot would be presented with

Figure 6.2 SPSS for Windows (v. 22–23) syntax and frequencies for the three distress variables to be used with Cochran's *Q* test.

```
***hospitalized children with cancer-20 cases.sav***

COMPUTE filter_$=(group=1).                                   (5)
VARIABLE LABELS filter_$ 'group=1 (FILTER)'.
VALUE LABELS filter_$ 0 'Not Selected' 1 'Selected'.
FORMATS filter_$ (f1.0).
FILTER BY filter_$.
EXECUTE.

FREQUENCIES VARIABLES=distress_child_T1 distress_child_T2
distress_child_T3                                             (6)
 /ORDER=ANALYSIS.

*Nonparametric Tests: Related Samples.
NPTEST                                                        (7)
 /RELATED TEST(distress_child_T1 distress_child_T2 distress_child_T3)
  COCHRAN(SUCCESS=LIST(1) COMPARE=PAIRWISE)                   (8)
 /MISSING SCOPE=ANALYSIS USERMISSING=EXCLUDE (9)
 /CRITERIA ALPHA=0.05 CILEVEL=95.
```

distress_child_T1 intervention distress

		Frequency	Percent	Valid Percent	Cumulative Percent
Valid	.00 no, no distressed	1	10.0	10.0	10.0
	1.00 yes, distressed	(9)	90.0	90.0	100.0
	Total	10	100.0	100.0	

distress_child _T2 distress immediately post intervention

		Frequency	Percent	Valid Percent	Cumulative Percent
Valid	.00 no, no distressed	7	70.0	70.0	70.0
	1.00 yes, distressed	(3)	30.0	30.0	100.0
	Total	10	100.0	100.0	

distress_child_T3 distress 3 days post intervention

		Frequency	Percent	Valid Percent	Cumulative Percent
Valid	.00 no, no distressed	4	40.0	40.0	40.0
	1.00 yes, distressed	(6)	60.0	60.0	100.0
	Total	10	100.0	100.0	

Figure 6.3 SPSS for Windows (v. 22–23) output for Cochran's *Q* test.

Hypothesis Test Summary

	Null Hypothesis	Test	Sig.	Decision
1	The distributions of preintervention distress, distress immediately post intervention and distress 3 days post intervention are the same for the specified categories.	Related-Samples Cochran's Q Test (10)	.011	Reject the null hypothesis.

Asymptotic significances are displayed. The significance level is .05.

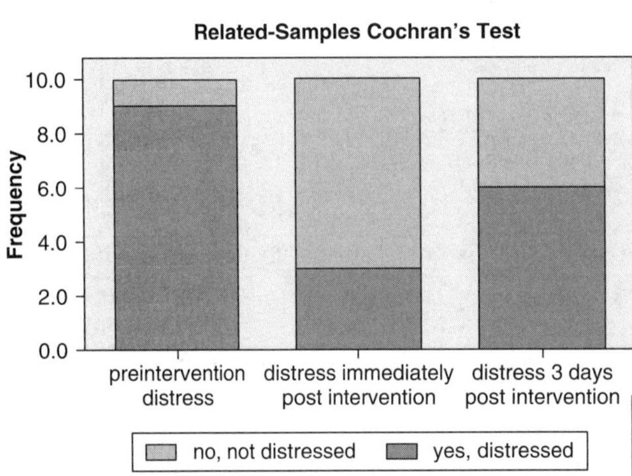

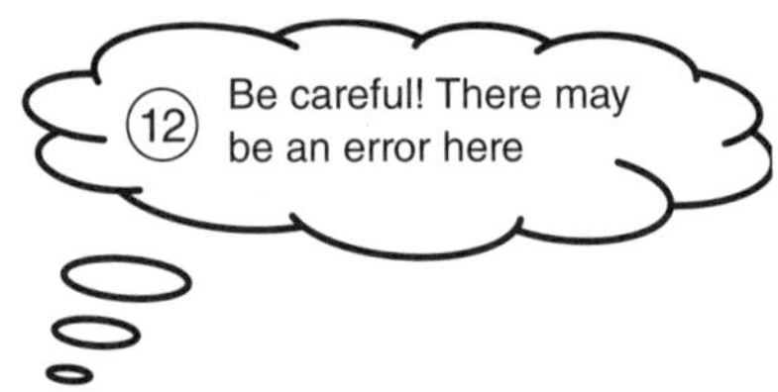

Total N	10
Test Statistic (11)	9.000
Degrees of Freedom	2
Asymptotic Sig. (2-sided test)	.011

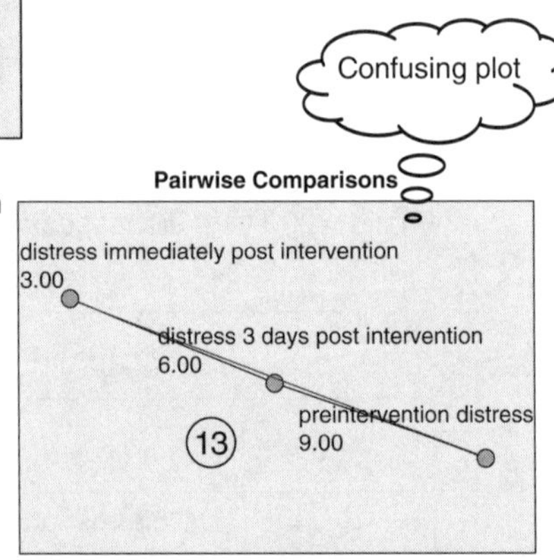

Each node shows the sample number of successes.

Sample1-Sample2	Test Statistic	Std. Error	Std. Test Statistic	Sig.	Adj.Sig.
distress immediately post intervention -distress 3 days post intervention	-.300	.200	-1.500	.134	.401
distress immediately post intervention -preintervention distress	.600	.200	3.000	.003	.008 (14)
distress 3 days post intervention-preintervention distress	.300	.200	1.500	.134	.401

Each row tests the null hypothesis that the Sample 1 and Sample 2 distributions are the same.
Asymptotic significances (2-sided tests) are displayed. The significance level is .05.

the time elements on the X-axis and the number of "successes" (1) on the Y-axis. In this plot of pairwise comparisons, however, it appears that the number of "successes" has been plotted along the X-axis. This makes it look as though we have a straight line.

Because of the risk of increased Type I error, the researcher may opt to adjust the alpha for these tests. One conservative adjustment is Bonferroni's inequality (adjusted $\alpha' = \alpha/k$ where k = the number of post hoc tests to be performed and α equals the original alpha level [.05]). In our hypothetical intervention study, we have three potential pairwise comparisons regarding distress: preintervention versus immediate postintervention, preintervention versus 3 days postintervention, and immediate postintervention versus 3 days postintervention. It should be noted that we are not obliged to choose all three comparisons. We might in fact choose only two of the three potential comparisons (e.g., pre- to immediate postintervention and post- to 3 days postintervention). In that case, the Bonferroni adjustment would be made for two rather than three comparisons.

In this example, however, we are interested in all three comparisons. Our adjusted α', therefore, is .017 (i.e., $\alpha/k = .05/3 = .017$). We will reject the null hypothesis of no differences between the two time periods if $p < .017$. Examining the pairwise comparisons in Figure 6.3, there are only two time periods that were statistically significantly different from one another: preintervention distress and distress immediately postintervention ($p = .008$) (14).

Looking at the distributions for the three time periods, what would we conclude? It appears that the number of children in the staff-initiated intervention who reported feeling distressed declined significantly from pre- to immediate postintervention but then began to rise 3 days following the conclusion of the intervention; however, the rise in number of distressed children did not return to baseline.

Using Internet Resources to Determine the Outcome of Cochran's *Q* Test

A search of the currently available statistical resources in the public domain did not produce an Internet site that listed Cochran's *Q* test as an available procedure. Other websites did list this test, but those sites either required a download to a computer (e.g., EPI Stat) or restricted the researcher to a temporary download with subsequent request for purchase (e.g., http://www.xlstat.com and www.medcalc.org). The interested reader is referred to one site, http://statpages.org, which lists Internet resources and downloads in the public domain that hopefully, one day, will allow on-site analyses of data using the Cochran's *Q* test.

Presentation of Results

Table 6.3 presents a format that might be used to present the results of the Cochran's *Q* test. This material could also be presented in the text as follows:

> The results of Cochran's *Q* test indicate that there was a significant change in the distress levels for the children from the staff-initiated intervention group over the three time periods ($p = .01$). To determine where the differences lay, post hoc tests were undertaken using a Bonferroni correction (two-tailed $\alpha = .017$) to accommodate for the increased risk of Type I error. These analyses indicated that

Table 6.3 Suggested Presentation of Cochran's *Q* Test Results

	Reported Distress?		*Cochran's Q*	
Time Period	*Yes*	*No*	χ^2	p
Pretest[a]	9	1	9.00	.01
Immediately postintervention	3	7		
3 days postintervention	6	4		

[a]Significantly different from immediately postintervention, $p = .008$.

the significant decreases in the reported distress for the children in the staff-initiated intervention occurred from pretest to immediately postintervention ($p = .008$). Although the children's distress started to return to baseline, no other significant changes between time periods were obtained.

Advantages, Limitations, and Alternatives of Cochran's *Q* Test

Cochran's *Q* test has the advantage of examining change in categorical data over multiple observations. A disadvantage to this test is that it does not evaluate the extent of change, only whether a change has occurred. It also does not consider the trajectory of possible changes. The test is not very accurate when the sample size is small and does not allow for comparisons across groups, because this is a test for use with dependent observations. A somewhat unsatisfactory solution is to run a Cochran's *Q* test on each of the two groups independently and to compare the results. Unfortunately, this approach does not allow the researcher to assess group-by-time interaction.

Because Cochran's *Q* test is intended for use with dichotomous data, it has no parametric equivalent. If the data to be analyzed are at least ordinal level of measurement, the Friedman test is preferable to Cochran's *Q* test, especially when the sample size is small and the data are ordered (Siegel & Castellan, 1988). Myers, DCecco, White, and Borden (1982) reported that Cochran's *Q* test had problems with sample sizes of less than 16 but gave accurate Type I error rates for larger samples, even under conditions of extreme heterogeneity of covariance.

Examples From Published Research

Kyrgiou, M., Koliopoulos, G., Martin-Hirsch, P., Arbyn, M., Prendiville, W., & Paraskevaidis, E. (2006). Obstetric outcomes after conservative treatment for intraepithelial or early invasive cervical lesions: Systematic review and meta-analysis. *Lancet, 367*(9509), 489–498.

Rentinck, I. C. M., Gorter, J. W., Ketelaar, M., Lindeman, E., & Jongmans, M. J. (2009). Perceptions of family participation among parents of children with cerebral palsy followed from infancy to toddler hood. *Disability & Rehabilitation, 31*(22), 1828–1834. doi: 10.1080/09638280902822286

Robinson, J. G., Wang, S., Smith, B. J., & Jacobson, T. A. (2009). Meta-analysis of the relationship between non-high-density lipoprotein cholesterol reduction and coronary heart disease risk. *Journal of the American College of Cardiology, 53*(4), 316–322.

Schrager, S. M., Wong, C. F., Weiss, G., & Kipke, M. D. (2011). Human immunodeficiency virus testing and risk behaviors among men who have sex with men in Los Angeles County. *American Journal of Health Promotion, 25*(4), 244–247. doi: 10.4278/ajhp.090203-ARB-43

THE FRIEDMAN TEST

In Chapter 5, the Wilcoxon signed-ranks test was presented as a useful technique for analyzing continuous data that have been collected on a single sample across two time periods or conditions. It also could be used when subject pairs are matched and randomly assigned as pairs to an experimental or control group. The Friedman test extends the Wilcoxon signed-ranks test to include (1) more than two time periods of data collection or conditions or (2) groups of three or more matched subjects, with a subject from each group being randomly assigned to one of the three or more conditions.

The Friedman test examines the ranks of the data generated during each time period or condition to determine whether the variables share the same underlying distribution. This nonparametric test is analogous to the parametric repeated-measures analysis of variance (ANOVA) without a comparison group.

An Appropriate Research Question for the Friedman Test

Numerous examples from the health care research literature illustrate the variety of situations to which the Friedman test can be applied. Philip, Ayyangar, Vanderbilt, and Gaebler-Spira (1994) used the Friedman test to evaluate the effects of rehabilitation on the functional outcomes of 30 children after treatment for primary brain tumors. The same test was used by Loerakker et al. (2012) to evaluate plasma variations of biomarkers for muscle damage in male nondisabled and spinal cord–injured subjects. Similarly, Kaartinen and colleagues (2012) used this test in their investigation of whether autonomic arousal during eye contact, as measured by skin conductance responses, was associated with the level of social skills among children with autism spectrum disorder. McCain (1992) used the same test to assess the effectiveness of three interventions designed to facilitate inactive awake states in 20 preterm infants. In each of these examples, the authors elected to use the Friedman test because their data did not meet the assumptions of a parametric test.

In our hypothetical intervention example, suppose we had collected information concerning the 10 children's fatigue levels not only at preintervention and immediately postintervention following the staff-initiated intervention but also 3 days postintervention. An example of a research question that could be answered with the Friedman test is as follows:

> What are the differences in the self-reported fatigue levels of the 10 children who took part in the staff-initiated intervention across the three time periods (i.e., preintervention, immediate postintervention, and 3 days postintervention)?

Null and Alternative Hypotheses

Table 6.4 presents an example of null and alternative hypotheses, generated from the research question presented earlier, that would be appropriate for a Friedman test. Note that because this test is nonparametric, the focus of attention is on medians, not the means. In addition, the alternative hypothesis presented in Table 6.4 is nondirectional. If the alternative hypothesis had been directional, planned comparisons would have been a more powerful approach to analyzing the data. Overall tests of significance followed by post hoc tests are used when the researcher is not certain of direction and prefers to explore rather than predict outcomes.

Overview of the Procedure

To undertake a Friedman test, the data are first cast into a two-way table with N rows and k columns. As with Cochran's Q test, N represents the number of subjects or matched sets of subjects and k represents the number of conditions or data collection periods. For example, if there were six sets of four matched subjects that were going to be randomly assigned to one of four conditions, $N = 6$ and $k = 4$. In our hypothetical intervention example, because we have 10 subjects whose self-reported fatigue was measured at three time periods, $N = 10$ and $k = 3$. Table 6.5 presents the fatigue data for the 10 children in the intervention group across the three periods of time. The data set that we will be using for the Friedman test is hospitalized children with cancer-20 cases (study.sagepub.com/pett2e).

Note that the data in Table 6.5 for each row (i.e., for each matched set or subject) have been ranked from lowest to highest and their ranked columns summed (1). If the null hypothesis of no differences between the conditions or time periods is true, the sum of the ranks for each column (R_j) should be no different from that which would be expected by chance (i.e., $N[k + 1]/2$) (Siegel & Castellan, 1988). In our example, if there are no differences between the children's self-reported preintervention, immediate postintervention,

Table 6.4 Example of Null and Alternative Hypotheses for a Friedman Test

Null Hypothesis
H_0: There will be no differences among the median self-reported fatigue scores at preintervention, immediate postintervention, and 3 days postintervention for the 10 children who took part in the staff-initiated intervention.
Alternative Hypothesis
H_a: There will be at least one difference among the median fatigue scores at preintervention, immediate postintervention, and 3 days postintervention for the 10 children who took part in the staff-initiated intervention.

Table 6.5 Frequencies of Self-Reported Fatigue Data for the 10 Children in the Intervention Group

	Preintervention		*Immediate Postintervention*		*3 Days Postintervention*		
ID	*Score*	*Rank* $R(X_{ij})$	*Score*	*Rank* $R(X_{ij})$	*Score*	*Rank* $R(X_{ij})$	$R(X_{ij})^2$
1	7	3	5	1	6	2	$3^2 + 1^2 + 2^2 = 14$
2	4	2	4	2	4	2	$2^2 + 2^2 + 2^2 = 12$
3	6	3	5	1.5	5	1.5	$3^2 + 1.5^2 + 1.5^2 = 3.5$
4	3	1	6	3	4	2	14
5	6	3	3	1	4	2	14
6	7	3	3	1	6	2	14
7	6	3	5	1.5	5	1.5	13.5
8	7	3	5	1	6	2	14
9	5	3	4	1.5	4	1.5	13.5
10	7	3	5	1	6	2	14
(1) $\Sigma R(X_{ij})$[a]		27		14.5		18.5	$\Sigma R(X_{ij})^2 = 136.5$

[a] $\Sigma R(X_{ij})$ represents the sum of the ranks within each column, preintervention, immediate postintervention and 3 days postintervention

and 3 days postintervention fatigue, the sum of the ranks for each of these three time periods should be equal to 20 (10[3 + 1]/2 = 20). If the null hypothesis is not true, then the sum of the ranks would vary from column to column. Our sums for the ranks in Table 6.5—27, 14.5, and 18.5—are not equal. Are these differences sufficiently large to reject the null hypothesis?

The Friedman test examines the rank totals of each time period or condition to determine the extent to which these totals differ from their expected sums using the following formula (Conover, 1999):

$$F_r = \frac{12}{Nk(k+1)} \sum_{j=1}^{k} \left(R_j - \frac{N(k+1)}{2} \right)^2$$

where

R_j = the sum of the ranks for column j,

N = the number of subjects, and

k = the number of time periods or conditions.

Conover (1999) points out that because an exact distribution for this test is difficult to find, an approximation to the distribution is typically used. This approximation is the χ^2 distribution with $df = k - 1$.

When there are ties among the ranks for a given row, Conover (1999) offers an adjustment to the formula, which accounts for the presence of ties. That is, let A equal the sum of the squares of the ranks including ties and C equal the "correction factor" (p. 370):

$$A = \sum_{i=1}^{n}\sum_{j=1}^{k}\left[R\left(X_{ij}\right)\right]^2$$

$$C = nk\left(k+1\right)^2 / 4$$

Then the adjusted for ties formula for the Friedman test would be as follows:

$$F_{r(adj)} = \frac{(k-1)\sum_{j=1}^{k}\left(R_j - \frac{N(k+1)}{2}\right)^2}{A - C}$$

Like the overall F test in ANOVA, if the obtained value of the Friedman statistic is significant, the researcher can conclude that at least one condition or time period is statistically significantly different from another.

Because we have several ties in our ranked fatigue data (see Table 6.5), we would need to use the adjusted Friedman test, $F_{r(adj)}$. To obtain this adjusted F, we need to first calculate A and C. From Table 6.5, we can see that A, the sum of the squared ranks for each subject across all three time periods, is as follows:

$$A = \sum_{i=1}^{n}\sum_{j=1}^{k}\left[R\left(X_{ij}\right)\right]^2 = \sum\left(14 + 12 + 13.5 + \ldots + 13.5 + 14\right) = 136.5$$

The value of C, the "correction" factor, would be

$$C = \frac{nk\left(k+1\right)^2}{4} = \frac{10(3)(3+1)^2}{4} = \frac{10(3)(16)}{4} = \frac{480}{4} = 120$$

With A and C, as well as the information obtained in Table 6.5, we can now calculate $F_{r(adj)}$:

$$F_{r(adj)} = \frac{(k-1)\sum_{j=1}^{k}\left(R_j - \frac{N\left(k+1\right)}{2}\right)^2}{A - C}$$

$$= \frac{(3-1)\sum_{j=1}^{3}\left(R_j - \frac{10\left(3+1\right)}{2}\right)^2}{136.5 - 120}$$

$$= \frac{2[(27-20)^2 + (14.5-20)^2 + (18.5-20)^2]}{16.5}$$

$$= \frac{2[49 + 30.25 + 2.25]}{16.5} = 9.879$$

If the assumptions of the Friedman test have been met, our critical χ^2 value with $df = 3 - 1 = 2$ and $\alpha = .05$ is 5.99 (see Appendix A, Table A.2, for the critical values of the χ^2 distribution). Because this value is smaller than our obtained $F_{r(adj)}$ of 9.879, the null hypothesis will be rejected. Our conclusion is that at least one of our time periods is statistically significantly different from each other. To determine where those differences lie, post hoc comparisons would need to be undertaken. These post hoc tests will be discussed in detail below.

Critical Assumptions of the Friedman Test

The Friedman test shares the assumptions of the Wilcoxon signed-ranks test but extends these assumptions to include more than two conditions or periods of data collection.

1. *The data to be analyzed are at least ordinal level of measurement.* Our data, the measures of self-reported fatigue at three points in time, meet this assumption because these Likert-type scales are ordinal level of measurement.

2. *The data from a randomly selected sample are either (a) multiple observations from a single sample across more than two time periods or conditions or (b) blocks of matched subjects in which the subjects from a given block are each randomly assigned to one of the three or more conditions.* This assumption implies that the researcher either has collected repeated measures on a single sample for more than two time periods or has matched sets of subjects who have been randomly assigned to three or more given conditions. The fatigue data consist of multiple observations across three time periods from a single sample of 10 children who took part in the staff-initiated intervention. These data, although not from a randomly selected sample, do meet the assumption of paired observations.

3. *The subjects or blocks of subjects are independent; that is, the results within one block do not have an influence on the results within the other blocks.* This third assumption means that no subject appears more than once and, therefore, does not appear within more than one block (or row). This would also imply that subjects who might have an undue influence on each other (e.g., husbands and wives, or twins) are not in separate blocks. Because our blocks (or rows) consist of single subjects and none of the subjects are related, our data meet this assumption.

Computer Commands

Figure 6.4 presents the SPSS for Windows (v. 22–23) commands used to generate the Friedman test using the data set, hospitalized children with cancer-20 cases (study.sagepub.com/pett2e).

Only the children in the staff-initiated intervention group were selected by using the commands, *Data . . . Select Cases . . . If the condition is satisfied (Group = 1).* Then, the dialog boxes for the Friedman test are opened by selecting the same items from the menu as for Cochran's *Q* test: *Analyze . . . Nonparametric Tests . . . Related Samples . . . Customize Analysis . . .* (1). After having moved the three fatigue variables into the *Fields* dialog box (2), the Friedman test was selected from the *Settings . . . Choose Tests . . .* menu (3). To obtain multiple comparisons of the three time periods, select *All pairwise comparisons . . .* in the *Multiple comparisons* dialog box (4).

Computer-Generated Output

Figure 6.5 presents the syntax commands and computer-generated output that were obtained from SPSS for Windows (v. 22–23). As with the previous tests, only the 10 children from the staff-initiated intervention group (Group = 1) were selected for this analysis

Figure 6.4 SPSS for Windows (v. 22–23) commands for the Friedman test.

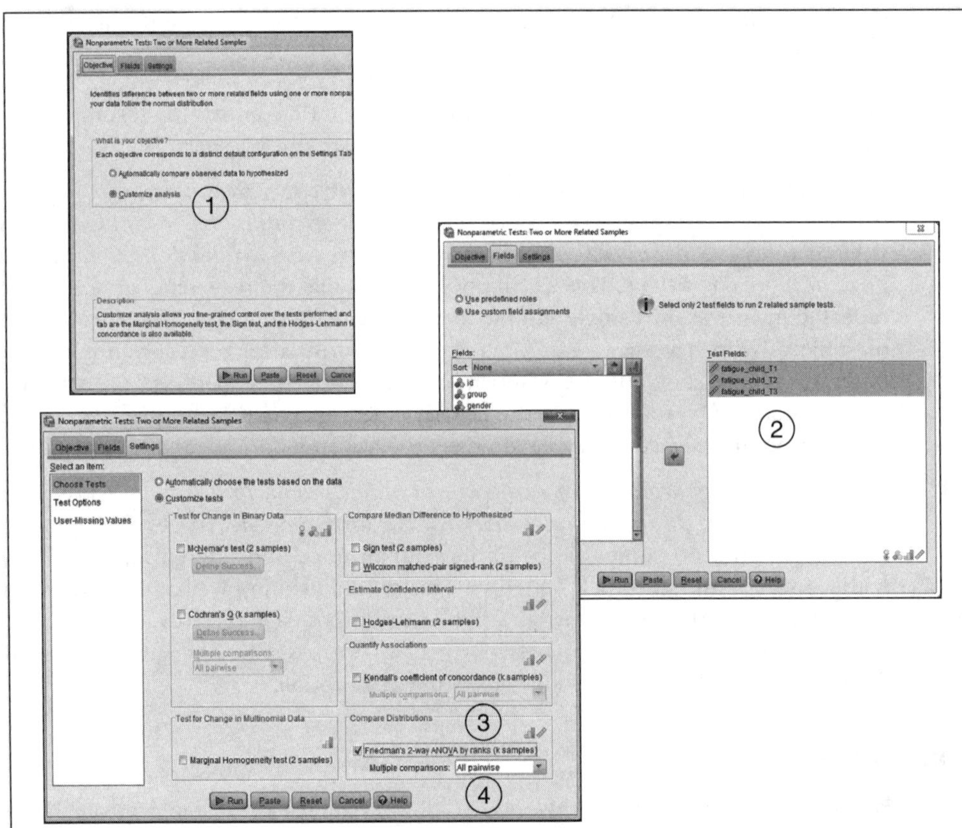

Reprints Courtesy of International Business Machines Corporation, © International Business Machines Corporation

Figure 6.5 SPSS-generated syntax commands and output for the Friedman test.

```
***Data set: hospitalized children with cancer-20 cases.sav***

COMPUTE filter_$=(group = 1).   (5)
VARIABLE LABELS filter_$ 'group = 1 (FILTER)'.
VALUE LABELS filter_$ 0 'Not Selected' 1 'Selected'.
FORMATS filter_$ (f1.0).
FILTER BY filter_$.
EXECUTE.

*Nonparametric Tests: Related Samples.
NPTESTS
 /RELATED TEST(fatigue_child_T1 fatigue_child_T2 fatigue_child_T3)
 FRIEDMAN(COMPARE=PAIRWISE)   (6)
/MISSING SCOPE=ANALYSIS USERMISSING=EXCLUDE (7)
 /CRITERIA ALPHA=0.05  CILEVEL=95.
```

Hypothesis Test Summary

	Null Hypothesis	Test	Sig.	Decision
1	The distributions of pre-intervention fatigue, immediate post-intervention fatigue and 3-days post-intervention fatigue are the same.	Related-Samples Friedman's Two-Way Analysis of Variance by Ranks	(8) .007	Reject the null hypothesis.

Asymptotic significances are displayed. The significance level is .05.

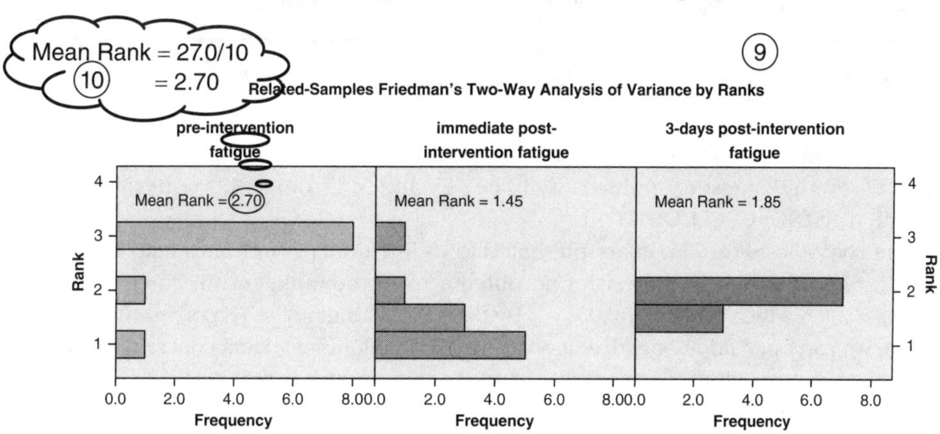

(Continued)

Figure 6.5 (Continued)

Total N	10
Test Statistic	9.879 (11)
Degrees of Freedom	2
Asymptotic Sig. (2-sided test)	.007

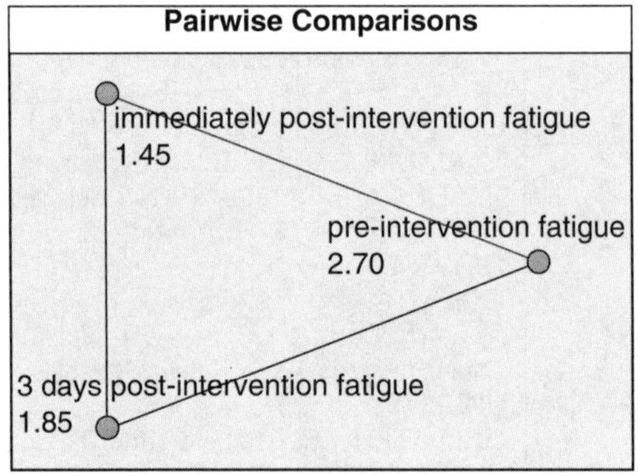

(13)

Each node shows the sample average rank.

Sample1-Sample2	Test Statistic	Std. Error	Std. Test Statistic	Sig.	Adj.Sig.
immediate post-intervention fatigue-3-days post-intervention fatigue	-.400	.447	-.894	.371	1.000
immediate post-intervention fatigue-pre-intervention fatigue	1.250	.447	2.795	.005	(12) .016
3-days post-intervention fatigue-pre-intervention fatigue	.850	.447	1.901	.057	.172

(14) p>0.05

Each row tests the null hypothesis that the Sample 1 and Sample 2 distributions are the same.
Asymptotic significances (2-sided tests) are displayed. The significance level is .05.

(5). The syntax commands also indicate that the Friedman test has been requested (6) and that any missing values will be excluded from all requested analyses ("USERMISSING=EXCLUDE") (7).

The Hypothesis Test Summary presented to us in Figure 6.5 indicates that, at $\alpha = .05$, we should reject the null hypothesis of no differences in the ranks for the three time periods since $p = .007$, which is less than .05 (8). By double-clicking on the Hypothesis Test Summary figure, we can open additional dialog boxes to obtain additional detail concerning the results. For example, the output for the *Related-Samples Friedman's Two-Way Analysis of Variance by Ranks* is presented (9). It continues to be a mystery (to me at least) as to why the Friedman test is considered a "Two-Way Analysis of Variance by Ranks" since the test only considers changes in the same sample across time and is not able to undertake a between-group comparison (e.g., between the staff-initiated intervention and usual-care groups).

The mean ranks for the three time periods, 2.70, 1.45, and 1.85, for the children in the staff-initiated intervention group presented in the table are the averages of the summed ranks that we obtained in Table 6.5 (e.g., 27.0/10 = 2.70) (10). These values indicate that the children's average ranks for their fatigue scores were highest at preintervention (2.70), decreased immediately following the intervention (1.45), and then increased somewhat 3 days postintervention (1.85).

The computer-generated χ^2 value for the Friedman test was 9.879 with $df = 2$ (11). This is the same value as that which we obtained when we hand-calculated the Friedman test using the F test, which adjusted for ties. As indicated earlier, to determine whether this value is significant, it is necessary to compare the obtained significance level, $p = .007$ (8), to our prestated alpha level (e.g., .05). If the obtained significance is lower than this prestated alpha, we will reject the null hypothesis of no differences among the average ranks for the three time periods. Because this is an overall test and not directional, we can examine the significance level directly without dividing it in half as we did for the directional Wilcoxon test in Chapter 5. The resulting p value, .007, indicates that our null hypothesis can be rejected because .007 is less than our stated level of alpha (.05). We can conclude, therefore, that at least one of the average ranks for the three time periods is significantly different from one of the others. Now we are in a position to undertake the post hoc comparison tests to determine where the differences are located.

Post Hoc Comparisons to Determine Differences in the Ranks

Once a determination has been made that the overall Friedman test is significant, post hoc tests can be undertaken that compare the differences in average ranks for all possible pairs (or certain conditions against a baseline) to determine where the differences lie. The null hypothesis of no differences in mean ranks of the pairs being examined (e.g., Time 1 vs. Time 2, Time 1 vs. Time 3, etc.) will be rejected if the absolute value of these differences is greater than a specified critical value.

Two slightly different post hoc comparisons have been suggested to determine the differences in average ranks among the time periods or conditions. The first approach has been suggested by Conover (1999). The second approach is that which is presented in SPSS for Windows (v. 22–23). Given that the two approaches generate slightly different results, they are discussed in more detail here.

Conover (1999) provides the following formula to undertake multiple comparisons of the pairwise differences in ranks between conditions (or time periods) i and j:

$$\left[R_j - R_i\right] > t_{\left(1-\frac{\alpha}{2}\right)}\sqrt{\frac{(A-C)2N}{(N-1)(k-1)}\left(1-\frac{F_{r(adj)}}{N\left(N(k-1)\right)}\right)}$$

where R_j, R_i, A, C, N, k, and $F_{r(adj)}$ were defined above (see Overview of the Procedure) and, assuming that $\alpha = .05$, the t test statistic, $t_{(1-\alpha/2)}$, is obtained from a $t_{0.975}$ distribution with $(n-1)(k-1)$ degrees of freedom. Any two conditions (or time periods) whose differences in ranks are greater than this generated value will be considered statistically significantly different from one another. Note that Conover's (1999) formula examines the sum of the ranks, R_j and R_k, not their average values.

Table A.3 in Appendix A presents the critical values for the t distribution with varying degrees of freedom. Note that this critical value of the t is the upper critical value when $\alpha = .05$. From Table A.3, we can see that the critical value for $t_{0.975}$ with $df = (10-1)(3-1) = 18$ is 2.101.

For our data, with $t = 2.101$, $A = 136.5$, $C = 120$, $N = 10$, $k = 3$, and $F_{r(adj)} = 9.879$, the critical value of the difference in ranks can be calculated as follows:

$$\left[R_j - R_i\right] > t_{(1-\alpha/2)}\sqrt{\frac{(A-C)2N}{(N-1)(k-1)}\left(1-\frac{F_{r(adj)}}{N(N(k-1))}\right)}$$

$$\left[R_j - R_i\right] > 2.101\sqrt{\frac{(136.5-120)2(10)}{(10-1)(3-1)}\left(1-\frac{9.879}{10(10(3-1))}\right)}$$

$$\left[R_j - R_i\right] > 2.101\sqrt{\frac{(330)}{(18)}\left(1-\frac{9.879}{200}\right)}$$

$$\left[R_j - R_i\right] > 2.101\sqrt{(18.33)(0.9506)}$$

$$> 2.101\sqrt{(17.42)}$$

$$> 2.101(4.17) = 8.76$$

We will reject the null hypothesis of no difference in the ranks if and only if the absolute value of the difference in ranks is greater than 8.76.

Our ranks for the three time periods (preintervention, immediately postintervention, and 3 days postintervention) were 27, 14.5, and 18.5, respectively (Table 6.5). Therefore, the absolute value of these differences would be $|27 - 14.5| = 12.5$, $|27 - 18.5| = 8.5$, and $|14.5 - 18.5| = 4.0$. It appears that the only statistically significant difference in ranks for our intervention group occurred from preintervention to immediately postintervention (12.5). Since the rank at immediately postintervention (14.5) was lower than that at preintervention (27), we can conclude that the children's fatigue scores decreased from pre- to immediate postintervention.

Comparing post hoc differences in average ranks using SPSS for Windows.

Figure 6.5 provides us with the post hoc differences in the ranks of fatigue for the children in the staff-initiated intervention. As with the Conover (1999) approach, only one comparison, preintervention fatigue and immediate postintervention fatigue, was statistically significant: The children's fatigue levels declined from preintervention to immediate postintervention ($P = .016$) (12). The value for the generated test statistic (1.25), however, was different from that which was obtained for the Conover statistic (12.5). Notice that the difference is 12.5/10 = 1.25, suggesting that the test statistic being examined in SPSS is the average ranked difference.

In SPSS, a standardized test statistic (test statistic/standard error = standardized test statistic) (13) was used to evaluate statistical significance, not the chi-square test that Conover (1999) used. Let's examine how these test statistics were obtained using SPSS. To do this, we need to go to the SPSS algorithms that were used to obtain the pairwise post hoc comparisons for the Friedman test.

The algorithm for undertaking pairwise comparisons in SPSS (v. 22–23) is slightly different from the Conover (1999) approach. That is, to test the null hypothesis that there is no difference in the average ranks between two time periods, the test statistic is

$$T_{jk} = \frac{R_j - R_k}{n}$$

where R_j = the sum of the ranks for Time *j*. R_k = the sum of the ranks for Time *k*, and n = the sample size for the pair.

The *standardized statistic*, T^*_{jk}, is obtained from the following formula:

$$T^*_{jk} = \frac{T_{jk}}{\sigma} = \frac{\frac{R_j - R_k}{n}}{\sigma}$$

where the standard error of $\sigma = \sqrt{\frac{k(k+1)}{6n}}$ and k = the number of time periods we are examining. According to the SPSS for Windows algorithm, T^*_{jk} is distributed approximately as a z statistic. Turning to Table A.1 in Appendix A for the z distribution, we can see that, with a two-tailed $\alpha = .05$, the critical value of that z statistic would be $|1.96|$. Therefore, we will reject the null hypothesis of no difference between the pair of ranks if and only if $|T^*_{jk}| > |1.96|$.

Calculating T^*_{jk} for the pairwise comparison between immediate postintervention versus preintervention fatigue, we would obtain the following results:

$$T^*_{jk} = \frac{\frac{R_j - R_k}{n}}{\sqrt{\frac{k(k+1)}{6n}}} = \frac{2.70 - 1.45}{\sqrt{\frac{3(3+1)}{(6)(10)}}} = \frac{1.25}{\sqrt{0.20}} = \frac{1.25}{0.447} = 2.795$$

Since 2.795 is greater than 1.96, we can conclude that this pairwise comparison is statistically significant. Examining the differences in the average ranks indicates that, indeed, the average ranks of the fatigue scores of the children who participated in the staff-initiated intervention declined from preintervention to immediate postintervention. No other values for T^*_{jk} were statistically significant, as we can see from Figure 6.5 (14).

Using Internet Resources to Determine the Outcome of the Friedman Test

One of the better Internet resources currently available to determine the outcome of the Friedman test without having to calculate the statistic by hand or use SPSS for Windows is the website http://www.socr.ucla.edu/htmls/SOCR_Analyses.html (Figure 6.6). We have used this site in Chapter 5 to calculate the Wilcoxon signed-ranks test. To reiterate, this is not the only site that is available to calculate the Friedman test but is illustrative of what is possible using free websites available in the public domain.

After accessing the website and the spreadsheet (Figure 6.6), we will first click on the SOCR *Analyses* button and then indicate that we would like to undertake the Friedman test (e.g., *Friedman's test*) (15). Next, using the Excel workbook (Hospitalized Children with Cancer-20 cases.xlsx) that is available on the website study.sagepub.com/pett2e, highlight and copy the Fatigue_T1, Fatigue_T2, and Figure_T3 data for the group that we are interested in evaluating (e.g., the staff-initiated intervention or Group = 1). Bring the data for these 10 cases over into the www.socr.ucla.edu spreadsheet (16), and, using the *Paste* button paste the values that will be used for the Friedman test into the SOCR spreadsheet presented on the website (Figure 6.6). Note that the data of interest in this example are only those children who were in the staff-initiated intervention. If desired, you can also change the variable names from C1, C2, and C3 to Fatigue_t1, Fatigue_t2, and Fatigue_t3.

By clicking on the *Calculate* button (17), the output for the Friedman test is generated (Figure 6.6) (18). Note that the resulting χ^2 statistic (8.15) and p value (.017) (19) are lower than the hand-calculated and SPSS-generated values (9.87 and .007, respectively) (Figure 6.5). The reason for this is that this website currently does not adjust for ties in the data. Nevertheless, it is still low enough to reject the null hypothesis. Since it does not appear that this website provides us automatically with post hoc comparisons, we would have to undertake these comparisons using the Wilcoxon signed-ranks test (see Chapter 5 for details).

Presentation of Results

Table 6.6 offers a tabular presentation of the results of the Friedman test using the post hoc comparisons generated in SPSS for Windows. These data could also be presented in the text as follows:

> The results of the Friedman test indicate that there was a statistically significant difference in the median fatigue levels of the 10 children who took part in the staff-initiated intervention over the three time periods (p = .007). Post hoc analyses indicated that there were significant decreases in the children's reported fatigue from preintervention (*Md* = 6.0) to immediately postintervention (*Md* = 4.5) (p = .016). No other significant pairwise differences between time periods were obtained.

Figure 6.6 Output for Friedman test generated from the website www.socr.ucla.edu.

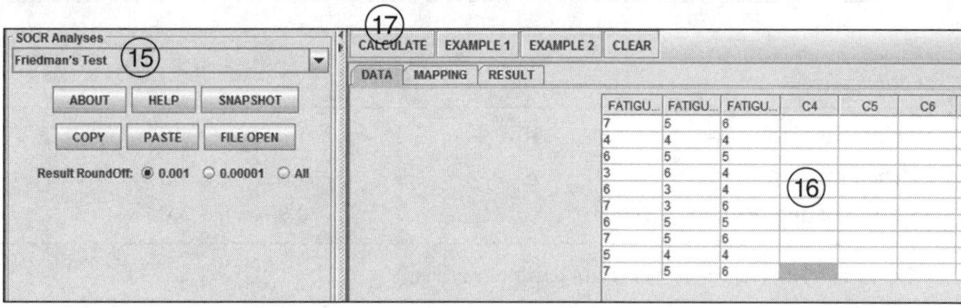

Result of Two Independent Friedmen's Test:
Groups Included = FATIGUE_T1 FATIGUE_T2 FATIGUE_T3

Total Number of Cases = 30
Number of Groups = 3
Group Size = 10

	FATIGUE_T1	FATIGUE_T2	FATIGUE_T3
1	7.0 (7.0)	5.0 (5.0)	6.0 (6.0)
2	4.0 (4.0)	4.0 (4.0)	4.0 (4.0)
3	6.0 (6.0)	5.0 (5.0)	5.0 (5.0)
4	3.0 (3.0)	6.0 (6.0)	4.0 (4.0)
5	6.0 (6.0)	3.0 (3.0)	4.0 (4.0)
6	7.0 (7.0)	3.0 (3.0)	6.0 (6.0)
7	6.0 (6.0)	5.0 (5.0)	5.0 (5.0)
8	7.0 (7.0)	5.0 (5.0)	6.0 (6.0)
9	5.0 (5.0)	4.0 (4.0)	4.0 (4.0)
10	7.0 (7.0)	5.0 (5.0)	6.0 (6.0)
Average	2.7	1.45	1.85

(18)

Grand Average = 2.000
Degrees of Freedom = 2
Sum of Squares = .815
Chi-Square Statistics = 8.150 (19)
P-Value = .017

Advantages, Limitations, and Alternatives to the Friedman Test

The Friedman test is a versatile technique that can be used both with randomized block designs and with multiple observations of a single sample. It is especially useful when the dependent data being analyzed are continuous but their distributions are skewed.

Table 6.6 Suggested Presentation of Friedman Test Results

					Friedman	
Fatigue Scores	N	M	SD	Md	χ^2	p
Preintervention[a]	10	5.8	1.4	6.0		
Immediate postintervention	10	4.5	1.0	5.0	9.879	.007
3 days postintervention	10	5.0	0.9	5.0		

[a]Significantly different from immediate postintervention, $p = .016$.

There are, however, several potential drawbacks to this test. As indicated with the Wilcoxon test (Chapter 5), although the Friedman test is used to assess medians, it really is based on an assessment of ranks. Therefore, it is possible to obtain differences in directions between medians and mean ranks. It is also conceivable that the medians do not change but that the Friedman test yields a significant result. The researcher needs to carefully examine both the medians and mean ranks to be certain that the results make intuitive sense.

Although it is often referred to as the "Friedman two-way ANOVA by ranks," the Friedman test is restricted to within-group comparisons only. It is not possible to use this test for between-group comparisons across multiple time periods or conditions. This is a major disadvantage in clinical research because it is not possible to make experimental-control group comparisons. While it is possible to analyze each of the groups independently and compare their results, there does not appear to be a nonparametric test available in the more popular statistical packages that provide a repeated-measures group-by-time interaction analysis with independent groups.

Parametric and nonparametric alternatives to the Friedman test.

The parametric counterpart to the Friedman test is the within-subjects repeated-measures ANOVA. There has been some question about the relative efficiency of the Friedman test compared to the *F* test for the repeated-measures ANOVA. Recall from Chapter 3 that the *power efficiency* of a test refers to the increase in sample size that is necessary to make one test (e.g., the Friedman test) as powerful as its rival (e.g., the *F* test) given a constant alpha level and fixed sample size for the rival test. Siegel and Castellan (1988) indicate that, compared to the *F* test, the power efficiency of the Friedman test is 64% when $k = 2$, increases to 80% for $k = 5$, and increases further to 87% for $k = 10$, where k = the number of time periods. This means that the discrepancy in sample size requirements decreases as the number of time periods or conditions increases. Hettmansperger (1984) argues that the Friedman test does not have as high a power efficiency relative to the *F* test in ANOVA as the Wilcoxon signed-ranks test does with the paired *t* test. Zimmerman and Zumbo (1993) conducted a computer simulation to compare the Friedman test, the Wilcoxon signed-ranks test, repeated-measures ANOVA, and repeated-measures ANOVA on ranks. These authors conclude that an ANOVA based on ranks may have more potential than the Friedman test in its sensitivity.

Two additional nonparametric tests to which the Friedman test is functionally related are Kendall's coefficient of concordance (W) and the Quade test (Conover, 1999; Quade, 1979; Siegel & Castellan, 1988). Kendall's coefficient of concordance will be examined in detail in Chapter 9. It is a simple modification of the Friedman test and can be used in the same situations for which the Friedman test is applicable. It has been used primarily as an assessment of "agreement in ranking" rather than as a test of differences among medians. The Quade test (Conover, 1999; Quade, 1979; Theodorsson-Norheim, 1987), like the Friedman test, is a *k*-sample extension of the Wilcoxon signed-ranks test but weights the raw data within each block. It is said to be more powerful for a small number of treatment conditions, while the Friedman test may be more powerful when the number of treatments is five or more (Theodorsson-Norheim, 1987). Unfortunately, this test is not available in SPSS for Windows. A perusal of available websites indicates that several programmers have written programs that allow for the calculation of the Quade test in Excel.

Summary

In this chapter, we have examined two nonparametric tests that are useful for assessing differences among observations across more than two time periods or conditions: Cochran's *Q* test and the Friedman test. To determine which of these two tests would be most appropriate for a specific set of data, it would be useful to review briefly the characteristics of the two tests.

Cochran's *Q* test is a useful statistical technique that can be used when the researcher is interested in evaluating change in dichotomous data across more than two time periods or conditions. It also can be used to examine agreement among raters or to evaluate relative difficulty of items on a test.

When the outcome data that are being evaluated across multiple time periods or conditions have some continuity attached to their meanings (i.e., they are at least at the ordinal level of measurement), the Friedman test is the preferred nonparametric statistic. It is a very versatile and robust statistic that can be used both with multiple measurements on a single sample (e.g., pretest, posttest, and follow-up) and on randomized block designs in which matched subjects in a block are randomly assigned to one of *k* conditions.

Both Cochran's *Q* and the Friedman test are overall tests of significance. Post hoc tests are needed, therefore, to determine where the specific differences among the groups lie. A disadvantage to both of these tests is that they can accommodate only within-subjects (or blocks) measurements. They are not useful for evaluating between-group differences, although some accommodations can be made to analyze such data. In the next two chapters, we will examine tests for independent groups. Chapter 7 will present nonparametric statistics that can be used with two independent groups: the Fisher exact test, the chi-square test, the median test, and the Wilcoxon-Mann-Whitney test. In Chapter 8, we will examine tests that accommodate more than two independent groups: the chi-square test for *k* independent samples and the Kruskal-Wallis one-way analysis of variance by ranks.

TEST YOUR KNOWLEDGE

Here is a "test" of your knowledge on the main points regarding the various nonparametric statistics that have been discussed in this chapter. You will want to reread the chapter should you find that you cannot recall their content.

1. What are the main differences between the Cochran's *Q* and Friedman tests, and when would you consider using each of these nonparametric tests?
2. What are the critical assumptions of each of these two nonparametric tests? Did the distress and fatigue data that were used in this chapter meet those assumptions?
3. What are the advantages/disadvantages to each of these two tests, and what nonparametric/parametric tests might you use instead?
4. Why was it necessary to separate out the staff-initiated intervention group from the usual-care group when running the nonparametric tests discussed in this chapter?
5. Why is it a bit of a misnomer to label this test statistic as the "Friedman two-way ANOVA by ranks"?

COMPUTER EXERCISES

The following computer exercises should enable you to build on your skills in using SPSS for Windows, Excel, and/or Internet-based programs.

1. Using either the SPSS for Windows data set (hospitalized children with cancer-20 cases.sav) or the Excel spreadsheet (hospitalized children with cancer-20 cases.xlsx) made available to you at study.sagepub.com/pett2e, undertake the Cochran's *Q* and Friedman test for the preintervention, postintervention, and 3 days postintervention distressed (*distressed_T1*, *distressed_T2*, and *distressed*_T3) and fatigue data (*fatigue_T1*, *fatigue_t2*, and *fatigue_T3*) for the usual-care group (Hint: be sure to select only those cases for whom Group = 0). Set a two-tailed alpha at .05. For the Friedman test, request post hoc comparisons.
   a. Looking at your results in Question 1, what was your decision with regard to the null hypotheses for these two tests? Were there any statistically significant differences in your post hoc comparisons?

b. Compare the results that you have obtained for the usual-care group with that of the staff-initiated intervention as detailed in this chapter. Were the results for the two groups different or similar? What conclusions would you draw from your results?

2. Twenty participants, ages 48 to 49 years, who were enrolled in a workplace health maintenance plan attended a 3-hour educational workshop addressing the need for routine colorectal cancer screening after age 50. None of the participants had previously undergone colorectal cancer screening. Prior to the workshop, the participants were asked to indicate, on a 7-point scale (1 = *very unlikely* to 7 = *very likely*) the extent to which they would be likely to obtain a routine colonoscopy once they reached age 50. This same question was asked again immediately following the workshop and 1 month later. Because the researchers did not have sufficient evidence to support their expectation that the educational workshop would increase the participants' perceived likelihood that they would undergo a colonoscopy screening once they reached age 50, they decided to proceed with an overall test of significance followed by post hoc tests.

   a. What nonparametric statistical test would you use to analyze these data?

   b. State the null and alternative hypotheses for this analysis.

   c. Is this a one- or a two-tailed test? Please justify your answer.

   d. Using the SPSS for Windows data set provided to you at study.sagepub.com/pett2e (colorectal cancer screening workshop data.sav), undertake your analysis of these data using $\alpha = .05$. Alternatively, use an available website (e.g., http://www.socr.ucla.edu/htmls/SOCR_Analyses.html) to undertake your analyses using the Excel data from the SAGE website (colorectal cancer screening workshop data.xlsx).

   e. Based on the results you have obtained, were the participants more likely to seek a colonoscopy once they reached age 50? Justify your answer.

   f. Create a table and written paragraph that would reflect your results.

Visit **study.sagepub.com/pett2e** to access SAS output, SPSS datasets, SAS datasets, and SAS examples.

CHAPTER 7

Tests for Two Independent Samples

- Fisher's exact test
- Chi-square test of independence
- Mann-Whitney *U* test

In Chapters 5 and 6, we examined nonparametric tests that could be used when the data to be analyzed are dependent; that is, the data either are generated from repeated observations of a single sample or are obtained from matched samples. In health care research, we are often interested in comparing the outcomes obtained among groups or samples that are independent of one another, such as intervention and control groups, males and females, or persons of differing marital status. Two groups are considered *independent* if membership in one group excludes the possibility of membership in the second group. For example, a remarried respondent cannot also be listed as divorced, or a member of an intervention group cannot be a member of the control group. Two ways that independent samples can be obtained are (1) they are randomly drawn from mutually exclusive populations, such as a population of males and a population of females, or (2) they are randomly assigned to only one of several possible conditions, such as an experimental or control group.

In this chapter, we will examine three nonparametric tests that are available when the independent or predictor variable is *dichotomous;* that is, this variable is made up of two mutually exclusive groups or *independent samples* and there are no repeated measures. Two of the tests, Fisher's exact test and the chi-square test of independence, are used when both the independent and dependent variables are at the nominal level of measurement. The third test, the Wilcoxon-Mann-Whitney *U* test, is used when the independent variable is nominal and the dependent variable is at least at the ordinal level of measurement.

It should be noted that all these tests are used when the data are collected during one time period. The only time these tests can be used for repeated measures is when a difference score (e.g., Time 1 – Time 2) is calculated and these obtained difference scores are compared between the groups.

FISHER'S EXACT TEST

Fisher's exact test is used to analyze data for which both the independent and dependent variables are dichotomous. It is especially useful when sample sizes are so small that the chi-square test for independent samples is inappropriate (McNemar, 1969). For example, in SPSS for Windows, Fisher's exact test is the default in SPSS for Windows for the chi-square test of independence when the expected value of a 2 × 2 contingency table for every cell is less than 5, or when the total sample size is less than 20. Regardless of statistical package, Fisher's exact test should be the preferred approach for a 2 × 2 table unless all cells have expected frequencies ≥ 5. The main purpose of such a test is to examine whether two populations differ from each other in the proportion of subjects who fall into one of two classifications. For example, we might be interested in comparing males and females with regard to their success (+) or failure (–) in treatment.

An Appropriate Research Question for Fisher's Exact Test

Fisher's exact test has been used extensively in clinical research. A quick review of the health care literature for the 5-year period 2008–2013, for example, indicated that more than 500 peer-reviewed clinical studies had included a Fisher's exact test in their statistical analyses. Both the sample sizes and the research purposes varied considerably. For example, in the genetic counseling field, Pastore, Morris, and Karns (2008) used this statistic to evaluate women's emotional reactions to a Fragile X permutation test. Bontempi, Mugno, Bulmer, Danvers, and Vancour (2009) used Fisher's exact test to examine gender differences in the relationship between human immunodeficiency virus/sexually transmitted disease testing and condom use among 1,500 undergraduate students. In women's health, Stone et al. (2011) used Fisher's exact test to compare pregnancy outcomes after bariatric surgery for 102 women who remained obese at conception to those who were not obese, and in health psychology, Klosky et al. (2013) used the same test to evaluate risky sexual behaviors among 307 adolescent survivors of childhood cancer. Other studies that have used the same statistic to examine health outcomes include Bhambhani et al. (2010); Cerulli, Talbot, Tang, and Chaudron (2011); and Collado, Faulks, Nicolas, and Hennequin (2013).

Suppose, in our hypothetical intervention study, that we were interested in comparing the children in our staff-initiated intervention and usual-care groups with regard to their immediate postintervention distress (yes or no) following the planned intervention. An example of a research question that could be answered using Fisher's exact test would be as follows:

> Is the proportion of children expressing distress immediately following the intervention lower in the staff-initiated intervention group than the usual-care group?

Null and Alternative Hypotheses

Table 7.1 illustrates the null and alternative hypotheses that would be suitable for use with a Fisher's exact test given the research question outlined above. Note that the alternative hypothesis is directional. We are predicting that there will be differences in proportions of distress between the staff-initiated intervention and usual-care groups in favor of the group that received the intervention. Because the alternative hypothesis is directional, we will be undertaking a one-tailed Fisher's exact test.

Table 7.1 Example of Null and Alternative Hypotheses Suitable for Fisher's Exact Test and the Chi-Square Test for Two Independent Samples

Null Hypothesis
H_0: The proportion of children in the staff-initiated intervention group who express distress immediately following the intervention will be no different from that of the usual-care group; that is, the two variables, group membership and postintervention distress, are independent.
Alternative Hypothesis
H_a: A smaller proportion of children who take part in the staff-initiated intervention will express distress immediately following the intervention compared to the children in the usual-care group; that is, the two variables, group membership and postintervention distress, are associated.

If, on the other hand, we had been examining preintervention distress, we would most likely posit a nondirectional alternative hypothesis since we would like to know whether our random assignment to groups was effective in creating similar groups, at least with regard to the children's distress prior to the intervention. In that case, we would undertake a two-tailed Fisher's exact test.

Overview of the Procedure

To undertake Fisher's exact test, the dichotomous data to be analyzed are first cast into a 2 × 2 contingency table similar to Table 7.2, in which entries represent frequencies, not scores.

Table 7.2 Format for a 2 × 2 Contingency Table for Fisher's Exact Test

	Dependent Variable		
Independent Variable	*0*	*1*	*Total*
0	a	b	$a + b$
1	c	d	$c + d$
Total	$a + c$	$b + d$	N

Next, the probability is calculated of obtaining an arrangement of numbers in the four cells exactly like, or more disproportionate than, what was obtained in the original 2 × 2 table given similar row and column totals. For small sample sizes (e.g., $N \leq 15$), the hypergeometric distribution is employed, using the following formula (Conover, 1999; Siegel & Castellan, 1988):

$$p = \frac{(a+b)!(c+d)!(a+c)!(b+d)!}{n!a!b!c!d!}$$

where

p = the probability of obtaining the *exact* arrangement of variables presented in Table 7.2, and

! = factorial sign, e.g., $a! = a(a-1)(a-2)\ldots 1$.

Fisher's exact test can become quite tedious to calculate by hand because p values need to be calculated not only for the exact frequencies but also for frequencies *more extreme* than what was obtained given similar row and column totals. This total generated p value is then compared to the preset alpha level (e.g., $\alpha = .05$). If this generated p value is less than the alpha, the null hypothesis that the generated arrangement of cell frequencies occurred purely by chance is rejected.

Calculating Fisher's exact test for the distress data.

Table 7.3 presents that data that we have obtained for our distress data. The data set that we are using is hospitalized children with cancer-20 cases.sav (study.sagepub.com/pett2e). Two of the 10 children in the usual-care group and 7 of the children in the staff-initiated intervention reported "no distress" immediately postintervention. Are these differences in proportions, 2/10 and 7/10, large enough such that we can reject the null hypothesis of equal proportions? To answer this question, we need to undertake a Fisher's exact test.

Table 7.3 The 2 × 2 Contingency Table Used to Examine the Effects of the Intervention on Postintervention Distress Using Fisher's Exact Test

	Postintervention Distress[a]		
Group[b]	*No*	*Yes*	*Total*
Usual care	2	8	10
Staff-initiated intervention	7	3	10
Total	9	11	20

[a]0 = not distressed, 1 = distressed.

[b]0 = usual care, 1 = staff-initiated intervention.

Luckily, our sample size is small enough such that we can generate the probability of obtaining cell discrepancies as large as or larger than what we have obtained in Table 7.3. There are also available a number of open access websites (e.g., www.danielsoper.com and www.vassarstats.net) that provide calculators with which we can obtain exact probability values for Fisher's exact test, especially when our sample size is small (e.g., less than 15). We will use one of those websites when we examine Internet resources for calculating a Fisher's exact test.

To calculate Fisher's exact test for the distress data by hand, we would need to first cast our values into 2 × 2 tables that reflect cell discrepancies equal to or greater than that which is in Table 7.3. That means that we want to find those exact probabilities when d = 3, 2, or 1 since we have a directional alternative hypothesis (Table 7.1). Table 7.4 presents a list of the possible discrepancies. Note that we do not have a $d = 0$ because then we would have too many children (n = 11) assigned to the usual care group, not the designated n = 10.

Next we need to calculate the exact probability of obtaining such tables and sum those probabilities. Table 7.4 indicates that, when $d = 3$, $p = .0325$. When $d = 2$, p = change to: .00268, and when $d = 1$, $p = .000059$. The sum of these three probabilities is .034889. Given a one-tailed $\alpha = .05$, we would reject the null hypothesis of equal proportions since $p < \alpha$, or $.034889 < .05$. According to Fisher's exact test, a smaller proportion of children in the staff-initiated intervention reported distress compared to the children in the usual-care group.

An alternative to Fisher's exact test for larger sample sizes is the chi-square test for two independent samples, a test that will be reviewed later in this chapter. This statistic is the default in SPSS for Windows when the sample size is sufficiently large (i.e., when all expected cell values in a 2 × 2 table are greater than 5).

Fisher's exact test is usually considered to be a one-tailed test because it examines results that are as extreme as or more extreme than the obtained values in a specific direction (Hays, 1994; Siegel & Castellan, 1988). Hays (1994) suggests that when all row and column totals are equal, the two-tailed significance level can be obtained by doubling the p value. When the marginal totals are not equal (e.g., $[a + b] \neq [c + d]$), a different procedure must be used to obtain a two-tailed significance level. SPSS for Windows does not restrict Fisher's exact test to a one-tailed test but presents both one- and two-tailed probability values, adjusting for unequal marginal totals when necessary.

Critical Assumptions of Fisher's Exact Test

1. *Both independent and dependent variables are dichotomous, with two mutually exclusive categories.* Both variables being analyzed need to be dichotomous, with two mutually exclusive categories. In our hypothetical intervention study, both the grouping and distress variables are dichotomous, with two independent categories. If these variables were not dichotomous, their levels could be collapsed to meet this assumption.

2. *The data to be analyzed have been obtained from a random sample and represent frequencies, not scores.* As with all nonparametric statistical tests, the assumption is that the data have been obtained from a randomly selected sample. For this test, it is assumed

Table 7.4 Presentation of 2 × 2 Tables Reflecting Cell Discrepancies for Cell $d \le 3$ (From Table 7.3)

Group	Distressed?		
	No (0)	*Yes (1)*	*Total*
Usual care (0)	2 a	b 8	10
Staff-initiated intervention (1)	7 c	d 3	10
Total	9	11	20

$$p_{d=3} = \frac{(a+b)!(c+d)!(a+c)!(b+d)!}{n!a!b!c!d!}$$

$$p_{d=3} = \frac{(10)!(10)!(9)!(11)!}{20!2!8!7!3!} = 0.03215$$

Group	Distressed?		
	No (0)	*Yes (1)*	*Total*
Usual care (0)	1 a	b 9	10
Staff-initiated intervention (1)	8 c	d 2	10
Total	9	11	20

$$p_{d=2} = \frac{(a+b)!(c+d)!(a+c)!(b+d)!}{n!a!b!c!d!}$$

$$p_{d=2} = \frac{(10)!(10)!(9)!(11)!}{20!1!9!8!2!} = 0.00268$$

Group	Distressed?		
	No (0)	*Yes (1)*	*Total*
Usual care (0)	0 a	b 10	10
Staff-initiated intervention (1)	9 c	d 1	10
Total	9	11	20

$$p_{d=1} = \frac{(a+b)!(c+d)!(a+c)!(b+d)!}{n!a!b!c!d!}$$

$$p_{d=1} = \frac{(10)!(10)!(9)!(11)!}{20!0!10!9!1!} = 0.000059$$

$$p_{d\le3} = p_{d=3} + p_{d=2} + p_{d=1}$$

$$p_{d\le3} = 0.03215 + 0.00268 + 0.000059$$

$$p_{d\le3} = 0.034889$$

that the values in each cell of the 2 × 2 table represent numbers of subjects, not scores. Our hypothetical data are presented as counts, not scores. While the 20 children were randomly assigned to the two treatment conditions, they were selected from a sample of convenience of children from a given hospital who were hospitalized for cancer. While it is rare that random sampling and random assignment co-occur, it is important that we be aware that using a sample of convenience potentially affects the generalizability of our results (i.e., the population we can generalize to).

3. *Because this is an exact test of probability, it is necessary to know the number of cases in the marginal totals before the data are analyzed.* Some statisticians have argued that Fisher's exact test is appropriate only when the marginal totals for both the independent and dependent variables are known (Daniel, 2000). This requirement suggests that the study needs to be experimental in design because the researcher has control over the types of subjects entered into the study. For example, a researcher might want to be certain that a similar proportion of randomly assigned intervention or control group subjects possess a particular characteristic of interest (e.g., high blood pressure). In this case, both sets of marginal totals for group membership (intervention, control) and blood pressure (high, normal) could be fixed prior to the study.

Even with an experimental design, however, this assumption is not easily met. In our hypothetical study, we would need to know prior to collecting our data not only the number of children assigned to the staff-initiated intervention and usual-care groups but also the total number of children in each group who answered "yes" or "no" to the question concerning distress immediately postintervention. This achievement is hardly realistic, given that the distress variable is not being manipulated, we hope, by the researcher. This assumption, therefore, is very restrictive, particularly in descriptive studies.

Computer Commands

Figure 7.1 presents the SPSS for Windows (v. 22–23) commands that were used to generate Fisher's exact test using the data set, hospitalized children with cancer-20 cases (study.sagepub.com/pett2e). This dialog box was obtained by selecting the following items from the menu: *Analyze . . . Descriptive Statistics . . . Crosstabs*. The two dichotomous variables, type of intervention (*Group*) and immediate postintervention distress (*Distress*_T2) are placed in the rows and columns (1). To obtain Fisher's exact test, the *Chi-Square* was selected from the *Statistics* menu in this dialog box (2). Observed and expected values (3) as well as row and column percentages (4) also were requested under the *Cells* subcommand in the *Crosstabs* dialog box.

Computer-Generated Output

Figure 7.2 presents the syntax commands and computer-generated output for Fisher's exact test that was generated from SPSS for Windows. The syntax commands (5) indicate that the command *Crosstabs* has been used to generate Fisher's exact test through its *Statistics = Chisq* subcommand (6). The generated table is set up such that, as requested in the syntax commands, the following values will be presented in the table: the count, expected value, row percentage, and column percentage (7).

The *Case Processing Summary* (8) indicates that we have 20 cases that we are examining with no missing data. Next we are presented with the 2 × 2 table that compares the two groups, staff-initiated intervention with the usual-care group, regarding their distress immediately postintervention (9). The first row of information in the table,

Figure 7.1 SPSS for Windows (v. 22–23) commands for generating Fisher's exact test.

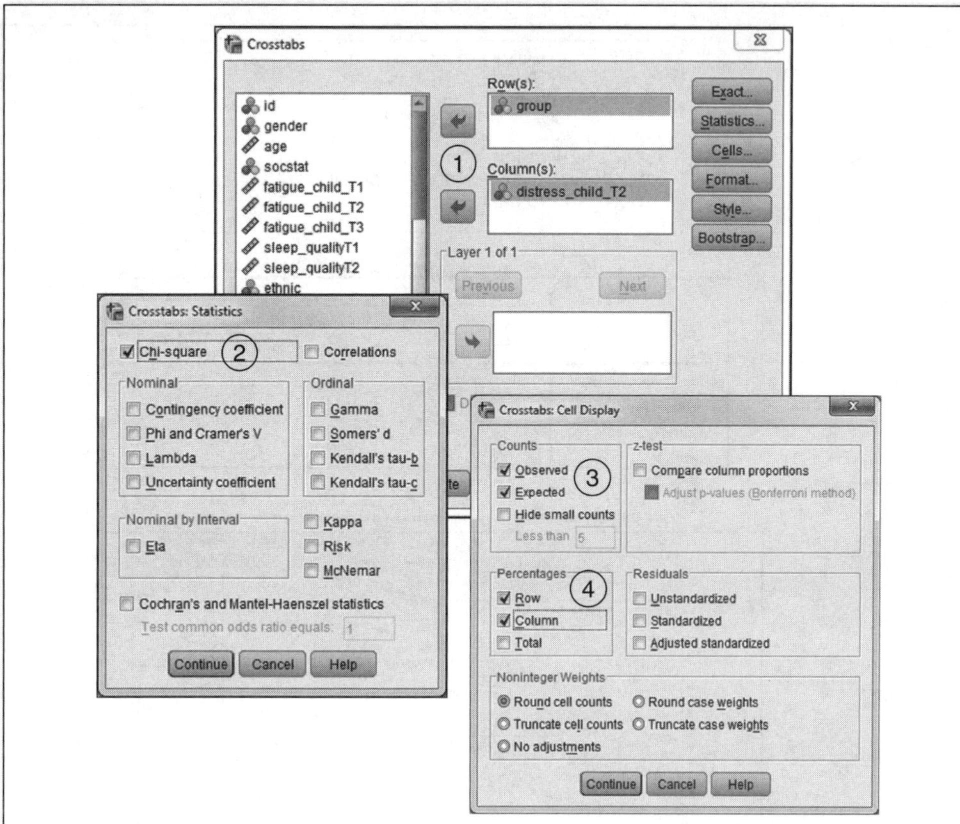

Count (10), represents the number of children in each cell. These are the same values that are presented in Table 7.3. The second row of values, *Expected Count* (11), indicates the number of children who would be expected in the particular cell if the null hypothesis were true: that the two variables, group membership and distress immediately postintervention, were completely independent. The third and fourth rows, *% within staff-initiated intervention vs. usual care* and *% within distress immediately postintervention* (12), represent the row and column percentages expressed as a percentage of all cases in that particular row or column.

For example, from Figure 7.2, of the 11 children who expressed distress immediately postintervention, 3 children (27.3%) (13) were from the staff-initiated intervention group compared to 8 children (72.7%) from the usual-care group (14). In contrast, the expected values for each of these two cells were 5.5, suggesting that the two variables, group membership and distress immediately postintervention, are not independent. Looking at

Figure 7.2 SPSS for Windows (v. 22–23) generated output for Fisher's exact test.

```
*** Data set: hospitalized children with cancer-20 cases***

CROSSTABS (5)
 /TABLES=group BY distress_child_T2
 /FORMAT=AVALUE TABLES
 /STATISTICS=CHISQ (6)
 /CELLS=COUNT EXPECTED ROW COLUMN (7)
 /COUNT ROUND CELL.
```

Case Processing Summary (8)

	Cases					
	Valid		Missing		Total	
	N	Percent	N	Percent	N	Percent
staff-initiated intervention vs. usual care * distress immediately post intervention	20	100.0%	0	0.0%	20	100.0%

staff-initiated intervention vs. usual care * distress immediately post intervention Crosstabulation (9)

			distress immediately post intervention		
			no, not distressed	yes, distressed	Total
staff-initiated intervention vs. usual care	usual care group (11) (12)	Count (10)	2	8	10
		Expected Count	4.5	(14) 5.5	10.0
		% within staff-initiated intervention vs. usual care	20.0%	(15) 80.0%	100.0%
		% within distress immediately post intervention	22.2%	72.7%	50.0%
	staff-initiated intervention	Count	7	3	10
		Expected Count	4.5	(13) 5.5	10.0
		% within staff-initiated intervention vs. usual care	70.0%	(15) 30.0%	100.0%
		% within distress immediately post intervention	77.8%	27.3%	50.0%
Total		Count	9	11	20
		Expected Count	9.0	11.0	20.0
		% within staff-initiated intervention vs. usual care	45.0%	55.0%	100.0%
		% within distress immediately post intervention	100.0%	100.0%	100.0%

Chi-Square Tests

	Value	df	Asymp. Sig. (2-sided)	Exact Sig. (2-sided)	Exact Sig. (1-sided)
Pearson Chi-Square	5.051[a]	1	.025		
Continuity Correction[b]	3.232	1	.072		
Likelihood Ratio	5.300	1	.021		
Fisher's Exact Test				(17) .070	(16) .035
Linear-by-Linear Association	4.798	1	.028		
N of Valid Cases	20				

a. 2 cells (50.0%) have expected count less than 5. The minimum expected count is 4.50. (18)

b. Computed only for a 2x2 table

the third row of values, it is apparent that 30% (3 of 10) of the children in the staff-initiated intervention group indicated they were distressed immediately postintervention compared to 80% (8 of 10) of the children in the usual-care group (15).

To determine whether the differences in proportions between the groups are significant, we need to look at the information presented for Fisher's exact test (16). Because the one-tailed generated p value for this statistic, .035, is less than our stated alpha (.05), the null hypothesis of independence of the two variables, group membership and distress immediately postintervention, is rejected. This computer-generated one-tailed p value, .035, is the same as the one-tailed p value that had been hand-calculated in Table 7.4. The conclusion to be drawn is that the children in the staff-initiated intervention group were less likely to express distress immediately postintervention than the children in the usual-care group.

Notice that the two-tailed significance for Fisher's exact test is also presented ($p = .07$) (17). Because there were equal numbers of children in the intervention and usual-care groups ($n = 10$), this value is, as Hays (1994) suggests, double the one-tailed p value. Had the numbers of children in each group been unequal (e.g., 10 children in the staff-initiated intervention group and only 9 children in the usual-care group), the two-tailed significance value would not have been twice the one-tailed value. Also, had our alternative hypothesis been nondirectional, we would not have been able to reject the null hypothesis of equal proportions since $.07 > .05$. In addition, we have been given the message that "2 cells (50%) have expected count less than 5" (18). As we will see later in this chapter, this would be a problem if we were to run a chi-square test on these data.

SPSS for Windows offers additional tests for contingency tables when the chi-square tests are requested. These tests include the Pearson chi-square, the chi-square test with a Yates correction, the likelihood ratio, and the Mantel-Haenszel test for linear association. Interpretation of these tests will be presented later in this chapter and in Chapter 8.

Internet Resources for Generating Fisher's Exact Test

A number of currently available open access Internet resources provide calculators with which one can obtain exact probability values for Fisher's exact test (e.g., www.danielsoper.com and www.vassarstats.net). For this current example, we will use vassarstats.net to generate the exact probability values for our data.

To generate a Fisher's exact test for our data via an open access website, we would go to the website (e.g., www.vassarstats.net). In this particular website, we would click on *Frequencies* . . . and indicate that we want to generate a 2 × 2 table for cross-categorized frequency tables (Version 1). This will open the 2 × 2 Data Entry table presented in Figure 7.3 (19).

After entering our values into the data entry table (Note: be careful that the data entered reflect the cells presented in Table 7.4), all we need to do is click on *Calculate*. . . . The exact one- and two-tailed probability values are presented (20). These are exact values, .035 and .07, as that which we obtained from our hand calculation (Table 7.4) and SPSS for Windows (Figure 7.2). This was so much easier than calculating the probability values by hand!

Figure 7.3 Internet-generated results for Fisher's exact test.

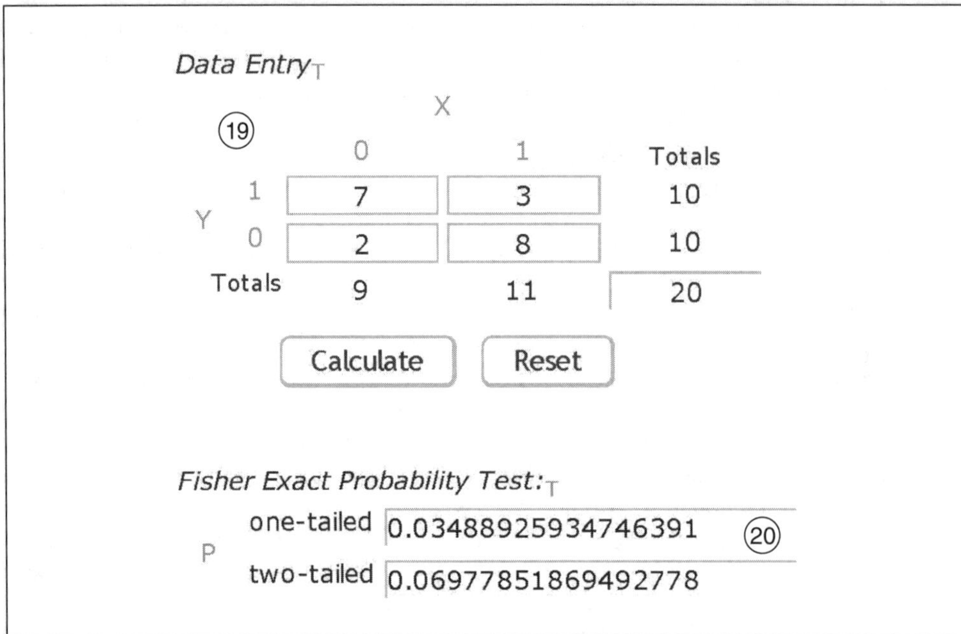

Presentation of Results

Table 7.5 is a suggested presentation of the results obtained from Fisher's exact test. The findings presented in this table could be interpreted and addressed in the text using the following statement:

> The results of Fisher's exact test indicate that significantly fewer of the 10 children in the staff-initiated intervention ($n = 3$) expressed distress immediately postintervention than did the 10 children in the usual-care group ($n = 8$) ($p = .035$).

Advantages, Limitations, and Alternatives to Fisher's Exact Test

Fisher's exact test is an extremely useful and powerful statistic if the independent and dependent variables are both dichotomous. It is especially useful if either the sample size or the expected value of a particular cell is small (i.e., $N \leq 20$ or expected values < 5). If the sample size is larger than 20, calculation of the test by hand quickly becomes unwieldy and tedious. In that situation, an open access Internet resource could be used. Alternatively, Siegel and Castellan (1988) suggest that when the sample size is greater

Table 7.5 Suggested Presentation of Fisher's Exact Test Results

	Distress Immediately Postintervention						
	Yes		*No*		*Total*		
Group Membership	N	%	N	%	N	%	p[a]
Staff-initiated intervention	3	27.3	7	77.8	10	50.0	
Usual care	8	72.7	2	22.2	10	50.0	.035
Total	11	55.0	9	45.0	20	100.0	

[a]The *p* value is for a one-tailed Fisher's exact test.

than 15, the approximation of the chi-square test should be used. Fisher's exact test cannot be used when the variables being considered are continuous or are categorical with more than two levels.

Several critics of Fisher's exact test have indicated that the test is too conservative (Hirji, Tan, & Elashoff, 1991; Overall & Hornick, 1982), that it is less likely to correctly reject the null hypothesis. In response to this criticism, both Hirji et al. (1991) and Overall and Hornick (1982) present modified versions of Fisher's exact test that are purported to be more likely to correctly reject the null hypothesis than the unmodified version.

Parametric and nonparametric alternatives to Fisher's exact test.

Because Fisher's exact test deals with 2 × 2 tables in which the variables being examined are at the nominal level of measurement, there is no parametric equivalent to this test. The chi-square test for two independent samples is a nonparametric alternative to Fisher's exact test when the sample size is sufficiently large or when the categorical variables have more than two levels. Camilli (1990), however, suggests that Barnard's (1945) 2 × 2 test is theoretically superior to the chi-square test and "all of its corrected cousins." (p. 135). He further concludes that Fisher's exact test is the most rational choice.

Berry and Mielke (1987) present an approach to using Fisher's exact test with 3 × 2 cross-classification tables and, as indicated, there have been suggested modified versions of Fisher's exact test (Hirji et al., 1991; Overall & Hornick, 1982) that appear to be less conservative than the unmodified version. Lowry (www.vassarstats.net) presents a Freeman-Halton (Freeman & Halton, 1951) extension of the Fisher's exact probability test for 2 × 3, 3 × 2, and 3 × 3 tables.

Examples From Published Research

Bhambhani, Y., Mactavish, J., Warren, S., Thompson, W. R., Webborn, A., Bressan, E., . . . Vanlandewijck, Y. (2010). Boosting in athletes with high-level spinal cord injury: Knowledge, incidence and attitudes of athletes in paralympic sport. *Disability & Rehabilitation, 32*(26), 2172–2190. doi: 10.3109/09638288.2010.505678

Bontempi, J. B., Mugno, R., Bulmer, S. M., Danvers, K., & Vancour, M. L. (2009). Exploring gender differences in the relationship between HIV/STD testing and condom use among undergraduate college students. *American Journal of Health Education, 40*(2), 97–105.

Cerulli, C., Talbot, N. L., Tang, W., & Chaudron, L. H. (2011). Co-occurring intimate partner violence and mental health diagnoses in perinatal women. *Journal of Women's Health, 20*(12), 1797–1803. doi: 10.1089/jwh.2010.2201

Collado, V., Faulks, D., Nicolas, E., & Hennequin, M. (2013). Conscious sedation procedures using intravenous midazolam for dental care in patients with different cognitive profiles: A prospective study of effectiveness and safety. *PLoS ONE, 8*(8), e71240.

Goetz, A. M., Squier, C., Wagener, M. M., & Muder, R. R. (1994). Nosocomial infections in the human immunodeficiency virus-infected patient: A two year survey. *American Journal of Infection Control, 22,* 334–339.

Graff-Radford, N. R., Godersky, J. C., & Jones, M. P. (1989). Variables predicting surgical outcome in symptomatic hydrocephalus in the elderly. *Neurology, 39,* 1601–1604.

THE CHI-SQUARE TEST FOR TWO INDEPENDENT SAMPLES

The chi-square test for two independent samples (χ^2) is one of the most commonly used nonparametric statistics in health care research. Like Fisher's exact test, this test can be used to assess 2 × 2 contingency tables when both the independent and dependent variables are at the nominal level of measurement. Whereas Fisher's exact test is typically used for small samples ($n \leq 20$), the chi-square test is used when the total sample size is greater than 20 and the expected values for each cell are greater than 5. The chi-square test for two independent samples can also be used when the dependent variable has more than two categories. In Chapter 8, we will examine a chi-square test of association in which both independent and dependent variables are categorical with more than two levels.

An Appropriate Research Question for the Chi-Square Two-Sample Test

The chi-square test for two independent samples (sometimes abbreviated as the *chi-square test* or χ^2 test) has been used in numerous clinical research projects. For example, Anders and Evans (2010) used the chi-square test for two independent samples in their comparison of Pub Med versus Google Scholar literature searches in respiratory care. Robl, Jewell, and Kanotra (2012) used the same statistic to assess the effect of parental involvement on problematic social behaviors among school-aged children in Kentucky. Siegler et al. (2011) also used this test to evaluate the influence of heart size on the accuracy of the electrocardiogram during an exercise stress test.

In our hypothetical study with only 20 children, the chi-square two-sample test would not be appropriate since two of the four cells of the 2 × 2 table have cells with expected frequencies of less than 5 (4.5) (Figure 7.2, (18)). This is a violation of one of the assumptions of this test. To use the chi-square test, it would be necessary to increase the sample size. For the purposes of examining how the chi-square test might be used with these data, therefore, the number of children in our hypothetical intervention study has been magically increased from 20 to 30. This data file, hospitalized children with cancer-30 cases.sav, can be found on the SAGE website (study.sagepub.com/pett2e). A research question that could be answered using this chi-square test for two independent samples is similar to that for Fisher's exact test:

> What is the association between group membership (i.e., staff-initiated intervention vs. usual care) and the children's expressed distress (yes, no) immediately following the intervention?

Null and Alternative Hypotheses

The wording of the null hypothesis for the chi-square test for two independent samples is similar to that of Fisher's exact test (Table 7.1). It would state that the two variables, group membership and distress immediately following the intervention, are independent. For a chi-square test, however, the alternative hypothesis is nondirectional. Therefore, the alternative hypothesis would state that the two variables are dependent but does not predict a direction.

Overview of the Procedure

To undertake a chi-square test for two independent samples, the frequency data are first cast into a $2 \times k$ table (where k = the number of levels of the dependent variable). In our example, we would generate a 2×2 table because the variables, group membership and children's distress immediately postintervention, are dichotomous. Next, the frequency of cases that fall within a particular cell is compared to the frequency that would be expected by chance if the two variables, group membership and distress, were independent. The expected number of cases in a particular cell (Exp_{ij}) is the product of the marginal totals for a particular row (R_i) and column (C_j) divided by the total sample size (N):

$$Exp_{ij} = (R_i)(C_j) / N$$

From these data, a chi-square statistic (χ^2) is generated using the following formula:

$$\chi^2 = \sum_{i=1}^{r} \sum_{j=1}^{c} \frac{(Obs_{ij} - Exp_{ij})^2}{Exp_{ij}}$$

where

Obs_{ij} = the observed number of cases for a particular cell located in the ith row and jth column,

Exp_{ij} = the expected number of cases for the same cell if the variables were independent, and

$\sum\sum$ = an indication that the fraction is summed across all rows (r) and columns (c).

If the data meet the assumptions of the chi-square test for two independent samples, this statistic is asymptotically distributed as a χ^2 with $(r - 1)(c - 1)$ degrees of freedom. If the resulting χ^2 statistic is sufficiently large, the null hypothesis of independence of variables is rejected.

This χ^2 statistic, however, is distributed approximately as a χ^2 *only* if the expected frequencies are sufficiently large. A general rule of thumb is that if the degrees of freedom are equal to 1 (e.g., it is a 2 × 2 contingency table), all expected frequencies for the table should be ≥ 5. For larger tables ($df > 1$), no more than 20% of the cells should have expected frequencies less than 5.

Calculating the chi-square test for the distress data.

To undertake a chi-square test for two independent samples, the dichotomous data to be analyzed are first cast into a 2 × 2 contingency table similar to Table 7.6, in which entries represent frequencies, not scores. Remember that we are now using the data set, hospitalized children with cancer-30 cases.sav (study.sagepub.com/pett2e).

Table 7.6 The 2 × 2 Contingency Table Used to Examine the Effects of the Intervention on Postintervention Distress Using the Chi-Square Test for Two Independent Samples

	Postintervention Distress[a]				
	No		*Yes*		
Group[b]	*Observed*	*Expected*	*Observed*	*Expected*	*Total*
Usual care	4	7	11	8	*15*
Staff-initiated intervention	10	7	5	8	*15*
Total	14		16		*30*

[a]0 = not distressed, 1 = distressed.

[b]0 = usual care, 1 = staff-initiated intervention.

(1) Exp = (R*C) /N =(15*16)/30 = 8

Table 7.6 indicates that 10 children in the staff-initiated intervention group expressed no distress immediately postintervention compared to only 4 children in the usual-care group. If the two variables were independent, the expected number of children in each nondistressed group would be 7 ($Exp_{ij} = [R_i][C_j]/N = [15][14]/30 = 7$). The expected number of children in the distressed groups would be 8 ($Exp_{ij} = [15][16]/30 = 8$) (1). The reason that the expected row frequencies are identical in each column is because there are equal numbers of children in each group ($n = 15$). As a result, the numerator and denominator are the same for the expected row frequencies in each column, (14*15)/30 and (16*15)/30, respectively.

To determine whether the differences between the observed and expected values are sufficiently large to reject the null hypothesis of independence of variables, we need to calculate the chi-square statistic and evaluate its significance level. If the significance level (p value) is less than our prestated alpha level, we will reject the null hypothesis of independence of the two variables, group membership and distress immediately postintervention. Alternatively, we will reject the null hypothesis if and only if our calculated χ^2 value is greater than the critical value of the χ^2 at the given α (e.g., $\alpha = .05$). To summarize the rule of thumb:

$$\textit{Reject } H_o \textit{ if and only if actual } \chi^2 > \textit{critical } \chi^2 \textit{ or } p < \alpha$$

Using the formula outlined above, we can calculate the following chi-square statistic:

$$\chi^2 = \sum_{i=1}^{r} \sum_{j=1}^{c} \frac{(Obs_{ij} - Exp_{ij})^2}{Exp_{ij}} = \frac{(4-7)^2}{7} + \frac{(11-8)^2}{8} + \frac{(10-7)^2}{7} + \frac{(5-8)^2}{8} = 4.82$$

Is this calculated χ^2 value, 4.82, large enough to reject the null hypothesis of no association between group membership and immediate postintervention distress? To determine this, we would need to find the critical value of this chi-square statistic, given our prestated alpha level (e.g., $\alpha = .05$).

Table A.2 in Appendix A provides us with the critical points of the chi-square distribution at various degrees of freedom (df). Given our 2 × 2 table, our $df = (r - 1)(c - 1) = (2 - 1)(2 - 1) = 1$. Since Table A.2 presents the cumulative probability of the chi-square distribution (the area under the curve that lies to the left of the area for our stated alpha; e.g., .05), we would look for that cumulative probability value that is equal to $(1 - \alpha)$ or $(1 - .05 = .95)$. This value, .95, is in the fourth-to-last column in Table A.2. Since our $df = 1$, the critical value for our $\chi^2 = 3.84$. Please note that this critical value, 3.84, will always be the same for any table that has $df = 1$ and $\alpha = .05$.

Since our actual χ^2 (4.82) > critical χ^2 (3.84), we can reject the null hypothesis and conclude that there is an association between the two variables, group membership and postintervention distress. The two variables are dependent in that it appears that fewer children in the staff-initiated intervention ($n = 5$) expressed distress immediately postintervention than did the children in the usual-care group ($n = 11$). The strength of this relationship will be discussed when we examine the computer printout.

Critical Assumptions of the Chi-Square Test for Two Independent Samples

1. *The data being analyzed must be frequency data, not scores.* Like Fisher's exact test, the data being examined must consist of counts, not scores. Our data, group membership and children's distress, meet this assumption. They are each coded 0s and 1s and represent frequencies, not scores.

2. *The variables being examined are categorical, with mutually exclusive levels.* For the chi-square test for two independent samples, the independent variable must be

dichotomous. The dependent variable, however, may have more than two levels. Each observation must be assigned to one and only one cell. This means that the cells are mutually exclusive, and no subject has contributed to more than one cell. Because both the group membership (staff-initiated intervention, usual care) and distress immediately postintervention (yes, no) variables are dichotomous, with mutually exclusive levels, this assumption is met.

3. *The observations must be independent of one another.* This assumption implies that no pair of observations can have any influence on another pair of observations. This is not a test for repeated observations of the same subject. Because, in our hypothetical study, each subject has only one pair of values, group membership and expressed distress, this assumption has been met.

The assumption of independence for the chi-square test is very important because if the observations are associated in any way, they can have dramatic effects on the researcher's decision regarding the null hypothesis. Violation of the assumption of independence could occur when a subject is asked to provide multiple responses to a particular question. For example, in our hypothetical study, a mother might be requested to list all the prescription drugs her child is taking, or a record might be kept of the types of side effects the child is experiencing. In both instances, although the types of drugs taken and side effects could be listed in a contingency table, the cells are no longer independent because the respondent's information could appear multiple times in the table. A chi-square test of independence therefore would be inappropriate. Several authors (Agresti & Liu, 2001; Bilder & Loughin, 2004) have suggested approaches to assessing marginal independence between two categorical variables with multiple responses.

4. *If the two variables being examined are dichotomous, resulting in a 2×2 contingency table with* df = *1, all expected frequencies for the table should be at least 5. For larger tables where* df > *1, no more than 20% of the cells should have expected frequencies of less than 5.* This rule is important because, as indicated earlier, the chi-square statistic is distributed approximately as a χ^2 *only* if the expected frequencies are sufficiently large. We will examine the extent to which the data from our hypothetical study meet this rule when we examine the computer printout.

Computer Commands

As with Fisher's exact test, the *Analyze . . . Descriptive Statistics . . . Crosstabs* commands in the SPSS for Windows (v. 22–23) menu will generate the chi-square test for two independent samples (Figure 7.1). Once the *Crosstabs* dialog box has been selected, open the *Statistics* menu and click on the boxes for the chi-square test and measures of association for 2×2 tables, such as the phi coefficients. Other useful information can be obtained by opening the *Cells* menu and requesting observed and expected frequencies, row and column percentages, and unstandardized and standardized residuals.

Computer-Generated Output

Figure 7.4 presents the syntax commands and computer-generated output for the chi-square test for two independent samples obtained from the SPSS for Windows (v. 22–23) *Crosstabs* commands. The syntax commands outline all that we have requested. In the printout, we are presented with the actual frequency (*Count*), expected frequency (*Expected*), percentages expressed in terms of row totals (*Row*), column totals (*Column*), unstandardized residuals (*Resid*), and standardized residuals (*Sresid*) (2). As we will see later in this discussion, the standardized residuals are especially helpful in determining which cells are influencing the outcomes observed.

Figure 7.4 Syntax and SPSS for Windows-generated output for the chi-square two-sample test.

```
***Data set: hospitalized children with cancer-30 cases.sav***

    CROSSTABS
      /TABLES=group BY distress_t2
      /FORMAT=AVALUE TABLES
      /STATISTICS=CHISQ PHI
      /CELLS=COUNT EXPECTED ROW COLUMN RESID SRESID (2)
      /COUNT ROUND CELL.
```

group intervention vs. usual care grps * distress_t2 distress immediately post-intervention Crosstabulation

			distress_t2 distress immediately post-intervention		
			.00 not distressed	1.00 distressed	Total
group intervention vs. usual care grps	.00 usual care	Count	(3) 4	11	15
		Expected Count	7.0	(5) 8.0	15.0
		% within group intervention vs. usual care grps	(4) 26.7%	73.3%	100.0%
		% within distress_t2 distress immediately post-intervention	28.6%	68.8%	50.0%
		Residual	(6) -3.0	3.0	
		Std. Residual	-1.1	1.1	
	1.00 staff-initiated intervention	Count	(3) 10	5	15
		Expected Count	7.0	(5) 8.0	15.0
		% within group intervention vs. usual care grps	(4) 66.7%	(8) 33.3%	100.0%
		% within distress_t2 distress immediately post-intervention	71.4%	31.2%	50.0%
		Residual	(10) 3.0	-3.0	
		Std. Residual	1.1	-1.1	
Total		Count	14	16	30
		Expected Count	14.0	16.0	30.0
		% within group intervention vs. usual care grps	46.7%	53.3%	100.0%
		% within distress_t2 distress immediately post-intervention	100.0%	100.0%	100.0%

Residual = Observed − Expected = 4 − 7 = −3.0

$$\text{Std Residual} = \frac{\text{Observed} - \text{Expected}}{\sqrt{\text{Expected}}}$$

Chi-Square Tests

	Value	df	Asymp. Sig. (2-sided) (9)	Exact Sig. (2-sided) (7)	Exact Sig. (1-sided)
Pearson Chi-Square	4.821[a]	1	.028		
Continuity Correction[b]	3.348	1	.067		
Likelihood Ratio	4.963	1	.026		
Fisher's Exact Test				.066	.033
Linear-by-Linear Association	4.661	1	.031		
N of Valid Cases	30				

a. 0 cells (0.0%) have expected count less than 5. The minimum expected count is 7.00.

b. Computed only for a 2x2 table

Symmetric Measures

		Value	Approx. Sig.
Nominal by Nominal	Phi (11)	-.401	.028
	(12) Cramer's V	.401	.028
	Contingency Coefficient	.372	.028
N of Valid Cases		30	

a. Not assuming the null hypothesis.

b. Using the asymptotic standard error assuming the null hypothesis.

Figure 7.4 indicates that 10 children in the staff-initiated intervention group expressed no distress immediately postintervention compared to only 4 children in the usual-care group (3). If the two variables were independent, the expected number of children in each nondistressed group would be 7 (Expected Count (Exp_{ij}) = $[R_i][C_j]/N$ = [15][14]/30 = 7) (4). The expected number of children in the distressed groups if the null hypothesis were true would be 8 (Expected Count (Exp_{ij}) = [16][15]/30 = 8) (5). The unstandardized residuals (*Residual*) represent the difference between what we actually obtained in a given cell compared to what would have been expected if the null hypothesis were true. From Figure 7.4, we can see that the differences between the actual count (*Count*) and the expected count (*Expected Count*) (i.e., the *Residuals*) are either −3.0 or +3.0 for all of our cells (6).

To determine whether the differences between the observed and expected values are sufficiently large to reject the null hypothesis of independence of variables, we need to examine the generated Pearson chi-square and its significance level. If the significance level (Note: in SPSS for Windows, *Asymp Sig* = the *p* value) is less than our prestated alpha level (e.g., $\alpha = .05$), we will reject the null hypothesis. In our case, the χ^2 value is 4.82, the same as that which we obtained above (7). Because the generated *p* value (.028) for this χ^2 is less than our prestated alpha ($\alpha = .05$), we will reject the null hypothesis. The conclusion to be drawn is that the two variables, group membership and the children's distress immediately postintervention, are significantly associated or dependent.

Notice that in addition to the *Count* and *Expected Count,* we are also presented with the *% within group intervention vs. usual care groups* and *% within distress immediately postintervention*. This first percent reports the row percentages in the table while the second percent reports the column percents. Looking at the row percents presented in Figure 7.4, it appears that fewer children in the staff-initiated intervention group (n = 5, 33.3%) (8) expressed distress immediately following the intervention than did the children in the usual-care group (n = 11, 73.3%).

Hinkle, Wiersma, and Jurs (2003) point out that the chi-square distribution (χ^2) is a continuous distribution with no breaks in its continuity. A serious problem occurs, therefore, when the expected frequencies in any of the cells for a 2 × 2 table are less than 5 because the resulting sampling distribution for this χ^2 could depart substantially from continuity. To improve the approximation to a χ^2 distribution when categorical data are being analyzed, an adjustment to the χ^2 has been suggested: the Yates correction for continuity (Cochran, 1954). The Yates correction factor for continuity is as follows:

$$\chi^2 = \sum\sum \frac{(Obs_{ij} - Exp_{ij} - .5)^2}{Exp_{ij}}$$

Although the Yates correction has the advantage of making adjustments for the fact that there are categorical data, there are distinct disadvantages to its use. Hinkle et al. (2003) warn that, for a 2 × 2 table, the generated χ^2 value with the Yates correction is extremely conservative. This results in a substantial loss of power and a tendency to incorrectly fail to reject the null hypothesis. For that reason, these authors recommend ignoring the continuity correction for 2 × 2 tables. Siegel and Castellan (1988) recommend using the

Yates correction when the sample size is ≥ 40 because the correction considerably improves the approximation to the χ^2 distribution.

In Figure 7.4, we can see that the problem raised by Hinkle and colleagues (2003) has occurred in our hypothetical study. The Yates continuity correction has resulted in a more conservative χ^2 value (3.348) that is no longer significant ($p = .067$) (9) at our level of alpha. If we had used the χ^2 value that was corrected for continuity, therefore, we would have failed to reject the null hypothesis and would have, perhaps falsely, concluded that the two variables, group membership and distress immediately postintervention, were independent (i.e., not associated).

Analyzing Residuals to Determine Which Cells Are Influencing the Outcome

The chi-square statistic is an overall test of independence between two variables. Given a significant result, this statistic does not indicate which cells appear to be major contributors to the observed differences. Several approaches can be used to determine which cells are influencing the outcomes observed. In Chapter 8, we will examine an approach suggested by Siegel and Castellan (1988) to analyze directions of influence in tables that are larger than 2 × 2. In this chapter, we will examine the standardized residuals to determine which cells appear to be influencing the value of the χ^2 statistic obtained.

The difference between the actual and expected values represents the *residual* (i.e., what is "left over"). In SPSS for Windows, it is possible to request three types of residuals: unstandardized, standardized, and adjusted unstandardized. Because unstandardized residuals are influenced by the size of the sample, Hinkle et al. (2003) suggest that the *standardized* residuals be used to examine which cell(s) appear to be influencing the outcomes observed. To obtain a standardized residual for each category, a value similar to a z statistic is obtained. The difference between the observed and expected values of a cell is obtained and divided by the square root of the expected value:

$$Std.\ Residual = \frac{(Observed - Expected)}{\sqrt{Expected}}$$

For Cell 3 in the table presented in Figure 7.4, the standardized residual would be $(10 - 7)/2.645 = 1.1$ (10). How big does a standardized residual need to be in order to influence the chi-square value? The general rule is that a cell that has a standardized residual that is greater than the absolute value of 2 is one that is influencing the chi-square statistic. The reason for this is that by standardizing the residual, we are treating the residual like a z score from a standard normal distribution where 95% of the values would lie within −2 and +2 standard deviations of the mean (0). Any value $>|2|$, therefore, could be considered to be an "outlier" and implies that the cell in question is an important contributor to the significant χ^2 value (Haberman, 1984; Hinkle et al., 2003).

In our hypothetical example, all the absolute values of the standardized residuals are similar (1.1), and no value exceeds 2. We would conclude, therefore, that there is no one cell that is unduly influencing the generated χ^2 value.

Determining the Strength of Association Between Two Variables

The generated χ^2 statistic and its p value provide little information concerning the strength of the association between the two variables being examined. It is also not possible to compare χ^2 values across studies of different sample sizes (or table sizes) because the size and interpretation of the statistic is directly influenced by the size of the sample and degrees of freedom: For a given degree of freedom, an increase in sample size will most likely increase the value of the χ^2. It is possible, therefore, to obtain statistically significant results from the chi-square test for two independent samples that may or may not be of clinical interest to the researcher.

Several commonly used measures of association that are generated from the chi-square statistic provide the researcher with information concerning the strength of the association between two categorical variables (e.g., the phi coefficient, the contingency coefficient, and Cramér's V). One useful statistic for 2 × 2 tables is the *phi coefficient*. This statistic is examined in greater detail in Chapter 9. In Chapter 10, the use of odds ratios to evaluate strength of association will be addressed. These statistics, along with logistic regression, are commonly used in medical and public health studies and are increasingly being reported in social science research. In this chapter, the interpretation of the phi coefficient in view of a significant χ^2 statistic will be discussed briefly.

The phi coefficient.

When a significant χ^2 for a 2 × 2 contingency table has been obtained, the phi coefficient can be used to determine the strength of association between the two variables. This coefficient is obtained by taking the square root of a significant χ^2 value that has been divided by the total sample size:

$$\phi = \sqrt{\frac{\chi^2}{N}}$$

For a 2 × 2 table, the values for the phi coefficient range between 0 and 1.00, with 0 indicating no relationship and 1.00 indicating a perfect relationship. If the categories of the independent and dependent variables in the 2 × 2 table have been coded 0 and 1, the phi coefficient is related to the Pearson product-moment correlation: $\phi = |r_{xy}|$ (Chapter 9). For interpretive purposes, therefore, the strength of relationship between two categorical variables could be viewed in a context similar to what Hinkle et al. (2003) suggest for a Pearson r (Table 7.7); that is, phi coefficients that range from 0 to .49 suggest a relationship that is of weak or low strength, .50 to .69 is a relationship of moderate strength, .70 to .89 indicates a strong relationship, and .90 to 1.00 suggests a very strong relationship.

The phi coefficient for our hypothetical study (Figure 7.4, (11)) was calculated as follows:

$$\phi = \sqrt{\frac{\chi^2}{N}} = \sqrt{\frac{4.82}{30}} = .40$$

Table 7.7 Suggested Rule of Thumb for Interpreting the Phi Coefficient for 2 × 2 Tables

Size of Phi Coefficient	r^2	*Strength of Association*
.90 to 1.00	.81 – 1.00	Very strong
.70 to .89	.49 – .80	Strong
.50 to .69	.25 – .48	Moderate
.30 to .49	.09 – .24	Low
.00 to .29	.00 – .08	Weak

According to the Hinkle et al. (2003) criteria (Table 7.7), the strength of association between group membership and children's distress immediately postintervention is, at best, low. Notice, too, that the phi presented in Figure 7.4 is –.40, not +.40. The reason for the negative value is that, for a 2 × 2 table, the phi coefficient is equal to the Pearson correlation coefficient so that in SPSS for Windows, its sign matches that of the correlation coefficient (–.40).

The contingency coefficient and Cramér's *V*.

When one dimension of the table is greater than 2 (i.e., 2 × *k*), the value of the phi coefficient may not lie between 0 and 1 because the χ^2 value can be greater than the sample size. In that instance, the use of the *contingency coefficient* (*C*) has been suggested, where

$$C = \sqrt{\frac{\chi^2}{\chi^2 + N}}$$

Although the value of this contingency coefficient will always lie between 0 and 1, it will never attain the upper limit of 1, and its maximum value depends on the number of rows and columns in the table (Conover, 1999). That is,

$$C_{max} = \sqrt{\frac{L-1}{L}}$$

where L = the smaller of the number of rows and columns.

That would mean that, for a 4 × 4 table, the maximum value for C would be 0.87 since $L = 4$. For that reason, Cramér (1946) developed *Cramér's V*, a variant of the contingency coefficient:

$$V = \sqrt{\frac{\chi^2}{N(L-1)}}$$

where

N = the sample size, and

L = the smaller of the number of rows and columns.

This statistic will always range between 0 and 1 and, for a 2 × 2 table, will have the same value as the phi coefficient. In our hypothetical study (Figure 7.4), the phi coefficient and Cramér's V (11) have the same value since $(L - 1) = (2 - 1) = 1$ so Cramér's V simplifies to the phi coefficient. The contingency coefficient, .372 (12), is slightly smaller because of the larger denominator, $\sqrt{\chi^2 + N}$ versus $\sqrt{\chi^2}$. Note that all of the coefficients are significant at the same level as the χ^2 statistic ($p = .028$, (7)).

Internet Resources for Generating the Chi-Square Test

As with the Fisher's exact test, there are a number of currently available open access Internet resources that provide calculators with which one can obtain a chi-square test (e.g., www.danielsoper.com and www.vassarstats.net). For this current example, we will use www.vassarstats.net to generate the chi-square test.

This statistic was very easy to generate from this website. Once in the vassarstats website, click on *Clinical Research Calculators . . . Chi-Square, Cramer's V, and Lambda.* From there, select the number of rows and columns (two each) and then the values for the four cells (4, 11, 10, and 5). Clicking on the *Calculate* button will generate the results obtained in Figure 7.5.

Figure 7.5 Internet-generated chi-square test for two independent samples.

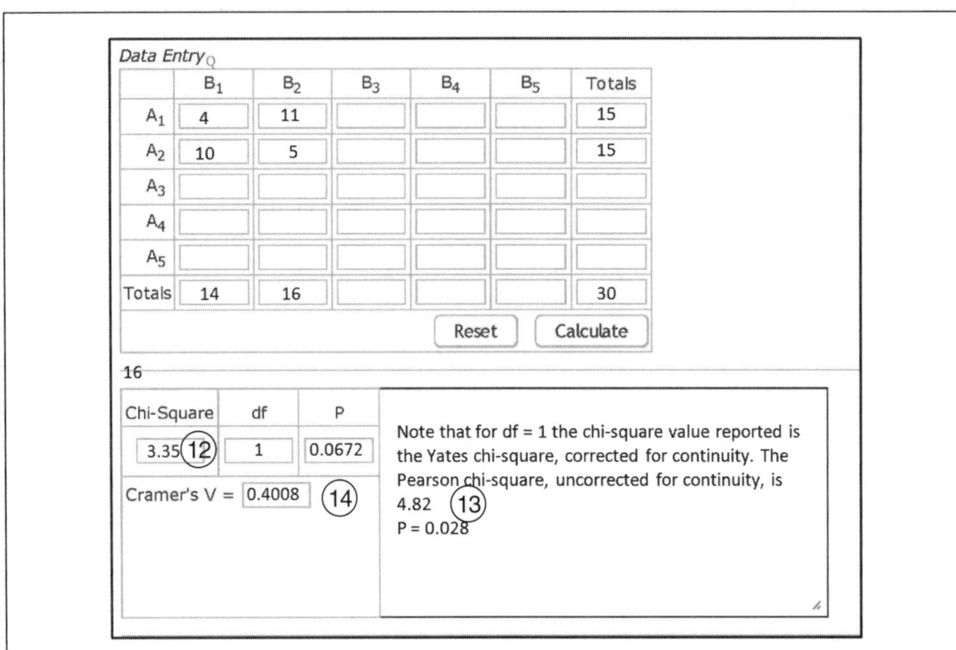

SOURCE: Retrieved from www.vassarstats.net

As Figure 7.5 indicates, we are presented with two chi-square values: the Yates chi-square statistic, which has been corrected for continuity (3.35) (12), and the Pearson chi-square uncorrected for continuity (4.82) (13). Both values are similar, thank goodness, to those that were generated in SPSS for Windows. We are also presented with Cramér's *V*, which is the same as the phi for a 2 × 2 table (.4008) (14).

Presentation of Results

Table 7.8 suggests a table that could be used to present the results obtained from the chi-square test for two independent samples.

Table 7.8 Suggested Presentation of Results for the Chi-Square Test for Two Independent Samples

	Distress Immediately Postintervention							
	Yes		*No*		*Total*			
Group	N	%	N	%	N	%	χ^2	p[a]
Staff-initiated intervention	5	33.3	10	66.7	15	50		
Usual care	11	73.3	4	26.7	15	50	4.82	.03
Total	16	53.3	14	46.7	30	100		

[a]Phi = .401.

These results could also be interpreted and presented in the text as follows:

The results of the chi-square test for two independent samples indicate that the 15 children in the intervention group expressed a lower rate of distress immediately postintervention (n = 5, 33.3%) than did the 15 children in the control group (n = 11, 73.3%) (χ^2 = 4.82, p = .03). The strength of the relationship between group membership and distress immediately postintervention fear was low (ϕ = .40), suggesting that other factors besides the staff-initiated intervention may be influencing children's distress immediately postintervention.

Advantages, Limitations, and Alternatives to the Chi-Square Test for Two Independent Samples

The chi-square test for two independent samples is a very popular test that is easily understood and interpreted, especially when the data are cast into a 2 × 2 table. When the contingency table is larger, it is more difficult to determine which cells are most strongly influencing the significant χ^2. In Chapter 8, we will examine ways to partition larger contingency tables to determine where the major influences lie. Two additional disadvantages to the chi-square test for two independent samples are its sensitivity to departure from the assumption concerning expected frequencies, especially for 2×2 tables, and its insensitivity to order in the categorical variables.

Since the chi-square test for two independent samples is used when both independent and dependent variables are categorical, there is no parametric alternative to this test. Because the chi-square test is extremely sensitive to both sample size and expected frequencies, Cochran (1954) and Siegel and Castellan (1988) recommend that if the sample size is ≤ 20 and the data to be analyzed are in a 2×2 table, Fisher's exact test should be used instead of the chi-square test for independent samples. If the sample size is between 20 and 40, the chi-square test could be used for a 2×2 table if all the expected values in the cells are greater than 5. If there are cells that have expected frequencies less than 5, Fisher's exact test is recommended. When the sample is greater than 40, it is recommended that the Yates correction be used for 2×2 tables (Cochran, 1954; Ludbrook & Dudley, 1994; Siegel & Castellan, 1988).

These recommendations are not universally accepted, however. Campbell (2007), for example, has observed that the expected value of 5, the classically accepted minimum expected value for 2×2 tables, is somewhat arbitrary, a position also suggested by Cochran (1952). Campbell points out that there is lack of agreement as to the optimal measure of choice for "smaller" or "larger" sample sizes. He further argues that the boundary between "large" and "small" sample sizes is unclear and that there is a lack of consensus as to which versions of the chi-square or Fisher's exact test should be used. To address this issue, Campbell examined computer-simulated results from a comparison of seven tests of 2×2 tables in terms of their Type I errors (i.e., the probability of incorrectly rejecting the null hypothesis). He concluded that, when all expected values for a 2×2 table are at least 1, the researcher should use a chi-square test that is adjusted by a factor of $(N - 1)/N$. Fisher's exact test would be the preferred measure otherwise (Campbell, 2007).

For $2 \times k$ or larger tables, both Cochran (1954) and Siegel and Castellan (1988) indicate that the chi-square test can be used if no more than 20% of the cells have expected frequencies of less than 5. If the data do not meet this assumption, it is possible to collapse cells so that a smaller table is generated. The choice of which cells should be collapsed together, however, requires thoughtful consideration, a discussion of which can be found in Chapter 8.

As indicated above, for 2×2 tables, the phi statistic generated from the χ^2 is related to the Pearson product-moment correlation provided that the cells for these categorical variables are coded as 0s and 1s. A correlation coefficient that is generated from these data can be interpreted as a Pearson product-moment correlation. For $2 \times k$ tables, however, the chi-square test for two independent samples is not sensitive to order. For that reason, other nonparametric tests may be better alternatives when the dependent variable has some presumed order. In Chapter 8, we will examine the use of a Mantel-Haenszel chi-square test when the categorical data have some presumed order. In the final sections of this chapter, we will examine the use of the Wilcoxon-Mann-Whitney *U* test when the dependent variable is ordinal.

Examples From Published Research

Anders, M. E., & Evans, D. P. (2010). Comparison of PubMed and Google Scholar literature searches. *Respiratory Care, 55*(5), 578–583.

Robl, J., Jewell, T., & Kanotra, S. (2012). The effect of parental involvement on problematic social behaviors among school-age children in Kentucky. *Maternal & Child Health Journal, 16,* 287–297. doi: 10.1007/s10995-012-1187-4

Siegler, J. C., Rehman, S., Bhumireddy, G. P., Abdula, R., Klem, I., Brener, S. J., . . . Heitner, J. F. (2011). The accuracy of the electrocardiogram during exercise stress test based on heart size. *PLoS ONE, 6*(8), e23044. doi: 10.1371/journal.pone.0023044

THE WILCOXON-MANN-WHITNEY *U* TEST

Fisher's exact test and the chi-square test for two independent samples are used when both the independent and dependent variables being examined are categorical. Because these two tests are not sensitive to order, they are not ideal measures to use when the dependent variable has some order to it. The next test that we will examine is the Wilcoxon-Mann-Whitney *U* test. This powerful nonparametric test is very useful when the dependent variable to be examined is at least ordinal level of measurement and either it does not meet the assumptions of a parametric test or the researcher wishes to generalize to more than just a "normally distributed" population.

This nonparametric test for two independent samples was independently developed by both Wilcoxon (1945) (the Wilcoxon *W* ranked sum statistic) and Mann and Whitney (1947) (the Mann-Whitney *U* statistic), thus the origins of its current name, the Wilcoxon-Mann-Whitney *U* test (Conover, 1999; Neter, Wasserman, & Whitmore, 1993). This test is not to be confused with the Wilcoxon signed-ranks test (Chapter 5), which is used with dependent samples. To avoid possible confusion, this test will be referred to in this chapter as the *Mann-Whitney test.*

The Mann-Whitney test is used when the researcher wants to determine whether two independent samples are from the same population. It tests the null hypothesis that the two population probability distributions are the same (i.e., $F_1(x) = F_2(x)$). The Mann-Whitney test has particularly strong power when the alternative hypothesis states that there is a location shift in the two distributions, that the distribution in one group differs from the distribution in the second group by some value of theta (i.e., $F_1(x) = F_2(x + \theta)$). If data differences are assumed to arise from this location shift, then a statistically significant Mann-Whitney test implies differences in medians and all other matching quantiles in the two populations (Conover, 1999; Fagerland & Sandvik, 2009).

An Appropriate Research Question for the Mann-Whitney Test

The Mann-Whitney test is often used to compare two groups with regard to a given criterion that is measured on at least an ordinal scale, such as depression, wellness, or age. This test also can be used to compare change scores for two populations to determine whether these change scores come from the same population. That is, the researcher may want to compare the changes in a dependent variable (e.g., perceived quality of life) in two groups (e.g., intervention and control) across two periods of time. To do this, the researcher first creates a new variable (e.g., QOLDIFF, the difference between quality of life at Time 2 and Time 1) that represents a change score (e.g., QOLDIFF = QOL2 – QOL1). The Mann-Whitney test is then run on the new dependent variable, QOLDIFF, and the independent variable (GROUP), which is dichotomous.

In our hypothetical example, we might be interested in comparing the staff-initiated intervention and usual-care groups of 20 hospitalized children with cancer regarding the children's self-reported evaluations of the intensity of their fatigue immediately following the intervention. The data set that we will be using is hospitalized children with cancer-20 cases.sav (study.sagepub.com/pett2e). This variable, intensity of fatigue immediately postintervention, has been measured on a 7-point ordinal scale on which 1 = *not at all fatigued* and 7 = *extremely fatigued.* A possible research question that could be answered using the Mann-Whitney test is as follows:

> Do the children who receive the staff-initiated intervention designed to reduce nocturnal sleep awakenings (intervention group) report lower intensity of fatigue immediately postintervention than the children who do not receive the intervention (usual-care group)?

Null and Alternative Hypotheses

The Mann-Whitney test is another of the most commonly used nonparametric tests in the health care research literature. A cursory search of the Medline, CINAHL, and PsychInfo databases for the 5-year period 2008–2013, for example, yielded more than 17,000 peer-reviewed research publications—from a variety of disciplines and using a broad range of sample sizes—that reported using at least one Mann-Whitney test in their statistical analyses. These projects included a randomized controlled trial of a car safety seat insert to reduce hypoxia in 78 term infants (McIntosh, Tonkin, & Gunn, 2013); a national cross-sectional survey comparing health-related quality of life, work status, and health care utilization and costs according to hip and knee joint disease severity among 1,157 Australian citizens (Ackerman, Ademi, Osborne, & Liew, 2013); an intervention designed to test the effects of a population-based self-efficacy message card campaign on compliance with a tobacco-free university campus policy (Fallin et al., 2013); and, interestingly, a study designed to characterize changes in eyebrow slope among 100 women with increasing age to better direct brow rejuvenation (Delyzer & Yazdani, 2013).

In our hypothetical study of the impact of a staff-initiated intervention on fatigue levels of children who have been hospitalized with cancer, we have indicated from our research question that we are interested in comparing the staff-initiated intervention and usual-care groups with regard to their reported intensity of fatigue immediately postintervention. An example of null and alternative hypotheses that could be answered using a Mann-Whitney test is given in Table 7.9. Note that the alternative hypothesis is directional; therefore, our Mann-Whitney test will be one-tailed.

Table 7.9 Example of Null and Alternative Hypotheses Suitable for Use With the Mann-Whitney Test

Null Hypothesis
H_0: There will be no difference between the staff-initiated intervention and usual-care group of hospitalized children with regard to the distributions of the intensity of their fatigue scores immediately postintervention; that is, the two groups come from the same population (i.e., $F_{\text{staff-initiated}}(x) = F_{\text{usual care}}(x)$).
Alternative Hypothesis
H_a: The distribution of intensity of fatigue scores immediately postintervention for the hospitalized children receiving the staff-initiated intervention will be lower than that of the children in the usual-care group; that is, $F_{\text{staff-initiated}}(x) = F_{\text{usual care}}(x - \theta)$.

We also could have compared the change in intensity of fatigue scores from preintervention to immediately postintervention for the intervention and usual-care groups. If we had chosen that route, we would have needed to first create a new variable to represent the change scores. In SPSS for Windows, this is accomplished by clicking on the commands *Transform . . . Compute* and defining a new variable (e.g., Fatigue_Chg = Intensity_Fatigue_T1 – Intensity_Fatigue_T2). The Mann-Whitney test is then run on this new variable, Intensity_Fatigue_Chg.

Overview of the Procedure

To calculate a Mann-Whitney test, the data for both groups are first combined into a single sample, and their scores on the dependent variable are ranked from lowest to highest without regard to their position on the independent variable. Tied observations are assigned the average of the tied ranks. Next, the independent groups are separated out, and the sum of the assigned ranks for each group is calculated. If the null hypothesis that the groups come from the same population is true, the sum of the ranks for both groups should be similar. If the sum of the ranks for one group is very different from the other, there is evidence to suspect that the two samples did not come from the same population. The null hypothesis is rejected if the sum of the ranks for one group is sufficiently larger than that for the second group.

The statistic that is generated to determine whether the null hypothesis is to be rejected is the U statistic. This statistic takes into account both the measure of central tendency and the distribution of the scores and is defined as the smaller of U_1 and U_2, where

$$U_1 = n_1 n_2 + \frac{n_1(n_1+1)}{2} - R_1$$

$$U_2 = n_1 n_2 + \frac{n_2(n_2+1)}{2} - R_2$$

where

n_1 = the number of observations in Group 1,

n_2 = the number of observations in Group 2,

R_1 = the sum of the ranks assigned to Group 1, and

R_2 = the sum of the ranks assigned to Group 2.

The sampling distribution of this *U* statistic is known and, like the *t* distribution or the chi-square distribution, can be used for testing hypotheses. When the sample size is large, this *U* distribution quickly approaches a normal distribution with a mean, $\mu_u = (n_1 n_2)/2$, and standard deviation, $\sigma_u = \sqrt{(n_1 n_2)(n_1 + n_2 + 1)/12}$. There is, however, some disagreement in the literature as to how large is "large." Neter et al. (1993) indicate that the approximation is adequate when both groups have sample sizes of 10 or more. Hinkle et al. (2003) argue that each group should have a sample size larger than 20.

The decision rule for the Mann-Whitney test is that, for small sample sizes, the null hypothesis is rejected if the obtained value of *U* (the smaller of U_1 or U_2) is *smaller* than the critical value of *U* at the predetermined level of alpha (e.g., $\alpha = .05$). Table A.4 (a–c) in Appendix A presents the critical values of *U* for various one- and two-tailed levels of alpha. We will examine how to interpret this table when we calculate the Mann-Whitney *U* test for our data.

For larger sample sizes, a *z* statistic is generated (Hinkle et al., 2003; Neter et al., 1993; Siegel & Castellan, 1988):

$$z = \frac{U - \mu_u}{\sigma_u} = \frac{U - n_1 n_2 / 2}{\sqrt{n_1 n_2 (n_1 + n_2 + 1)/12}}$$

The null hypothesis is rejected if the absolute value of the obtained *z* value is *greater* than the absolute value of the critical *z* at the prespecified alpha level. The reason for this apparent contradiction in rejection rules between the small and large sample statistics is that the *U* statistic for smaller sample sizes examines the *minimum* value of U_1 or U_2 and compares its minimum value to a critical minimum value that would occur if the null hypothesis were true. In contrast, for larger samples, the generated *z* statistic is compared to a critical *z* value at a prespecified alpha level.

Calculating the Mann-Whitney *U* statistic for the intensity of fatigue data.

Table 7.10 presents the actual values and ranks for the intensity of fatigue data broken down by the usual-care group (0) and the staff-initiated intervention (1). First, the data for all 20 children have been ordered from lowest to highest (i.e., from 1–20) (1), their ranks were determined (2), and then those ranks were separated out by groups (3) and summed (4). Since the mid-rank is used for tied data, the ranks for the two 3s are 1.5 since they occupy positions 1 and 2 in the rankings (5). The four values of "4" have been ranked 4.5 since they occupied positions 3 through 6 ([3 + 4 + 5 + 6]/4 = 4.5) (6).

Table 7.10 Actual Values and Their Rankings by Group: The Mann-Whitney *U* Test

Intensity of Fatigue Immediately Postintervention					*Ranking of Data*		
Group[1]	*Value*	(3) *Rank*	*Sum of Ranks*	*Mean Ranks*	(1) *Lowest to Highest*	(2) *Actual Rank*	*Rank Position*
0	6	17			3	1.5	(5) 1
0	5	10.5			3	1.5	2
0	7	20			4	4.5	(6) 3
0	6	17			4	4.5	4
0	4	4.5			4	4.5	5
0	6	17			4	4.5	6
0	6	17			5	10.5	7
0	5	10.5			5	10.5	8
0	5	10.5	(4)		5	10.5	9
0	5	10.5	R_1 = 134.50	13.45	5	10.5	10
1	5	10.5			5	10.5	11
1	4	4.5			5	10.5	12
1	5	10.5			5	10.5	13
1	6	17			5	10.5	14
1	3	1.5			6	17	15
1	3	1.5			6	17	16
1	5	10.5			6	17	17
1	4	4.5			6	17	18
1	4	4.5	(4)		6	17	19
1	5	10.5	R_2 = 75.50	7.55	7	20	20

[1]Usual-care group = 0, staff-initiated intervention = 1.

By separating out the groups and summing their ranks in Table 7.10, we obtain the values of R_1 = 134.50 and R_2 = 75.50 (4). To calculate U_1 and U_2, we would use the formulas offered above:

$$U_1 = n_1 n_2 + \frac{n_1(n_1+1)}{2} - R_1 = (10)\,(10) + \frac{10(10+1)}{2} - 134.5 = 20.50$$

$$U_2 = n_1 n_2 + \frac{n_2(n_2+1)}{2} - R_2 = (10)\,(10) + \frac{10(10+1)}{2} - 75.50 = 79.50$$

The minimum of the two ranks, U, therefore, is 20.50.

To determine if our U (20.50) is sufficiently small enough for us to reject the null hypothesis of no difference between the two groups with regard to the intensity of their self-reported fatigue levels immediately postintervention, we need to turn to Table A.4 in Appendix A. Notice there are three tables offered for the critical values for the Mann-Whitney U test depending on the level of α that we have chosen and whether the test is directional or nondirectional. Let us assume that $\alpha = .05$. Because our alternative hypothesis is directional, we will use Table A4.A for the one-tailed directional test when $\alpha = .05$. Table 7.11 presents a snippet of that table to show how to determine the critical value of the U statistic.

Table 7.11 Example of Determining the Critical Value of the Mann-Whitney *U* Test Using Table A.4A

Table A.4 Critical values for the Wilcoxon/Mann-Whitney Test (U)
A. 2 tailed (non-directional) $\alpha = .10$;
1-tailed (directional) $\alpha = .05$

	n_2															
n_1	1	2	3	4	5	6	7	8	9	10	11	12	13	14	15	16
1	-	-	-	-	-	-	-	-	-	-	-	-	-	-	-	-
2	-	-	-	-	0	0	0	1	1	1	1	2	2	2	3	3
3	-	-	0	0	1	2	2	3	3	4	5	5	6	7	7	8
4	-	-	0	1	2	3	4	5	6	7	8	9	10	11	12	14
5	-	0	1	2	4	5	6	8	9	11	12	13	15	16	18	19
6	-	0	2	3	5	7	8	10	12	14	16	17	19	21	23	25
7	-	0	2	4	6	8	11	13	15	17	19	21	24	26	28	30
8	-	1	3	5	8	10	13	15	18	20	23	26	28	31	33	36
9	-	1	3	6	9	12	15	18	21	24	27	30	33	36	39	42
10	-	1	4	7	11	14	17	20	24	27	31	34	37	41	44	48
11	-	1	5	8	12	16	19	23	27	31	34	38	42	48	50	54
12	-	2	5	9	13	17	21	26	30	34	38	42	47	51	55	60
13	-	2	6	10	15	19	24	28	33	37	42	47	51	56	61	65

Given that there were 10 children in both the intervention and usual-care groups, to find the critical value of U, we need to go to the row in which $n_1 = 10$ and across to the column where $n_2 = 10$ (Table 7.11). Where the two intersect, we will find that critical value ("27"). Because our calculated U (20.50) is smaller than that critical value (27), we will reject the null hypothesis that the two groups are similar with regard to their intensity of fatigue levels immediately postintervention. We can conclude that the children in the staff-initiated intervention reported lower intensity of fatigue than did the children in the usual-care group.

Obtaining a Confidence Interval for the Median of the Differences for the Mann-Whitney Test

As indicated earlier, the Mann-Whitney test is a test of differences in distributions of two groups. If we can assume that the distributions for the two groups are similar except for their location shift, then we can feel comfortable in positing that the test also provides a point estimate for comparing the differences in medians between two groups (e.g., the differences in median intensity of fatigue scores immediately postintervention between the staff-initiated intervention and usual-care groups). While this single-point estimate and its corresponding p value is informative, building a confidence interval (*interval estimate*) around the differences in medians provides more useful information than a single estimate alone (Newson, 2006; Zhou & Dinh, 2005).

A 95% confidence interval defines a range of values such that the population parameter of interest (in this case, a median difference between two groups) will fall within this range in 95% of samples (Field, 2009). This means that if we were to resample the population 100 times, the "true" value in the population for the statistic we are examining (aka *the population parameter*) would lie between the two values 95 out of 100 times. These confidence intervals are built around the sample statistic (e.g., the median difference between two groups). In our example, we could state the following: "There is a 95% probability that the true population median difference in intensity of fatigue immediately postintervention between the usual-care group and our staff-initiated intervention falls between _____ and _____."

There are several suggested approaches to obtaining a $(1 - \alpha)\%$ confidence interval for the median of the differences for two independent groups (Conover, 1999; Curtis & Marascuilo, 1992; Lehmann, 2006; Newson, 2006; Sprent & Smeeton, 2001). One approach that is available in SPSS for Windows (v. 18 and above) is the Hodges-Lehmann estimator of location based on ranks (and its confidence interval) (Hodges & Lehmann, 1963; Newson, 2006, 2007). An alternative approach, also available in SPSS for Windows, is to undertake a t test (and subsequent confidence interval) on the ranked data (Conover, 1999). In this section, we will examine how the Hodges-Lehmann confidence interval for the median of the differences is obtained. Later, when we generate the SPSS for Windows output for the Mann-Whitney test, we will compare the Hodges-Lehmann confidence interval with that which is generated from the independent t test on the ranked data.

Sprent and Smeeton (2001) offer a clear explanation of how to calculate a Hodges-Lehmann confidence interval when using the Mann-Whitney test to examine the median of the differences in two independent samples. To do this, the raw scores are first ordered from lowest to highest for each group. The set of ranked raw scores from one group is then placed in the first row of a table; the ranked data from the second group are placed in the first column of said table. Table 7.12 provides an example of such a table for the intensity of fatigue data immediately postintervention for the usual-care and staff-initiated intervention groups.

Once the scores for the two groups are placed into the first row and column of the table, the scores of one group (e.g., the usual-care group) are subtracted from the scores of the second group (e.g., staff-initiated intervention) with the differences placed in the body of the table. In Table 7.12, for example, for cell 1, the first score in row 1 ("3") is subtracted from the first score in column 1 ("4") (7). This procedure is continued for all available cells. In our example, we have 100 cells (Table 7.12).

The next step is to eliminate the most extreme low and high values to determine which low and high values are remaining. To do this, we need to first identify the critical value for the Mann-Whitney U at our given level of α. Let us assume that we are

Table 7.12 Approach to Calculating the 95% Confidence Interval for the Mann-Whitney *U* Test ($U_{cv} = 23$)

Staff-initiated Intervention Group: Intensity of Fatigue scores-T2	Usual Care Group: Intensity of Fatigue scores-T2									
	4	5	5	5	5	6	6	6	6	7
3	1	2	2	2	2	3	3	3	3	4
3	1	2	2	2	2	3	3	3	3	4
4	0	1	1	1	1	2	2	2	2	3
4	0	1	1	1	1	2	2	2	2	3
4	0	1	1	1	1	2	2	2	2	3
5	−1	0	0	0	0	1	1	1	1	2
5	−1	0	0	0	0	1	1	1	1	2
5	−1	0	0	0	0	1	1	1	1	2
5	−1	0	0	0	0	1	1	1	1	2
6	−2	−1	−1	−1	−1	0	0	0	0	1

(7) 4 – 3 = 1

(8) Min value = 0

(9) Max value = 2

(10) Median = 1

calculating a 95% confidence interval. That would mean that our two-tailed $\alpha = .05$. Turning to Table A.4 (b) in Appendix A, the critical value for U when $n_1 = n_2 = 10$ is 23. That means that the 23 highest and lowest values are those that lie beyond $\alpha = .025$ on each side of the U distribution. Therefore, we will eliminate the 23 most extremely low and 23 most extremely high values and then identify the remaining minimum and maximum values. These will represent the lower and upper bounds for the 95% confidence interval for the median of the differences. We can also obtain the median value for these 100 difference scores by rank-ordering the differences and then determining the median value for those differences.

The 23 most extremely low and high values are presented as the shaded values in the lower and upper quadrants of Table 7.12. The values that are remaining are presented along the diagonal of the table. Examining the remaining unshaded values indicates that the minimum and maximum values that are not extreme are the values of 0 (8) and 2 (9), respectively. The median of these 100 differences is the midpoint of all 100 ranked values (i.e., the value that lies between the 50th and 51st ranked difference score). The 50th and 51st value for our ranked differences is 1 (10).

How would we interpret these values of 0, +2, and +1? The point estimate for the median of the difference scores is +1.0. Because this value is positive (i.e., usual-care group – staff-initiated intervention group > 0), that means that the usual-care group had higher fatigue scores than did the staff-initiated intervention. We could also say that there is a 95% probability that the true median of the difference scores in the population lies between 0 and +2.

But wait! Typically, we would say that if the value of 0 was contained in this interval, we could not reject the null hypothesis that there are no median differences between the two groups. Yet, in our calculated example above, we found that, per the Mann-Whitney test, there *were* statistically significant differences between the group medians, or mean ranks ($p < .05$), between the usual-care and staff-initiated intervention groups. Is this conflicting evidence?

The answer appears to lie mainly in the discrete nature of ordinal-level data that have a restricted range of 1 to 7. That means that the largest (and smallest) differences could only be $|6|$. In addition, there were 23 ties (i.e., $x - y = 0$) in the data (Table 7.12), and therefore 0s were not always extreme cases. Also, there *is* a difference in interpretation between the *differences in medians* between two independent groups (per the Mann-Whitney test) and the *median differences* among the scores per the Hodges-Lehmann estimation. When we examine the confidence intervals for the ranked data per the independent t test, we will see a confirmation of this conflicting evidence.

Critical Assumptions of the Mann-Whitney Test

1. *The independent variable is dichotomous, and the scale of measurement for the dependent variable is at least ordinal.* The Mann-Whitney test is used when there are two groups and the dependent variable being examined is at least at the ordinal level of measurement. The grouping variable for our hypothetical study has two levels (staff-initiated intervention, usual care), and our intensity of fatigue variable immediately

postintervention is measured on a 7-point ordinal Likert-type scale. We have, therefore, met this assumption.

2. *The data consist of a randomly selected sample of independent observations from two independent groups.* It is assumed that the data have been randomly selected, that there are no repeated observations, and that the two levels of the independent variable are mutually exclusive. In our hypothetical study, the independent variable, group membership, consists of two mutually exclusive groups. The dependent variable, intensity of fatigue immediately postintervention, consists of observations of the 20 children wherein no subject appears more than once in the data set and there are no repeated observations. However, even though the children were randomly assigned to the staff-initiated intervention and usual-care groups, the initial preintervention sample was one of convenience. For that reason, we would want to be cognizant of the implications that such a sample of convenience will have on the generalizability of our findings. If, for example, our original sample of convenience consisted of middle-class Caucasian children, could we generalize our findings to children of other social status and ethnicity?

3. *The population distributions of the dependent variable for the two independent groups share a similar unspecified shape but with a possible difference in measures of central tendency.* The Mann-Whitney test assumes that the two levels of the independent variable share a similar shape with regard to the distribution of the dependent variable. This shape need not be bell shaped or normal. This assumption is important if we want to draw conclusions about the differences in the medians of our two groups. In our hypothetical intervention study, we will need to examine the extent to which our data have similarity of distribution shapes. We will check this assumption using the Kolmogorov-Smirnov (K-S) two-sample goodness-of-fit test (Chapter 4) when we undertake the computer analysis of the Mann-Whitney test.

Computer Commands

To obtain a Mann-Whitney test in SPSS for Windows (v. 22–23), click on the following items in the drop-down menu: *Analyze . . . Nonparametric Tests . . . Independent Samples*. That will open the dialog box presented in Figure 7.6. The dependent variable is *Intensity of fatigue immediately postintervention* (*Intensity_fatigue_t2*), and the independent variable is our grouping variable (*Group*) (11). The two levels of this categorical independent variable are defined by clicking on the *Define Groups* subcommand and indicating that all members of Group 1 (the usual-care group) have been assigned the value of 0 and all members of Group 2 (the staff-initiated intervention group) have been assigned the value of 1. The *Mann-Whitney* test is selected from the *Customize tests* menu (12). We will also ask for the Hodges-Lehmann confidence interval for the median difference (13). Even though we have a one-tailed test with α = .05, we will maintain the 95% two-tailed confidence interval. Technically, we (and you) might have elected to lower this confidence interval to 90% to reflect that there is α = .05 on both sides of the confidence interval (14).

Figure 7.6 SPSS for Windows (v. 22–23) dialog boxes for generating the Mann-Whitney test.

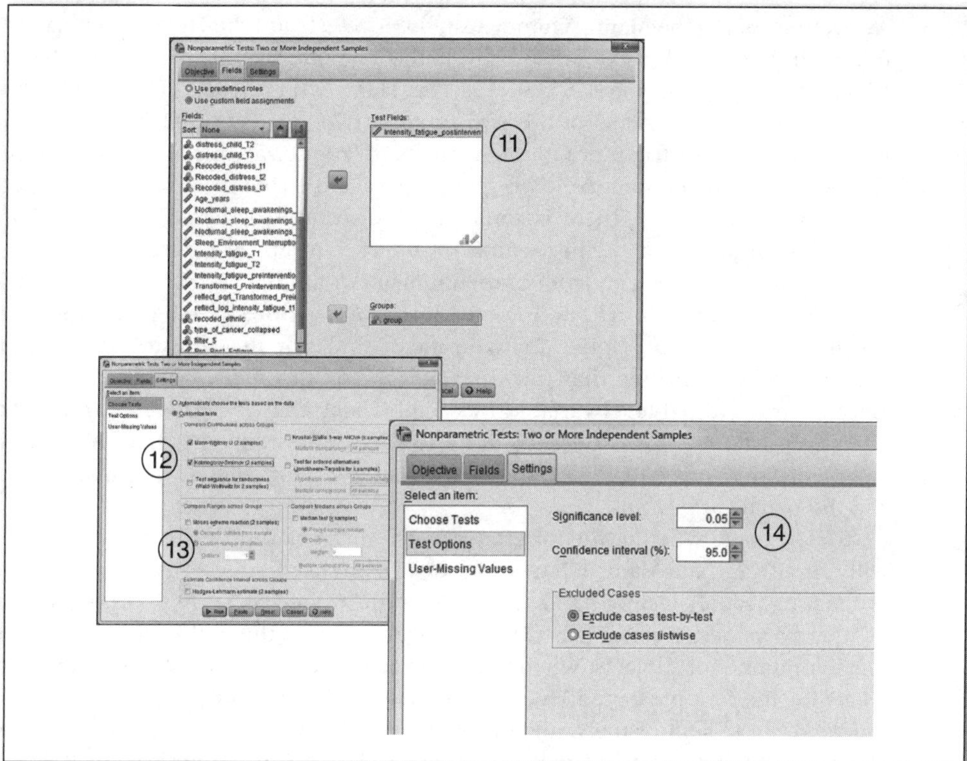

Assessing the Shapes of the Distributions

Assumption 3 of the Mann-Whitney test states that the population distributions of the dependent variable for the two independent groups share a similar but unspecified shape. We saw in Chapter 4 that there are two ways to assess the extent to which our data meet this assumption: (1) examine visually the histograms of the dependent variable within the various levels of the independent variable or (2) use the K-S two-sample test to check for similarity of distributions. The K-S two-sample test is quite easy to generate here because it uses the same SPSS for Windows dialog box as the Mann-Whitney test. To ascertain the extent to which our data meet Assumption 3, we merely need to select the *Kolmogorov-Smirnov* test (12) in addition to the *Mann-Whitney* from the *Customize tests* group (Figure 7.6).

Computer-Generated Output for the Mann-Whitney Test

The computer-generated output for the K-S and Mann-Whitney tests is presented in Figure 7.7. We are first presented with the syntax for these tests. The syntax indicates that we are requesting the Mann-Whitney test, the K-S test, and the Hodges-Lehman 95% confidence interval (15). Next we are given the Hypothesis Test Summary of the Mann-Whitney test (16) and the K-S test (17). The Mann-Whitney test indicates that there are differences in the medians of the two groups (two-tailed $p = .023$), while the K-S test indicates that the distributions of the intensity of fatigue variable are similar for the usual-care and staff-initiated intervention groups ($p = .400$). That means that we can conclude that, per Assumption 3, there is similarity of distributions across the two groups. This finding is supported by the histograms for the two groups in Figure 7.7 (18).

In Figure 7.7, the *mean rank* of the intensity of fatigue variable is presented instead of the *sum of the ranks* (R_1 and R_2) to allow comparisons of ranks even if the groups are not equal in size. Notice that the mean rank for the staff-initiated intervention group (7.55) is smaller than the mean rank for the usual-care group (13.45) (19). Because this ordinal-level variable was scored such that 1 = *not at all fatigued* and 7 = *extremely fatigued,* the difference in these mean ranks suggests that the staff-initiated intervention group had lower intensity of fatigue immediately postintervention than did the usual-care group.

To determine whether the difference in the mean ranks for the two groups is statistically significant, the Mann-Whitney U statistics are used. As we saw when we calculated the Mann-Whitney test by hand, the presented U value (20.5) (20) represents the smaller of the two values, U_1 and U_2. W (75.5) (21) is the sum of the ranks for the group with the smaller number of subjects. When the group sizes are equal, W represents the sum of the ranks for the first presented level of the dichotomous variable (R_1). In our hypothetical study, W is the sum of the ranks for the usual-care group (R_1) because it was assigned the value of 0 in the *Value Labels* subcommand in SPSS for Windows (i.e., 0 = usual care, 1 = staff-initiated intervention).

Because the total sum for any set of consecutive integers from 1 to N is $[N(N + 1)/2]$ (Siegel & Castellan, 1988), R_2 is obtained easily by subtracting R_1, from this total sum:

$$R_2 = \frac{N(N+1)}{2} - R_1 \frac{20(20+1)}{2} - 75.5 = 210 - 75.5 = 134.5$$

R_1 and R_2 can also be obtained directly from the computer printout (Figure 7.7) by multiplying the mean rank for a particular group by its sample size; for example, 13.45(10) = 134.5.

Given this information, we can then reconstruct our values for U_1 and U_2 using the formulas outlined above and can see that $U = 20.5$ because that is the minimum of U_1 and U_2.

$$U_1 = n_1 n_2 + \frac{n_1(n_1+1)}{2} - R_1 = (10)(10) + \frac{10(10+1)}{2} - 134.5 = 20.50$$

$$U_2 = n_1 n_2 + \frac{n_2(n_1+1)}{2} - R_2 = (10)(10) + \frac{10(10+1)}{2} - 75.50 = 79.50$$

Figure 7.7 Computer-generated output for the Mann-Whitney test (SPSS for Windows, v. 22–23).

```
***Data set: hospitalized children with cancer-20 cases

NPTESTS
 /INDEPENDENT TEST (Intensity_fatigue_T2) GROUP (group) MANN_WHITNEY
  KOLMOGOROV_SMIRNOV HODGES_LEHMANN
 /MISSING SCOPE=ANALYSIS USERMISSING=EXCLUDE (15)
 /CRITERIA ALPHA=0.05 CILEVEL=95.
```

Hypothesis Test Summary

	Null Hypothesis	Test	Sig.	Decision
1	The distribution of Child's self-report immediately post intervention is the same across categories of staff-initiated intervention vs. usual care.	Independent-Samples Mann-Whitney U Test (16)	.023[1]	Reject the null hypothesis.
2	The distribution of Child's self-report immediately post intervention is the same across categories of staff-initiated intervention vs. usual care.	Independent-Samples Kolmogorov-Smirnov Test (17)	.400	Retain the null hypothesis.

Asymptotic significances are displayed. The significance level is .05.

[1]Exact significance is displayed for this test.

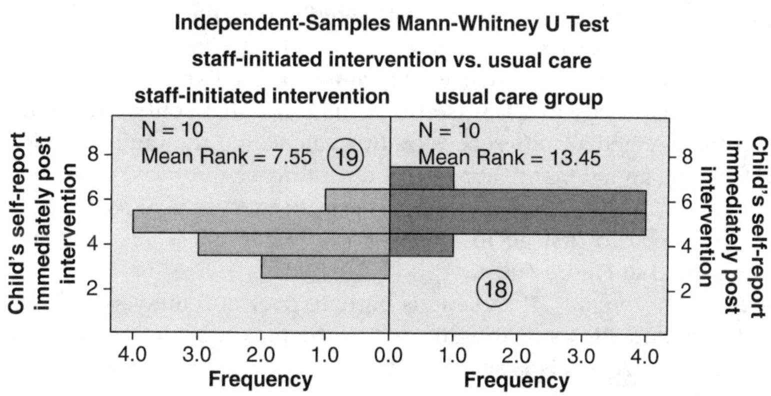

Total N		20
Mann-Whitney U	(20)	20.500
Wilcoxon W	(21)	75.500
Test Statistic		20.500
Standard Error		12.644
Standardized Test Statistic	(23)	-2.333
Asymptotic Sig. (2-sided test)		.020
Exact Sig. (2-sided test)	(22)	.023

Confidence Interval Summary

Confidence Interval Type	Parameter	Estimate	95% Confidence Interval	
			Lower	Upper
Independent-Samples Hodges-Lehman Median Difference	Difference between medians of Child's self-report immediately post intervention across categories of staff-initiated intervention vs. usual care.	1.000	.000	2.000 (24)

In SPSS for Windows, the exact two-tailed significance level of U is presented when the sample size is less than 30 (22). For larger sample sizes, a two-tailed z statistic with corrections for ties is used (23). If the sample were large with many ties, we might want to use the results obtained from the z statistic.

Because the sample size for this hypothetical study is small ($N = 20$), we will use the exact two-tailed significance level of U to determine the statistical significance of our test. Since the alternative hypothesis is directional, it will be necessary to divide this two-tailed p value in half to determine whether this p value is less than the prestated alpha level. In our hypothetical study, the one-tailed p value (.023/2 = .012) (22) is less than $\alpha = .05$. The null hypothesis that the two groups come from the same population therefore is rejected. We conclude, therefore, that the children in the staff-initiated intervention group had statistically significantly lower intensity of fatigue scores immediately postintervention than did the children in the usual-care group. This is the same conclusion that we reached when we calculated the Mann-Whitney test by hand.

The 95% Confidence Interval for the Differences in Medians

Figure 7.7 also provides us with the Hodges-Lehmann estimate and the 95% confidence interval for the difference in medians between the usual-care and staff-initiated intervention groups (24). Similar to what we calculated above, the median difference in scores between the two groups was presented as a 1 along with the lower (.000) and upper (2.000) limits of the 95% confidence interval for the median differences.

Earlier in this discussion, it was also pointed out that confidence intervals could be obtained for the median differences by first calculating the ranks for the raw data and then calculating an independent t test (and confidence intervals) on the ranks (Conover, 1999; Zimmerman, 2012). This is relatively easy to execute in SPSS for Windows. To rank the data, we need to first go to *Transform . . . Rank Cases. . . .* This opens the dialog boxes presented in Figure 7.8.

The *intensity_fatigue_T2* variable is brought over into the variable list (25). Clicking on the *Ties* button allows us to indicate that the rank assigned to ties will be the mean of the tied ranks (26). This is similar to the approach that we used in Table 7.10.

Figure 7.8 also presents the dialog boxes for obtaining the independent t test. This box was obtained by clicking on the following commands in the drop-down main menu: *Analyze . . . Compare Means . . . Independent-Samples T Test . . .* and bringing over the newly created rank of intensity of fatigue variable (*Rintensi*) into the test variable list (27). Our grouping variable will be the *Group* variable that has two levels: usual care (0) and staff-initiated intervention (1) (28). By clicking *OK . . .*, we are presented with the SPSS-generated output in Figure 7.9.

Figure 7.9 first presents us with the syntax that was used to generate the ranked intensity of fatigue variable for Time 2 (*Rintensi*) (29) and the independent t test. Notice that the "Means" of the rank of intensity of fatigue variable (30) is the same as the mean ranks (13.45 and 7.55) presented in Figure 7.7 (19). Next we are presented with the SPSS-generated output for the independent t test. Even though this is a textbook on nonparametric statistics, we need to briefly examine the meaning of the results of this t test. For the interested reader,

Figure 7.8 SPSS dialog boxes for ranking raw data and generating the 95% confidence interval for the median differences using the independent t test.

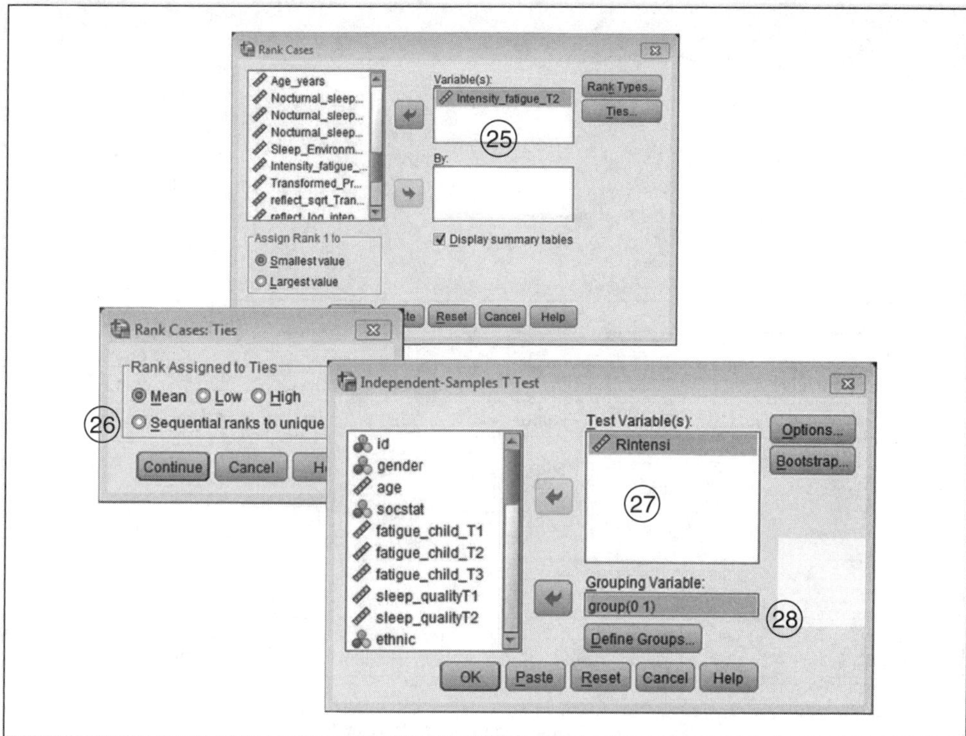

there are many useful texts that present easy-to-read but still in-depth discussions of this parametric test (e.g., Field (2013); Kellar and Kelvin (2012); Salkind (2012)).

The SPSS-generated output for the independent samples t test consists of two separate tests: *Levene's test for equality of variances* in the two groups (an important assumption of the t test) and the *t test for equality of means*. Let us assume that $\alpha = .05$. The null hypothesis for Levene's test of equality of variances is that the variances in two (or more) groups are equal. The alternative hypothesis is that the variances are not equal. Because it is a goodness-of-fit-test, we would prefer *not* to reject the null hypothesis ($p > \alpha$ or $p > .05$) so that we can examine the t test when *equal variances are assumed* (i.e., the t test presented on the first line of our t test output). If Levene's test is statistically significant ($p < .05$), then we cannot assume equal variances and must turn to the second row to obtain the t test for unequal variances.

Figure 7.9 indicates that the p value (*sig*) for Levene's test was .917 (31), which is clearly > .05. Our conclusion is that the variances for the two groups (usual care and staff-initiated intervention) are equal. The t test that we will examine, therefore, is one in which equal variances are assumed (i.e., row 1 of the output). That two-tailed significance is $p = .015$

Figure 7.9 SPSS output for generating ranked data and calculating a 95% confidence interval for the differences in medians using the independent *t* test.

```
***Data set: hospitalized children with cancer-20 cases***

RANK VARIABLES=Intensity_fatigue_T2 (A)
 /RANK
 /PRINT=YES
 /TIES=MEAN.

T-TEST GROUPS=group(0 1)
 /MISSING=ANALYSIS
 /VARIABLES=RIntensi
 /CRITERIA=CI(.95).
```

Created Variables[a]

Source Variable	Function	New Variable	Label
Intensity_fatigue_T2[b]	Rank	RIntensi (29)	Rank of Intensity_fatigue_T2

a. Mean rank of tied values is used for ties.
b. Ranks are in ascending order.

Group Statistics

	staff-initiated intervention vs. usual care	N	(30) Mean	std. Deviation	Std. Error Mean
Rank of Intensity_fatigue_T2	usual care group	10	13.45000	4.810001	1.521056
	staff-initiated intervention	10	7.55000	5.002499	1.581929

Independent Samples Test

		Levene's Test for Equality of Variances		t-test for Equality of Means						
									95% Confidence Interval of the Difference	
		F	Sig.	t	df	Sig. (2-tailed)	Mean Difference	Std. Error Difference	Lower	Upper
Rank of Intensity_fatigue_T2	Equal variances assumed	.011	.917 (31)	2.686	18	(32) .015	5.900000	2.194564	1.289392	10.510608
	Equal variances not assumed			2.686	17.972	.015	5.900000	2.194564	1.288884 (33)	10.511116

(one-tailed $p = .015/2 = .0075$) (32), which indicates that the usual-care group reported higher average ranks of intensity of fatigue immediately postintervention (13.45) than did the staff-initiated intervention.

While that conclusion supports our findings from the Mann-Whitney test, we are most interested in examining the 95% confidence interval for the difference in the mean ranks of the two groups, 1.29 and 10.51 (33). These two values indicate that the true difference in mean ranks in intensity of fatigue in the population lies between 1.29 and 10.51 with 95% probability. Since 0 (what the null hypothesis stated the differences in mean ranks to be) did not fall in that interval, we can reject the null hypothesis that there were no differences between the usual-care and staff-initiated intervention groups regarding the mean ranks of the intensity of fatigue variable immediately postintervention.

Figure 7.10 Results of the Internet-generated Mann-Whitney test.

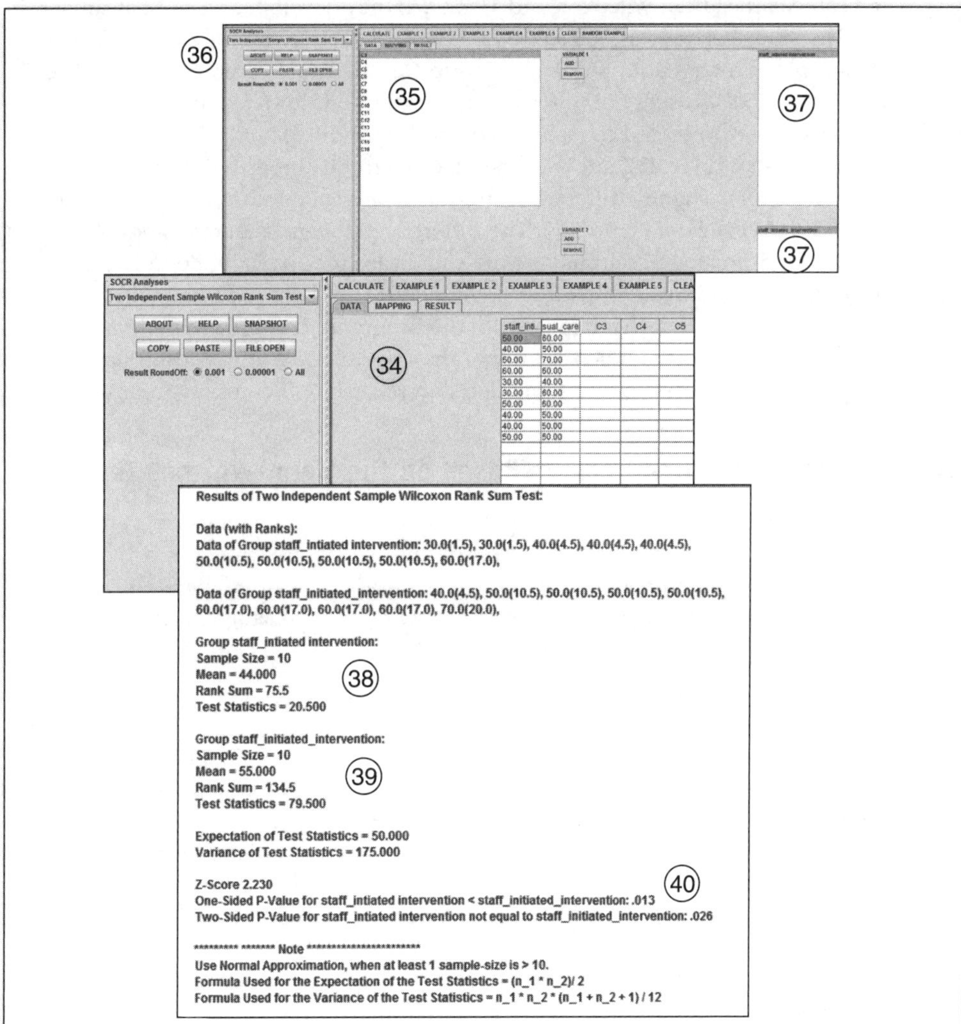

SOURCE: www.socr.ucla.edu/htmls/ana/TwoIndependentSampleWilcoxonRankSum_Analysis.html.

Internet Resources for Generating the Mann-Whitney Test

There are a number of open access Internet resources available to generate a Mann-Whitney test. Not many sites, however, will generate the $(1 - \alpha)\%$ confidence interval for the median difference between two groups. One website that currently provides a calculator for the Mann-Whitney test but not the confidence interval is www.socr.ucla.edu. Figure 7.10 presents the table from that website that we used to input the unranked intensity of fatigue data for the usual care (C1) and staff-initiated intervention groups (C2) (34). This dialog box was obtained by clicking on the *Mapping* button (35), selecting the independent samples Wilcoxon rank sum test (36) and *Adding* variables C1 and C2 into the analysis box (37).

Note that the resulting output in Figure 7.10 is that of the Wilcoxon rank sum test. As indicated earlier, both Wilcoxon and Mann Whitney developed this test at similar times with similar, though not always exact, results. Here we are given the output for Group C1 (the staff-initiated intervention) (38) and Group C2 (the usual-care group) (39). The *Rank Sum* (75.5) and *Test Statistics* (20.5) for Group C1 (the staff-initiated intervention group) are the same as those presented for the *Wilcoxon W* and the *Mann-Whitney U* in Figure 7.7 (20) (21). The z statistic (2.23) and one-sided p value for the median differences between C1 and C2 (.013) (40) is slightly different from our SPSS-generated z statistic (–2.33) and p value (.023/2 = .0115) from Figure 7.7. The difference in signs is understandable since Group 1 for the SPSS-generated output was the usual-care group (0) while the staff-initiated intervention group (1) was group C1 in Figure 7.10. The slight differences in the z statistic and p values, however, may have to do with the programs' handling of tied ranks and, perhaps, the website's use of the Wilcoxon rather than the Mann-Whitney test. Despite minor differences, both tests arrive at the same decision regarding the null hypothesis.

Obtaining an Effect Size Measure Based on the Mann-Whitney Test

There have been several suggested approaches to calculating effect size measures (and their confidence intervals) that are based on the Mann-Whitney test (Newcombe, 2006). An effect size that estimates the degree of separation between two frequency distributions can be obtained by dividing U by the product of the two sample sizes (Newcombe, 2006):

$$\text{Effect size}\ (\text{ES}) = \hat{\theta} = \frac{U}{(n_1)(n_2)}$$

In our example, our effect size equals .205 (20.5/100 = .205) since $U = 20.5$, and $n_1 = n_2 = 10$. To obtain a 95% confidence interval for this degree of separation between the two frequency distributions (staff-initiated intervention vs. usual-care group), Newcombe (2006) refers the reader to an Excel program on his website. Because websites change often, the interested reader is referred to the Cardiff University website (www.cardiff.ac.uk; type in Prof. Robert Newcombe's name or use http://medicine.cf.ac.uk/person/prof-robert-gordon-newcombe/research/) and, hopefully, you will be referred to Newcombe's "Resources" page. There you will find several Excel files that can be used to generate confidence intervals for the Mann-Whitney U.

Table 7.13 presents the results of calculating the effect size and its confidence interval for the Mann-Whitney U using Newcombe's Excel file. According to this output, with an

Table 7.13 Calculation of the Effect Size and Confidence Interval for the Mann-Whitney *U* Statistic

Spreadsheet GENERALISEDMW.

This spreadsheet calculates confidence limits for theta = U/mn by 40 interval bisections.

Uses method 5 of Newcombe RG (2006).

Confidence intervals for an effect size measure based on the Mann-Whitney statistic

Part 2: Asymptotic methods and evaluation. Statistics in Medicine 25, 559-573.

The spreadsheet displays point and interval estimates on both theta and delta (corresponding standardised difference) scales.

Displays Gaussian curves separated by delta hat, delta lower and delta upper SDs.

Degrees of separation beyond .000001 < theta < .999999 (corresponding to |delta| > 6.7224) are displayed truncated to this degree of separation.

To use, replace input values for **m**, **n** and **U/mn** in **bold** as appropriate.

Calculated U/mn from SPSS etc. can be pasted into cell F20.

Two-sided confidence level required		**95%**	
Data: m = 10		**n = 10**	**U/mn = 0.2050**
		Corresponding U = 20.5	
		Confidence limits	
Results:	**Point estimate**	**Lower**	**Upper**
Theta	0.2050	0.0772	0.4635
Delta	−1.1652	−2.0138	−.1297

SOURCE: Professor Robert Newcombe at Cardiff University, http://medicine.cf.ac.uk/primary-care-public-health/resources/

effect size of .205 and a sample size of 10 in each group, our 95% confidence interval for our effect size would be .077 to .464. How would we interpret this effect size and confidence interval? Since θ can range between 0 and .99 (Table 7.13), we could treat these results like the phi coefficient (Table 7.7) and conclude that, at best, the effect size for the differences between the distributions is weak.

Presentation of Results

Table 7.14 is a suggested presentation of the results of the Mann-Whitney test. Note that we have presented the z statistic from Figure 7.7 (–2.33) and the one-tailed p value for that z statistic (p = .023/two-tailed = .011). Because the sample size is less than 30, it would also be possible to omit the z statistic and simply present the p value for the U statistic, as we did for Fisher's exact test (Table 7.4). These data could also be interpreted and presented in the text as follows:

> The results of the Mann-Whitney test indicate that the 10 hospitalized children in the staff-initiated intervention group reported statistically significantly lower intensity of fatigue immediately postintervention than the 10 children in the usual-care group ($z = -2.33$, one-tailed $p = .01$). The effect size of the differences in the two distributions was weak ($\theta = .205$, 95% CI: .08–.46).

Table 7.14 Suggested Presentation of Mann-Whitney Test Results

	Staff-Initiated Intervention			*Usual Care*			*Mann-Whitney*[a]	
	N	*Mean*	*Median*	N	*Mean*	*Median*	z	p[b]
Intensity of fatigue immediately postintervention	10	4.4	4.5	10	5.0	5.0	−2.33	.011

[a]Effect size (θ) = .205; 95% CI: .08, .46.

[b]The p value is for a one-tailed test.

Advantages, Limitations, and Alternatives to the Mann-Whitney Test

The Mann-Whitney test is a very powerful test, especially when the outcome data being analyzed have a nonnormal distribution with outliers. Relative to the independent t test, the Mann-Whitney test has excellent asymptotic efficiency, especially when the sample sizes are equal (Gibbons & Chakraborti, 1991; Hettmansperger, 1984). This means that as the sample size increases, it quickly approaches the power of the independent t test. Siegel and Castellan (1988) indicate that when the Mann-Whitney test is applied to data that meet the assumptions of the t test, the power efficiency of the Mann-Whitney test approaches 95.5% as N increases and is close to 95% for moderate-size samples. This means that, even with moderate or small sample sizes, the Mann-Whitney test is nearly as powerful as the independent t test in being able to correctly reject the null hypothesis.

The parametric counterpart to the Mann-Whitney test is the independent t test. As indicated, the independent t test is more powerful than the Mann-Whitney test when the assumptions for this parametric test are met. When the assumptions are not met (e.g., the data are not distributed normally), the Mann-Whitney test is the more powerful test, especially when the tails of the distribution are heavy and there are outliers present in the data (Conover, 1999; Zimmerman & Zumbo, 1993). It is also important that the two distributions are similar except for differences in position. Fagerland and Sandvik (2009) caution about the lack of robustness of the Mann-Whitney test, especially when the two distributions have different degrees of skewness.

A nonparametric alternative that could be used if the shapes of the distributions are not similar is the median test (Chapter 8). When the distributions are similar, however, the median test is not as powerful as the Mann-Whitney test. Alternatively, the nonparametric permutation test is a flexible alternative that compares two populations (Butar & Park, 2008; Collingridge, 2013; Good, 1995, 2005). These tests are especially useful when the distribution of the dependent variable in the population is unknown. Permutation tests were originally proposed by R. A. Fisher (1935) but were found to be quite cumbersome computationally for all but small samples. Recently, however, these tests have become more popular thanks to the availability of inexpensive powerful computers.

A *t* test on the ranks of the data is also a useful alternative to the Mann-Whitney test. Zimmerman (2012), however, warns about the accuracy of this rank-order procedure. In a set of simulations comparing the Wilcoxon-Mann-Whitney with the rank transformations and *t* tests, Zimmerman reported that the decision to accept/reject the null hypothesis and resulting *p* values were dependent on the sample size, significance level, and the shape of the distributions.

Examples From Published Research

Ackerman, I. N., Ademi, Z., Osborne, R. H., & Liew, D. (2013). Comparison of health-related quality of life, work status, and health care utilization and costs according to hip and knee joint disease severity: A national Australian study. *Physical Therapy, 93*(7), 889–899. doi: 10.2522/ptj.20120423

Becker, P. T., Grunwald, P. C, Moorman, J., & Stuhr, S. (1993). Effects of developmental care on behavioral organization in very low birth weight infants. *Nursing Research, 42,* 214–220.

Fallin, A., Johnson, A. O., Riker, C., Cohen, E., Rayens, M. K., & Hahn, E. J. (2013). An intervention to increase compliance with a tobacco-free university policy. *American Journal of Health Promotion, 27*(3), 162–169. doi: 10.4278/ajhp.110707-QUAN-275

McIntosh, C. G., Tonkin, S. L., & Gunn, A. J. (2013). Randomized controlled trial of a car safety seat insert to reduce hypoxia in term infants. *Pediatrics, 132*(2), 326–331. doi: 10.1542/peds.2013-0127

McMurdo, M. E., & Rennie, L. M. (1994). Improvements in quadriceps strength with regular seated exercise in the institutionalized elderly. *Archives of Physical Medicine and Rehabilitation, 75,* 600–603.

Summary

In this chapter, we have examined three nonparametric tests that can be used when the independent variable is at the nominal level of measurement: Fisher's exact test, the chi-square test for two independent samples, and the Wilcoxon-Mann-Whitney *U* test (also called the Mann-Whitney test). We have also seen how another two-sample test, the Kolmogorov-Smirnov test, can be used to assess the similarity of shapes of distributions and examined two different approaches to obtaining a confidence interval for differences in medians between two independent samples.

Both Fisher's exact test and the chi-square test for two independent samples are used when the dependent variable is categorical. Fisher's exact test is used with 2×2 contingency tables, whereas the chi-square test is useful for $2 \times k$ contingency tables. Neither of these two tests has a parametric alternative because the data being examined are categorical.

When the data are at least ordinal level of measurement, the Mann-Whitney test is preferred because it is sensitive to order in the data. This is a test for independent samples for which the dependent variable is at least at the ordinal level of measurement. The Mann-Whitney test is a very powerful test and is almost as powerful as its parametric counterpart, the independent *t* test. It is a particularly useful test when the data do not meet the assumptions of a *t* test, especially when the sample is small, the group sizes are unequal, and/or the tails of the distributions are large. One of the assumptions of a Mann-Whitney test, however, is that the distributions of the two independent samples are similar in shape. When this assumption is not met, the median test can be used in its place.

The next chapter extends discussion to nonparametric tests that can be used when the independent variable has more than two levels. The four tests that will be examined are the chi-square test for *k* independent samples, the Mantel-Haenszel chi-square test for ordered categories, the median test, and the Kruskal-Wallis one-way ANOVA.

TEST YOUR KNOWLEDGE

Here is a "test" of your knowledge on the main points regarding the various nonparametric statistics that have been discussed in this chapter. You will want to reread the chapter should you find that you cannot recall their content.

1. What are the main differences between Fisher's exact test, the chi-square test for two independent samples, and the Mann-Whitney test, and when would you consider using each of these nonparametric tests?
2. What are the critical assumptions of each of these three nonparametric tests? Did the distress and intensity of fatigue data that were used in this chapter meet those assumptions?
3. What are the advantages/disadvantages to each of these two tests, and what nonparametric/parametric tests might you use instead?
4. Why was it necessary to increase the sample size for the chi-square test for two independent samples?
5. Why is it that we only looked at one point in time (immediately following the intervention) in order to compare the usual-care and staff-initiated intervention groups? What could we have done if we had wanted to use a pre-post intervention comparison between the two groups?

COMPUTER EXERCISES

The following computer exercises should enable you to build on your skills in using SPSS for Windows, Excel, and/or Internet-based programs.

1. Using either the SPSS for Windows data set (hospitalized children with cancer-20 cases.sav) or the Excel spreadsheet (hospitalized children with cancer-20 cases.xlsx) made available to you at study.sagepub.com/pett2e, undertake Fisher's exact test, the chi-square test for two

independent samples for the preintervention distress (*distressed_T1*), and the Mann-Whitney test for the preintervention intensity of fatigue (*intensity_fatigue*_T1) variables using the variable, *Group,* as the independent variable. Set a two-tailed alpha at .05.

a. Looking at your results in Question 1, what was your decision with regard to the null hypotheses for these three tests?
b. Compare the results that you have obtained for the preintervention variables with those of the immediate postintervention variables as detailed in this chapter. Were the pre- and postintervention results different or similar? What conclusions would you draw from your results?

2. A group of researchers was interested in examining the impact of a daily automated telephone intervention to improve glycemic control and lower perceived severity of diabetes in older overweight women with Type 2 diabetes. A convenience sample of 40 overweight women with Type 2 diabetes (ages 50 and older) were recruited from a primary care clinic at an urban medical center in the Intermountain West. The 40 women were randomly assigned in equal numbers to either the telephone intervention ($n = 20$) or usual-care group ($n = 20$). The duration of the telephone intervention was 90 days.
3. Prior to the telephone intervention (Time 1) and upon completion of the study (Time 2), all participants were asked to indicate the approximate number of days that they had experienced being on "the blood sugar rollercoaster" (i.e., fluctuating blood sugars from too high to too low and vice versa) in the previous two weeks. The researchers hypothesized that those women who participated in the automated telephone intervention would report a decrease in the number of days of being on the blood sugar rollercoaster than would the usual-care group. The data set that you can use for this analysis is Type II diabetes.sav (or Type II diabetes.xlsx) which can be found on the SAGE website, study.sagepub.com/pett2e.

a. Using SPSS for Windows (or Excel), create a variable that reflects the differences between the participants' number of rollercoaster days at Time 1 versus Time 2 (e.g., Days_on_coaster__Diff = Days_on_coaster_T1 − Days on_coaster_T2). What nonparametric statistical test would you use to analyze these data?
b. State the null and alternative hypotheses for this analysis.
c. Is this a one- or a two-tailed test? Please justify your answer.
d. Using the SPSS for Windows data set provided to you undertake your analysis of these data using $\alpha = .05$. Alternatively, use an available website (e.g., http://www.socr.ucla.edu) to undertake your analyses using the Excel data from the SAGE website (Type II diabetes.xlsx).
e. Rank the difference scores and, using an independent *t* test, generate the 95% confidence interval for the differences in the ranked Roller_coaster_Diff scores. Based on the results you have obtained, did the telephone intervention have an effect on lowering of the number of blood sugar rollercoaster days compared to the usual-care group? Justify your answer.
f. Create a table and written paragraph that would reflect your results.

(Continued)

(Continued)

4. In the same study that was described in Question 2 (Type II diabetes.sav), the participants were asked at the conclusion of the intervention whether they had needed insulin during the 14-day intervention period. The following table presents the responses of the women in the two groups, automated telephone intervention and usual-care groups, regarding their need for insulin.

	Group		
Need for Insulin?	*Automated Telephone*	*Usual Care*	*Total*
Yes	7	14	22
No	13	6	18
Total	20	20	40

   a. Enter these data into an SPSS for Windows data file (or Excel spreadsheet). If you are having trouble entering the data, you can find the variables in the Type II data sets listed in Question 3.
   b. What nonparametric statistical test would you use to analyze these data?
   c. State the null and alternative hypotheses for this analysis.
   d. Is this a one- or a two-tailed test? Please justify your answer.
   e. Using SPSS for Windows, another statistical package of your choosing, Excel, or an alternative website (e.g., www.vassarstats.net), undertake your analysis of these data using $\alpha = .05$. Be sure to obtain the standardized residuals and phi coefficient for these data.
   f. What are the actual and critical values of your statistical test? Based on those values, what is your decision relative to your null hypothesis?
   g. What do the standardized residuals tell you about your results (i.e., which group had the greater need for insulin during the intervention period)?
   h. Interpret your phi coefficient.
   i. Create a table and written paragraph that would reflect your results.

Visit **study.sagepub.com/pett2e** to access SAS output, SPSS datasets, SAS datasets, and SAS examples.

CHAPTER 8

Assessing Differences Among Several Independent Groups

- Chi-square test for *k* independent samples
- Mantel-Haenszel chi-square test for trends
- Median test
- Kruskal-Wallis one-way ANOVA test by ranks
- Two-way ANOVA by ranks

In Chapter 7, we examined nonparametric tests that would be suitable when the independent variable was dichotomous and the dependent variable was at any level of measurement. When the dependent variable is categorical, the Fisher's exact test or the chi-square test for two independent samples can be used. When it is at least ordinal level of measurement, the Mann-Whitney test is the test of choice.

In all forms of health care research, there are often more than two independent groups that are being compared. Subjects may be assigned randomly to one of three intervention conditions, or three patient groups having different diagnoses may be compared with regard to an outcome variable. A second independent categorical variable such as gender or intervention group might also be included. If the dependent variable is continuous and there are nominal-level independent variables, the parametric tests that are commonly used to assess such data are one- and two-way ANOVAs (analyses of variance). A number of assumptions, however, are associated with the F statistics generated from these tests that potentially could be violated. For example, within each of the independent groups, there may be unequal cell sizes. Perhaps the dependent variable is not normally distributed or the variances are not equal. The dependent variable may also be at less than the interval level of measurement, or the researcher may want to generalize beyond a normally distributed population. If these are issues, the researcher may want to consider nonparametric alternatives to the available parametric tests.

In this chapter, we will examine some nonparametric statistics for more than two independent groups. Five tests will be presented in detail: the chi-square test for *k* independent groups, the Mantel-Haenszel chi-square test for ordered categories, the median test, the Kruskal-Wallis one-way ANOVA by ranks, and the two-way ANOVA by ranks. We will also examine ways to assess strength of association for these tests and determine the influences of different cells when faced with significant results.

THE CHI-SQUARE TEST FOR *K* INDEPENDENT SAMPLES

In Chapter 7, we examined a chi-square test for two independent samples. For this test, the independent variable was nominal level of measurement but dichotomous, and the dependent variable was also nominal with two or more levels. The chi-square test for *k* independent samples is merely an extension of this test. It can be used when *both* the independent and dependent variables are nominal, typically with more than two levels. This test also can be used when the researcher wants to examine the effects of several independent variables (e.g., gender and diagnosis) on a nominal-level outcome variable (e.g., posthospital adjustment: poor, moderate, or excellent). Some researchers would argue that posthospital adjustment has order to its categories and therefore should be treated as an ordinal-level variable. This particular variable has been deliberately selected for analysis in this example so that we can compare the results obtained from the chi-square test with those of the Mantel-Haenszel chi-square test. The latter test takes advantage of the ordered categories.

An Appropriate Research Question for the Chi-Square Test

The chi-square test for *k* independent samples (referred to herein as the *chi-square test*) is one of the most popular nonparametric tests and has been used in a myriad of studies. For example, this test was used by Kothari, Zielinski, James, Charoth, and Luz (2014) to examine the effects of a Healthy Start Program on birth weights of racially diverse infants. Stork, Brown, Reilly, Secreti, and Brown (2006) used both the chi-square for independent samples and the Mantel-Haenszel chi-square test for trends in their investigation of emergency department treatment of viral gastritis in children using two different intravenous medications.

In our hypothetical study, we might be interested in assessing the relationship between the hospitalized child's cancer diagnosis (solid tumor, acute myeloid leukemia, lymphoma, or sarcoma) with the nurses' assessments of the child's sleep quality immediately postintervention (poor, moderate, very good). While it could be argued that the sleep quality variable is measured at the ordinal level, we will be treating it as a nominal-level variable. Given these two nominal-level variables, the following research question would be appropriate for use with a chi-square test:

> What is the relationship between a child's cancer diagnosis (solid tumor, acute myeloid leukemia, lymphoma, or sarcoma) and the nurse's assessment of the child's sleep quality immediately postintervention (poor, moderate, or very good)?

To evaluate this relationship, let us assume that we have collected data on 72 hospitalized children with cancer who have been randomly assigned to either the staff-initiated intervention or a usual-care group. Why do we now have 72 children and not the 20 and 30 children discussed in previous chapters? The reason for the increase in sample size is that, as you will see shortly, with a smaller sample, we would not have met a critical assumption related to the expected values of the chi-square test for *k* independent samples. These data (hospitalized children with cancer-72 cases.sav) can be found on the SAGE website (study.sagepub.com/pett2e).

Null and Alternative Hypotheses

Table 8.1 presents examples of possible null and alternative hypotheses generated from our research question that would be suitable for use with a chi-square test. Note that, like the chi-square test for two independent samples (Chapter 7), these hypotheses address independence of variables and are nondirectional.

Table 8.1 Example of Null and Alternative Hypothesis Suitable for Use With the Chi-Square Test for *k* Independent Samples

Null Hypothesis
H_0: There is no association between a child's cancer diagnosis and a nurse's assessment of the child's sleep quality immediately postintervention; that is, the two variables, cancer diagnosis and the child's sleep quality, are independent.
Alternative Hypothesis
H_a: There is an association between a child's cancer diagnosis and a nurse's assessment of the child's sleep quality immediately postintervention; that is, the two variables, cancer diagnosis and the child's sleep quality, are associated.

Overview of the Procedure

The chi-square test for *k* independent samples proceeds in the same way as the chi-square two-sample test from Chapter 7. First, the frequency data are placed into an $r \times c$ contingency table where r = the number of levels of the independent variable and c = the number of levels of the dependent variable. In our hypothetical example, because there are four levels for the cancer diagnosis variable and three levels for the sleep quality variable, ours would be a 4×3 contingency table. Table 8.2 presents the data for our diagnosis and sleep quality data.

Next, using the formula outlined in Chapter 7, the number of cases that would be expected in each of the cells if the null hypothesis of independence of variables were true is calculated. From these data, a chi-square statistic (χ^2) is generated by

Table 8.2 The 4 × 3 Contingency Table Used to Examine the Association Between Hospitalized Children's Cancer Diagnosis and Postintervention Sleep Quality Immediately Postintervention Using the Chi-Square Test for *k* Independent Samples

	Post-intervention Sleep Quality						
	Poor		*Moderate*		*Very good*		
Cancer diagnosis	*Observed*	*Expected*	*Observed*	*Expected*	*Observed*	*Expected*	*Total*
Solid tumor	4	6.33	8	6.60	7	6.07	19
Acute myeloid leukemia	8	6.00	5	6.25	5	5.75	18
Lymphoma	6	6.33	2	6.59	11	6.07	19
Sarcoma	6	5.33	10	5.56	0	5.11	16
Total	24		25		23		72

(1) Exp = (R*C) /N =(19*23)/72 = 6.07

comparing the observed frequencies with the expected frequencies in each cell using the following formula:

$$\chi^2 = \sum_{i=1}^{r} \sum_{j=1}^{c} \frac{(Obs_{ij} - Exp_{ij})^2}{Exp_{ij}}$$

where

Obs_{ij} = the observed number of cases for a cell in the *i*th row and *j*th column,

Exp_{ij} = the expected number of cases for the same cell if the null hypothesis were true,

Exp_{ij} = (Row total*Column Total)/Total *N* of cases = $(R)*(C)/N$, and

$\Sigma\Sigma$ = a double summation of the fraction across all rows (r) and columns (c).

If the data meet the assumptions of the chi-square test, this generated χ^2 statistic is distributed as a χ^2 with $(r - 1)(c - 1)$ degrees of freedom. The null hypothesis of independence of variables is rejected in favor of the alternative hypothesis if the generated χ^2 is greater than the critical value of the χ^2 at the specified alpha level and designated number of degrees of freedom. Alternatively, in examination of a computer printout, the null hypothesis is rejected if the generated significance level (p) is less than alpha (e.g., $\alpha = .05$).

Calculating the chi-square test for the diagnosis and sleep quality data.

Table 8.2 presents the observed and expected values obtained for the diagnosis and sleep quality data generated for the 72 hospitalized children. Notice that the expected number of children in the lymphoma/very good sleep quality was 6.07 (i.e., Exp = $(R^*C)/N$ = (19*23)/72 = 6.07) ①. The expected values for all of the 12 cells could easily be calculated in the same manner.

Once the observed and expected values for each cell in Table 8.2 have been obtained, a chi-square test can easily be calculated:

$$\chi^2 = \sum_{i=1}^{r}\sum_{j=1}^{c} \frac{(Obs_{ij} - Exp_{ij})^2}{Exp_{ij}} = \frac{(4-6.33)^2}{6.33} + \frac{(8-6.60)^2}{6.60} + \frac{(7-6.07)^2}{6.07} + \ldots + \frac{(10-5.56)^2}{5.56} + \frac{(0-5.11)^2}{5.11}$$

$$= 0.859 + 0.298 + 0.142 + \ldots + 3.556 + 5.111 = 18.292$$

To determine whether there is an association between cancer diagnosis and sleep quality, we would need to compare the actual value of our chi-square statistic with that of the critical value at a given level of alpha (e.g., $\alpha = .05$) and the degrees of freedom for our table. Since ours is a table with four rows and three columns, our degrees of freedom would be $(r - 1)(c - 1)$ or $(4 - 1)(3 - 1) = 6$. Our decision rule, therefore, is that we will reject the null hypothesis of no association between the two nominal-level variables if and only if our actual χ^2 is greater than a critical value of a χ^2 with $df = 6$.

The critical value of a χ^2 with $df = 6$ can be found in Appendix A, Table 2. After locating the row for our degrees of freedom (e.g., $df = 6$), we would then proceed across to the column where the cumulative probability = .95 (remember, we are looking for the critical value of the χ^2 such that .05 lies to the *right* of that critical value, or 1 – .95 = .05). That critical value would be 12.6. Given that our actual χ^2, 18.292, is larger than the critical value of the χ^2, we will reject the null hypothesis and conclude that there is an association between type of cancer diagnosis and postintervention sleep quality of the hospitalized children.

Critical Assumptions of the Chi-Square Test

The critical assumptions of the chi-square test for *k* independent samples are similar to those for the chi-square test for two independent samples in Chapter 7.

1. *Both the independent and dependent variables are categorical.*
2. *The data consist of frequencies, not scores.*
3. *Each randomly selected observation can be classified into only one category for the independent variable(s) and only one category for the dependent variable. There are no repeated observations and no multiple response categories.*

Our data partially meet all three of these assumptions because the two variables, type of cancer diagnosis and postintervention sleep quality, are categorical, and the data consist of frequencies that occupy mutually exclusive categories. The data which were drawn from a sample of convenience were randomly assigned to the treatment conditions. As was pointed out in Chapter 7, we will want to assess the extent to which our results are generalizable.

4. *If the degrees of freedom are greater than 1, no more than 20% of the cells may have expected frequencies of less than 5, and no cell should have an expected frequency of less than 1.*

The rule given in Assumption 4 is particularly important for a contingency table that is larger than 2 × 2. For example, in order for a 4 × 3 table to meet this rule, the total sample size must be at least 60 subjects if the marginal totals for all levels of the independent and dependent variables are equal. It would be larger if the marginal totals are not equal. Notice, too, that this assumption addresses *expected values,* not observed values.

In our hypothetical study, we started out with only 20 subjects. With such a small sample size, we would clearly fail to meet this important rule. If the data do not meet this rule, a possible solution would be to create a smaller table by combining the cells of the dependent and/or independent variables. For example, we might collapse our categorical variables to *poor* versus *good* sleep quality. The decision to collapse certain cells must be undertaken carefully so that the combined cells make intuitive sense given the research questions of the study.

Because this is a hypothetical study, we have the liberty of increasing our sample size without worrying about its consequences (e.g., cost and feasibility). Let us assume instead that there were 72 children enrolled in the study. These data can be found on the SAGE website (study.sagepub.com/pett2e hospitalized children with cases-72 cases.sav). This larger sample size increases the likelihood that the rule in Assumption 4 will be met. This assumption will be assessed in detail when we examine the computer printouts.

Computer Commands

Figure 8.1 presents the SPSS for Windows commands that are used to generate the chi-square test for *k* independent samples. This dialog box is opened by clicking on *Analyze . . . Descriptive Statistics . . . Crosstabs* in the menu. To obtain the chi-square test, the *Statistics* box is opened and the desired statistics are selected (e.g., *Chi-Square tests* to assess independence and *Cramér's V* to evaluate the strength of association (2)). Additional cell information (e.g., observed and expected frequencies and standardized residuals (3)) can be obtained by opening the *Cells* dialog box.

Note in Figure 8.1 that the row variable in this hypothetical example is the independent variable, cancer diagnosis (*type_of_cancer*) (4), whereas the column variable is the dependent variable, nurses' assessments of the children's postintervention sleep quality (*sleep_quality_T2*) (5). A second independent variable, such as gender, could have been

Figure 8.1 SPSS for Windows (v. 22–23) dialog boxes used to generate a chi-square test for *k* independent samples.

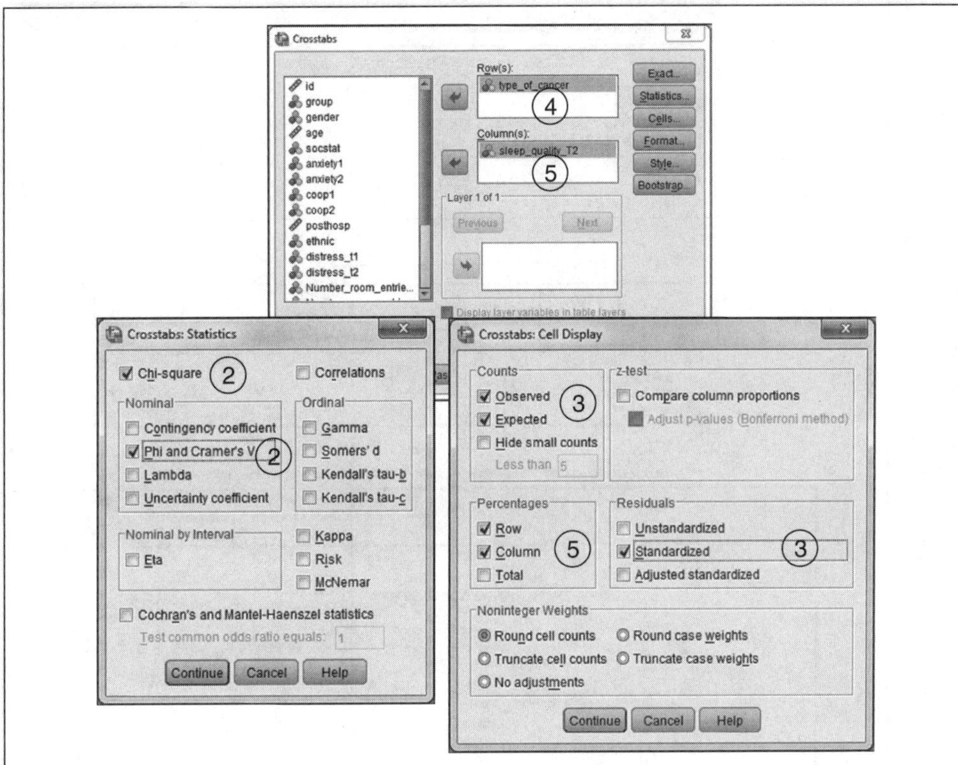

selected by clicking on the variable *gender* and moving it into the *Layer* box. It is important, however, to be parsimonious regarding layers, because each additional independent variable will increase sample size requirements.

Computer-Generated Output

Figure 8.2 presents the syntax commands and computer-generated printout from SPSS for Windows (v. 22–23) for the chi-square test for the 72 children in our hypothetical study. Because our syntax commands (6) were nearly identical to those for the chi-square test for two independent samples, this printout is very similar to that presented in Chapter 7.

First, we are given *Case Processing Summary,* which indicates the number of valid and missing cases that we have for this analysis. For this analysis, we have 72 cases (7) with no missing values. Next, we are presented with a crosstabs table that presents the

Figure 8.2 SPSS for Windows (v. 22–23) generated output for the chi-square test for *k* independent samples.

Data set: hospitalized children with cancer-72 cases.sav

(6)

```
CROSSTABS
/TABLES=type_of_cancer BY sleep_quality_T2
/FORMAT=AVALUE TABLES
/STATISTICS=CHISQ PHI
/CELLS=COUNT EXPECTED ROW COLUMN SRESID
/COUNT ROUND CELL.
```

Case Processing Summary

	Cases					
	Valid		Missing		Total	
	N	Percent	N	Percent	N	Percent
type of cancer of the child * sleep quality immediately following intervention	(7) 72	100.0%	0	0.0%	72	100.0%

type of cancer of the child * sleep quality immediately following intervention Crosstabulation

			sleep quality immediately following intervention			
			Poor sleep quality	Moderate sleep quality	Very good sleep quality	Total
type of cancer of the child	solid tumor	Count	4	8	7	19
	(8)	Expected Count	6.3	6.6	6.1	19.0
		% within type of cancer of the child	21.1%	42.1%	36.8%	100.0%
		% within sleep quality immediately following intervention	16.7%	32.0%	30.4%	26.4%
		Std. Residual	-.9	.5	.4	
	acute myeloid leukemia	Count	8	5	5	18
		Expected Count	6.0	6.3	5.8	18.0
		% within type of cancer of the child	44.4%	27.8%	27.8%	100.0%
		% within sleep quality immediately following intervention	33.3%	20.0%	21.7%	25.0%
		Std. Residual	.8	-.5	-.3	
	lymphoma	Count	6	2	(9) 11	19
		Expected Count	6.3	6.6	6.1	19.0
		% within type of cancer of the child	31.6%	10.5%	(10) 57.9%	100.0%
		% within sleep quality immediately following intervention	25.0%	8.0%	(11) 47.8%	26.4%
		Std. Residual	-.1	-1.8	(16) 2.0	
	sarcoma	Count	6	10	0	16
		Expected Count	5.3	5.6	5.1	16.0
		% within type of cancer of the child	37.5%	62.5%	0.0%	100.0%
		% within sleep quality immediately following intervention	25.0%	40.0%	0.0%	22.2%
		Std. Residual	.3	1.9	(17) -2.3	
Total		Count	24	25	23	72
		Expected Count	24.0	25.0	23.0	72.0
		% within type of cancer of the child	33.3%	34.7%	31.9%	100.0%
		% within sleep quality immediately following intervention	100.0%	100.0%	100.0%	100.0%

Chi-Square Tests

	Value	df	Asymp. Sig. (2-sided)
Pearson Chi-Square	18.292[a]	6	.006
Likelihood Ratio (13)	23.207	6	(14) .001
Linear-by-Linear Association	1.572	1	.210
N of Valid Cases	72		

a. 0 cells (0.0%) have expected count less than 5. The minimum expected count is 5.11. (12)

Symmetric Measures

		Value	Approx. Sig.
Nominal by Nominal	Phi	.504	.006
(15)	Cramer's V	.356	.006
N of Valid Cases		72	

actual frequency (*Count*) for each cell (8), the expected frequency for the cell under the null hypothesis of independence of variables (*Expected Count*), the percentages expressed in terms of row totals (*% within type of cancer of the child)*, column totals (*% within sleep quality immediately following the intervention*), and, finally, the standardized residuals (*Std. Residual*). For example, in row 3, column 3, there are 11 children (9) who have been diagnosed with lymphoma whose nurse reported that the child appeared to have very good postintervention sleep quality. The expected value for any cell is the product of the cell's row and column totals divided by the total sample size. For the cell that occupies row 3, column 3, we would have expected (19)(23)/72 = 6.1 children to occupy that cell if the null hypothesis of independence of variables were true. The difference between the actual frequency (11) and the expected value (6.1) suggests that the two variables, type of cancer diagnosis and sleep quality immediately postintervention, may not be independent.

Additional cell information can be gleaned from the printout. For example, looking at the row percentage for that same cell (10), 57.9% or 11 of the 19 hospitalized children who had been diagnosed with lymphoma were rated by their nurses to have had "very good" sleep quality following the intervention. Concerning the column percentages for that same cell (11), 47.8% or 11 of the 23 children who were rated by their nurses as having "very good" sleep quality immediately postintervention were children with a cancer diagnosis of lymphoma.

We can now examine the printout to determine the extent to which we have met Assumption 4: with $df > 1$, no more than 20% of the cells may have expected frequencies less than 5. The computer printout in Figure 8.2 indicates that 0 cells (0.0%) have expected frequencies of less than 5 (12). Given that we have met the requirement of Assumption 4, we will proceed with the test. Had we not met that assumption, we could have collapsed some cells so that we had a 3 × 3 table instead. The problem, however, would be that the collapsing of cells would need to make intuitive sense. Would it make sense, for example, to collapse solid tumors and lymphomas together even if their distributions regarding sleep quality were somewhat similarly distributed?

The generated χ^2 statistic can now be examined to determine whether the null hypothesis of independence of variables should be rejected. We had decided earlier that we would reject the null hypothesis of no association between the two variables since the actual χ^2 value presented in Figure 8.2 (18.292) (13) exceeds the critical value of our χ^2 (12.6) given in Appendix A, Table 2 for $df = 6$ and $\alpha = .05$. This decision is confirmed since the nondirectional p value for this calculated χ^2 statistic, .006 (14), is less than $\alpha = .05$. The conclusion to be reached, therefore, is that there is a significant association between the children's cancer diagnosis and nurses' evaluations of the children's sleep quality immediately postintervention; that is, the two variables, type of cancer of the child and children's sleep quality immediately following the intervention, are dependent.

Determining the Strength and Meaning of a Significant Association

The chi-square test is nondirectional. It tells us whether or not the variables under consideration are associated but tells us nothing about the strength of the association or which cells appear to be influencing the outcome observed. The Cramér's V statistic (Chapter 7) enables the reader to determine the strength of the association between the variables. There are two other useful approaches to ascertaining which cells have the most impact on the outcome: (1) examination of the standardized residuals (Hinkle, Wiersma, & Jurs, 2003) and (2) partitioning the $r \times c$ contingency table into smaller 2×2 independent subtables to determine where the differences are occurring (Siegel & Castellan, 1988).

Determining strength of association.

Once a significant association has been found between two categorical variables via the chi-square test, the next task is to determine the strength of this relationship. The computer printout in Figure 8.2 reports two measures of association: the phi coefficient and Cramér's V statistic. The phi coefficient is used for 2×2 tables, and Cramér's V statistic is used for contingency tables that are larger than 2×2. As indicated in Chapter 7, the formula for Cramér's V statistic is

$$V = \sqrt{\chi^2 / N(L - 1)}$$

where

χ^2 = the generated chi-square statistic,

N = the total number of cases,

L = the minimum number of rows or columns in the contingency table.

This Cramér statistic ranges from 0 to 1, where 0 implies no relationship and 1 a perfect relationship. Its significance level will be the same as for the χ^2 statistic.

The computer printout in Figure 8.2 indicates that Cramér's $V = .356$ (15). That is,

$$V = \sqrt{\chi^2 / \mathrm{N}(\mathrm{L} - 1)} = \sqrt{18.292 / 72(3 - 1)} = .356$$

Using the guidelines outlined in Chapter 7 (Table 7.7) for the strength of association for the phi/Cramér's V coefficient, we would conclude that the strength of the relationships between type of cancer diagnosis and quality of sleep immediately postintervention is weak.

Determining cell influences: Examining residuals.

There are several approaches to determining which cells most strongly influence the χ^2 value. One of the easiest approaches is to examine the sizes of the standardized residuals for each cell (see Chapter 7 for details). Cells that have standardized residuals greater than 2 in absolute value are categories that are major contributors to the significant χ^2 value (Hinkle et al., 2003).

In Figure 8.2, two cells have standardized residuals that come close to meeting this criterion: those children diagnosed with lymphoma whose sleep quality was rated as "very good" (16) (standardized residual = +2.0) and those children diagnosed with sarcoma whose sleep quality was also rated "very good" (17) (standardized residual = −2.3). Comparing the actual and expected frequencies for the lymphoma/"very good" sleep quality cell, there were more children with lymphoma who were rated by nurses to have "very good" sleep quality (n = 11) than would have been expected by chance (n = 6.1). In contrast, fewer children with sarcoma were rated by nurses to have "very good" sleep quality (n = 0) than would have been expected by chance (n = 5.1).

Partitioning the contingency table.

A second approach to examining cell influences is to subpartition the contingency table into a series of 2 × 2 independent subtables (Siegel & Castellan, 1988). The degrees of freedom available for the chi-square analysis dictate how many tables can be set up: There can be one independent 2 × 2 table for each degree of freedom (i.e., six 2 × 2 tables if $df = 6$). Because of the limited number of comparisons that can be made, the researcher needs to identify carefully which comparisons are most meaningful to the study.

Although the partitioning approach may initially appear confusing and cumbersome, it is really quite straightforward. First, the contingency table is arranged in such a way that the most meaningful 2 × 2 comparisons of the categorical data are made given the research questions of the study (Siegel & Castellan, 1988). Because the variables being examined are nominal, there is no restriction as to the order in which the rows and columns are placed in the table.

Siegel and Castellan (1988) indicate that, for clarity of understanding, it is best to begin the 2 × 2 partitioning in the upper left-hand corner of the table and then collapse the rows and columns of the table in a systematic and meaningful fashion. Figure 8.3 outlines the procedure for collapsing a 4 × 3 table into six independent 2 × 2 tables. There are six 2 × 2 tables because, for a 4 × 3 table, there are 6 degrees of freedom ($df = [r - 1][c - 1] = [4-1][3-1] = 6$).

The lower right-hand cell of each 2 × 2 subtable to be created always consists of a single set of frequencies and serves as the foundation for the 2 × 2 partition (Figure 8.3A, cell 1). The upper left-hand cell in the 2 × 2 table consists of the sum of all frequencies that lie directly up and to the left of this foundation cell (Figure 8.3A, cell 2). The lower left cell of the 2 × 2 subtable consists of the sum of all frequencies that lie directly to the left of the foundation cell (cell 3), whereas the upper right cell is the sum of the frequency values that lie directly above the foundation cell (cell 4).

Figure 8.3 Partitioning a 4 × 3 contingency table.

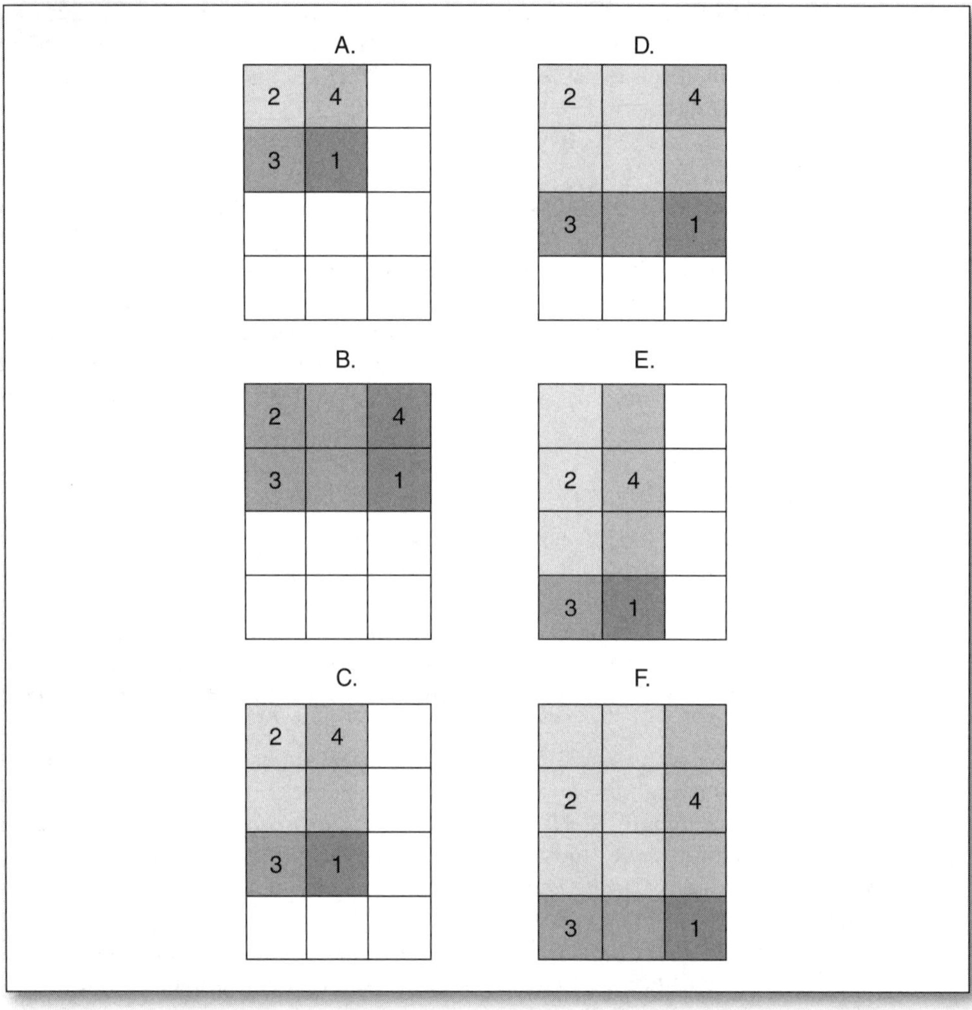

Following this pattern, the first partition consists of the four adjacent cells in the upper left-hand corner of the 4 × 3 table (Figure 8.3A). The second partition (Figure 8.3B) is begun by moving one cell to the right of the foundation cell identified in the first partition (Figure 8.3A, cell 1). The sum of all frequencies that lie in the cells directly above and to the left of this new foundation cell makes up cell 2 in the second 2 × 2 subtable. Cell 3 consists of the sum of the frequencies in the cells that lie directly to the left of cell 1, and cell 4 is made up of all frequencies that lie directly above cell 1.

The third partition (Figure 8.3C) is obtained by targeting the single cell directly below the foundation cell identified in the first partition as the new cell 1. Following the guidelines outlined above, cells 2, 3, and 4 can be obtained easily. A similar approach is taken for the last three partitions (Figure 8.3D,E).

Each of these six 2 × 2 subpartitions can now be treated as an independent 2 × 2 table each with one degree of freedom, and chi-square statistics can be calculated for each table. The resulting χ^2 values generated from the six 2 × 2 comparisons sum to the original χ^2 value. The calculations of these six chi-square statistics are tedious to perform by hand. While SPSS for Windows does not have the capability of partitioning contingency tables, we can easily generate these statistics using an online chi-square calculator.

Table 8.3 presents the partitioned 2 × 2 subtables for the 4 × 3 contingency table that examines the relationship between type of cancer diagnosis and the nurses' ratings of the children's postintervention fatigue. Note that 2 × 2 subpartition 1 (Table 8.3A) compares children with cancer diagnoses of *Solid Tumor* or *Leukemia* with regard to *Poor* or *Moderate* postintervention sleep quality. Subpartition 2 (Table 8.3B) compares children diagnosed with a *Solid Tumor* or *Leukemia* with regard to *Not Very Good* or *Very Good* postintervention sleep quality. Subpartition 3 (Table 8.3C) examines children with *Solid Tumor* or *Leukemia and Lymphoma* with regard to *Not Very Good* or *Very Good* postintervention sleep quality. Subpartitions D through E continue with similar sets of subpartitions.

Statistically analyzing the partitioned subtables.

To undertake the statistical analyses of these six 2 × 2 tables, we can make use of the chi-square interactive calculator programs that are freely available on the Internet. For this example, we will use http://www.quantpsy.org/chisq/chisq.htm, although any chi-square calculator will do. To illustrate the process, we will use Subpartition 6.

Figure 8.4 presents a screenshot obtained from having input the data obtained for Subpartition 6 into the chi-square matrix found on the quantpsy.org website. The chi-square value, 9.65, is statistically significant (p = .002). An examination of the observations in each of the four cells indicates that the sleep quality for those children with sarcoma was not "very good" compared to the nonsarcoma children (i.e., those with solid tumor, leukemia, or lymphoma).

Table 8.4 summarizes the chi-square test results obtained for all six subpartitions. Only Subpartition 6 is statistically significant. The sum of the chi-square values (18.36) is slightly larger than the total chi-square value (18.29) that we obtained in the computer-generated printout (Figure 8.2). The difference may be attributed to round-off differences in the two approaches.

Internet Resources for Generating the Chi-Square Test for *k* Independent Samples

As indicated in Chapter 7, a number of currently available open access Internet resources provide calculators with which one can obtain a chi-square test for independent samples. Currently, three sites (www.danielsoper.com, www.vassarstats.net, and

Table 8.3 Partitioning the 4 x 3 Contingency Table into Four Independent 2 x 2 Tables

A. Subpartition 1: Cancer Diagnosis (solid tumor, leukemia) vs. Postintervention Sleep Quality (Poor, Moderate)

	Postintervention Sleep Quality			
Cancer Diagnosis	*Poor*	*Moderate*	*Very Good*	*Total*
Solid tumor	4	8	7	19
Leukemia	8	5	5	18
Lymphoma	6	2	11	19
Sarcoma	6	10	0	16
Total	24	25	23	72

B. Subpartition 2: Cancer Diagnosis (solid tumor, leukemia) vs. Postintervention Sleep quality (Not very good [poor, moderate], Very good,)

	Postintervention Sleep Quality			
Cancer Diagnosis	*Poor*	*Moderate*	*Very Good*	*Total*
Solid tumor	4	8	7	19
Leukemia	8	5	5	18
Lymphoma	6	2	11	19
Sarcoma	6	10	0	16
Total	24	25	23	72

C. Subpartition 3: Cancer Diagnosis (Cancer Diagnosis (solid tumor +leukemia, lymphoma) vs. Sleep Quality (poor, moderate)

	Postintervention Sleep Quality			
Cancer Diagnosis	*Poor*	*Moderate*	*Very Good*	*Total*
Solid tumor	4	8	7	19
Leukemia	8	5	5	18
Lymphoma	6	2	11	19
Sarcoma	6	10	0	16
Total	24	25	23	72

D. Subpartition 4: Cancer Diagnosis (tumor + leukemia, lymphoma) vs. Sleep Quality (not very good [poor, moderate], very good)

Cancer Diagnosis	*Postintervention Sleep Quality*			*Total*
	Poor	*Moderate*	*Very Good*	
Solid tumor	4	8	7	19
Leukemia	8	5	5	18
Lymphoma	6	2	11	19
Sarcoma	6	10	0	16
Total	24	25	23	72

E. Subpartition 5: Cancer Diagnosis (non-sarcoma, sarcoma) vs. Sleep Quality (poor, moderate)

Cancer Diagnosis	*Postintervention Sleep Quality*			*Total*
	Poor	*Moderate*	*Very Good*	
Solid tumor	4	8	7	19
Leukemia	8	5	5	18
Lymphoma	6	2	11	19
Sarcoma	6	10	0	16
Total	24	25	23	72

F. Subpartition 6: Cancer Diagnosis (non-sarcoma, sarcoma) vs. Sleep Quality (not very good vs. very good)

Cancer Diagnosis	*Postintervention Sleep Quality*			*Total*
	Poor	*Moderate*	*Very Good*	
Solid tumor	4	8	7	19
Leukemia	8	5	5	18
Lymphoma	6	2	11	19
Sarcoma	6	10	0	16
Total	24	25	23	72

Figure 8.4 Obtaining a chi-square value for Subpartition 6. Output generated from http://www.quantpsy.org/chisq/chisq.htm.

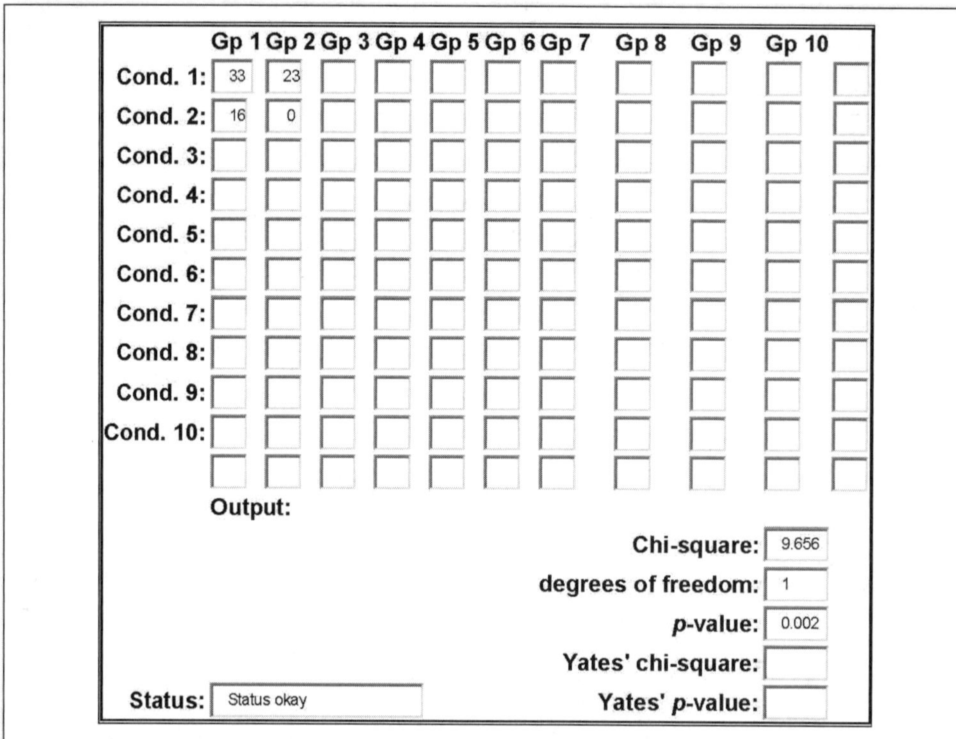

Table 8.4 Chi-Square Test Results for the Six Subpartitions

Subpartition	χ^2	*df*	*p*
1	1.98	1	0.15
2	0.34	1	0.56
3	1.78	1	0.18
4	3.36	1	0.07
5	1.25	1	0.26
6	9.65	1	0.002
Total	18.36	6	0.006

www.quantpsy.org) provide easy access to a chi-square calculator. Please refer to Chapter 7 for detailed information regarding how to use these sites.

Presentation of Results

Table 8.5 presents the results of the chi-square test for *k* independent samples in tabular form.

Table 8.5 Presentation of the Chi-Square Test Analyses of Children's Postintervention Sleep Quality in Table Form

	Postintervention Sleep Quality									
	Poor		*Moderate*		*Very Good*		*Total*			
Cancer Diagnosis	*N*	%	*N*	%	*N*	%	*N*	%	χ^2	p
Solid tumor	4	16.7	8	32.0	7	30.4	19	26.4	18.29	0.006
Acute myeloid leukemia	8	33.3	5	20.0	5	21.7	18	25.0		
Lymphoma	6	25.0	2	8.0	11	47.9	19	26.4		
Sarcoma	6	25.0	10	40.0	0	0.0	16	22.2		
Total	24	100.0	25	100.0	23	100.0	72	100.0		

These results also could be interpreted and presented in the text as follows:

The results of the chi-square test indicated a significant but weak association between the hospitalized children's cancer diagnosis and postintervention sleep quality (χ^2 = 18.29, p = .006, Cramér's V = .36). Examination of the standardized residuals and subpartitioning of the contingency table revealed that children with the diagnosis of sarcoma had poorer sleep quality than did children with other cancer diagnoses (χ^2 = 9.65, p = .002).

Advantages, Limitations, and Alternatives to the Chi-Square Test for *k* Independent Samples

The chi-square test for *k* independent samples is an extremely useful and flexible technique to be used when both the independent and dependent variables are categorical.

Because it is insensitive to order, the chi-square test is not the test of choice when either of the categorical variables has ordered levels. It is also improper to use this test when the data are not independent, for example, when there are multiple response categories, there are repeated observations, or the data are matched or paired samples.

There are no parametric alternatives to the chi-square test because it is intended for use with nominal-level data. When the data do not meet the assumptions of the chi-square test for *k* independent samples, the data could be collapsed into smaller contingency tables for use with Fisher's exact test or the chi-square test for two independent samples (Chapter 7). If either of the categorical variables has ordered levels, alternative nonparametric tests are the other tests reviewed in this chapter, especially the Mantel-Haenszel chi-square test for trends.

When one set of nominal-level data is to be evaluated with regard to the relative risk associated with a second nominal-level variable, the odds ratio (OR) is a useful statistic. When more than two categorical independent variables are being examined for their influence on a categorical dependent variable, two potentially useful approaches to data analysis are logistic regression and discriminant analysis. We will be examining both the odds ratio and logistic regression in greater detail in Chapter 10.

Examples From Published Research

Berry, J. G., Poduri, A., Bonkowsky, J. L., Zhou, J., Graham, D. A., Welch, C., . . . Srivastava, R. (2012). Trends in resource utilization by children with neurological impairment in the United States inpatient health care system: A repeat cross-sectional study. *PLoS Medicine, 9*(1), e1001158. doi: 10.1371/journal.pmed.1001158

Kothari, C. L., Zielinski, R., James, A., Charoth, R. M., & Sweezy Ldel, C. (2014). Improved birth weight for Black infants: Outcomes of a Healthy Start program. *American Journal of Public Health, 104*(Suppl. 1), S96–S104. doi: 10.2105/AJPH.2013.301359

Nokes, N. R., & Tucker, L. A. (2012). Changes in hip bone mineral density and objectively measured physical activity in middle-aged women: A 6-year prospective study. *American Journal of Health Promotion, 26*(6), 341–347. doi: 10.4278/ajhp.100622-QUAN-208

Stork, C. M., Brown, K. M., Reilly, T. H., Secreti, L., & Brown, L. H. (2006). Emergency department treatment of viral gastritis using intravenous ondansetron or dexamethasone in children. *Academic Emergency Medicine, 13*(10), 1027–1033.

THE MANTEL-HAENSZEL CHI-SQUARE TEST FOR TRENDS

It often happens in health care research that the categorical variables being examined have order to their levels (e.g., stages of disease, length of exposure, age levels, categories of social status, or quality of sleep) yet are not sufficiently ordinal to be treated as continuous variables. Use of the chi-square test for *k* independent samples with these data would result in loss of potentially valuable information because this test is insensitive to order. There is an extension of the chi-square test, the Mantel-Haenszel (M-H) chi-square test for trends, that takes order into account (Mantel, 1963; Mantel & Haenszel,

1959). It is, therefore, a useful test when the values assigned to the categories of both independent and dependent variables are ordered.

The M-H test has been used widely in epidemiologic case control studies in which there are stratified 2 × 2 tables and the researcher is interested in comparing the likelihood of the occurrence of an event (e.g., contracting cancer) given two groups who have been exposed versus unexposed to a risk factor (e.g., cigarette smoking) and who have been matched or paired with regard to certain characteristics (e.g., gender or age) (Altman, 1990; Armitage, Berry, & Matthews, 2008; Rothman, Greenland, & Lash, 2008). The focus of this presentation will be on the use of the M-H chi-square test to examine trends in data when at least one of the two categorical ordered variables has more than two levels and the data are not matched or paired.

An Appropriate Research Question for the Mantel-Haenszel (M-H) Chi-Square Test

Although the M-H test for stratified case control data has been used extensively in the epidemiology and medical literature, the M-H test for trends has been used more sparingly. Glazer, Morgenstern, and Doucette (1994) used the M-H test for trends to examine psychosocial, clinical, and medical correlates of race that might help to explain an observed association between race and incidence of tardive dyskinesia among a group of 398 seriously mentally ill outpatients. Zhang, Lee, Cowan, Fabsitz, and Howard (2011) used the same test to examine trends in coffee consumption and the incidence of Type 2 diabetes in men and women with normal glucose tolerance. Berry et al. (2012) used the M-H chi-square test to examine trends in inpatient resource utilization by children with neurological impairment, while Nokes and Tucker (2012) used this test to evaluate changes in hip bone mineral density and physical activity in middle-aged women.

In our hypothetical intervention study, there are several areas in which the M-H test could be used. In the previous example, we used the chi-square test for *k* independent samples to examine the association between two categorical variables, type of cancer diagnosis and postintervention sleep quality. Suppose instead we were interested not in cancer diagnosis but rather the nurses' assessments of the distress levels of the hospitalized children (low, medium, or high) and their postintervention sleep quality (poor, moderate, or very good).

Note that each of these variables has three levels that are ordered. If a chi-square test for *k* independent samples were used to determine whether there is an association between these two variables, it would be restricted in its ability to detect the degree of linearity between the two variables. The M-H chi-square test for trends can be used as an alternative. A research question that could be answered using this test would be as follows:

> Is there a linear trend associated with a nurse's evaluation of the hospitalized child's level of distress (low, medium, or high) and his or her postintervention sleep quality (poor, moderate, or very good)?

Null and Alternative Hypotheses

Table 8.6 presents an example of null and alternative hypotheses generated from our research question that would be suitable for use with an M-H chi-square test. Like the ordinary chi-square test, the M-H test is a nondirectional two-tailed test of significance. We will reject the null hypothesis of no linear trend if and only if the actual χ^2 is greater than its critical value or, similarly, if the obtained p value is less than our alpha (e.g., $\alpha = .05$).

Table 8.6 Example of Null and Alternative Hypotheses Suitable for Use With the Mantel-Haenszel Chi-Square Test

Null Hypothesis
H_0: There is no linear trend association between a nurse's assessment of a hospitalized child's level of distress (low, medium, or high) and that child's postintervention sleep quality (poor, moderate, or very good).
Alternative Hypothesis
H_a: There is a linear trend association between a nurse's assessment of a hospitalized child's level of distress (low, medium, or high) and that child's postintervention sleep quality (poor, moderate, or very good).

Overview of the Procedure

The data to be analyzed are first cast into an $r \times c$ contingency table in which there are two categorical variables whose levels are ordered. Unlike in the ordinary chi-square test, the order of placement of categories now is important because this is a test of linear trends. The M-H chi-square test should not be used with categorical data whose levels are not ordered. If the researcher suspects a nonlinear trend a priori, the categories could be reassigned category values based on the hypothesized trend.

The M-H chi-square test is easily calculated by hand and is readily available on free-access Internet sites and statistical computer packages. Conceptually, like the ordinary chi-square test, the M-H test for trends compares the actual frequencies in each cell with what would have been expected under the null hypothesis of no linear trend among the ordered categories (Armitage et al., 2008; Rothman et al., 2008). If the data meet the assumptions for a M-H chi-square test, this χ^2_{MH} is distributed as a χ^2 with $df = 1$(Armitage, 1955). This χ^2_{MH} has an easier formula (Norman & Streiner, 2008):

$$\chi^2_{MH} = \frac{[\sum(O_{ij} - E_{ij})]^2}{\sum \text{Var}(O_{ij} - E_{ij})} = r^2[W - 1) = r^2[n - 1)$$

where

O_{ij} = the observed value in cell *ij;*

E_{ij} = the expected value in cell *ij;*

$\text{Var}(O_{ij} - E_{ij})$ = the variance for the difference between the observed and expected values in cell *ij;*

W = sum of the weights assigned to each value in a cell; if no weight is assigned to the values, then W = the 1*sample size or *n;*

r^2 = the square of the Pearson product-moment correlation;

n = the total sample size.

From this formula, we can see that the M-H chi-square test for trends bears a strong resemblance to the Pearson correlation coefficient.

The decision rule will be to reject the null hypothesis of no linear trend in the ordered categories if the calculated χ^2_{MH} is greater than a critical value of the χ^2 with $df = 1$ at the specified alpha level. For example, if $\alpha = .05$, $\chi^2_{cv} = 3.84$ (Appendix A, Table A.2).

Critical Assumptions of the Mantel-Haenszel Chi-Square Test

The M-H chi-square test shares some of the assumptions of the ordinary chi-square test and has additional assumptions of its own.

1. *Both independent and dependent variables are categorical, with two or more levels.*
2. *The levels of both categorical variables are ordered.*
3. *The data consist of frequencies, not scores.*
4. *Each randomly selected observation can be classified into only one category for the independent variable(s) and only one category for the dependent variable. There are no repeated observations and no multiple response categories.*

Both articles (e.g., Cai and Zeng (2004); Charan and Biswas (2013); Kasiulevičius, Šapoka, and Filipavičiūtė (2006)) and free-access online calculators (e.g., Open Epi [www.openepi.com], EpiTools [http://epitools.ausvet.com.au/content.php?page=home], and www.danielsoper.com) are available to help the researcher to determine an adequate sample size for the M-H test when used with case control data. While no direct reference was located that addressed issues of adequate sample size when examining descriptive data for trends, because this is a chi-square test with $df = 1$, it would be reasonable to assume that the M-H test shares the following chi-square test requirement:

5. *No more than 20% of the cells may have expected frequencies of less than 5, and no cell should have an expected frequency of less than 1.*

The variables of interest in our hypothetical intervention study with 72 hospitalized children (children's distress and postintervention sleep quality) meet most of these requirements. The frequency data that have been generated are at the nominal level, ordered, with mutually exclusive categories. While the data for the 72 children have not been randomly selected, we will see from the output that none of the cells have expected frequencies less than 5.

Computer Commands

The computer commands to obtain the M-H chi-square test are quite straightforward and are similar to those for the ordinary chi-square test: *Analyze . . . Descriptive Statistics . . . Crosstabs.* In SPSS for Windows, the researcher is given the results of this test whenever *Chi-Square* statistics are requested from the *Statistics* dialog box (Figure 8.1). In this example, our independent variable is the children's *level of distress,* and the dependent variable is their *postintervention sleep quality*.

The Crosstabs procedure in SPSS for Windows that was used to obtain the chi-square test for independent samples includes the M-H test of linear trend among its chi-square test statistics. As indicated above, this test is calculated as $(W - 1)\ r^2$, where W = the sum of the case weights and r^2 is the squared Pearson correlation between the row and column variables. The test has 1 *df.* If no weight variable is designated, then all case weights equal 1.00, and W equals the sample size and the M-H chi-square = $(n - 1)\ r^2$ as outlined above. Norman and Streiner (2008) suggest that a nonparametric approach to obtaining this test would be to substitute a Spearman rho correlation in the formula in place of the Pearson *r.* As we will see, our results are similar, whichever correlation we choose to use.

The M-H test for trend will be printed in the "Chi-Square Tests" table and labeled "Linear-by-Linear Association." Note that this test will not be printed for any table in which either the row or column variable is a string variable. You can recode such a variable into a new numeric variable and use that numeric variable in the Crosstabs procedure.

Computer-Generated Output

Figure 8.5 presents the syntax commands and output for the M-H chi-square test for trends. Because the commands for this M-H test are identical to those of the ordinary chi-square test, the syntax commands and output are similar to Figure 8.2 with the only exception being that *Correlations* were also requested.

Because the Pearson correlation (r) between children's distress and their sleep quality immediately following the intervention is –.289 (Figure 8.5, (1)), the χ^2_{MH} could be calculated directly:

$$\chi^2_{MH} = r^2(n-1) = -.289^2(72-1) = 5.923$$

This value is similar to the χ^2_{MH} linear-by-linear value presented in Figure 8.4. If we had used the Spearman rho coefficient ($r_s = -.293$, Figure 8.4, (3)) the $\chi^2_{MH} = (-.293)^2$

Figure 8.5 Computer-generated output for the Mantel-Haenszel chi-square test for linear trends (SPSS for Windows, v. 22–23).

```
***Data set: hospitalized children with cancer-72 cases.sav***

CROSSTABS
  /TABLES=level_of_distress BY sleep_quality_T2
  /FORMAT=AVALUE TABLES
  /STATISTICS=CHISQ PHI CORR
  /CELLS=COUNT EXPECTED SRESID
  /COUNT ROUND CELL.
```

level_of_distress level of children's distress * sleep_quality_T2 sleep quality immediately following intervention Crosstabulation

			sleep_quality_T2 sleep quality immediately following intervention			
			1.00 Poor sleep quality	2.00 Moderate sleep quality	3.00 Very good sleep quality	Total
level_of_distress level of children's distress	1.00	Count	4	7	8	19
		Expected Count	6.3	6.6	6.1	19.0
		Std. Residual	-.9	.2	.8	
	2.00	Count	8	9	12	29
		Expected Count	9.7	10.1	9.3	29.0
		Std. Residual	-.5	-.3	.9	
	3.00	Count	12	9	3	24
		Expected Count	8.0	8.3	7.7	24.0
		Std. Residual	1.4	.2	-1.7	
Total		Count	24	25	23	72
		Expected Count	24.0	25.0	23.0	72.0

Chi-Square Tests

	Value	df	Asymp. Sig. (2-sided)
Pearson Chi-Square	7.601[a]	4	(6) .107
Likelihood Ratio	8.221	4	.084
Linear-by-Linear Association (2)	5.923	1	(4) .015
N of Valid Cases	72		

a. 0 cells (0.0%) have expected count less than 5. The minimum expected count is 6.07.

Symmetric Measures

		Value	Asymp. Std. Error[a]	Approx. T[b]	Approx. Sig.
Nominal by Nominal	Phi	.325			.107
	Cramer's V	(5) .230			.107
Interval by Interval	Pearson's R (1)	-.289	.106	-2.524	.014[c]
Ordinal by Ordinal (3)	Spearman Correlation	-.293	.106	-2.562	.013[c]
N of Valid Cases		72			

a. Not assuming the null hypothesis.

b. Using the asymptotic standard error assuming the null hypothesis.

c. Based on normal approximation.

(71) = 6.095. Are these values sufficiently large to reject the null hypothesis given a two-tailed $\alpha = .05$?

To make that decision, we could compare our actual χ^2_{MH} (5.923 or 6.095) with $\chi^2_{cv} = 3.84$ with $df = 1$. Because both the Pearson *r*– and Spearman rho–generated M-H statistics are greater than the critical value, we can reject the null hypothesis and conclude that there is a linear relationship between the children's levels of distress and their postintervention sleep quality.

Given that we have the computer printout, we can see that the significance value (*p*) for this χ^2_{MH} is .015 (4), which is less than $\alpha = .05$, again indicating that the null hypothesis of no linear trend is to be rejected. The conclusion to be drawn, therefore, is that there is a significant inverse linear trend between the children's levels of distress and their postintervention sleep quality adjustment: As the hospitalized children's distress increases, their postintervention sleep quality declines.

Is this linear trend very strong? To determine the strength of this trend, we would look at Cramér's *V* in Figure 8.5 (.230, (5)). From Table 7.7 in Chapter 7, we can determine that it is of low strength. There are also no standardized residuals with values greater than $|2|$. Notice, however, that had we used the ordinary chi-square test ($p = .107$, (6)) instead of the test of trends, our results would not have been statistically significant.

Internet Resources for Generating the Mantel-Haenszel (M-H) Chi-Square Test for Trends

While Internet resources for either generating the ordinary chi-square test for *k* independent samples or the M-H chi-square test for case control studies are relatively easy to locate, no free-access source appears to be currently available for generating the M-H chi-square test for trends directly. Without a statistical computer package, it appears that we would first need to generate a Pearson *r* or Spearman rho for our data either using an Internet resource or Excel and then hand-calculate the M-H chi-square test for trends using the formula, $\chi^2_{MH} = (n - 1)r^2$. We will be reviewing how to use Internet resources and Excel to generate correlations in Chapter 9.

Presentation of Results

The results of the Mantel-Haenszel chi-square test for trends could be presented in a manner similar to that for the ordinary chi-square test (Table 8.5) with the χ^2_{MH} presented instead of the χ^2 value. These results also could be stated in the text:

> The results of the Mantel-Haenszel chi-square test for trends indicated a statistically significant but weak linear trend between the hospitalized children's level of distress and postintervention sleep quality ($\chi^2_{MH} = 5.92$, $p = .015$, Cramér's $V = .22$). As the children's level of distress increased, their postintervention sleep quality declined.

Advantages, Limitations, and Alternatives to the Mantel-Haenszel Chi-Square Test for Trends

The Mantel-Haenszel chi-square test for trends is an underused chi-square test that is very useful when the categorical variables to be examined have ordered levels. Because of its relationship to the Pearson *r*, the Mantel-Haenszel chi-square test for trends is sensitive to order and, unlike the ordinary chi-square test, is able to detect linear trends among ordered nominal-level variables. This makes the Mantel-Haenszel chi-square test a more powerful alternative to the ordinary chi-square test when the levels are ordered. It should not be used, however, when the levels of the nominal-level variable do not have order or when the basic assumptions of the ordinary chi-square test have been violated.

Because the variables that are being examined with the Mantel-Haenszel chi-square test for trends are nominal level of measurement, there is no parametric equivalent to this test. As with the ordinary chi-square test, the data can be collapsed into a smaller table should the sample size not be large enough to meet this test's assumptions. If both sets of data to be examined are ordinal, an alternative to this test is the Spearman rho. If one variable is categorical and the other continuous, the point biserial correlation, median test, or the Kruskal-Wallis test would be alternative nonparametric tests to consider.

Examples From Published Research

Berry, J. G., Poduri, A., Bonkowsky, J. L., Zhou, J., Graham, D. A., Welch, C., . . . Srivastava, R. (2012). Trends in resource utilization by children with neurological impairment in the United States inpatient health care system: A repeat cross-sectional study. *PLoS Medicine, 9*(1), e1001158. doi: 10.1371/journal.pmed.1001158

Glazer, W. M., Morgenstern, H., & Doucette, J. (1994). Race and tardive dyskinesia among outpatients at a CMHC. *Hospital and Community Psychiatry, 45,* 38–42.

Kothari, C. L., Zielinski, R., James, A., Charoth, R. M., & Sweezy Ldel, C. (2014). Improved birth weight for Black infants: Outcomes of a Healthy Start program. *American Journal of Public Health, 104*(Suppl. 1), S96–S104. doi: 10.2105/AJPH.2013.301359

Nokes, N. R., & Tucker, L. A. (2012). Changes in hip bone mineral density and objectively measured physical activity in middle-aged women: A 6-year prospective study. *American Journal of Health Promotion, 26*(6), 341–347. doi: 10.4278/ajhp.100622-QUAN-208

Zhang, Y., Lee, E. T., Cowan, L. D., Fabsitz, R. R., & Howard, B. V. (2011). Coffee consumption and the incidence of Type 2 diabetes in men and women with normal glucose tolerance: The Strong Heart Study. *Nutrition, Metabolism, and Cardiovascular Diseases, 21*(6), 418–423.

THE MEDIAN TEST

The median test is used when the independent variable is categorical, the dependent variable is at least at the ordinal level of measurement, and the researcher wants to examine differences between two or more groups with regard to their measures of central tendency, specifically the median (Conover, 1999). It answers the question as to whether two or more groups come from populations with identical distributions. The median test is particularly appropriate when the exact values of extreme scores have been truncated to above or below a certain cutoff point (Siegel & Castellan, 1988). It also can be used when the assumption of similarity of shapes of distributions of the Mann-Whitney *U* test (Chapter 7) has not been met.

Let us return to our sample of 30 children with cancer (data set: hospitalized children with cancer-30 cases.sav located on the website study.sagepub.com/pett2e). Suppose we were interested in comparing the hospitalized children's number of nocturnal awakenings immediately following the staff-initiated intervention (i.e., Day 2 of hospitalization) split out by the three different types of cancer diagnoses (solid tumors, lymphoma, and leukemia or sarcoma).

Now we have an independent variable (type of cancer diagnosis) that is nominal level of measurement and a dependent variable, number of nocturnal sleep awakenings, that is interval level of measurement. Because the dependent variable is continuous, we cannot use a chi-square test to evaluate the relationship between cancer diagnosis and number of nocturnal sleep awakenings. We would use instead either the median test or the Kruskal-Wallis one-way ANOVA by ranks.

An Appropriate Research Question for the Median Test

In recent years, the median test has not been used as much as it was in the past. This may be due, in part, to user-friendly statistical packages that have facilitated the use of more powerful nonparametric statistics, including the Mann-Whitney test and the Kruskal-Wallis one-way ANOVA by ranks.

Despite the lack of popularity of the median test, several recent studies have made use of this handy statistic. Williams et al. (2008), for example, used the median test to evaluate whether the distribution of scores on a Childhood Autism Spectrum Test (CAST) for their sample of boys and girls were drawn from populations with the similar medians. Jooste, Weight, and Lombard (2000) used a two-sample median test to evaluate the short-term effectiveness of mandatory iodization of table salt, at an elevated iodine concentration, on the iodine and goiter status of schoolchildren with endemic goiter, and Canto et al. (2000) used the median test to examine clinical characteristics and mortality rates among 142,445 patients with myocardial infarction but who did not experience chest pain.

In our hypothetical study, we could use the median test to answer a number of different research questions. A typical example would be the following:

> Are there differences among the hospitalized children with three different types of cancer diagnoses (solid tumors, lymphoma, and leukemia or sarcoma) with regard to their number of nocturnal awakenings immediately following the staff-initiated intervention (i.e., Day 2 of hospitalization)?

Null and Alternative Hypotheses

Table 8.7 presents examples of possible null and alternative hypotheses derived from our research question that would be suitable for the median test. Note that our alternative hypothesis is nondirectional, making this a two-tailed test. It is also possible to predict the direction of the medians. This would necessitate using either a one-tailed median test, if only two groups are involved, or a priori comparisons, if there are more than two groups.

Table 8.7 Example of Null and Alternative Hypotheses Suitable for Use With the Median Test

Null Hypothesis
H_0: There are no differences in medians among the hospitalized children in the three diagnostic groups (solid tumors, lymphoma, and leukemia or sarcoma) with regard to their number of nocturnal awakenings immediately following the staff-initiated intervention (i.e., Day 2 of hospitalization). That is, all three groups have similar underlying distributions of number of nocturnal awakenings.
Alternative Hypothesis
H_a: There are differences in medians among the hospitalized children in the three diagnostic groups (solid tumors, lymphoma, and leukemia or sarcoma) with regard to their number of nocturnal awakenings immediately following the staff-initiated intervention (i.e., Day 2 of hospitalization). That is, at least one of the groups is different from the other(s) with regard to its underlying distribution of number of nocturnal awakenings

Overview of the Procedure

To undertake a median test, the data are first considered as a single sample, and the combined *grand* median for the scores on the dependent variable is calculated. Next, the sample is separated into the various levels of the independent variable. If the null hypothesis is true and the samples share the same median, then we would expect that about half the observations within each level of the independent variable would be either above or equal to/below the *grand median.*

The next step is to classify the observations within each group according to whether observations lie above or equal to/below the grand median. These frequency counts are then arranged in a 2 × *c* contingency table where the two rows represent the two categories, *greater than* or *less than/equal to* the median, and the *c* columns are the levels of the independent variable. Finally, the observed number of observations above and equal to/below the median for each of the levels of the independent variable, Obs_{ij}, is compared to what would have been expected (Exp_{ij}) under the null hypothesis of equal medians. The difference between the observed and expected values is then squared, divided by the expected value, and summed across all cells.

The test statistic used to evaluate this 2 × *c* contingency table is the chi-square statistic:

$$\chi^2 = \sum_{i=1}^{2} \sum_{j=1}^{c} \frac{(Obs_{ij} - Exp_{ij})^2}{Exp_{ij}}$$

where

Obs_{ij} = the observed number of observations in a cell in row *i* and column *j*;

Exp_{ij} = the expected number of observations in the same cell if the medians were equal; if the data meet the assumptions of the median test, this chi-square statistic is distributed as a χ^2 with $(c - 1)$ degrees of freedom; and

c = the number of levels of the independent variable.

The decision rule is to reject the null hypothesis of equal medians if this calculated χ^2 value exceeds the critical χ^2 value at $df = (c - 1)$ and the prestated α level (e.g., $\alpha = .05$). Alternatively, when presented with computer printouts, the decision rule would be to reject the null hypothesis if the generated significance level (p) is less than the predetermined α level.

Calculating the median test for the diagnosis and sleep disturbance T2 data.

Table 8.8 presents the observed values obtained for the diagnosis and number of nocturnal sleep awakenings immediately following the intervention (Day 2) data generated for the 30 hospitalized children. This table was obtained in SPSS for Windows (v. 22–23) using the commands *Analyze . . . Nonparametric tests . . . Legacy Dialogs . . . k Independent Samples,* adding the independent (type_of_cancer_collapsed) and dependent (number_of_sleep_awakenings_T2) variables into the group and test variable list, respectively, and designating the median test.

Table 8.8 SPSS-Generated Table of Frequencies for the Median Test

Frequencies

		type_of_cancer_collapsed type of cancer collapsed 3 levels		
		1.00 solid tumor	2.00 lymphoma	3.00 leukemia, sarcoma
Nocturnal_sleep_awakenings_Day2 Number of nocturnal sleep awakenings-Day 2	> Median	6	5	0
	<= Median	4	8	7

(1) Exp = (*R***C*)/*N*=(11)(10)/30= 3.67

To obtain the expected number of children in each cell, we would calculate these values just as we did for the chi-square test of independence. That is, for the first cell, Exp = (Row total*Column total)/Total sample size = (11*10)/30 = 3.67) (1). The expected values for all of the 12 cells could easily be calculated in the same manner.

Once the observed and expected values for each cell in Table 8.8 have been obtained, a chi-square test can easily be calculated:

$$\chi^2 = \sum_{i=1}^{r}\sum_{j=1}^{c} \frac{(Obs_{ij} - Exp_{ij})^2}{Exp_{ij}} = \frac{(6-3.67)^2}{3.67} + \frac{(5-4.77)^2}{4.77} + \frac{(0-2.57)^2}{2.57}$$

$$+ . \frac{(4-6.33)^2}{6.33} + \frac{(8-8.23)^2}{8.23} + \frac{(7-4.43)^2}{4.43}$$

$$= 1.479 + .011 + 2.570 + .858 + .006 + 1.491 = 6.415$$

To determine whether the median number of postintervention nocturnal sleep awakenings for the three cancer diagnoses is similar, we would need to compare the actual value of our chi-square statistic, 6.415, with that of a critical value ($df = c - 1 = 3 - 1 = 2$) at a given level of alpha (e.g., $\alpha = .05$). According to the chi-square table in Appendix A (Table A.2), the critical value of a chi-square with $df = 2$ is 5.99 (remember that we are looking for that point on the cumulative probability distribution, .95, such that $\alpha = .05$ lies beyond that critical value). Given that our actual χ^2, 6.415, is larger than the critical value of the χ^2, 5.99, we will reject the null hypothesis of equality of medians and conclude that there is at least one median that is statistically different from the others. To determine which medians are different, we would need to run post hoc tests. We will do that when we examine the SPSS output.

Critical Assumptions of the Median Test

There are few assumptions associated with the median test, which makes it a user-friendly nonparametric test. Other than the fact that the data have been obtained from a random sample, the following assumptions apply:

1. *The independent variable is at the nominal level of measurement. The dependent variable is at least at the ordinal level of measurement.*

2. *The levels of the independent variable are independent of one another; that is, a respondent can belong to one and only one sample of observations.*

Our data from the hypothetical study meet all the assumptions except for its being a random sample. The independent variable, type of cancer diagnosis, is at the nominal level of measurement with three mutually exclusive levels, and the dependent variable, number of nocturnal awakenings at Day 2 postintervention, is at the interval level of measurement.

Computer Commands

Figure 8.6 presents the SPSS for Windows dialog boxes that are used to undertake the median test. These boxes were opened by choosing the following items from the menu: *Analyze . . . Nonparametric Tests . . . Independent Samples . . . Compare medians across groups* (1). By clicking on the *Fields* . . . box (2), we can place the independent (*type_of_cancer_collapsed*) (3) and dependent (*nocturnal_sleep_awakening_Day2*) (4) variables into their appropriate fields. Clicking on the *Settings* box (5) allows us to *Compare Medians across Groups* (6) and to choose all pairwise comparisons (7).

Computer-Generated Output

The syntax commands (8) and computer-generated output for the median test are presented in Figure 8.7. We are first presented with the Hypothesis Test Summary. The *Sig* or *p* value = .04 (9), which is less than our prestated α level (.05). This means that

Figure 8.6 SPSS for Windows dialog boxes used to generate the median test.

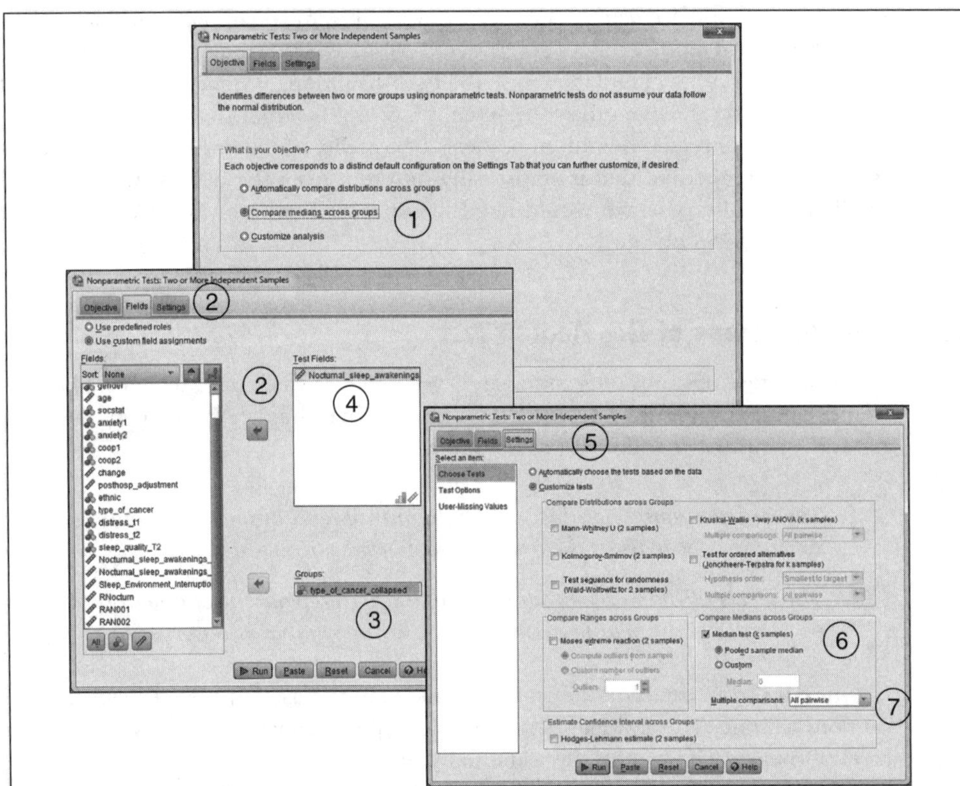

Figure 8.7 Computer output for the median test generated in SPSS for Windows (v. 22–23).

```
***Data set: hospitalized children with cancer-30 cases***

NPTESTS                                                    (8)
 /INDEPENDENT TEST (Nocturnal_sleep_awakenings_Day2) GROUP
  (type_of_cancer_collapsed) MEDIAN(TESTVALUE=SAMPLE
  COMPARE=PAIRWISE)
 /MISSING SCOPE=ANALYSIS USERMISSING=EXCLUDE
 /CRITERIA ALPHA=0.05 CILEVEL=95.
```

Hypothesis Test Summary

	Null Hypothesis	Test	Sig.	Decision
1	The medians of Number of nocturnal sleep awakenings-Day 2 are the same across categories of type of cancer collapsed 3 levels.	Independent-Samples Median Test (9)	.040	Reject the null hypothesis. (10)

Asymptotic significances are displayed. The significance level is .05.

Independent-Samples Median Test

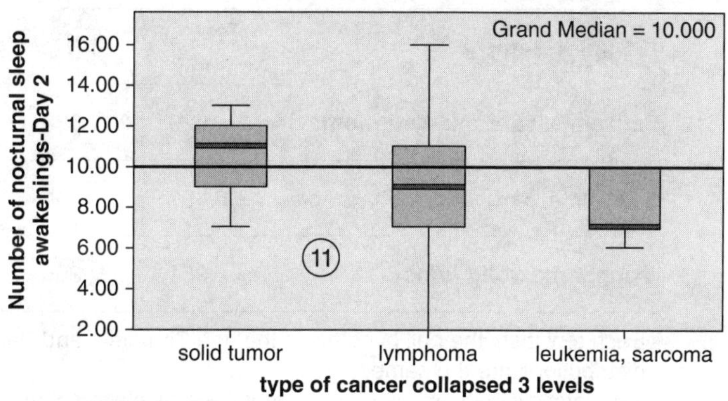

Total N	30
Median	10.000
Test Statistic	6.415
Degrees of Freedom	2
Asymptotic Sig. (2-sided test)	.040

1. More than 20% of the cells have expected values less than five.

(Continued)

Figure 8.7 (Continued)

Pairwise Comparisons of Type of Cancer Collapsed 3 Levels

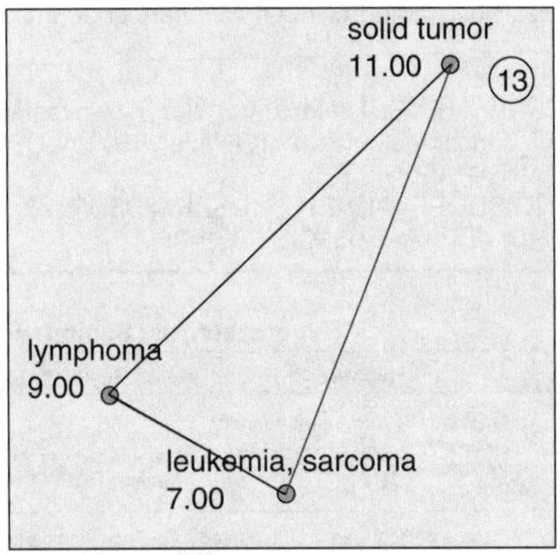

Each node shows the sample median of type of cancer collapsed 3 levels.

Sample1-Sample 2	Test Statistic	Sig.	Adj.Sig.
leukemia, sarcoma-lymphoma	.020	.888	1.000
leukemia, sarcoma-solid tumor	6.491	.011	(12) .033
lymphoma-solid tumor	1.051	.305	.916

Each row tests the null hypothesis that the Sample 1 and Sample 2 distributions are the same.
Asymptotic significances (2-sided tests) are displayed. The significance level is .05.

we would reject the null hypothesis and conclude, as we did earlier, that at least one median is different from the others.

Be cautious when interpreting the output.

Please note that, while the information presented to us in the *Decision box (Reject the null hypothesis)* (10) supports that decision, you, as the researcher, need to be careful not to "believe" all that is written. The *p* value that we are presented with (.040 (9)) represents a two-tailed *p* value. Suppose, for example, that we had an independent variable with two levels (e.g., the group intervention and that we had predicted that the staff-initiated intervention would have fewer postintervention nocturnal awakenings than the usual-care group). Suppose, too, that the generated *Sig* (i.e., the p value) was .07. The information that we would receive in the *Decision* box would be to *Retain the null hypothesis.* Yet this should not be our decision since our one-tailed directional p value would be .07/two-tailed = .035, a value that would be less than our $\alpha = .05$, assuming of course that the medians were in our predicted direction.

The boxplots presented in Figure 8.7 not only present the medians but also reflect the distributions of the dependent variable, number of nocturnal awakenings at Day 2. These data suggest that, while the distributions of the solid tumor, lymphoma, and leukemia/sarcoma groups are fairly compact, the lymphoma group has a more platykurtic, or spread-out, distribution (11).

By clicking on the *Pairwise Comparisons* button, we are also presented with the plots and pairwise comparisons of the distributions of the dependent variable, ***number of nocturnal awakenings_Day 2***, by type of cancer diagnosis. Some explanation of the generated output for these pairwise comparisons is in order. First, the total number of pairwise comparisons available to us is equal to $K(K-1)/2$, where K = the number of levels of the independent variable. In our example, our independent variable, type of cancer diagnosis, has three levels (solid tumor, lymphoma, and leukemia/sarcoma). Therefore, we will have 3 (3 – 1)/2 = 3 comparisons. These comparisons are multiple median tests in which only the pairs are considered, excluding the other levels of the independent variable.

In addition to the test statistic, which, for the median test, is a χ^2 value, we are given both an original p value (*Sig*) and an adjusted p value (*Adj. Sig*). Because there is increased potential for Type I error as a result of these multiple comparisons, the original significance level needs to be adjusted. For example, for the comparison between the leukemia/sarcoma and solid tumor groups, *Sig* = .011 and *Adj. Sig* = .033 (12). In SPSS for Windows, the formula for the adjusted p value is as follows:

$$p_{adj} = pK(K-1)/2$$

That would mean that the adjusted p value for the pairwise comparison of these two groups would be:

$$p_{adj} = (0.011)3(3-1)/2 = .033 \quad (12)$$

In addition to the table of pairwise comparisons, we are also presented with plots of the pairs. The yellow line indicates a statistically significant difference while the black line represents a nonstatistically significant difference. An examination of the plots and adjusted p values for all three pairwise comparisons (Figure 8.7) indicates that the median number of sleep awakenings at Day 2 for the solid tumor group (11.00) (13) is statistically significantly higher than the leukemia/sarcoma group (7.00) (adjusted $p = .033$) (12). No other statistically significant differences in pairs (adjusted p value >.05) were found.

Internet Resources for Generating the Median Test

To date, there does not appear to be available free online resources for directly calculating a median test for more than two groups. There are, however, several online resources for calculating the Kruskal-Wallis test, an alternative to the median test, which we will examine in the next section.

Presentation of Results

Table 8.9 is an example of how the results of the median test could be presented. To better describe the descriptive characteristics of the sample, means, medians, and ranges are presented. The table also indicates that the presented χ^2 value is the result of the median test in order to prevent confusion with other chi-square statistics. The results of this test could also be interpreted and presented in the text:

> The results of the median test indicate that there was a statistically significant difference among the three cancer diagnosis groups with regard to their median number of sleep awakenings at Day 2 of hospitalization ($p = .04$). Post hoc comparisons revealed that the median number of sleep awakenings at Day 2 for children with the diagnosis of solid tumors (11.0) was statistically significantly higher than the children in the leukemia/sarcoma group (7.00) ($p = .03$). No other statistically significant ($p > .05$) differences in pairs were found.

Table 8.9 Presentation of the Results of the Median Test Analyses of Number of Sleep Awakenings by Diagnosis of the Child

		# Sleep Awakenings: Day 2			*Median Test*		*Post-Hoc tests*	
Diagnosis	N	*Mean*	*Median*	*Range*	χ^2	p	*Group*	p
Solid tumor	10	10.5	11.0	7-13	6.92	0.04	$Mdn_1 > Mdn_3$	0.03
Lymphoma	13	9.1	9.0	2-16				
Leukemia, sarcoma	7	8.1	7.0	6-10				

Advantages, Limitations, and Alternatives to the Median Test

The median test has the advantage of being very straightforward and easy to apply, a characteristic that was especially welcomed during the precomputer era. It is a particularly useful test when the researcher does not know the exact values of all the scores, especially those at the extremes. The limitation of this test is that it considers only two possibilities for scores: They are either above or below/equal to the median. The size of the differences between the observed scores and the median is not taken into account. This results in the median test being a less powerful test than tests that do consider the size of differences, such as the Mann-Whitney test (Chapter 7) and the Kruskal-Wallis one-way ANOVA by ranks. Given that it is less powerful than these similar nonparametric statistics, Freidlin and Gastwirth (2000) have suggested that the median test be retired from general use.

There are two parametric alternatives to the median test: the *t* test when the independent variable is dichotomous and the one-way ANOVA when the independent variable has more than two levels. The nonparametric alternatives to the median test are the Mann-Whitney test for two groups and the Kruskal-Wallis one-way ANOVA for more than two groups. When the exact range of values for the dependent variable is known, the Mann-Whitney and Kruskal-Wallis tests are the preferred nonparametric tests because they take into account the size of the differences between the observed scores and the grand median.

Examples From Published Research

Canto, J. G., Shlipak, M. G., Rogers, W. J., Malmgren, J. A., Frederick, P. D., Lambrew, C. T., . . . Kiefe, C. I. (2000). Prevalence, clinical characteristics, and mortality among patients with myocardial infarction presenting without chest pain. *Journal of the American Medical Association, 283*(24), 3223–3229.

Jeffery, P. K., Wardlaw, A. J., Nelson, F. C., Collins, J. V., & Kay, A. B. (1989). Bronchial biopsies in asthma: An ultrastructural, quantitative study and correlation with hyperreactivity. *American Review of Respiratory Disease, 140,* 1745–1753.

Jooste, P. L., Weight, M. J., & Lombard, C. J. (2000). Short-term effectiveness of mandatory iodization of table salt, at an elevated iodine concentration, on the iodine and goiter status of schoolchildren with endemic goiter. *American Journal of Clinical Nutrition, 71*(1), 75–80.

Williams, J. G., Allison, C., Scott, F. J., Bolton, P. F., Baron-Cohen, S., Matthews, F. E., & Brayne, C. (2008). The Childhood Autism Spectrum Test (CAST): Sex differences. *Journal of Autism & Developmental Disorders, 38*(9), 1731–1739.

THE KRUSKAL-WALLIS ONE-WAY ANOVA BY RANKS

While the median test is used to determine whether *k* independent samples come from a population with a common median, the Kruskal-Wallis (K-W) one-way ANOVA by ranks is used to determine whether the distributions of the dependent variable are similar among the *k* levels of the independent variable. Thus, it is asking a different kind of question from the median test: *Are the distributions similar across all levels of the independent variable?* If the shapes of the distributions of the dependent variable for each level of the independent variable are similar (except for their measures of central tendency), then the K-W does indeed test for differences in medians.

Like the median test, the K-W test can be used when the independent variable is nominal level of measurement, with more than two levels, and the dependent variable is at least ordinal. It is considered to be more powerful than the median test when the distributions of the dependent variable are similar across the levels of the independent variable because it makes more complete use of the information contained in the observations (Kruskal & Wallis, 1952; Sprent & Smeeton, 2001). The K-W test ranks the values instead of merely noting them as being above or below the median. It is interesting that the K-W test was derived from the one-way ANOVA, with the actual observations being replaced by their ranks (Kruskal, 1952).

An Appropriate Research Question for the Kruskal-Wallis (K-W) Test

Numerous studies in the health care field have used the K-W test. In fact, since 2000, more than 12,000 peer-reviewed research articles in CINAHL, Medline, and PsycINFO have reported either having used the K-W test in a wide variety of settings or reporting on the test's characteristics. For example, Benyamini, Gerber, Molshatzki, Goldbourt, and Drory (2014) used the K-W test in a 13-year follow-up after a first myocardial infarction to evaluate recovery of self-rated health as a predictor of recurrent ischemic events. The K-W test was used by Ng et al. (2014) in their placebo-controlled trial that evaluated dose response to vitamin D supplementation in African Americans. Kydd, Touhy, Newman, Fagerberg, and Engstrom (2014) also used the K-W test to explore the attitudes of nurses and nursing students in Scotland, Sweden, and the United States toward working with older people. Chumbler et al. (2013) used the same test to evaluate postdischarge quality of care and age disparities among Veterans Administration (VA) ischemic stroke patients, and Barfield and Malone (2013) used the K-W test to examine perceived exercise benefits and barriers among power wheelchair soccer players.

In our hypothetical study, a research question that could be addressed using the K-W one-way ANOVA by ranks could be as follows:

> Are the distributions among the hospitalized children with three different types of cancer diagnoses (solid tumors, lymphoma, and leukemia or sarcoma) similar with regard to their number of nocturnal awakenings at Day 3 of their hospitalization?

Null and Alternative Hypotheses

Table 8.10 presents the null and alternative hypotheses for the K-W test. The null hypothesis states that the distributions for the three diagnosis groups are identical with similar medians. The alternative hypothesis states that the distributions are not identically located: At least one of the distributions is different from another and comes from a population with a different median.

Overview of the Procedure

To calculate a K-W test, the data for the entire sample are first ranked from lowest to highest. The smallest score in the sample is given a rank of "1," and the highest score is given the rank of *N*, where *N* represents the total sample size. Next, the scores in the separate cells are replaced by their rankings, and the average sum of the ranks for each cell is calculated. If the null hypothesis that the independent groups have similar underlying population distributions is true, the average sum of the ranks for each

Table 8.10 Example of Null and Alternative Hypotheses Suitable for Use With the Kruskal-Wallis Test

Null Hypothesis
H_0: There are no differences among the hospitalized children in the three diagnostic groups (solid tumors, lymphoma, and leukemia or sarcoma) with regard to their distributions of number of nocturnal awakenings at Day 3 of hospitalization. That is, all three groups have identical underlying distributions of number of nocturnal awakenings at Day 3 with similar medians.
Alternative Hypothesis
H_a: There are differences in the distributions among the hospitalized children in the three diagnostic groups (solid tumors, lymphoma, and leukemia or sarcoma) with regard to their number of nocturnal awakenings at Day 3 of hospitalization. That is, at least one of the groups is different from the other(s) with regard to its underlying distribution and median number of nocturnal awakenings at Day 3.

group should be the same. If the discrepancy between the average ranks for the independent groups is sufficiently large, the null hypothesis will be rejected.

There are a number of different formulae available to calculating the K-W test, all of which will produce similar results (Bewick, Cheek, & Ball, 2004; Conover, 1999; Siegel & Castellan, 1988). The formula (unadjusted for ties) for the K-W statistic that we will use compares the average rank for the separate cells to the average rank for the entire sample using the following formula (Siegel & Castellan, 1988):

$$\text{K-W} = \frac{12}{N(N+1)} \sum_{j=1}^{k} n_j(\bar{R}_j - \bar{R})^2$$

where

k = the number of groups,

n_j = the number of subjects in the jth group,

N = the total sample size,

$\bar{R}_j$ = the average of the ranks for the jth group, and

$\bar{R}$ = $(N + 2)/2$ = the average of the ranks for the entire sample.

When there are a number of ties in the data, a correction factor is added to the K-W formula:

$$\text{K-W}' = \frac{\text{K-W}}{1 - \frac{\sum_{j=1}^{g}(t_j^3 - t_j)}{N^3 - N}}$$

where

g = the total number of tied values,

t_j = the number of records tied at the jth value, and

N = total sample size.

Correcting for ties increases the value of the χ^2, which in turn enhances the likelihood that the null hypothesis will be rejected. Siegel and Castellan (1988) point out that if the number of ties is moderate (< 25%), there will be very little difference between the K-W and K-W′ statistics. Moreover, if the original K-W test is statistically significant, the adjusted K-W′ test will be as well.

If the data meet the assumptions of the Kruskal-Wallis one-way ANOVA by ranks and the sample size is sufficiently large (greater than five subjects per group), this K-W statistic is approximately distributed as a χ^2 with $df = (k - 1)$. The null hypothesis of equality of identical distributions will be rejected if the generated K-W statistic is greater than the critical value of the χ^2 at a prestated level of alpha (e.g., $\alpha = .05$) with $df = (k - 1)$. Alternatively, if presented with a computer printout, the null hypothesis will be rejected if the observed p value is less than the previously set α level.

Calculating the K-W test for the diagnosis and nocturnal awakenings (Day 3) data.

Table 8.11 presents the raw data for the number of nocturnal awakenings at Day 3 by the three levels of cancer diagnosis (solid tumor, lymphoma, and leukemia/sarcoma). The data set that we will be using is hospitalized children with cancer-30 cases.sav that can be found on the SAGE website (study.sagepub.com/pett2e). As indicated, the actual number of nocturnal awakenings at Day 3 is first sorted from lowest (3) to highest (15) ① and then ranked from 1 to 30 ②. Since the first three values are "3," their rank would be the average of the first three rankings (1, 2, and 3), or "2" ②. Similarly, the two values of "15" would occupy the 29th and 30th spots so their shared ranked value would be 29.5 ③. The ranks for each group are then summed ④ and averaged ⑤.

Using the formula described above, we would obtain the following:

$$\text{K-W} = \frac{12}{N(N+1)} \sum_{j=1}^{k} n_j \left(\bar{R}_j - \bar{R} \right)^2$$

$$= \frac{12}{30(30+1)} [10(20.60 - 15.5)^2 + 13(14.96 - 15.5)^2]$$

$$+7(9.21 - 15.5)^2$$

$$= \frac{12}{930} [260.1 + 3.791 + 276.949]$$

$$= 6.978$$

Table 8.11 Calculating the Kruskal-Wallis Test for the Diagnosis and Nocturnal Awakenings (Day 3) Data

	#Nocturnal Awakenings-Day 3							
		Actual Values		*Ranked Values by Diagnosis*				
Diagnosis[a]	*Actual Values*	*Sorted*	*Ranked*	*Group*	*Rank*	*Group*	*Sum of Ranks*	*Mean Rank* ($\bar{R}_j$)
1	8	(1) 3	(2) 2	1	7.5	1: (4)	206.0	(5) 20.60
1	13	3	2	1	13.5			
1	6	3	2	1	19			
1	12	4	4	1	19			
1	10	5	5.5	1	21.5			
1	12	5	5.5	1	24.5			
1	12	6	7.5	1	24.5			
1	12	6	7.5	1	24.5			
1	11	7	9.5	1	24.5			
1	10	7	9.5	1	27.5			
2	3	8	13.5	2	2	2:	194.5	14.96
2	15	8	13.5	2	2			
2	7	8	13.5	2	4			
2	3	8	13.5	2	9.5			
2	7	8	13.5	2	9.5			
2	4	8	13.5	2	13.5			
2	8	9	17	2	13.5			
2	15	10	19	2	13.5			
2	10	10	19	2	19			
2	11	10	19	2	21.5			
2	8	11	21.5	2	27.5			

(Continued)

Table 8.11 (Continued)

	#Nocturnal Awakenings-Day 3							
		Actual Values		Ranked Values by Diagnosis				
Diagnosis[a]	*Actual Values*	*Sorted*	*Ranked*	*Group*	*Rank*	*Group*	*Sum of Ranks*	*Mean Rank* ($\bar{R}_j$)
2	13	11	21.5	2	29.5			
2	8	12	24.5	2	29.5			
3	5	12	24.5	3	2	3:	64.5	9.21
3	5	12	24.5	3	5.5			
3	8	12	24.5	3	5.5	$\bar{R} = \frac{206.0 + 194.5 + 64.5}{30} = 15.5$		
3	9	13	27.5	3	7.5			
3	8	13	27.5	3	13.5			
3	3	15	(3) 29.5	3	13.5			
3	6	15	29.5	3	17			

[a]1 = solid tumor, 2 = lymphoma, 3 = leukemia/sarcoma.

Since 28 of 30 observations or 10 ranked values (2, 5.5, 7.5, 9.5, 13.5, 19, 21.5, 24.5, 27.5, and 29.5) were ties (Table 8.11), we will use the K-W test for ties:

$$\text{K-W}' = \frac{\text{K-W}}{1 - \frac{\sum_{j=1}^{g}(t_j^3 - t_j)}{N^3 - N}}$$

where, from Table 8.11, we can obtain

g = 10 ranked values with ties;

t_j (the number of tied observations/ranked values) = 3, 2, 2, 2, 6, 3, 2, 4, 2, 2; and

N = total sample = 30.

Table 8.11 indicates that there were 6 instances where 2 values were tied (e.g., '5'), 2 instances where 3 values were tied (e.g., '3'), 1 instance where 4 values were tied ('12'), and 1 instance in which 6 values were tied ('8'). Given this information, the correction factor is computed as follows:

$$1 - \frac{\sum_{j=1}^{g}\left(t_j^3 - t_j\right)}{N^3 - N} = 1 - \frac{6\left(2^3 - 2\right) + 2(3^3 - 3) + (4^3 - 4) + (6^3 - 6)}{30^3 - 30}$$

$$= 1 - \frac{36 + 48 + 60 + 210}{26,970} = 0.9868$$

For our data, the K-W test adjusted for ties would be

$$\text{K-W}' = \frac{\text{K-W}}{\textit{correction factor}} = \frac{6.978}{0.9868} = 7.07$$

As indicated, the K-W is distributed as a χ^2 with $df = k - 1$ or, in our case, $3 - 1 = 2$. According to Table A.2 in Appendix A, the critical value of the χ^2 with $df = 2$ when $\alpha =$ .05 is 5.99. Our conclusion is, therefore, that we will reject the null hypothesis of similarity of distributions since our actual χ^2 value corrected for ties, 7.07, is greater than 5.99. At least one of the distributions is statistically significantly different from the other. To determine which distribution is different, we would need to run post hoc tests. We will do that when we run these same analyses in SPSS for Windows.

Critical Assumptions of the Kruskal-Wallis Test

The Kruskal-Wallis test shares many of the assumptions of the Mann-Whitney test (Chapter 7) but extends these assumptions to more than two independent groups.

1. *The data have been collected from a randomly selected set of observations.*
2. *The dependent variable is at least ordinal level of measurement.*
3. *The independent variable is nominal, with more than two levels.*
4. *There is independence of observations within each group and between groups. There are no repeated measures or multiple response categories.*
5. *The shapes of the distributions of the dependent variable within each of the groups are similar except for a possible difference in measure of central tendency of at least one of the groups.*

The data from our hypothetical study partially meet these assumptions in that the dependent variable, number of nocturnal awakenings at Day 3, is interval level of measurement, the independent variable is categorical with three levels, and there are no repeated measures or multiple response categories. The similarity in shapes of the distributions for the three diagnosis groups can be determined by examining the histograms generated in the *Explore* command as outlined in Chapter 3. As we will see in Figure 8.8, the shapes of the three distributions in our analysis are not exactly similar; the distribution for the lymphoma group is more platykurtic than the other two. This is also not a random sample.

Computer Commands

The Median and Kruskal-Wallis tests are generated from the same dialog boxes in SPSS for Windows (Figure 8.6). These dialog boxes are opened by choosing the following items from the menu: *Analyze . . . Nonparametric Tests . . . Independent Samples . . . Customize analysis . . .*, inserting the dependent variable, *Nocturnal_sleep_awakenings_Day 3,* into the *Test field* and the independent variable (e.g., *type_of_cancer_collapsed*) into the *Group* field. If the null hypothesis is rejected, post hoc comparisons will also be performed.

Computer-Generated Output

Figure 8.8 presents the syntax commands (6) and computer-generated output for the K-W one-way ANOVA by ranks. The medians for the three cancer diagnosis groups are presented by the dark line going through each of the boxplots. These lines indicate that the children in the leukemia/sarcoma group had the lowest median for number of nocturnal awakenings at Day 3 of hospitalization (7), whereas the children diagnosed with sarcoma had the highest median number of nocturnal awakenings at Day 3 (8).

In the printout, we are also presented with the χ^2 (7.066 (9)) and *p* value (p = .029 (10)) for the K-W test. Note that the test has been adjusted for ties (11). This χ^2 value is similar to that which we obtained from the hand-calculated data (7.07).

To determine whether the K-W statistic is sufficiently large to reject the null hypothesis of similarity of distributions, we will reject the null hypothesis of similarity of distributions and equal medians if and only if our obtained *p* value (.029) is less than our prestated alpha (e.g., α = .05). Because .029 is less than .05, we will reject the null hypothesis of similarity of distributions and conclude that at least one of the groups has a significantly different distribution (and median) than the others.

Determining Which Groups Are Significantly Different

Like the one-way ANOVA, the Kruskal-Wallis test is an omnibus test in that, given a significant result, the test does not indicate where the differences are among the groups. To determine which groups are significantly different from one another, it is necessary to undertake post hoc comparisons. Two post hoc procedures are commonly used when a statistically significant K-W is obtained: the Dunn multiple-comparisons procedure and the use of the Mann-Whitney test to assess differences among the groups.

The Dunn multiple-comparisons procedure.

The Dunn procedure (Dunn, 1964) is a very effective, though somewhat conservative, post hoc approach to testing pairwise comparisons among groups. The procedure uses ranks based on all groups of the independent variable rather than just the two groups being compared. As with the post hoc procedure used for the median test, the *p* value for each of the pairwise comparisons is adjusted: $p_{adj} = pK(K - 1)/2$, where p = the original *p* value and K = the number of groups being compared. SPSS for Windows (v. 22–23) uses this procedure to undertake post hoc comparisons when the K-W test is found to be statistically significant.

Figure 8.8 Computer-generated printout for the Kruskal-Wallis one-way ANOVA by ranks.

```
***Data set: hospitalized children with cancer-30 cases***
                                    (6)
NPTESTS
 /INDEPENDENT TEST (Nocturnal_sleep_awakenings_Day3) GROUP
  (type_of_cancer_collapsed) KRUSKAL_WALLIS(COMPARE=PAIRWISE)
 /MISSING SCOPE=ANALYSIS USERMISSING=EXCLUDE
 /CRITERIA ALPHA=0.05 CILEVEL=95.
```

Hypothesis Test Summary

	Null Hypothesis	Test	Sig.	Decision
1	The distribution of Number of nocturnal sleep awakenings-Day 3 is the same across categories of type of cancer collapsed 3 levels.	Independent-Samples Kruskal-Wallis Test	.029	Reject the null hypothesis.

Asymptotic significances are displayed. The significance level is .05.

Independent-Samples Kruskal-Wallis Test

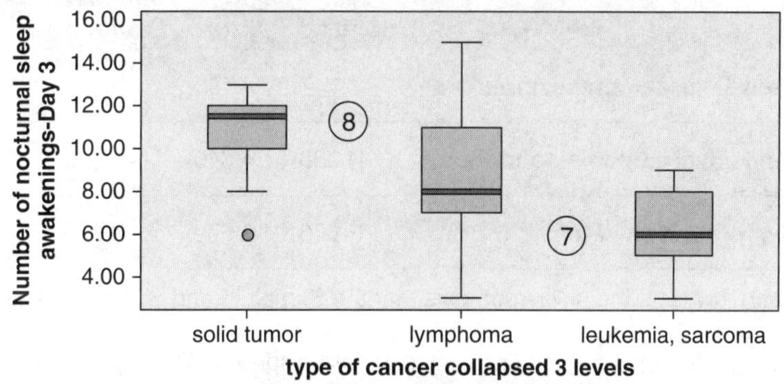

Total N	30	
Test Statistic	7.066	(9)
Degrees of Freedom	2	
Asymptotic Sig. (2-sided test)	.029	(10)

1. The test statistic is adjusted for ties. (11)

(Continued)

Figure 8.8 (Continued)

Pairwise Comparisons of type of cancer collapsed 3 levels

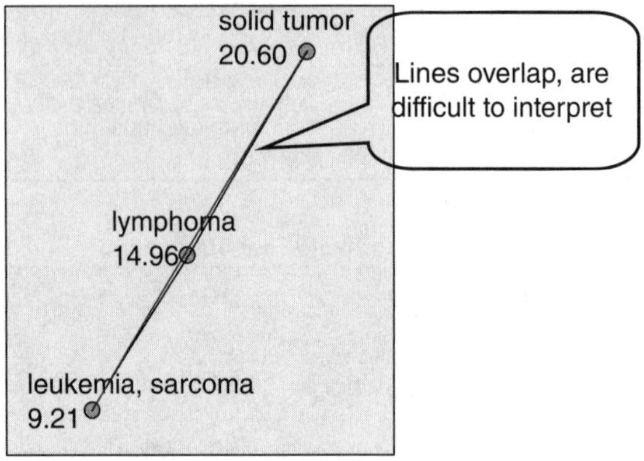

Each node shows the sample median of type of cancer collapsed 3 levels.

Sample1-Sample 2	Test Statistic	Std. Error	Std. Test Statistic	Sig.	Adj.Sig.	
leukemia, sarcoma-lymphoma	5.747	4.100	1.402	.161	.483	
leukemia, sarcoma-solid tumor	11.386	4.310	2.642	.008	.025	(12)
lymphoma-solid tumor	5.638	3.679	1.533	.125	.376	

Each row tests the null hypothesis that the Sample 1 and Sample 2 distributions are the same.
Asymptotic significances (2-sided tests) are displayed. The significance level is .05.

Once a determination has been made that there is at least one significant difference among the groups being tested (i.e., the Kruskal-Wallis test is significant), the differences in the mean ranks between the groups are computed pairwise. Next, a standard deviation (σ_{ij}) for each of these comparisons is calculated. From these values, a *t* statistic for each pairwise comparison is generated by dividing the absolute difference in ranks between each of the pairs by its standard deviation. This *t* statistic, which is distributed approximately normally, is compared to the standard normal *z* distribution. If the resulting *t* statistic at $\alpha/2$ is sufficiently large, the null hypothesis of no differences between the ranks is rejected. This *t* statistic is calculated as follows:

$$T_{ij} = \frac{|D_{ij}|}{\sigma_{ij}} = \frac{|\overline{R}_i - \overline{R}_j]}{\sigma_{ij}}$$

where

$|\bar{R}_i - \bar{R}_j|$ = the absolute value of the difference in mean ranks between Groups *i* and *j*;

$$\sigma_{ij} = \sqrt{A\left(\frac{1}{n_i} + \frac{1}{n_j}\right)}$$

$$A = \left[\frac{N(N+1)}{12} - \frac{\Sigma_{j=1}^{g}(t_j^3 - t)}{12(N-1)}\right]$$

N = the total sample size;

t_j, (the number of tied observations/ranked values) = 3, 2, 2, 2, 6, 3, 2, 4, 2, 2 for our data;

n_i = the sample size for Group *i;* and

n_j = the sample size for Group *j*.

In our hypothetical example, there are three pairwise comparisons to be made: Group 1 versus Group 2, Group 1 versus Group 3, and Group 2 versus Group 3. Since the value of *A* in the above equation will remain the same for all three comparisons, we can calculate it now:

$$A = \left[\frac{30(30+1)}{12} - \frac{6(2^3 - 2) + 2(3^3 - 3) + (4^3 - 4) + (6^3 - 6)}{12(30-1)}\right]$$

$$A = \left[77.5 - \frac{330}{348}\right] = (77.5 - 0.9482) = 76.5517$$

Table 8.12 presents the additional calculations and final *t* values for each of these comparisons. The SPSS for Windows output presented to us in Figure 8.8 also presents the pairwise comparisons by type of cancer both in the form of a plot and in a table of values. Unfortunately, the plot that has been generated for us is difficult to interpret because it appears to be a straight line going through all three cells.

Table 8.12 indicates that the *t* values for the three comparisons are 1.53, 2.64, and 1.40, respectively. To determine which pairs, if any, are significantly different from one another, it is necessary to compare the obtained *t* statistic for each of the three comparisons with the absolute value of a critical *z* at a predetermined two-tailed level of alpha (e.g., $\alpha = .05$). The null hypothesis of similarity of mean ranks for the pair of comparisons will be rejected if the absolute value of the *t* statistics is greater than the critical *z*.

Adjusting the α level (or *p* values) to accommodate pairwise comparisons.

What α should be used to examine these pairwise comparisons? We could use an unadjusted α (e.g., α = .05) and compare it to our unadjusted *p* value that we obtained

Table 8.12 Calculations for the Dunn Multiple Comparison Procedure

		Mean Rank Difference	*Standard Deviation of Differences*	t *Statistic*
Group	*Comparison*	$\lvert \bar{D} \rvert = \bar{R}_i - \bar{R}_j$	$\sigma_{ij} = \sqrt{A\left(\frac{1}{n_i} + \frac{1}{n_j}\right)}$	$T_{ij}^{*} = \frac{\lvert D \rvert}{\sigma_{ij}}$
1 vs.2	Solid tumor vs. lymphoma	|20.60 – 14.96| = 5.64	$\sigma_{12} = \sqrt{76.5517\left(\frac{1}{10} + \frac{1}{13}\right)} = 3.68$	$\frac{5.64}{3.68} = 1.53$
1 vs. 3	Solid tumor vs. leukemia, sarcoma	|20.60 – 9.21| = 11.39	$\sigma_{13} = \sqrt{76.5517\left(\frac{1}{10} + \frac{1}{7}\right)} = 4.312$	$\frac{11.39}{4.312} = 2.64$
2 vs. 3	Lymphoma vs leukemia, sarcoma	|14.96 – 9.21| = 5.75	$\sigma_{23} = \sqrt{76.5517\left(\frac{1}{13} + \frac{1}{7}\right)} = 4.102$	$\frac{5.75}{4.102} = 1.40$

in SPSS for Windows in Figure 8.8. That would be similar to comparing the critical value of our t ($|1.96|$ if $\alpha = .05$). Our conclusion would be that we would reject the null hypothesis of similarity of distributions if and only if our $p < \alpha$, or if the absolute value of the actual t statistic is greater than our critical value. Using these criteria, we would conclude that the only pair that was statistically significantly different from each other was the solid tumor and sarcoma/leukemia groups (12).

Because there are multiple comparisons being made on the same sample, we will need to adjust our α level to accommodate a potentially inflated Type I error. SPSS for Windows uses an adjusted p value: $p_{adj} = pK(K - 1)/2$, where p = our generated p value and K = the number of levels of the independent variable. We could also adjust the α level using Bonferroni's inequality, $\alpha' = \alpha/k$, where k = the number of tests being conducted. A third approach would be to use a slightly more liberal step-down approach suggested by Holms (Holland & Copenhaver, 1988; J. Stevens, 2009).

To illustrate the differences between the three approaches, we will use both the adjusted p value given to us in SPSS for Windows and the Bonferroni approach for the Dunn procedure. Then we will use the Holms step-down procedure to evaluate the Mann-Whitney post hoc comparisons.

Adjusting the p value is easy if we have the computer output that was presented in Figure 8.8. Only one of the three adjusted p values was statistically significant ($p_{adj} = pK(K - 1/2 = .008(3)(2)/2 = .024$ (12)). That is, the children diagnosed with solid tumors had a statistically significantly higher median number of nocturnal sleep awakenings at Day 3 than did the children diagnosed with leukemia or sarcoma. No other pairs were statistically significantly different from the other.

Using Bonferroni's inequality with $\alpha = .05$, we would obtain $\alpha' = \alpha/k = .05/3 = .016$. Comparing $\alpha = .016$ with our unadjusted p values from Figure 8.8 (.161, .008, and .125), the only pairwise difference that was statistically significant would be, again, the leukemia/sarcoma versus solid tumor pair. Dunn (1964) and Neave and Worthington (1988) suggest that, when undertaking post hoc comparisons, α should be more liberal than the usual $\alpha = .05$ (e.g., .10 or .20) so that any differences between groups can be detected. These authors point out that multiple comparisons should be made only once a significant overall test has been obtained at the usual α (e.g., $\alpha = .05$). This gives a good protection against inflated error when using a more liberal α for the post hoc tests.

Pairwise comparisons using the Mann-Whitney test.

An alternative test for post hoc comparisons that is readily available in statistical computer packages and in free Internet sites is the Mann-Whitney (M-W) test (for details of the Mann-Whitney test, see Chapter 7). This particular M-W test can be obtained in SPSS for Windows by selecting the following items from the SPSS menu: *Analyze . . . Nonparametric tests . . . Legacy Dialogs . . . 2 Independent Samples.* The groups to be compared (e.g., 1 vs. 2, 1 vs. 3, 2 vs. 3) can be specified by highlighting the independent (grouping) variable, clicking on the *Define Range* dialog box, and selecting the comparison groups (e.g., 1 vs. 3). Please note that we are using the legacy dialog box to generate the M-W test because the nominal-level variable, type of cancer, has three levels, and it is only through the *Legacy Dialogs . . .* command that we can specify the groups that we want to compare.

The result of comparing Groups 1 and 3 and its significance level (p values) is presented in Figure 8.9. The two remaining comparisons, Group 1 versus 2 ($p = .186$) and Group 2 versus 3 ($p = .275$), were not statistically significant ($p > .05$) and are not presented in Figure 8.9. Note that this p value is not corrected for ties and has not been adjusted for the inflated Type I error created as a result of undertaking three tests on the same set of data.

The Holms step-down procedure for post hoc comparisons.

The Holms step-down procedure will be used here to illustrate a third approach to adjusting for inflated Type I error. Using this procedure, the generated p values for the Mann-Whitney post hoc tests are first ranked from lowest to highest ($p_1, < p_2 < p_3 < \ldots p_i$). These p values are then compared to $\alpha/(k - i + 1)$, where α = the prestated alpha level (e.g., .10), k = the number of post hoc tests generated, and i = the index of the particular p value that is being compared. The null hypothesis for a particular test will be rejected if $p_i < \alpha/(k - i + 1)$.

Table 8.13 presents the results of the Holms procedure for the three post hoc tests in our hypothetical study. These results indicate that the only significant difference among the groups is between the solid tumor and leukemia/sarcoma groups because .002 < .033 (13). This result suggests that the hospitalized children with solid tumors had a statistically significantly higher median number of nocturnal awakenings compared to the children diagnosed with leukemia or sarcoma. The significance values for the other comparisons were both greater than our adjusted alpha levels, indicating that no other groups were significantly different. This is the same conclusion we reached using the Dunn multiple-comparison procedure.

Figure 8.9 Mann-Whitney post-hoc test comparing children diagnosed with solid tumors and those with leukemia/sarcoma generated in SPSS for Windows (v. 22–23).

```
***Data set: hospitalized children with cancer-30 cases.sav***

NPAR TESTS
 /M-W= Nocturnal_sleep_awakenings_Day3 BY type_of_cancer_collapsed(1 3)
 /MISSING ANALYSIS.
```

Ranks

	type_of_cancer_collapsed type of cancer collapsed 3 levels	N	Mean Rank	Sum of Ranks
Nocturnal_sleep_awakenings_Day3 Number of nocturnal sleep awakenings-Day 3	1.00 solid tumor	10	11.95	119.50
	3.00 leukemia, sarcoma	7	4.79	33.50
	Total	17		

Test Statistics[a]

	Nocturnal_sleep_awakenings_Day3 Number of nocturnal sleep awakenings-Day 3
Mann-Whitney U	5.500
Wilcoxon W	33.500
Z	-2.909
Asymp. Sig. (2-tailed)	.004
Exact Sig. [2*(1-tailed Sig.)]	.002[b]

a. Grouping Variable: type_of_cancer_collapsed type of cancer collapsed 3 levels

b. Not corrected for ties.

Table 8.13 Results of the Holms Step-down Procedure to Adjust for Type 1 Error When Undertaking Multiple Comparisons

I	*Group*	*Comparison*	*Obtained p value*[a]	$\alpha/(k - i + 1)$
1	1 vs. 3	Solid tumor vs. leukemia/ sarcoma	.002	.10/(3 – 1 + 1) = .033 (13)
2	1 vs. 2	Solid tumor vs. lymphoma	.186	.10/(3 – 2 + 1) = .05
3	2 vs. 3	Lymphoma vs. leukemia/ sarcoma	.275	.10/(3 – 3 + 1) = .10

Internet Resources for Generating the Kruskal-Wallis Test

A number of free Internet resources could be used to generate the K-W test. One current resource is www.vassasrstats.net. Once on the website, we click on *Ordinal* tests to obtain the K-W test. Next, we are asked for k (the number of levels of the independent variable [e.g., $k = 3$ for our variable, types of cancer diagnosis]) and, then, upon request, we indicate the number of observations for each of the cells (e.g., 10, 13 and 7). Once we have identified the number of cases in each of the cells, we can copy and paste the raw data (e.g., from Excel) into the *Raw Data* list. After deleting any empty values at the end of each column, we *import data to data cells*. Figure 8.10 presents the imported data and generated output from this Internet resource. Notice that the test statistic, H, is the same as our hand-calculated value that was not adjusted for ties (6.97) and that p = .0307 (14). The "*" indicates that if the sample sizes in each of the cells is at least 5, the sampling distribution of the generated statistic, H, is distributed as a chi-square with $df = k - 1$. If any of the *ns* in the cells are less than 5, then the sampling distribution of H and the p value are an approximation of the chi-square distribution.

Presentation of Results

The results of the Kruskal-Wallis test could be presented in a table similar to that used for the median test (Table 8.9). Instead of the χ^2 value for the median test, however, the K-W χ^2 value is presented with its corresponding p value (e.g., 6.37, $p = .04$). The results, along with the post hoc comparisons, also could be presented in the text as follows:

> The results of the Kruskal-Wallis test indicate that there were significant differences among the three cancer diagnosis groups with regard to the children's number of nocturnal sleep awakenings at Day 3 of their hospitalization ($\chi^2_{K\text{-}W} = 7.07$, $p = .03$). Post hoc analyses using the Dunn procedure indicated that the hospitalized children diagnosed with solid tumors had a higher median number of nocturnal sleep awakenings at Day 3 than the children diagnosed with leukemia/sarcoma ($p = .025$). No other groups had significantly different median nocturnal sleep awakenings at Day 3.

Figure 8.10 Output for the Kruskal-Wallis test generated from www.vassarstats.net.

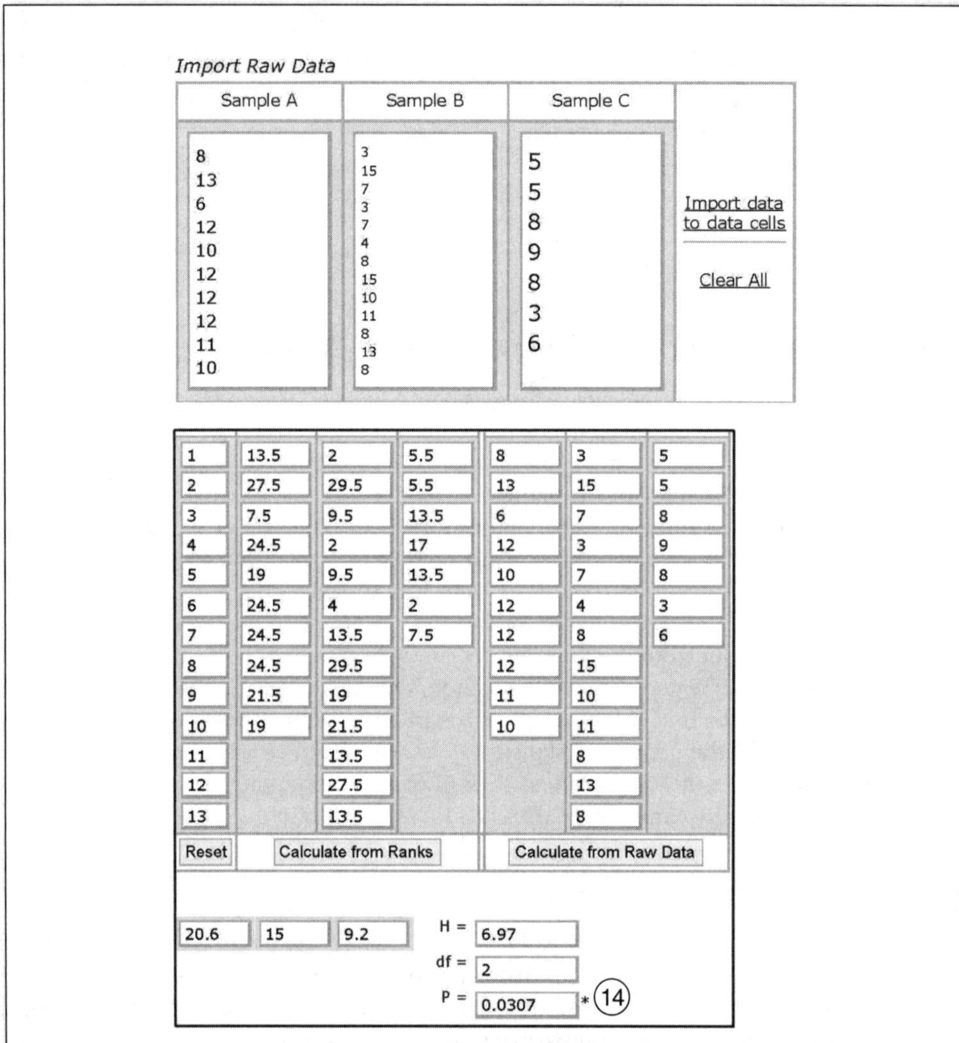

SOURCE: ©Richard Lowry 1998–2014. All rights reserved. Retrieved form www.vassarstats.net

Advantages, Limitations, and Alternatives to the Kruskal-Wallis Test

The Kruskal-Wallis one-way ANOVA by ranks is a simple test to understand and use. Like the one-way ANOVA, the K-W test does not require equal sample sizes. It is also one of the most popular and powerful of the nonparametric tests for continuous data.

The parametric alternative to the Kruskal-Wallis test is the one-way ANOVA. This test assumes normality of distributions within each level of the independent variable and equality of variances among levels of the independent variable. The ANOVA is more powerful than the K-W test when its more stringent assumptions have been met. Although the ANOVA is robust with regard to normality of distributions, it is less reliable when the assumption of equal variances has been violated. Moreover, the K-W test has power that is almost equal to that of the ANOVA for normal distributions and is more powerful than the parametric statistic when the distribution of the data is skewed (Dexter, 1994; Gibbons, 1985; Neave & Worthington, 1988). Daniel (2000) reports that the asymptotic efficiency of the K-W test relative to the F test for the one-way ANOVA is .955 if the distribution of the dependent variable within the groups is normal and not less than .864 when the shapes of the distributions are similar. Alternative nonparametric tests that could be used in place of the K-W test are those that were reviewed in this chapter: the median test, the Mantel-Haenszel chi-square test, and the chi-square test for k independent samples.

Examples From Published Research

Barfield, J. P., & Malone, L. A. (2013). Perceived exercise benefits and barriers among power wheelchair soccer players. *Journal of Rehabilitation Research & Development, 50*(2), 231–238. doi: 10.1682/JRRD.2011.12.0234

Benyamini, Y., Gerber, Y., Molshatzki, N., Goldbourt, U., & Drory, Y. (2014). Recovery of self-rated health as a predictor of recurrent ischemic events after first myocardial infarction: A 13-year follow-up. *Health Psychology, 33*(4), 317–325. doi: 10.1037/a0031371

Kydd, A., Touhy, T., Newman, D., Fagerberg, I., & Engstrom, G. (2014). Attitudes towards caring for older people in Scotland, Sweden and the United States. *Nursing Older People, 26*(2), 33–40. doi: 10.7748/nop2014.02.26.2.33.e547

Ng, K., Scott, J. B., Drake, B. F., Chan, A. T., Hollis, B. W., Chandler, P. D., . . . Fuchs, C. S. (2014). Dose response to vitamin D supplementation in African Americans: Results of a 4-arm, randomized, placebo-controlled trial. *American Journal of Clinical Nutrition, 99*(3), 587–598. doi: 10.3945/ajcn.113.067777

Packer, T. L., Sauriol, A., & Brouwer, B. (1994). Fatigue secondary to chronic illness: Postpolio syndrome, chronic fatigue syndrome, and multiple sclerosis. *Archives of Physical Medicine and Rehabilitation, 75*, 1122–1126.

THE TWO-WAY ANOVA BY RANKS

What statistical approaches could we use if we have a continuous dependent variable that is not normally distributed, perhaps has unequal variances with two (or more) independent variables that are nominal level of measurement? Because there are two independent variables (and their interaction), we would not be able to consider the K-W test without some manipulation since the K-W test assumes there is only a single independent nominal-level variable.

Several potential approaches to undertaking a nonparametric two-way ANOVA have been suggested when the dependent variable is not normally distributed and, perhaps, when there is not homogeneity of variance. These include (1) transforming a nonnormally distributed dependent variable to one that more closely resembles a normal distribution, (2) constructing Wald-type or weighted *F* statistics based on ranks for assessing the main effects and their interaction (Akritas, 2011; Akritas & Arnold, 1994; Akritas, Arnold, & Brunner, 1997; Akritas, Stavropoulos, & Caroni, 2009), or (3) using a distribution-free procedure that rank transforms the original data and then performs a two-way ANOVA on the ranks using either *F* or chi-square statistics (Akritas & Brunner, 2003; Conover & Iman, 1981; Puri & Sen, 1985).

Data transformations. Commonly used transformations for severely skewed data include the log, square root, and inverse transformations. Chapter 3 of this textbook and Tabachnick and Fidell (2013) present more in-depth discussion of these transformations. These will not be the focus of the present discussion since we are focusing on nonparametric alternatives to the parametric two-way ANOVA.

Use of Wald-type and weighted *F* statistics. In response to concerns about the nonlinear nature of rank transformations and their subsequent inability to perform successfully under certain conditions, Akritas and Arnold (1994) introduced Wald and, subsequently, weighted *F*-type statistics based on ranks (Akritas et al., 2009). Unfortunately, this very promising theoretical approach to nonparametric analyses of factorial designs has not as yet become readily available (via statistical computer packages) to researchers whose primary focus is on the practical application of nonparametric statistics in real-world settings.

Rank-transformed tests. Distribution-free tests include the many nonparametric tests that are based on replacing the original data with their ranks. There has been much discussion in recent years about the best approach to obtaining a two-way ANOVA using ranked data. Two approaches to the two-way ANOVA that make use of ranked data are the rank tests (Puri & Sen, 1985) and the rank transform tests (Conover & Iman, 1976, 1981). The main difference between these two approaches is in the authors' choice of final statistic to determine significance (Toothaker & Newman, 1994). Each approach first ranks all of the dependent variable data from 1 to *N* (where N = the total sample size). These ranked data then serve as the dependent variable in a two-way ANOVA. From this analysis, the sums of squares for rows, columns, and rows × columns interaction are obtained. Finally, the statistics are computed.

For the Puri and Sen (1985) rank test, the test statistics for the rows (r), columns (c), and their interaction (r × c) are as follows (Toothaker & Newman, 1994): $(N-1)SS_r/SS_{total}$, $(N-1)SS_c/SS_{total}$, and $(N-1)SS_{r \times c\ interaction}/SS_{total}$. The distributions of these three statistics are asymptotically distributed as chi-square statistics with $df_r = J-1$, $df_c = K-1$, $df_{r \times c} = (J-1)(K-1)$, respectively, where J = #rows and K = #columns.

Rank transform tests (Conover & Iman, 1981) use the same approach as the Puri and Sen (1985) rank test, but their statistics are slightly different. Conover and Iman (1981) suggest that the parametric two-way ANOVA be applied to the rank-transformed data, and the ANOVA *F* tests are then applied to the ranks (Akritas, 1990; Conover, 1999; Conover & Iman, 1981; Puri & Sen, 1985; Toothaker & Newman, 1994): $F_r = MS_r/MS_w$, $F_c = MS_c/MS_w$, and $F_{r \times c} = MS_{r \times c}/MS_w$. The distributions of these *F* statistics are asymptotically distributed as an *F* statistic with degrees of freedom of $df_r = J-1$, $df_c = K-1$, $df_{r \times c} = (J-1)(K-1)$, respectively, in the numerator of the F statistic and $df_w = JK(n - 1)$ in the denominator (Toothaker & Newman, 1994).

An Appropriate Research Question for the Two-Way ANOVA by Ranks

Despite the flurry of articles written prior to 2000 that discussed the potential use of the two-way ANOVA with rank-transformed data, this approach has hardly been used in recent years. For example, a search of the research literature cited in CINAHL, Medline, and PsycInfo for the years 2000–2014 yielded only one verifiable reference to its use. Other references indicated the use of a nonparametric ANOVA, but on closer examination, it was apparent that the statistics the researchers used were the one-way Kruskal-Wallis and Friedman tests. None of these references used a two-way or higher design.

Why would this potentially useful two-way ANOVA by ranks be ignored in preference to the parametric two-way ANOVA or other nonparametric tests? One possible explanation is that researchers have preferred to use data transformations (e.g., the log and square root) to generate a more normally distributed dependent variable. The second possibility is that writers of statistical textbooks have elected not to include the two-way ANOVA by ranks in their discussion of nonparametric tests but rather have focused on the Kruskal-Wallis and Friedman tests (Akritas, 2014).

A third explanation is that rank transformations of the dependent variable may have problems. That is, while rank statistics are robust against outliers and have good power properties (Akritas & Brunner, 2003) and may also have sufficient robustness and power when assessing the main effects in a two-way layout, they may produce mixed results when assessing for interaction (Blair, Sawilowsky, & Higgins, 1987; Conover, 1999; Thompson, 1991; Thompson & Ammann, 1989; Toothaker & Newman, 1994). It is also apparent from a review of the nonparametric statistics literature that there is not universal agreement as to the best strategy for rank transforming the dependent variable using the two-way ANOVA by ranks.

Regardless of the reasons for the exclusion, this nonparametric competitor to the parametric two-way ANOVA offers an alternative to the challenges that arise when trying to identify an appropriate transformation that produces a more normally distributed dependent variable. So, let's examine the results we would obtain if we used the rank (Puri & Sen, 1985) and rank transform approaches (Conover & Iman, 1976) to the two-way ANOVA.

Null and Alternative Hypotheses

Suppose we wanted to examine not only the impact of the child's cancer diagnosis but also the group intervention and their interaction on the number of nocturnal sleep awakenings of the hospitalized children at Day 3 of their hospitalization. The data set that we will use for this example is hospitalized children with cancer-20 cases.sav which can be found on the SAGE website: study.sagepub.com/pett2e. Table 8.14 presents the null and alternative hypotheses that would be suitable for the two-way ANOVA by ranks. Note that we will be examining the hypotheses for group, diagnosis, and group × diagnosis interaction.

Table 8.14 Example of Null and Alternative Hypotheses Suitable for Use With the Two-Way Analysis of Variance by Ranks

Null and Alternative Hypotheses:
Group Intervention
H_0: There are no differences among the hospitalized children in the two groups (staff-initiated intervention and usual-care groups) with regard to their distributions of number of nocturnal awakenings at Day 3 of hospitalization. That is, the two groups have identical underlying distributions of number of nocturnal awakenings at Day 3 with similar medians.
H_a: There are differences in between the hospitalized children in the two groups (staff-initiated intervention vs. usual care) with regard to their distributions and median number of nocturnal awakenings at Day 3 of hospitalization.
Diagnosis
H_0: There are no differences among the hospitalized children in the three diagnostic groups (solid tumors, lymphoma, and leukemia or sarcoma) with regard to their distributions of number of nocturnal awakenings at Day 3 of hospitalization. That is, all three groups have identical underlying distributions of number of nocturnal awakenings at Day 3 with similar medians.
H_a: There are differences in the distributions among the hospitalized children in the three diagnostic groups (solid tumors, lymphoma, and leukemia or sarcoma) with regard to their number of nocturnal awakenings at Day 3 of hospitalization. That is, at least one of the groups is different from the other(s) with regard to its underlying distribution and median number of nocturnal awakenings at Day 3.
Group x Diagnosis Interaction
H_0: There is no group x diagnosis interaction with regard to the hospitalized children's distributions of number of nocturnal awakenings at Day 3 of hospitalization. That is, all 6 groups have identical underlying distributions of number of nocturnal awakenings at Day 3 with similar medians.
H_a: There is a group x diagnosis interaction with regard to the distributions among the hospitalized children with regard to their number of nocturnal awakenings at Day 3 of hospitalization. That is, at least one of the 6 groups is different from the other(s) with regard to its underlying distribution and median number of nocturnal awakenings at Day 3.

Overview of the Procedure

To calculate the two-way ANOVA by ranks, the data for the entire sample are first ranked from lowest to highest. As with the K-W test, the smallest score in the sample is given a rank of "1," and the highest score is given the rank of *N*, where *N* represents the total sample size. Next, the ranked data for the dependent variable are submitted to the parametric two-way ANOVA along with the two independent variables, group intervention and cancer diagnosis. In this example, we will compare the two approaches to ranking suggested by Puri and Sen (1985) and Conover and Iman (1981). For these comparisons, we will focus on the computer-generated output rather than produce the two-way ANOVA by ranks results "by hand" as we have done for the other nonparametric statistics presented in the chapter. The reason for this is that hand calculation of a two-way ANOVA is cumbersome and would not add substantially to the discussion. For those who are interested, there are excellent statistics books that describe the two-way ANOVA in depth (e.g., Field (2013); Hinkle et al. (2003); Sheskin (2003); J. P. Stevens (2013)).

Critical Assumptions of the Two-Way ANOVA by Ranks

The assumptions of the two-way ANOVA by ranks are similar to the parametric two-way ANOVA but without the assumption of a normal distribution of the dependent variable.

1. *The data have been collected from a randomly selected set of observations.*
2. *The dependent variable is at least ordinal level of measurement.*
3. *The independent variables are nominal level of measurement each with two or more levels.*
4. *There is independence of observations within each group and between groups. There are no repeated measures or multiple response categories.*
5. *The shapes of the distributions of the dependent variable within each of the groups are similar except for a possible difference in measure of central tendency of at least one of the groups.*

The data from our hypothetical study of 30 hospitalized children with cancer partially meet these assumptions in that the dependent variable, number of nocturnal awakenings at Day 3, is interval level of measurement, and the two independent variables, group intervention and cancer diagnosis, are nominal level of measurement. There are also no repeated measures or multiple response categories. The similarity in shapes of the distributions for the two independent variables can be determined by examining the plots and coefficients generated in the *Explore* command as outlined in Chapter 3 (see Figure 8.12). This is also not a random sample.

Computer Commands

To undertake a two-way ANOVA by ranks, it is first necessary to create a variable that represents the rank of the dependent variable, *nocturnal_sleep_awakening_day3*. To accomplish that in SPSS (v. 22–23), click on the commands *Transform . . . Rank cases. . . .* Next, indicate the variable that is to be ranked (*nocturnal_sleep_awakening_day3*). Figure 8.11 presents the dialog boxes that were used to generate the rank-transformed variable. Note that the ranked data have been requested (1) with ties being assigned the average of the tied ranks (2).

Figure 8.11 Transforming a dependent variable into its ranks in SPSS for Windows (v. 22–23).

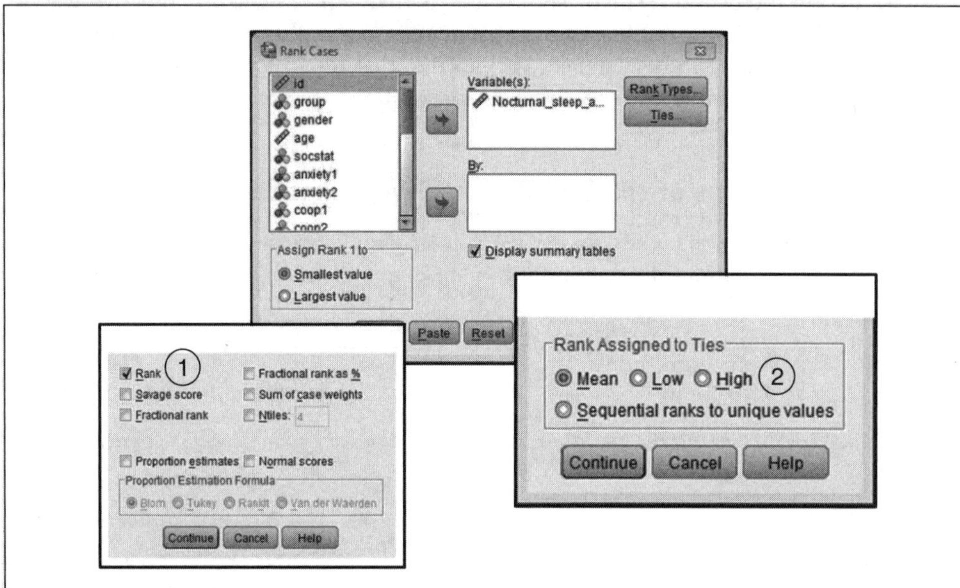

Figure 8.12 presents the plots of the rank-transformed dependent variable using the *Explore . . .* command in SPSS for Windows. The shapes of the distributions within each of our independent variables (*cancer diagnosis* and *type of intervention*) are not exactly similar. It appears that the distribution of the dependent variable for the lymphoma group is more platykurtic than the other two; there is also an outlier within the solid tumor group.

Figure 8.13 presents the commands used to obtain the two-way ANOVA by ranks in SPSS for Windows (v. 22–23). These windows were opened by clicking on *Analyze . . . General Linear Model . . . Univariate. . . .* The newly created ranked variable, *RNocturn*, is the dependent variable and the two independent variables, *Group* and *type_of_cancer_collapsed,* are the fixed factors (3). By clicking on *Model . . .* we can indicate that we are requesting the full model, including the interaction (4). In *Options . . .* we have requested the estimated marginal means for the rank-transformed data, the descriptive statistics, estimates of effect size, observed power, and homogeneity tests (5). By clicking on *Post hoc . . .* we can indicate that we want two post hoc tests for our diagnosis variable: the more liberal least significance difference (LSD) test and the more conservative Tukey test (6). While we are unable to undertake post hoc tests for our dichotomous group intervention variable, we can easily determine which group (intervention vs. usual care) is different from the other by examining the descriptive statistics. Finally, by clicking on *Plots . . .* we can plot the average ranks of the cells by

Figure 8.12 Generating the plots of the rank-transformed dependent variable using the *Explore* command in SPSS for Windows (v. 22–23).

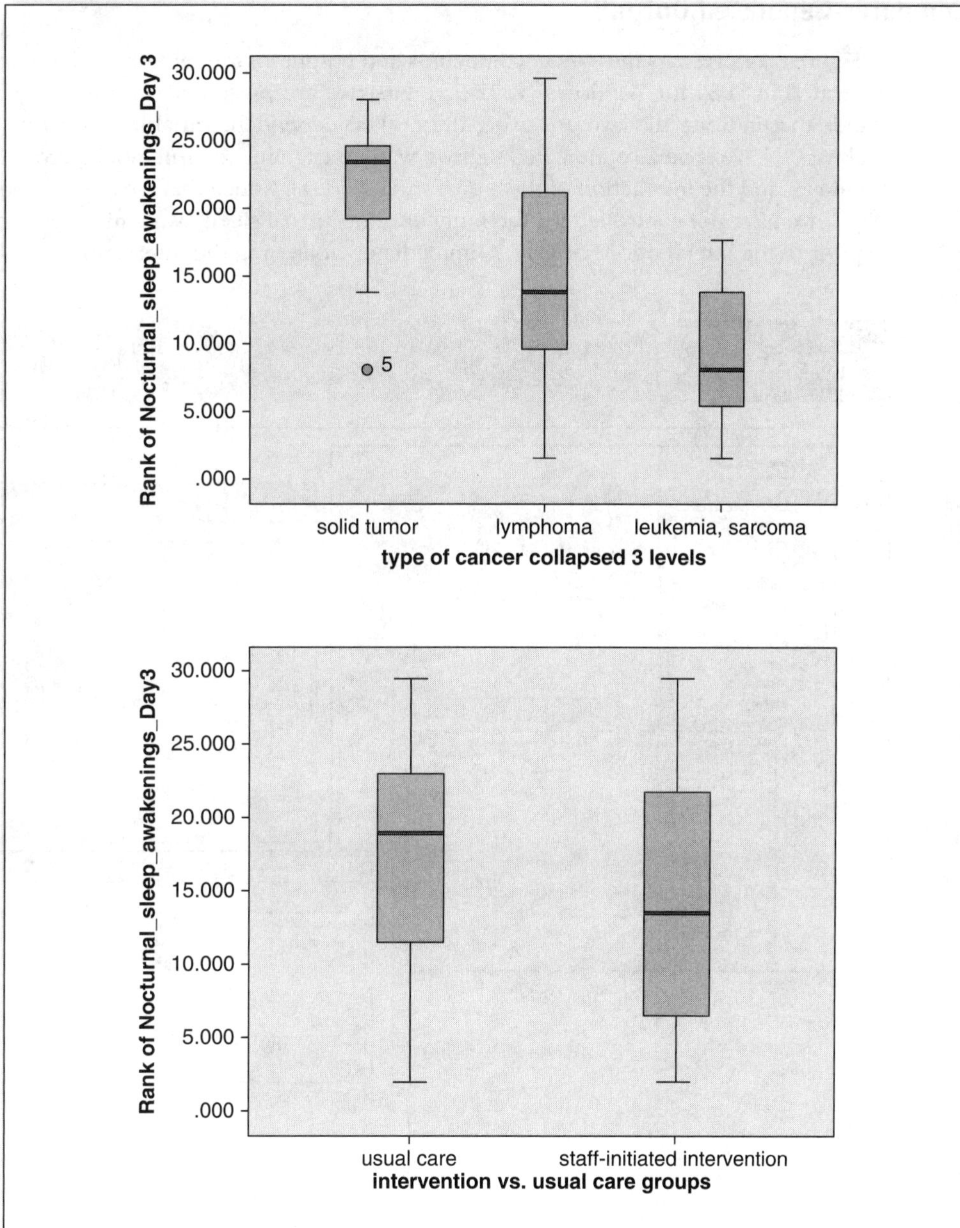

placing the diagnosis variable along the horizontal axis with separate lines for the group intervention variable (7).

Computer-Generated Output

Figure 8.14 presents the syntax commands and output for the two-way ANOVA by ranks generated in SPSS for Windows (v. 22–23). First we are presented with the syntax commands that indicate that we are using the ranked dependent variable, *RNocturn,* in our analysis (8). We have also indicated that we want to examine the full model, group, cancer diagnosis, and the interaction of these two variables (9). Notice that we are just looking at Day 3; we have not controlled for the number of nocturnal sleep awakenings at either Day 1 (prior to the intervention) or Day 2 (immediately following the intervention).

Figure 8.13 Dialog boxes used to generate the two-way ANOVA by ranks in SPSS for Windows (v. 22–23).

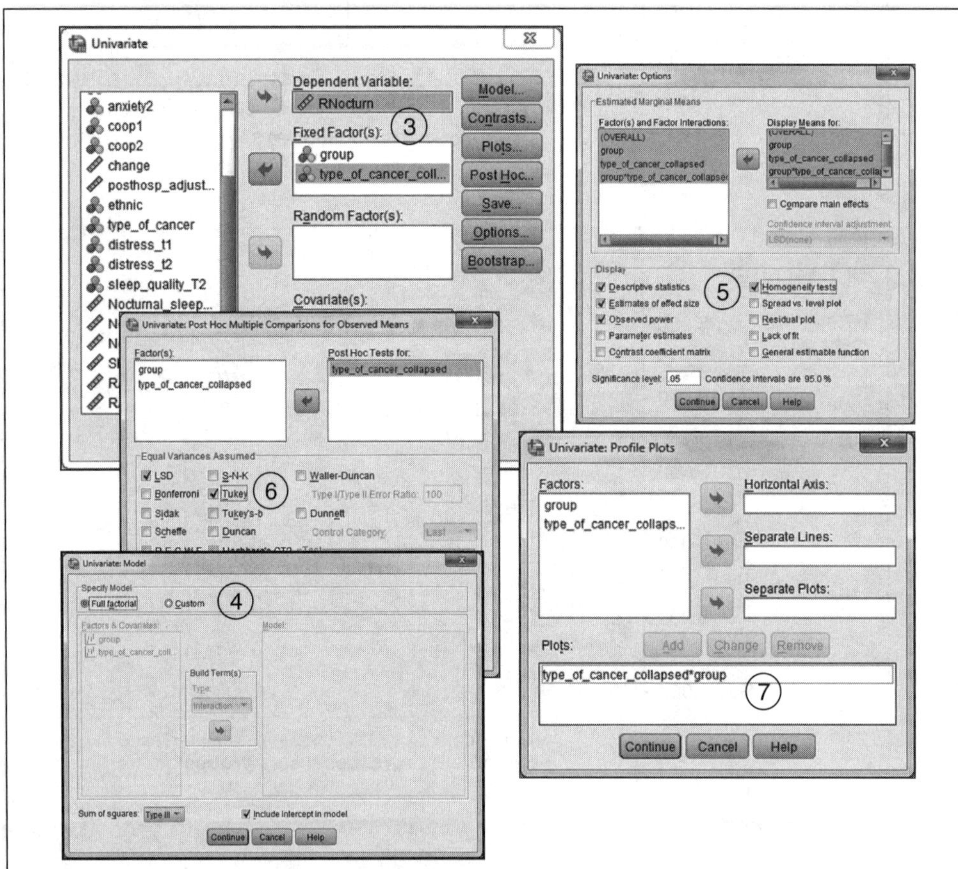

Figure 8.14 Syntax commands and computer-generated output for the two-way ANOVA by ranks generated in SPSS for Windows (v. 22–23).

```
***Data set: hospitalized children with cancer-30 cases.sav***

UNIANOVA RNocturn BY group type_of_cancer_collapsed (8)
 /METHOD=SSTYPE(3)
 /INTERCEPT=INCLUDE
 /POSTHOC=type_of_cancer_collapsed(TUKEY LSD)
 /PLOT=PROFILE(type_of_cancer_collapsed*group)
 /EMMEANS=TABLES(OVERALL)
 /EMMEANS=TABLES(group)
 /EMMEANS=TABLES(type_of_cancer_collapsed)
 /EMMEANS=TABLES(group*type_of_cancer_collapsed)
 /PRINT=OPOWER ETASQ DESCRIPTIVE
 /CRITERIA=ALPHA(.05)
 /DESIGN=group type_of_cancer_collapsed group*type_of_cancer_collapsed. (9)
```

Descriptive Statistics

Dependent Variable: RNocturn Rank of Nocturnal_sleep_awakenings_Day3

group intervention vs. usual care grps	type_of_cancer_collapsed type of cancer collapsed 3 levels	Mean	Std. Deviation	N
.00 usual care	1.00 solid tumor (10)	22.37500	2.657536	4
	2.00 lymphoma	16.83333	8.310385	9
	3.00 leukemia, sarcoma	4.75000	3.889087	2
	Total	16.70000	8.465898	15
1.00 staff-initiated intervention	1.00 solid tumor (10)	19.41667	7.670832	6
	2.00 lymphoma	10.75000	12.990381	4
	3.00 leukemia, sarcoma	11.00000	5.220153	5
	Total	14.30000	9.147209	15
Total (11)	1.00 solid tumor	20.60000	6.113737	10
	2.00 lymphoma	14.96154	9.837135	13
	3.00 leukemia, sarcoma	9.21429	5.476139	7
	Total	15.50000	8.745442	30

Levene's Test of Equality of Error Variances[a]

Dependent Variable: RNocturn Rank of Nocturn

F	df1	df2	Sig.
1.734	5	24	.165

(12)

Tests the null hypothesis that the error variance of the dependent variable is equal across groups.

a. Design: Intercept + group + type_of_cancer_collapsed + group * type_of_cancer_collapsed

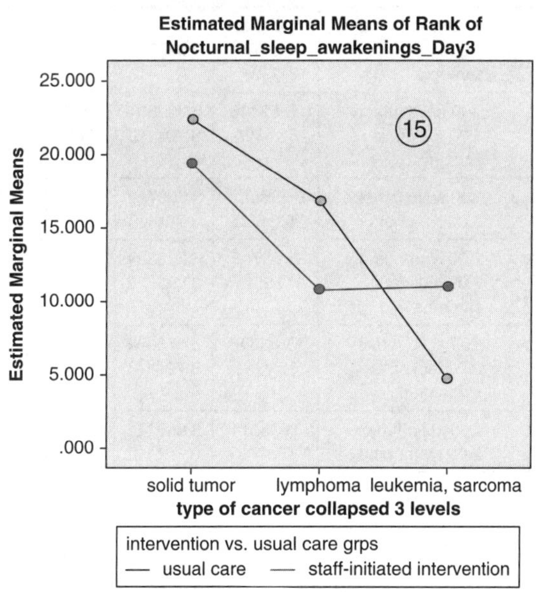

(Continued)

Figure 8.14 (Continued)

Tests of Between-Subjects Effects

Dependent Variable: RNocturn Rank of Nocturnal_sleep_awakenings_Day3

Source	Type III Sum of Squares	df	Mean Square	(13) F	Sig.	Partial Eta Squared	Noncent. Parameter	Observed Power[b]
Corrected Model	719.729[a]	5	143.946	2.306	.076	.324	11.529	.636
Intercept	4903.488	1	4903.488	78.546	.000	.766	78.546	1.000
group	5.274	1	5.274	.084	.774	.004	.084	.059
type_of_cancer_collapsed	639.729	2	319.865	5.1 24	.014	.299	10.247	.772
group * type_of_cancer_collapsed	145.1 06	2	72.553	1.162	.330	.088	2.324	.231
Error	1498.271	24	62.428					
Total	9425.500	30						
Corrected Total	2218.000	29						

a. R Squared = .324 (Adjusted R Squared = .184)
b. Computed using alpha = .05

Multiple Comparisons

Dependent Variable: RNocturn Rank of Nocturnal_sleep_awakenings_Day3

	(I) type of cancer collapsed 3 levels	(J) type of cancer collapsed 3 levels	Mean Difference (I-J)	Std. Error	Sig.	95% Confidence Interval Lower Bound	95% Confidence Interval Upper Bound
Tukey HSD	1.00 solid tumor	2.00 lymphoma	5.63846	3.323394	.227	-2.66101	13.93793
	(14)	3.00 leukemia, sarcoma	11.38571*	3.893722	.020	1.66197	21.10946
	2.00 lymphoma	1.00 solid tumor	-5.63846	3.323394	.227	-13.93793	2.66101
		3.00 leukemia, sarcoma	5.74725	3.704110	.286	-3.50297	14.99748
	3.00 leukemia, sarcoma	1.00 solid tumor	-11.38571*	3.893722	.020	-21.10946	-1.66197
		2.00 lymphoma	-5.74725	3.704110	.286	-14.99748	3.50297
LSD	1.00 solid tumor	2.00 lymphoma	5.63846	3.323394	.103	-1.22069	12.49761
	(14)	3.00 leukemia, sarcoma	11.38571*	3.893722	.007	3.34947	19.42196
	2.00 lymphoma	1.00 solid tumor	-5.63846	3.323394	.103	-12.49761	1.22069
		3.00 leukemia, sarcoma	5.74725	3.704110	.134	-1.89765	13.39216
	3.00 leukemia, sarcoma	1.00 solid tumor	-11.38571*	3.893722	.007	-19.42196	-3.34947
		2.00 lymphoma	-5.74725	3.704110	.134	-13.39216	1.89765

Based on observed means.
The error term is Mean Square (Error) = 62.428.
*.The mean difference is significant at the .05 level.

Let's look at the descriptive statistics that have been generated for the rank-transformed variable. From Figure 8.14, it appears that the ranked sleep awakening variable for the staff-initiated intervention (14.3, (10)) is slightly lower than that of the usual-care group (16.7). It also appears that ranked values for children diagnosed with lymphoma (14.9) are lower than that of the children diagnosed with solid tumors (20.0) (11).

Based on the output that we have generated in SPSS, can we reject the null hypothesis for group, diagnosis, and diagnosis × group interaction? To determine this, we need to turn to both Levene's test for equality of error variances and then the tests of between-subjects effects. In a two-way ANOVA for ranks or for the original data, it is assumed that there is equality of variances. Levene's test provides us with that information. The null hypothesis for Levene's test is that the variances are equal; the alternative hypothesis states that the variances are not equal. We will reject the null hypothesis of equal variances if and only if the p value for Levene's test (*Sig*) is less than a prestated level of α (e.g., .05). The p value for Levene's test in Figure 8.14 is .165 (12), a value that is less than .05. Therefore, we cannot reject the null hypothesis of equal variances. Are we happy about that? You betcha.

Now we need to determine whether we have any statistically significant main or interaction effects for our rank-transformed dependent variable. As mentioned, we will examine two approaches to determining those outcomes: the Conover and Iman (1981) and the Puri and Sen (1985) rank transform approaches. Since the Conover and Iman approach follows that which we are presented with in the printout, let us examine those results first.

Conover-Iman rank transform.

Turning to the tests of between-subjects effects in Figure 8.14, we are presented with F statistics: .084, 5.124, and 1.162 for group, diagnosis, and group × diagnosis interaction, respectively (13). These values were obtained by following a protocol similar to Conover and Iman (1981):

$$F_{group} = \frac{Mean\ Square_{group}}{Mean\ Square_{within}} = \frac{5.274}{62.428} = 0.084$$

$$F_{diagnosis} = \frac{Mean\ Square_{diagnosis}}{Mean\ Square_{within}} = \frac{319.865}{62.428} = 5.124$$

$$F_{group*diagnosis} = \frac{Mean\ Square_{group*diagnosis}}{Mean\ Square_{within}} = \frac{72.553}{62.428} = 1.162$$

Using the Conover-Iman rank-transform approach, these F statistics are distributed as F's with $df = r - 1$, $c - 1$, and $(r - 1)(c - 1)$ in each of the numerators and $df = JK(n - 1)$ in the denominator. These are the same values that we obtain in the Tests of Between Subjects Effects in Figure 8.14. That is, the p values for group, cancer diagnosis, and group × cancer diagnosis interaction are .774, .014, and .330 respectively. These values would lead us to conclude that, per the Conover and Iman (1981) approach to rank-transformed data, there was no statistically significant group or group × diagnosis interaction effect for the rank-transformed number of nocturnal sleep awakenings at Day 3. Examining the post hoc tests and plots for the statistically significant variable, diagnosis, it appears that the solid tumor group had statistically significantly higher average ranks than did the leukemia/sarcoma group (Tukey: $p = .02$; LSD: p = .007 (14)). Looking at the plot of these mean ranks, Figure 8.14 (15), we might have thought there was a group × diagnosis interaction effect given the crossover lines, but that effect was not statistically significant ($p = .330$).

The Puri-Sen approach.

The Puri-Sen approach (Puri & Sen, 1985) calculates the statistics slightly differently and uses chi-square statistics to determine statistical significance:

$$F_{group} = (N-1)\frac{Sum\ of\ Squares_{group}}{Sum\ of\ Squares_{total}} = (29)\frac{5.274}{2218} = 0.069$$

$$F_{diagnosis} = (N-1)\frac{Sum\ of\ Squares_{diagnosis}}{Sum\ of\ Squares_{total}} = (29)\frac{639.729}{2218} = 8.364$$

$$F_{group*diagnosis} = (N-1)\frac{Sum\ of\ Squares_{group*diagnosis}}{Sum\ of\ Squares_{total}} = (29)\frac{145.106}{2218} = 1.897$$

According to Puri and Sen, the distributions of these three statistics are asymptotically distributed as chi-square statistics with $df_r = J - 1$, $df_c = K - 1$, $df_{r \times c} = (J - 1)(K - 1)$, respectively, where J = #rows and K = #columns. In our example, $df_{group} = 2 - 1 = 1$, $df_{diagnosis} = 3 - 1 = 2$, and $df_{group \times diagnosis} = (2 - 1)(3 - 1) = 2$. Table A.2 in Appendix A presents the critical values of the χ^2 for $df = 1$ and $df = 2$. Assuming $\alpha = .05$, we are looking at the cumulative probability of .95. These critical values would be 3.84 and 5.99, respectively. We will reject the null hypothesis of no differences in the rank-transformed dependent variable if and only if our actual statistics are greater than their critical value.

What are our conclusions regarding these statistics? It appears that it is only with *Diagnosis* that we can reject the null hypothesis of no differences in mean ranks since the actual χ^2 value, 8.364, is greater than its critical value (5.99). These conclusions are similar to that which we obtained using the Conover-Iman approach. In fact, they are the same conclusions that we would have reached had we used the parametric two-way ANOVA: $F_{group} = .56$ ($p = .814$), $F_{diagnosis} = 4.518$ ($p = .022$), and $F_{group \times diagnosis} = 1.103$ ($p = .348$).

Internet Resources for Generating the Two-Way ANOVA by Ranks

Several open access resources could be used to generate a two-way ANOVA using a rank-transformed dependent variable. One such site, www.vassarstats.net, offers a relatively straightforward approach to entering the ranked data. First, one identifies the number of rows or levels for independent variable 1 (e.g., *group* with two levels) followed by the number of columns or levels for independent variable 2 (e.g., *diagnosis* with three levels). Next we are requested to enter the rank-transformed data for each of the generated six cells (Figure 8.15). It is easiest to cut and paste the ranked data from a spreadsheet such as Excel.

The results presented to us in Figure 8.15 support our previous calculations: We must retain the null hypotheses for both group and group × diagnosis interaction. There is, however, a statistically significant difference among the diagnosis groups: At least one of

Figure 8.15 Output generated for the two-way ANOVA by ranks using a free-access Internet resource

Data Entry

	Col 1	Col 2	Col 3
Row 1	19 21.5 24.5 24.5	4 9.5 13.5 13.5 13.5 19 21.5 27.5	2 7.5
Row 2	7.5 13.5 19 24.5 24.5 27.5	2 2 9.5 29.5	5.5 5.5 13.5 13.5 17

ANOVA Summary

Source	SS	df	MS	F	P
Rows	43.2	1	43.2	0.69	0.4144
Columns	540.44	2	270.22	4.33	0.0248
r × c	136.09	2	68.05	1.09	0.3523
Error	1498.27	24	62.43		
Total	2218	29			

SOURCE: Retrieved from www.vassarstats.net

the mean ranks is different from the others. Given our previously obtained post hoc tests, it appears that the children diagnosed with solid tumors had a higher number of nocturnal sleep awakenings than did the leukemia/sarcoma group.

Presentation of Results for the Two-Way ANOVA by Ranks

The results of the two-way ANOVA by ranks analysis could be presented in a table similar to that which is presented in Table 8.15. These results could also be summarized as follows:

The results of the two-way analysis of variance by ranks indicated that there were no statistically significant intervention group ($p = .77$) or intervention group × diagnosis effects ($p = .33$). There was, however, a statistically significant diagnosis effect ($p = .001$). That is, the mean rank of the number of nocturnal awakenings for those children diagnosed with solid tumors was significantly higher than those children diagnosed with leukemia/sarcoma (Tukey: $p = .02$).

Table 8.15 Presentation of the Results for the Two-Way ANOVA by Ranks

	Rank transform-#Sleep Awakenings					
Group	N	*Mean Rank*	*SS Source*	F	p	*Post Hoc Tests*
Usual Care						
Solid tumor	4	22.4	Group	0.084	0.77	Solid tumor > Leukemia/ Sarcoma
Lymphoma	9	16.8	Diagnosis	5.124	0.01	
Leukemia, Sarcoma	2	4.8	Group × Diagnosis	1.162	0.33	
Total	15	16.7				
Staff-initiated Intervention						
Solid tumor	6	19.4				
Lymphoma	4	10.8				
Leukemia, Sarcoma	5	11.0				
Total	15	14.3				
Total						
Solid tumor	10	20.6				
Lymphoma	13	14.9				
Leukemia, Sarcoma	7	9.2				
Total	30	15.5				

Advantages, Limitations, and Alternatives to the Two-Way ANOVA by Ranks

As indicated earlier, the use of the two-way ANOVA with rank-transformed data has had both supporters and critics. Advantages to the use of this approach are that it can accommodate the use of ordinal-level data for the dependent variable, does not assume normality of that distribution, is not affected by outliers, and is robust to errors that are not normally distributed (Conover & Iman, 1981; Sawilowsky, 1990). Conover (1999) has suggested that, in experimental designs where there is no nonparametric alternative, the researcher use the parametric ANOVA on the data and then use the same procedure on the rank-transformed data. If similar results are obtained, Conover recommends using the parametric tests. When the results are substantially dissimilar, he suggests examining the data closely for outliers, skewness, and other nonsymmetric abnormalities. These conditions, while unduly influencing the outcome of a parametric analysis, are less impactful on data that have been rank transformed.

A major limitation to the use of rank-transformed data is that this approach does not appear to perform well with more complex factorial designs. For example, even though there have been advocates who have pointed out that the rank-transformed procedure is an easy and convenient alternative to analysis of covariance (ANCOVA) (Conover & Iman, 1982), it is this author's opinion that the use of such an approach should be undertaken with caution.

The parametric alternative to the two-way ANOVA using transformed data would be to either transform the dependent variable using an alternate transformation (e.g., a log or square root transformation) or to run the two-way ANOVA on the original data. It is also possible to create a single new independent variable that represents the interaction between the two (or more) independent variables and run a Kruskal-Wallis test using this newly created variable.

Unfortunately, the alternative nonparametric measures suggested by Akritas et al. (2009) have not as yet been put in place for use with the more commonly used statistical packages. It is hoped that this omission will be corrected both by the nonparametricians and statistical software developers in the not so distant future. Several useful resources are available that provide the interested reader with in-depth discussions of the challenges of using rank transformations and the use of other approaches in factorial designs when data do not meet the assumptions of their parametric tests (e.g., Sawilowsky (1990); Thompson (1991); Toothaker and Newman (1994); Wang and Akritas (2004)).

Summary

In this chapter, we examined five nonparametric statistical tests that can be used when the independent variable had more than two groups: the chi-square test for k independent samples, the Mantel-Haenszel chi-square test for ordered categories, the median test, the Kruskal-Wallis test, and the two-way analysis of variance test by ranks. The first two of these tests are intended to be used when the dependent variable is categorical. The last two tests are to be used when the dependent variable is continuous. Table 8.16 outlines when each of these tests is most appropriately used given the level of measurement of the independent and dependent variables.

The chi-square coefficient is used when both the independent and dependent variables are nominal level. When either or both of the independent and dependent variables are ordinal level of measurement, it is best to use the Mantel-Haenszel chi-square test that takes advantage of the rank ordering of data. The median and Kruskal-Wallis tests are useful when the independent variable is nominal level with two or more levels, and, finally, the two-way ANOVA by ranks is a useful option to use when there are two or more nominal-level independent variables with an ordinal, interval, or ratio dependent variable. Should the researcher be concerned about the advisability of using rank-transformed data with the two-way ANOVA, an alternative could also be to create a new variable that represents the combination of the independent variables and conducting a Kruskal-Wallis on the newly created variable.

Table 8.16 Nonparametric Tests for Independent Groups That Would Be Suitable With Variables of Specific Levels of Measurement

		Dependent Variable		
		Nominal	*Ordinal*	*Interval/Ratio*
	Nominal ($k \geq 2$ levels)	Chi-Square	Mantel-Haenszel Chi-Square	Median test Kruskal-Wallis
Independent Variable	Nominal (Two or more independent variables)	Chi-Square	Two-Way ANOVA by Ranks	Two-Way ANOVA by Ranks
	Ordinal	Mantel-Haenszel Chi-Square	Mantel-Haenszel Chi-Square	–
	Interval/ratio	–	–	–

TEST YOUR KNOWLEDGE

1. Give an example from your area of research interest that would be suitable for the following nonparametric statistics (Note: in each instance, state the independent and dependent variables for your analysis and their levels of measurement):
   a. Chi-square test for k independent samples
   b. Mantel-Haenszel chi-square test
   c. Median test
   d. Kruskal-Wallis test
   e. Two-way ANOVA by ranks

2. For each of the examples that you have provided in Question 1, please provide a null and alternative research hypothesis that could be used with the statistics you have listed.
3. Why would a researcher decide to use a Mantel-Haenszel chi-square test in lieu of the more traditional chi-square test for independent samples? Please explain.
4. You are applying for funds to carry out a small-scale study of the impact of a staff-initiated intervention to reduce anxiety in 20 children hospitalized with cancer. As part of your statistical analyses, you have proposed to use a two-way ANOVA on your rank-transformed anxiety data to examine the impact of gender and diagnosis on the postintervention anxiety levels of the children. What would be two advantages and two disadvantages to using this approach? What alternative strategies could you use instead?

COMPUTER EXERCISES

Using the data posted on the SAGE website (study.sagepub.com/pett2e) hospitalized children with cancer-72 cases.xlsx please answer the questions that follow the research questions posted:

1. Is there an association between group membership (staff-initiated intervention vs. usual-care groups) and whether or not the hospitalized children are distressed prior to the intervention?
2. What is the relationship between the children's social status position and the nurses' evaluation of their sleep quality at Day 2 of the intervention?
   a. What is the statistical test you will use to answer each of these research questions?
   b. What alpha level have you chosen?
   c. Please state the null and alternative hypotheses for this research question.
   d. Undertake the analyses using a statistical computer package of your choice.
   e. Evaluate the strength of the relationship between these two variables and whether there are any cells that influence the statistic chosen.
   f. Summarize the results of your analyses of each of these questions.
   g. Choose an open access resource on the Internet to undertake your analyses as well. Do those results agree with your responses to a–f?
3. What are the differences between the three social status groups with regard to their parents' assessment of the children's immediate posthospital adjustment?
   a. What are the independent and dependent variable(s) in this analysis, and what are their levels of measurement?
   b. What is the statistical test you will use to answer this research question?

(Continued)

(Continued)

c. What alpha level have you chosen?

d. Please state the null and alternative hypotheses for this research question.

e. Undertake the analyses, including post hoc tests, using a statistical computer package of your choice.

f. Summarize the results of your analysis, including the direction of the results.

g. Choose an open access resource on the Internet to undertake your analyses as well. Do those results agree with your responses to f?

4. Using the same data set listed above, undertake a two-way ANOVA using rank-transformed data to examine the following research question:

   What are the effects of the group intervention, social status, and group × social status interaction on parents' assessments of their children's immediate posthospital adjustment?

   a. What are the independent and dependent variable(s) in this analysis, and what are their levels of measurement?

   b. How will you set up the data such that they are rank transformed?

   c. What alpha level have you chosen?

   d. Please state the null and alternative hypotheses for this research question.

   e. Undertake the analyses, including post hoc tests, using a statistical computer package of your choice.

   f. Summarize the results of your analysis, including the direction of the results.

   g. Choose an open access resource on the Internet to undertake your analyses as well. Do those results agree with your responses to f?

Visit **study.sagepub.com/pett2e** to access SAS output, SPSS datasets, SAS datasets, and SAS examples.

CHAPTER 9

Tests of Association Between Variables

- Phi coefficient
- Cramér's *V* coefficient
- Kappa coefficient
- Point biserial correlation
- Spearman rho correlation
- Kendall's tau

It frequently occurs in health care research that we are interested in measuring the degree of association or correlation between two variables. In our hypothetical study, for example, we might want to examine the relationship between a child's age and his or her level of anxiety prior to a staff-initiated intervention. Depending on the level of measurement of the two variables being examined, there are a number of nonparametric tests that can provide information about the extent of the relationship between variables. In this chapter, we will examine six bivariate measures of association: the phi, Cramér's *V*, and kappa coefficients for two categorical variables; the point biserial correlation for examining the relationship between a dichotomous and a continuous variable; and the Spearman rho rank-order correlation and Kendall's tau coefficients for two variables that are at least ordinal level of measurement.

THE PHI COEFFICIENT

It was pointed out in Chapter 8 that the phi coefficient is a useful statistic for determining the strength of relationship between two dichotomous variables after a chi-square test of association or Fisher's exact test for small samples has produced a significant result. In this section, we will examine this coefficient in greater depth.

An Appropriate Research Question for the Phi Coefficient

The phi coefficient serves a number of useful functions. It can be used when the researcher is interested in testing hypotheses about the degree and strength of the relationship between two variables that are dichotomous, such as gender (male, female) and test results (pass, fail). It is typically used after a significant result has been obtained from the chi-square test for two independent samples. It also has been used to assess the criterion-related validity of two autism rating scales (Eaves & Milner, 1993) and to evaluate the suitability of multiple-choice questions on examinations (Koeslag, Schach, & Melzer, 1987).

A number of examples in the health care literature demonstrate the versatility of the phi coefficient. Donlan and Lee (2010) used the phi coefficient to assess the strength of relationship between selected culture-bound syndromes and mental health among Mexican migrants in the United States. Kallert, Glöckner, and Schützwohl (2008) used the same statistic in their systematic review of outcomes related to acute involuntary versus voluntary psychiatric hospital admission. The phi coefficient was also used by Mansell et al. (2010) to evaluate the strength of association between previously documented concussions and experiencing concussive signs and symptoms following head impacts in 201 collegiate athletes. In a very different context, Meiser-Stedman, Smith, Glucksman, Yule, and Dalgleish (2007) used this same statistic to assess parent-child agreement for acute stress, posttraumatic stress, and other psychopathology among children and adolescents exposed to single-event trauma.

The hypothetical example from Chapter 7 will be used to illustrate the approach to evaluating the strength of the phi coefficient when the two variables of interest are at the nominal level of measurement. We will continue to use the same data set, hospitalized children with cancer-30 cases.sav, that can be found on the SAGE website, study.sagepub.com/pett2e. In Chapter 7 (Table 7.7), the chi-square test indicated that the two variables, group membership (intervention, control) and children's expressed distress immediately following the staff-initiated intervention (yes, no), were not independent ($\chi^2 = 4.82$, $p = .028$). We concluded, therefore, that the two variables were associated. Because the chi-square test for independence does not evaluate the strength of that association, we used the phi coefficient to determine this. A research question that could be answered using the phi coefficient, therefore, would be as follows:

> What is the strength of association between group membership (i.e., staff-initiated intervention vs. usual care) and the children's expressed distress (yes, no) immediately following the intervention?

Null and Alternative Hypotheses

Table 9.1 presents examples of null and alternative hypotheses generated from the research question outlined above that could be analyzed using the phi coefficient. Note that, as for the chi-square statistic, the null and alternative hypotheses for the phi coefficient reflect the association between two dichotomous variables.

Table 9.1 Example of Null and Alternative Hypotheses Suitable for Testing With a Phi Coefficient

Null Hypothesis
H_0: There is no association between the variables of group membership (staff-initiated intervention, usual care) and children's expressed distress (yes, no) immediately following the intervention.
Alternative Hypothesis
H_a: There is an association between the variables of group membership (staff-initiated intervention, usual care) and children's expressed distress (yes, no) immediately following the intervention.

Overview of the Procedure

To calculate the phi coefficient, the variables of interest are first arranged in a 2 × 2 table in which the data represent frequencies, not scores (Table 9.2). The variables, *X* and *Y*, represent the independent and dependent variables whose categories have been assigned the values of 0 and 1, and the values of *a* through *d* represent the frequencies for these categories.

From this 2 × 2 contingency table, a χ^2 statistic (Chapter 7) is calculated. The phi coefficient, ϕ, is obtained either directly from the 2 × 2 table or by taking the square root of the χ^2 value divided by the total sample size:

$$\varphi = \frac{(ad - bc)}{\sqrt{a + b)(c + d)(a + c)(b + d)}} = \sqrt{\chi^2 / N}$$

Because ϕ is based on a χ^2 value, the significance level for this coefficient is the same as for the χ^2 statistic. The null hypothesis of no association will be rejected if the calculated χ^2 value is greater than the critical χ^2 at $df = 1$ or, alternatively, if the generated p value is less than the prestated α level (e.g., .05).

Table 9.2 Example of a 2 × 2 Table Used to Calculate the Phi Coefficient

	Variable Y		
Variable X	*0*	*1*	*Total*
0	*a*	*b*	*a* + *b*
1	*c*	*d*	*c* + *d*
Total	*a* + *c*	*b* + *d*	*N*

The values for the phi coefficient for a 2 × 2 table typically range from 0 to 1.00. However, as we will soon see in Figure 9.2, when there is a negative correlation between the two variables of interest, phi may also be negative depending on the statistical package used. Should that happen, then the absolute value of phi should be evaluated. Also, when tables have dimensions that are larger than 2 × 2, phi may not lie between the values Of 0 and 1.00. For that reason, the phi coefficient is restricted to the analysis of 2 × 2 tables, and an extension of this statistic, Cramér's *V* coefficient, is used for larger tables.

If the values of the two dichotomous variables have been coded "0" and "1," the size of the phi coefficient and the Pearson product-moment correlation are identical. For that reason, the strength of relationship between two such categorical variables is interpreted in a context similar to that for the Pearson *r* (Table 7.7) (Hinkle, Wiersma, & Jurs, 2003). That is, values of ϕ above .90 indicate an extremely strong relationship, .70 to .89 a strong relationship, .50 to .69 a moderate relationship, .30 to .49 a low relationship, and below .30 a weak relationship.

Critical Assumptions of the Phi Coefficient

Because the phi coefficient is determined by the chi-square statistic, the critical assumptions of the chi-square test for two independent samples (Chapter 7) apply here. The variables are dichotomous (2 × 2 tables), and observations are independent and consist of frequencies, not scores. The data in our hypothetical study partially meet all these assumptions, with the exception of random selection. Both the independent and dependent variables (group membership and children's anxiety) have been measured on a nominal scale with two levels.

Computer Commands

In SPSS for Windows, the phi coefficient is generated from the same computer commands used for the chi-square test for two independent samples (Chapter 7). These are presented in Figure 9.1. The data set that we are using is hospitalized children with cancer-30 cases.sav which is found on the SAGE website (study.sagepub.com/pett2e). To obtain the phi coefficient, open the *Crosstabs Statistics* dialog box by clicking on *Analyze . . . Descriptive Statistics . . . Crosstabs. . . .* One of the variables (e.g., *Group*) is placed in the row cell, and the second variable (e.g., *Distress_t2*) is placed in the column cell. By clicking on *Statistics . . .*, several statistical options, including the phi coefficient, are presented for the analysis of the association between nominal variables (Figure 9.1).

Computer-Generated Output

The syntax commands, results of the chi-square test, and requested phi coefficient for our data already have been presented in Figure 7.4, but for ease of discussion, they are duplicated in Figure 9.2. The syntax commands indicate that the phi coefficient has been requested (1). The resulting analyses indicate that the obtained value of phi was $|-.40|$ (2). The generated *p* value for phi is the same as the χ^2 statistic (p = .028, (3)) and is less than

Figure 9.1 SPSS for Windows (v. 22–23) commands for the Phi and Cramér's *V* coefficients.

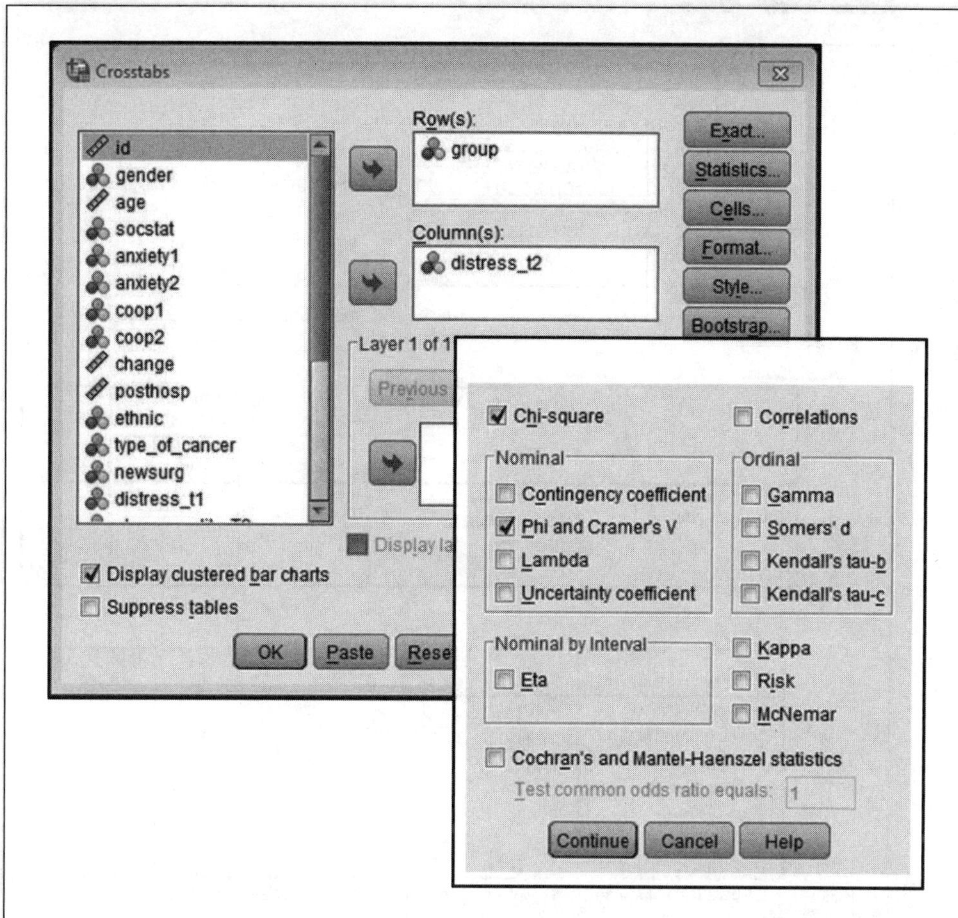

our prestated alpha (.05); therefore, this phi coefficient is statistically significant. It could also be obtained as follows:

$$\varphi = \sqrt{\chi^2 / N} = \sqrt{4.82 / 30} = .40$$

According to the Hinkle et al. (2003) criteria for assessing the strength of association (presented in Table 7.7), a phi coefficient of .40 is, at best, weak. Our conclusion would be, therefore, that there is a statistically significant but weak association between group membership and postintervention distress.

Figure 9.2 SPSS for Windows (v. 22–23) syntax commands and computer-generated output for the phi coefficient.

```
***Data set: hospitalized children with cancer-30 cases.sav***

CROSSTABS
  /TABLES=group BY distress_t2
  /FORMAT=AVALUE TABLES
  /STATISTICS=CHISQ PHI        (1)
  /CELLS=COUNT
  /COUNT ROUND CELL
  /BARCHART.
```

group intervention vs. usual care grps * distress_t2 distress immediately post-intervention Crosstabulation

Count

		distress_t2 distress immediately post-intervention		
		.00 not distressed	1.00 distressed	Total
group intervention vs. usual care grps	.00 usual care	4	11	15
	1.00 staff-initiated intervention	10	5	15
Total		14	16	30

Chi-Square Tests

	Value	df	Asymp. Sig. (2-sided)	Exact Sig. (2-sided)	Exact Sig. (1-sided)
Pearson Chi-Square	4.821[a]	1	(3) .028		
Continuity Correction[b]	3.348	1	.067		
Likelihood Ratio	4.963	1	.026		
Fisher's Exact Test				.066	.033
Linear-by-Linear Association	4.661	1	.031		
N of Valid Cases	30				

a. 0 cells (0.0%) have expected count less than 5. The minimum expected count is 7.00.

b. Computed only for a 2x2 table

Symmetric Measures

		Value	Approx. Sig.
Nominal by Nominal	Phi (2)	-.401	(3) .028
	Cramer's V	.401	.028
N of Valid Cases		30	

Internet Resources for Generating the Chi-Square Test

As indicated in Chapter 7, a number of currently available open access Internet resources provide calculators with which one can obtain a chi-square test and phi coefficient (e.g., www.danielsoper.com and www.vassarstats.net). For the chi-square example in

Chapter 7, we used www.vassarstats.net, the results of which are presented in Chapter 7, Figure 7.5. Notice that this site presents the results of the Cramér's *V* coefficient, which, for a 2 × 2 table, is the same as the phi coefficient.

Presentation of Results

The results of the statistical analysis using the phi coefficient could be presented along with results of the chi-square test of association (Table 7.8). They also could be presented in the text as follows:

> The results of the chi-square analysis indicate a significant but weak association between group membership (intervention, usual care) and the children's postintervention distress ($\varphi = .40$, $p = .03$).

Advantages, Limitations, and Alternatives to the Phi Coefficient

The phi coefficient offers a useful test for assessing the strength of relationship between two dichotomous variables when the chi-square test of association has been found to be significant. Because the phi coefficient takes into account sample size, it also allows the researcher to compare strengths of association across studies. A disadvantage to use of this statistic is that it can take on values greater than 1 when the table is larger than 2 × 2. For that reason, a related statistic, the Cramér's *V* coefficient, is recommended for use with larger tables.

When the data from the independent and dependent dichotomous variables are coded "0" and "1," the phi coefficient is equivalent to the absolute value of the Pearson product-moment correlation coefficient. Nonparametric alternatives to the φ coefficient are the contingency coefficient (Chapter 7), the Cramér's *V* coefficient (discussed below), and the Tetrachoric correlation (Hinkle et al., 2003). The Tetrachoric correlation is used when both dichotomous variables are assumed to have underlying continuity with a normal distribution (e.g., two items on a particular test). Because both the independent and dependent variables are nominal level of measurement, there are no parametric alternatives to the phi coefficient.

Examples From Published Research

Donlan, W., & Lee, J. (2010). Coraje, nervios, and susto: Culture-bound syndromes and mental health among Mexican migrants in the United States. *Advances in Mental Health, 9*(3), 288–302.

Eaves, R. C., & Milner, B. (1993). The criterion-related validity of the Childhood Autism Rating Scale and the Autism Behavior Checklist. *Journal of Abnormal Child Psychology, 21,* 481–491.

Kallert, T. W., Glöckner, M., & Schützwohl, M. (2008). Involuntary vs. voluntary hospital admission: A systematic literature review on outcome diversity. *European Archives of Psychiatry and Clinical Neuroscience, 258*(4), 195–209.

Mansell, J. L., Tierney, R. T., Higgins, M., McDevitt, J., Toone, N., & Glutting, J. (2010). Concussive signs and symptoms following head impacts in collegiate athletes. *Brain Injury, 24*(9), 1070–1074. doi: 10.3109/02699052.2010.494589

Meiser-Stedman, R., Smith, P., Glucksman, E., Yule, W., & Dalgleish, T. (2007). Parent and child agreement for acute stress disorder, post-traumatic stress disorder and other psychopathology in a prospective study of children and adolescents exposed to single-event trauma. *Journal of Abnormal Child Psychology, 35*(2), 191–201.

CRAMÉR'S *V* COEFFICIENT

When the contingency table is greater than 2 × 2, an alternative measure of strength of association is Cramér's *V* coefficient (Cramér, 1946). In some texts (Daniel, 1990; Siegel & Castellan, 1988), the Cramér statistic is referred to as *Cramér's C* coefficient. Other texts (Hays, 1994; Hinkle et al., 2003) and SPSS for Windows label this statistic *Cramér's V*. For consistency with the computer printouts being reviewed, the Cramér statistic will be referred to in this text as *Cramér's V*.

Cramér's *V* is a modified version of the phi coefficient that adjusts for the number of levels of the categorical variable, thus allowing the coefficient to retain its range of 0 and 1. When the contingency table is 2 × 2, Cramér's *V* has the same value as the phi coefficient.

An Appropriate Research Question for Cramér's *V* Coefficient

Like the phi coefficient, Cramér's *V* coefficient is useful when the researcher is interested in assessing the strength of association between two categorical variables once a χ^2 statistic has been determined to be significant. For example, Basta, Shacham, and Reece (2008) used Cramér's *V* after obtaining a significant chi-square to evaluate psychological distress and engagement in human immunodeficiency virus (HIV)–related services among 617 individuals seeking mental health care. Garrett et al. (2004) used the same statistic to evaluate the relationship between stages of change for smoking cessation, fruit and vegetable consumption, and physical activity in a health plan population. Cramér's *V* coefficient was also used by Hempton et al. (2011) to examine contrasting perceptions of health professionals and older adults in Australia regarding what constitutes elder abuse. It was also used by Van den Broeck, Himpens, Vanhaesebrouck, Calders, and Oostra (2008) in their examination of the influence of gestational age on type of brain injury and neuromotor outcome in high-risk neonates.

In Chapter 8, we used the chi-square test for *k* independent samples to examine the association between a child's cancer diagnosis (solid tumor, acute myeloid leukemia, lymphoma/sarcoma) and the nurse's assessment of the child's sleep quality immediately postintervention (poor, moderate, or very good). We will continue to use the same data set, hospitalized children with cancer-72 cases.sav (study.sagepub.com/pett2e). In that example, a statistically significant association was found between the child's cancer diagnosis and the child's adjustment (χ^2 = 18.29, p = .006). Given this significant result, we might be interested in assessing the strength of that significant relationship. Cramér's *V* coefficient can be of help with this analysis. A research question that would be suitable for use with Cramér's *V* is as follows:

> What is the strength of the relationship between a child's cancer diagnosis (solid tumor, acute myeloid leukemia, lymphoma/sarcoma) and the nurse's assessment of the child's sleep quality immediately postintervention (poor, moderate, or very good)?

Null and Alternative Hypotheses

Table 9.3 presents null and alternative hypotheses that would be suitable for use with the Cramér coefficient. Note that the hypotheses are similar to those of the chi-square test for *k* independent samples (Table 8.1) because Cramér's *V* is based on the χ^2 statistic.

Overview of the Procedure

The frequency data are first arranged in an $r \times c$ contingency table, and a χ^2 statistic is computed (Chapter 8). From this obtained χ^2 value, Cramér's *V* coefficient is obtained:

$$\text{Cramér's } V = \sqrt{\frac{\chi^2}{N(L-1)}}$$

where

L = the smaller of the number of rows or columns in the contingency table, and

N = the total sample size.

Because Cramér's *V* is based on the χ^2 statistic, its significance level is the same as that for the χ^2; that is, the null hypothesis is rejected if the calculated χ^2 is greater than the critical χ^2 with $df = (r - 1)(c - 1)$ or, alternatively, if the generated *p* value for the χ^2 is less than the predetermined level of α.

Like the phi coefficient for 2×2 tables, the value of Cramér's *V* can range between 0 and 1, with higher values indicating greater strength of association. A limitation to this statistic is that although a value of 0 indicates no association between the two variables, a value of 1 does not always imply a perfect relationship (Daniel, 1990; Siegel & Castellan, 1988). This perfect relationship occurs only when the contingency table being analyzed is square (i.e., there are as many rows as columns in the table).

If the contingency table has more rows than columns (or vice versa), a value of 1 for the Cramér coefficient would indicate that there is a perfect relationship in one direction

Table 9.3 Example of a Null and Alternative Hypothesis Suitable for Use With Cramér's *V* Coefficient

Null Hypothesis
H_0: There is no association between a child's cancer diagnosis and a nurse's assessment of the child's sleep quality immediately postintervention; that is, the two variables, cancer diagnosis and the child's sleep quality, are independent.
Alternative Hypothesis
H_a: There is an association between a child's cancer diagnosis and a nurse's assessment of the child's sleep quality immediately postintervention; that is, the two variables, cancer diagnosis and the child's sleep quality, are dependent.

(e.g., from the row to column variable) but not necessarily in the other (Siegel & Castellan, 1988). Siegel and Castellan (1988) also indicate that, except for 2 × 2 tables, values of Cramér's *V* are not directly comparable to the Pearson product-moment correlation; therefore, the guidelines offered for interpreting the strength of the phi coefficient (Table 7.7) do not necessarily apply to Cramér's *V*. Larger values of this coefficient, however, do indicate a greater degree of relationship between two categorical variables.

Critical Assumptions of Cramér's *V* Coefficient

Because Cramér's *V* coefficient is calculated from the χ^2 statistic, the requirements for this coefficient are similar to those for the χ^2 statistic for $r \times c$ independent groups outlined in Chapter 8; that is, assumptions are made that the variables being examined are categorical; the pairs of randomly selected observations are independent; the data being analyzed are frequency data, not scores; and the cells in the $r \times c$ contingency table are mutually exclusive and exhaustive. The selected data from our hypothetical study with 72 cases meet all these assumptions except for random selection.

Computer Commands

Similar to the phi coefficient, Cramér's *V* is generated in SPSS for Windows from the same computer commands used for the chi-square test of independence (Chapter 8). These are presented in Figure 9.1. To obtain Cramér's *V*, open the *Crosstabs Statistics* dialog box by clicking on *Analyze . . . Descriptive Statistics . . . Crosstabs. . . .* One of the variables (e.g., *Child's Diagnosis*) is placed in the row cell, and the second variable (e.g., the child's sleep quality immediately postintervention) is placed in the column cell. By clicking on *Statistics . . .*, several statistical options, including Cramér's *V*, are presented for the analysis of the association between nominal variables (Figure 9.1).

Computer-Generated Output

Figure 9.3 presents the syntax commands and computer-generated output for the Cramér's *V* coefficient that were obtained in SPSS for Windows (v. 22–23). Note that the syntax command *phi* will produce both the phi and Cramér's *V* coefficients (Figure 9.3 ①). Note, too, that we will be using the hospitalized children data set with 72 cases (study.sagepub.com/pett2e) to remain consistent with the results obtained in Chapter 8.

In the printout, we are presented with the chi-square statistic, the interpretation of which is presented in detail in Chapter 8. As requested, we are also presented with Cramér's *V* coefficient ②. This statistic was obtained as follows:

$$\text{Cramér's } V = \sqrt{\frac{\chi^2}{N(L-1)}} = \sqrt{\frac{18.292}{72(3-1)}} = 0.356$$

Figure 9.3 SPSS for Windows (v. 22–23) syntax commands and computer-generated output for Cramér's *V* coefficient.

```
***Data set: Hospitalized children with cancer-72 cases.sav***

CROSSTABS
 /TABLES=type_of_cancer BY sleep_quality_T2
 /FORMAT=AVALUE TABLES
 /STATISTICS=CHISQ PHI (1)
 /CELLS=COUNT
 /COUNT ROUND CELL.
```

Chi-Square Tests

	Value	df	Asymp. Sig. (2-sided)
Pearson Chi-Square	18.292[a]	6	(3) .006
Likelihood Ratio	23.207	6	.001
Linear-by-Linear Association	1.572	1	.210
N of Valid Cases	72		

a. 0 cells (0.0%) have expected count less than 5. The minimum expected count is 5.11.

Symmetric Measures

		Value	Approx. Sig.
Nominal by Nominal	Phi	.504	(3) .006
	Cramer's V	(2) .356	.006
N of Valid Cases		72	

As indicated, this coefficient has the same significance level (.006) as the χ^2 statistic from which it was derived (3). Because .006 is less than our prestated α level (.05), we will reject the null hypothesis of no association and conclude that there is a significant association between the child's cancer diagnosis and his or her sleep quality. Since the Cramér statistic can range between 0 and 1, the strength of this relationship (.356) according to our guidelines presented in Table 7.7 is low.

Presentation of Results

The Cramér statistic can be presented in a table similar to Table 8.5, along with the frequencies and χ^2 statistic. It could also be presented in the text as follows:

> The results of the chi-square analyses indicate a statistically significant but weak association between the hospitalized child's diagnosis and the nurse's assessment of the quality of his or her postintervention sleep quality ($\chi^2 = 18.29$, $p = .006$, Cramér's $V = .356$).

Chapter 8 also suggests potentially useful approaches to determining which cells in the contingency table appear to have the most influence on these results.

Advantages, Limitations, and Alternatives to the Cramér's *V* Coefficient

A major advantage to Cramér's *V* statistic is that it does not have many assumptions associated with it. A disadvantage of this statistic is that, unlike the phi coefficient, the Cramér coefficient does not bear any direct relationship to the Pearson correlation coefficient if the contingency table is larger than 2 × 2. Moreover, if the table is not square, the value of 1 for Cramér's *V* does not imply a perfect relationship between the two categorical variables. Cramér's *V* nevertheless does allow the researcher to compare tables of different sizes and tables based on different sample sizes but with the same number of dimensions.

If the contingency table being examined is 2 × 2 and the categories are coded "0" and "1," Cramér's *V* takes on the same value as the phi coefficient and shares the phi coefficient's relationship to the Pearson product-moment correlation, $V = \phi = |r|$. If the contingency table is larger than 2 × 2 and the categories are ordered and equally spaced, a nonparametric correlation such as Spearman's rho (discussed later in this chapter) might be considered. If there is no order to the categories, there is no parametric equivalent to Cramér's *V*, and there are few nonparametric alternatives to this test.

Examples From Published Research

Basta, T., Shacham, E., & Reece, M. (2008). Psychological distress and engagement in HIV-related services among individuals seeking mental health care. *AIDS Care, 20*(8), 969–976.

Garrett, N. A., Alesci, N. L., Schultz, M. M., Foldes, S. S., Magnan, S. J., & Manley, M. W. (2004). The relationship of stage of change for smoking cessation to stage of change for fruit and vegetable consumption and physical activity in a health plan population. *American Journal of Health Promotion, 19*(2), 118–127.

Hempton, C., Dow, B., Cortes-Simonet, E. N., Ellis, K., Koch, S., LoGiudice, D., . . . Ames, D. (2011). Contrasting perceptions of health professionals and older people in Australia: What constitutes elder abuse? *International Journal of Geriatric Psychiatry, 26*(5), 466–472. doi: 10.1002/gps.2549

Raggi, A., Leonardi, M., Antozzi, C., Confalonieri, P., Maggi, L., Cornelio, F., & Mantegazza, R. (2010). Concordance between severity of disease, disability and health-related quality of life in myasthenia gravis. *Neurological Sciences, 31*(1), 41–45.

Van den Broeck, C., Himpens, E., Vanhaesebrouck, P., Calders, P., & Oostra, A. (2008). Influence of gestational age on the type of brain injury and neuromotor outcome in high-risk neonates. *European Journal of Pediatrics, 167*(9), 1005–1009.

THE KAPPA COEFFICIENT

Researchers in health care often make use of clinical observations obtained from health care providers to evaluate client outcomes or to assign patients to diagnostic categories. It is important when undertaking such research to determine the extent to which the variability in the observed outcomes can be attributed to true variation in the characteristic that is being assessed or is, instead, the result of errors of measurement, including observer biases and disagreement. Researchers interested in partitioning out such variability would typically assess *interobserver agreement,* or the extent to which observers agree in their ratings or assignment to categories of the characteristic of interest.

Numerous approaches have been used to assess interobserver agreement. These approaches typically take the form of evaluating the percentage of agreement among observers. That is,

$$\text{percentage agreement} = \frac{\text{number of agreements}}{\text{number of agreements} + \text{number of disagreements}} * 100$$

where

number of agreements = the number of cases rated the same by two raters, and

number of disagreements = the number of cases rated differently by two raters.

Although percentage agreement gives a rough estimate of interobserver agreement, a major problem with this statistic is that it does not consider the fact that some of the observer agreement can be expected to occur purely by chance (Bakeman & Gottman, 1997). An advantage to the kappa coefficient is that it takes into account chance agreement.

For example, two or more practitioners might be asked to assign each of n patients to one of k diagnostic or outcome categories. The extent of their agreement could then be evaluated to determine the extent to which the practitioners agree on the placement of the patients in the particular categories. If the diagnostic or treatment conditions to which the patients are assigned are at the nominal level of measurement and if the researcher also wants to adjust for chance agreement, the kappa coefficient (Cohen, 1968) can be used to assess the extent of interobserver or interrater agreement.

The kappa coefficient (κ) (aka *Cohen's kappa*) represents a family of indexes of agreement that vary slightly from one another in their form and function. Extensive discussions of the various forms that these kappas can take can be found in Cohen (1960, 1968), Fleiss (1971), Krippendorff (2013), and Bakeman and Gottman (1997). Additional discussion regarding the use of the kappa coefficient can be found in Blackman and Koval (1993), P. F. Brennan and Hays (1992), R. L. Brennan and Prediger (1981), Feuerman and Miller (2008), Green (1981), Rigby (2000), and Sim and Wright (2005). This discussion will focus on a very basic form of kappa, an assessment of agreement between two observers. The interested reader is encouraged to seek out the references cited above for extensions of this discussion to $k \times k$ tables when there are more than two observers.

An Appropriate Research Question for the Kappa Coefficient

The kappa coefficient has been used in a variety of studies. Beach et al. (1992) used the kappa coefficient to evaluate the degree of agreement between spouses and patients recovering from acute myocardial infarctions concerning the couples' reporting of frequency of sexual activity. Capio, Sit, and Abernethy (2011) used a similar approach to compare two raters' process-oriented assessments of fundamental movement skills in children with cerebral palsy.

In our hypothetical study, suppose we were interested in comparing our two groups (staff-initiated intervention and usual care) of hospitalized children with cancer with regard to nurse evaluations of their sleep quality (poor, moderate, very good) immediately following the intervention. A convenient and economical approach would be to assign a single observer the task of evaluating a child's sleep quality. A serious drawback to this approach is that it would not be possible to determine whether the variability in sleep quality observed among the children in the two groups was a result of true differences among the children or instead resulted from observer bias. To assess the extent of this potential bias, we would want to include an additional observer of the children's sleep quality for at least a portion of the sample to determine the extent of interobserver agreement.

Assume, therefore, that two nurses were asked to assess the 30 participating children's sleep quality at Day 1 following the intervention. These data can be found in 'data set for calculating kappa.sav' (study.sagepub.com/pett2e). A research question that could be answered using the kappa coefficient would be as follows:

> To what extent do the two nurses agree in their assessment of the children's sleep quality at Day 1 following the intervention?

Null and Alternative Hypotheses

Table 9.4 presents an example of possible null and alternative hypotheses generated from our research question that would be suitable for use with the kappa coefficient. Because we are interested in the extent of *agreement,* not *disagreement,* between two raters, the research hypothesis is directional. We are testing the null hypothesis H_0: $\kappa \le 0$ against the one-tailed alternative hypothesis H_a: $\kappa > 0$. The reason for this directional test is that, in our research hypothesis, we are addressing *beyond chance* agreement and are not contemplating the depressing possibility that there could be *less than chance* agreement between the raters. The null hypothesis of no interobserver agreement beyond chance will be rejected if the significance of kappa is greater than the critical value of a z statistic at one-tailed alpha = .05. Using Table A.1 in Appendix A, we can determine that the critical value for a one-tailed z statistic for $\alpha = .05$ is +1.64. It is that z statistic for which the cumulative distribution function = 1 − .05 = .95.

Table 9.4 Example of Null and Alternative Hypotheses Appropriate for Use With the Kappa Statistic

Null Hypothesis
H_0: The two nurses do not agree on their evaluations of children's sleep quality (poor, moderate, or very good) at Day 1 postintervention.
Alternative Hypothesis
H_a: The two nurses do agree on their evaluations of children's sleep quality (poor, moderate, or very good) at Day 1 postintervention.

Overview of the Procedure

The basic form that kappa takes is as follows (Bakeman & Gottman, 1986):

$$\text{k} = \frac{\text{proportion of observed agreement} - \text{proportion of chance agreement}}{1 - \text{proportion of chance agreement}}$$

$$= \frac{P_o - P_c}{1 - P_c}$$

Given a square $r \times c$ contingency table, the proportion of observed agreement (P_0) is determined by summing the number of agreements that appear on the diagonal of the contingency table and dividing by the total number of paired observations (i.e., N = the number of observer agreements + the number of disagreements):

$$P_o = \frac{\text{number of agreements}}{N}$$

The proportion of chance agreement (P_c) for each cell on the diagonal is determined in a manner similar to that used for the chi-square statistic in Chapter 7. First, the row and column marginal totals for each cell on the diagonal are multiplied together; the result is divided by the total number of observations. This provides the number of observations that could have been expected to occur by chance in the particular cell on the diagonal. The proportion of chance agreement, P_c, is obtained by dividing this expected frequency by the total number of observations. Finally, these proportions are summed across all the cells on the diagonal to obtain the total proportion of chance agreement:

$$P_c = \sum_{i=1}^{k} \frac{\text{(row marginal) (column marginal)}}{N^2}$$

Given these two proportions, all that is needed is to plug in the values into the kappa formula. Values of kappa can theoretically range from −1 to +1. A negative value of kappa implies that the proportion of agreement resulting from chance is greater than the proportion of observed agreement, not a desirable situation. For that reason, alternative hypotheses are directional, with higher positive values of kappa indicating stronger interobserver agreement.

Let us suppose that two nurse observers rated 30 hospitalized children with cancer with regard to the quality of their sleep at Day 1 postintervention. Table 9.5 presents the results of their assessments. These data can also be found in the SPSS data file located on the SAGE website (study.sagepub.com/pett2e).

The first task is to calculate the probability of observed agreement between the two nurse observers (i.e., those values that appear on the diagonal of the table):

$$p_o = \frac{number\ of\ agreements}{N} = \frac{3+8+12}{30} = \frac{23}{30} = 0.7667$$

Next we would calculate the agreement that could occur purely by chance:

$$p_c = \sum_1^k \frac{(row\ marginal)(column\ marginal)}{N^2} = \frac{(6)(3)+(11)(12)+(13)(15)}{30^2}$$

$$= \frac{18+132+195}{900} = \frac{345}{900} = 0.3833$$

With these calculated probabilities, we can now calculate the kappa coefficient:

$$\kappa = \frac{p_o - p_c}{1 - p_c} = \frac{0.7667 - 0.3833}{1 - 0.3833} = \frac{0.3834}{0.6167} = 0.6217$$

The question we are now faced with is whether this kappa coefficient is such that we can say that the two nurse observers agree with regard to the children's sleep quality.

Table 9.5 Results of Interobserver Agreement on Children's Sleep Quality at Day 1 Postintervention Using the Kappa Coefficient

	Nurse Observer 2							
	Poor		*Moderate*		*Very Good*		*Total*	
Nurse Observer 1	N	p[a]	N	p	N	p	N	p
Poor	3	0.10	3	0.10	0	0.00	6	0.20
Moderate	0	0.00	8	0.27	3	0.10	11	0.37
Very good	0	0.00	1	0.03	12	0.40	13	0.43
Total	3	0.10	12	0.40	15	0.50	30	1.00

[a] *p* = probability of being in that particular cell (e.g., 3/30 = 0.10), the probability of both observers agreeing on the rating of "poor" for the sleep quality of three children.

Assessing the kappa coefficient.

There are two approaches to assessing a kappa coefficient: testing its level of significance (Bakeman & Gottman, 1997) and evaluating its magnitude using criteria suggested by Fleiss (1971). Siegel and Castellan (1988) indicate that, for large *N*, kappa is approximately normally distributed. To determine whether the obtained kappa is significantly greater than 0, the obtained kappa is divided by its standard error (i.e., the square root of its estimated variance) to produce a *z* statistic that is used for hypothesis testing:

$$\text{significance of } \kappa = z = \frac{\kappa}{\sqrt{\text{Var}(\kappa)}}$$

The null hypothesis that $\kappa \leq 0$ will be rejected if the value of this generated z statistic is greater than the critical value of *z* at the prestated one-tailed level of alpha (e.g., $z = 1.64$ at $\alpha = .05$).

The estimated variance of kappa is somewhat involved to calculate directly from a contingency table. Fleiss, Cohen, and Everitt (1969) and Bakeman and Gottman (1997) present the formula for calculating the estimated variance of kappa assuming that kappa = 0. The formula takes into account the number of rater assessments (*N*) and the row and column marginals. That is,

$$\widehat{Var}\left(\hat{\kappa}\right) = \frac{1}{N\left(1 - p_c\right)^2}\left\{\sum_{i=1}^{k} p_{i.}p_{.i}\left[1 - \left(p_{.i} + p_{i.}\right)\right]^2 + \sum_{\substack{i=1\\i \neq j}}^{k}\sum_{j=1}^{k} p_{i.}p_{.j}\left(p_{.i} + p_{j.}\right)^2 - p_c^2\right\}$$

where

N = the number of rater assessments or tallies,

p_c = the probability of chance agreement,

$p_{i.}$ = the probability that the subjects will be assigned to the *i*th row, and

p_j = the probability that the subjects will be assigned to the *j*th column.

Using this formula for the estimated variance and our calculated values for p_c and p_o, we can calculate the estimated variance for kappa when $k = 0$. To do that, it is easiest to break up that estimated variance into more doable parts:

$$\frac{1}{N\left(1 - p_c\right)^2} = \frac{1}{30\left(1 - 0.3833\right)^2} = 0.0876$$

Now using the probabilities presented for the marginals of Table 9.5, we can calculate the second part of the equation:

$$\sum_{i=1}^{k} p_{i.}p_{.i}\left[1 - \left(p_{.i} + p_{i.}\right)\right]^2$$

$$= (0.10)(0.20)\left[1 - (0.20 + 0.10)\right]^2 + (0.40)(0.37)\left[1 - (0.37 + 0.40)\right]^2$$

$$+ (0.43)(0.50)\left[1 - (0.50 + 0.43)\right]^2 = 0.0098 + 0.0078 + 0.0011 = 0.0187$$

The third part of the equation is a bit more complicated, but by carefully noting the appropriate *i's* and *j's* (with the *i's* not equal to the *j's*), we arrive at the following sum:

$$+\sum_{\substack{i=1 \\ i \neq j}}^{k}\sum_{j=1}^{k} p_{i.}p_{.j}\left(p_{.i}+p_{j.}\right)^2 = p_{1.}p_{.2}\left(p_{.1}+p_{2.}\right)^2 + p_{1.}p_{.3}\left(p_{.1}+p_{3.}\right)^2 + p_{2.}p_{.1}\left(p_{.2}+p_{1.}\right)^2$$

$$+p_{2.}p_{.3}\left(p_{.2}+p_{3.}\right)^2 + p_{3.}p_{.1}\left(p_{.3}+p_{1.}\right)^2 + p_{3.}p_{.2}\left(p_{.3}+p_{2.}\right)^2$$

$$=(0.20)(0.40)(0.10+0.37)^2+(0.20)(0.50)(0.10+0.43)^2$$

$$+(0.37)(0.10)(0.40+0.20)^2+(0.37)(0.50)(0.40+0.43)^2$$

$$+(0.43)(0.10)(0.50+0.20)^2+(0.43)(0.40)(0.50+0.37)^2$$

$$=0.0177+0.0281+0.0133+0.1274+0.0211+0.1302=0.3378$$

Next we need to calculate p_c^2, which in this case is $(.3833)^2$ or .1469. Now we are ready to use the estimated variance formula for kappa:

$$\widehat{Var}\left(\hat{\kappa}\right)=(.0876)[.0187+.3378-.1469]=.01836$$

Now we are ready to calculate the significance of kappa:

$$\text{significance of } \kappa = z = \frac{\kappa}{\sqrt{\text{Var}(\kappa)}} = \frac{0.6217}{\sqrt{0.01836}} = 4.58$$

Because our calculated z statistic (4.58) is greater than our critical value (1.64), we can reject the null hypothesis from Table 9.4 and conclude that the nurse observers did agree on their evaluations of children's sleep quality (poor, moderate, or very good) at Day 1 postintervention.

Although a significant z statistic indicates that the observers agree significantly more than would be expected by chance, this statistic does not indicate the strength of agreement. Even low values of kappa can be statistically significant. As Bakeman and Gottman (1997) point out, a significant kappa only indicates that the raters agree beyond chance. To further evaluate observer agreement, we need to examine the size of kappa itself.

Unfortunately, there is no gold standard with which to assess values of kappa. Based on their experiences with using kappa with numerous coding schemes, Bakeman and Gottman (1997) view kappas that are less than .70 with some concern. This may be a bit stringent, however. Fleiss (1971), for example, indicates that kappas of .40 to .60 are fair, .60 to .75 are good, and values greater than .75 are excellent. Using slightly different criteria, Landis and Koch (1977) suggest that values ≤ 0 indicate no agreement, .01 to .20 are slight, .21 to .40 are fair, .41 to .60 are moderate, .61 to .80 are substantial, and values greater than .81 are almost perfect. Sim and Wright (2005), in an excellent review of the use, interpretation, and sample size requirements for kappa, caution that these benchmarks are arbitrary, that the effects of weighting and number of assessment categories need to be taken into consideration when evaluating the magnitude of kappa. Krippendorff (2013) points out that there is no magical number for assessing reliability coefficients. Rather, the choice of an acceptable cutoff point for such a coefficient is a function of the potential costs of drawing invalid conclusions from unreliable data.

Critical Assumptions of the Kappa Coefficient

The critical assumptions for the kappa coefficient are as follows:

1. *The nominally scaled data are paired observations of the same phenomena (e.g., Observer 1 vs. Observer 2).*
2. *Observations are assigned to categories that are mutually exclusive and may or may not have order to them.*
3. *The resulting agreement or "confusion matrix" (Bakeman & Gottman, 1997) is symmetric (same number of rows and columns), such as 2 × 2 or 3 × 3.*

The data from our hypothetical study meet all these assumptions. The two nurse observers both evaluated the quality of sleep at Day 2 postintervention of the same group of 30 hospitalized children. The categories of sleep quality (poor, moderate, and very good) were mutually exclusive, ordered categories. The nurses' ratings resulted in the 3 × 3 agreement matrix presented in Table 9.5.

Computer-Generated Output

Fortunately, the value of kappa, its estimated variance, and the *z* statistic can be generated easily in SPSS for Windows (v. 22–23) using the *Crosstabs* commands that generated the chi-square test of independence. First, open the data set for the two nurse observers (data set for calculating kappa.sav located at study.sagepub.com/pett2e). Click on *Analyze . . . Descriptives . . . Crosstabs* . . . and indicate that the row variable is *sleep_quality_nurse_observer1* and the column variable is *sleep_quality_nurse_observer2*. Click on the kappa statistics under the *Statistics* subcommand.

Figure 9.4 presents the syntax commands and computer-generated output from SPSS for Windows (v. 22–23) for the kappa coefficient. The syntax commands indicate that, as requested, the kappa coefficient will be generated (1). The contingency table in Figure 9.4 indicates the frequency of agreement between the nurses with regard to the sleep quality at Day 1 of the 30 children. This agreement or "confusion matrix" is a 3 × 3 square contingency table in which the diagonal values (3, 8, and 12) (2) represent the number of exact agreements between Nurse Observer 1 and Nurse Observer 2. As indicated earlier in this section, the proportion of observed agreement, P_0, is .7667; the total proportion of chance agreement, P_c, is .3883; and the kappa coefficient (3) is .622, the same as that which was hand-calculated. Interobserver agreement has now been corrected for chance agreement and is considerably lower (.622) than the exact agreement (.7667). Bakeman and Gottman (1997) point out that these two values can be quite disparate if there are few coding categories and low marginal frequencies.

The "Approx. T^b" presented in Figure 9.4, 4.586 (4), is, thank goodness, similar to the *z* statistic that we hand-calculated to determine the significance of kappa (4.58) and it is statistically significantly greater than 0 (p = .000 (5)). Our conclusion, therefore, is similar to that which we concluded earlier: The nurse observers significantly agreed with one another beyond chance levels with regard to their evaluations of the children's postoperative recovery. The size of this kappa, .6216, fits Fleiss's (1971) characterization of inter-observer agreement as "fair to good."

Recall that this z statistic ("Approx.T") was obtained by dividing the kappa value (.622) by its standard error (i.e., the square root of its estimated variance) to produce a z statistic that we used for hypothesis testing:

$$\text{Significance of } \kappa = z = \frac{\kappa}{SE(\kappa)} = \frac{\kappa}{\sqrt{\text{Var}(\kappa)}}$$

Although the results of this calculation are presented in Figure 9.4 (4.586 (4)), this statistic cannot be directly obtained using the standard error presented to us (.122 (6)) because the denominator of this z statistic uses an asymptotic standard error assuming the null hypothesis to be true. Unfortunately, this value is not reported in the table.

Figure 9.4 Syntax and computer-generated output in SPSS for Windows (v. 22–23) for the kappa coefficient.

```
***Data set: Data set for calculating kappa.sav***

CROSSTABS
  /TABLES=Sleep_quality_nurse_observer1 BY Sleep_quality_nurse_observer2
  /FORMAT=AVALUE TABLES
  /STATISTICS=KAPPA  (1)
  /CELLS=COUNT
  /COUNT ROUND CELL.
```

Sleep_quality_nurse_observer1 Rater 1 -assessment of sleep quality Day 1 * Sleep_quality_nurse_observer2 Rater 2 Assessment of sleep quality Day 1 Crosstabulation

Count

		Sleep_quality_nurse_observer2 Rater 2 Assessment of sleep quality Day 1			
		1.00 Poor	2.00 Moderate	3.00 Very Good	Total
Sleep_quality_nurse_observer1 Rater 1 - assessment of sleep quality Day 1	1.00 Poor	3	3	0	6
	2.00 Moderate	0	8	3	11
	3.00 Very Good	0	1	12	13
Total		3	12	15	30

(2)

Symmetric Measures

		Value	Asymp. Std. Error[a]	Approx. T[b]	Approx. Sig.
Measure of Agreement	Kappa	.622	.122	4.586	.000
N of Valid Cases		30	(6)	(4)	(5)

(3)

a. Not assuming the null hypothesis.

b. Using the asymptotic standard error assuming the null hypothesis.

Instead, we are presented with an asymptotic standard error (.122) that *does not* assume the null hypothesis. This value (.122), is smaller than the standard error (.1355) that was used to calculate the significance of kappa (i.e., the "Approx. T" or what we have referred to as the "z statistic").

Assessing asymmetric tables.

Note that the table presented in the printout in Figure 9.4 is square: It has equal numbers of rows and columns. This allows us to use the standard *integer* mode for the *Crosstabs* command in SPSS for Windows. Suppose, however, that one of the marginal frequencies had been equal to zero (e.g., Nurse Observer 2 did not consider any of the children to have poor sleep quality, whereas Nurse Observer 1 did). If such a situation were to occur and the *Crosstabs* command had been selected from the menus, the computer would generate an asymmetric 3 × 2 table as in Figure 9.5. Is the kappa that is generated from this table accurate?

Figure 9.5 SPSS for Windows syntax commands and output for kappa when the table is asymmetric.

```
***Data set: Data set for calculating kappa when a row or column equals 0.sav***

CROSSTABS                                                        (7)
/Variables = Sleep_quality_nurse_observer1(1,3) Sleep_quality_nurse_observer2(1,3)
/TABLES=Sleep_quality_nurse_observer1 BY Sleep_quality_nurse_observer2
/FORMAT=AVALUE TABLES
/STATISTICS=KAPPA
/CELLS=COUNT
/COUNT ROUND CELL.
```

Sleep_quality_nurse_observer1 Rater 1 -assessment of sleep quality Day 1 * Sleep_quality_nurse_observer2 Rater 2 Assessment of sleep quality Day 1 Crosstabulation

Count

		Sleep_quality_nurse_observer2 Rater 2 Assessment of sleep quality Day 1			
		1.00 Poor	2.00 Moderate	3.00 Very Good	Total
Sleep_quality_nurse_observer1 Rater 1 - assessment of sleep quality Day 1	1.00 Poor	0	6	0	6
	2.00 Moderate	0	8	3	11
	3.00 Very Good	0	1	12	13
Total		0	15	15	30

Symmetric Measures

		Value	Asymp. Std. Error[a]	Approx. T[b]	Approx. Sig.
Measure of Agreement	Kappa	.444	.121	3.275	.001
N of Valid Cases		30			

a. Not assuming the null hypothesis.

b. Using the asymptotic standard error assuming the null hypothesis.

Should this asymmetric matrix occur—and it commonly does in the real world—it turns out that the generated kappa is, indeed, accurate. To be certain of its accuracy, we can switch to the syntax mode in SPSS for Windows to operate the *general* mode for *Crosstabs*. This means that all the *Crosstabs* syntax commands presented in Figure 9.5 need to be typed into the syntax box. In addition, prior to the */Tables* command, the variables and their potential ranges, for example, */Variables = Nurse_Observer1 (1,3) Nurse_Observer2 (1,3)* ⑦, need to be specified along with the remaining commands.

Figure 9.5 gives an example of the syntax commands and resulting printout when one of the row or column marginals is equal to zero. Note that commands have changed slightly to accommodate the apparent asymmetry in the table and to indicate to SPSS for Windows that we are in the *general* mode for *Crosstabs*. The resulting output, however, can be interpreted similar to that which we used in Figure 9.4.

Internet Resources for Generating the Kappa Coefficient

Several Internet sites currently provide useful resources for generating the kappa coefficient (e.g., http://justusrandolph.net/kappa/ and http://department.obg.cuhk.edu.hk / researchsupport/Cohen_Kappa_matrix.asp). A third site that is especially helpful is ReCal (Freelon, 2010), an open access website that focuses on various forms of interrater reliability. It can be accessed by going to http://dfreelon.org/utils/recalfront.

To generate a kappa statistic using this resource, it is necessary to first set up the data using a spreadsheet such as Excel. Each row represents the cases of interest; the columns represent the raters' numbered assessments of the cases. A header row is allowed, but the program will ignore it. For example, the Excel file for the two nurse observers' sleep quality assessments of the 30 hospitalized children (study.sagepub.com/pett2e) consists of a 30 (rows) by 2 (columns) Excel data file along with a header column identifying the observer. Each observer is assigned one of three values to the children's sleep quality: 1 = poor, 2 = moderate, and 3 = very good. Notice that there are no blank cells (e.g., missing data). Once this Excel file has been created, it needs to be saved as a ".csv" file (i.e., comma-separated values) (e.g., study.sagepub.com/pett2e file for calculating Cohens kappa.csv). It is this .csv file that is submitted to ReCal2 ("2" representing two raters).

Figure 9.6 presents the results that were obtained by submitting the .csv file to ReCal2. Notice that the obtained kappa using this resource (.622 ⑧) is similar to our hand-calculated value and that which we obtained in SPSS for Windows (Figure 9.4 ③). Note, too, that the ReCal resource also offers three additional interrater statistics: Fleiss's kappa (Fleiss, 1971), Krippendorff's alpha (Hayes & Krippendorff, 2007; Krippendorff, 2013), and Scott's Pi (Scott, 1955). All of these statistics have useful attributes. Unlike Cohen's kappa and Scott's Pi, for example, Fleiss's kappa and Krippendorff's alpha are not limited to two observers.

Presentation of Results

Table 9.6 is an example of a suitable presentation of the results of the analysis of interobserver agreement for the computer output presented in Figure 9.4. It is also possible to present the results in the text as follows:

Figure 9.6 Screenshot of online calculation of the kappa coefficient.

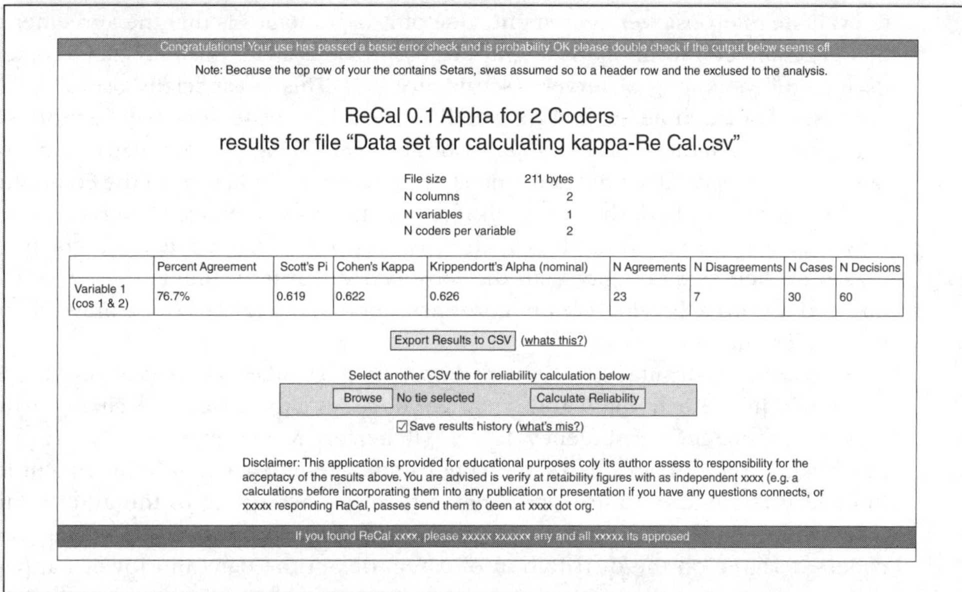

SOURCE: ReCal is © Deen Freelon All Rights Reserved. Retrieved from http://dfreelon.org/utils/recalfront/.

An evaluation of agreement between two nurse observers with regard to their assessments of 30 children's sleep quality at Day 1 postintervention was undertaken. The exact percentage agreement between the two observers was 77%. A kappa coefficient was used to correct for chance agreement among the observers. This resulted in a significant kappa of .62 ($z = 4.59$, $p < .0001$). The size of this kappa indicates that there was fair to good interobserver agreement (Fleiss, 1971).

Table 9.6 Results of Interobserver Agreement on Children's Sleep Quality at Day 1 Postintervention

	Nurse Observer 2				
Nurse Observer 1	*Poor*	*Moderate*	*Very Good*	*Total*	*kappa*
Poor	3	3	0	6	0.62*
Moderate	0	8	3	11	
Very good	0	1	12	13	
Total	3	12	15	30	

*$p < .001$.

Advantages, Limitations, and Alternatives to the Kappa Coefficient

The kappa coefficient is an extremely useful nonparametric statistic that can be used to evaluate interobserver agreement. One of its advantages is that the agreement matrix that is generated for this statistic graphically provides a clear display of agreements and disagreements among observers (see Figure 9.4). This is especially useful for training purposes. For example, the matrix can illustrate which observers may be more sensitive to the nuances in the coding or diagnostic scheme. The agreement matrix can also point out where observer disagreements most often occur. As indicated in the computer printout in Figure 9.4, six of the seven disagreements between Nurse Observer 1 and Nurse Observer 2 were situations in which Observer 1 evaluated the children lower with regard to their sleep quality than did Observer 2. Future training, therefore, might be directed toward achieving greater consensus among the raters concerning the meaning of these categories.

A serious disadvantage to Cohen's kappa in particular is that it is very sensitive to low totals in the marginals and small contingency tables because chance values are higher for smaller contingency tables (Bakeman & Gottman, 1997). Krippendorff (2013) also argues that Cohen's kappa does not take into account individual differences in coders' tendencies to use particular categories. According to the author, failure to take into account coder preferences has the effect of producing higher kappas when coders disagree on the distribution of categories in the data and lower kappas when they agree.

A number of refinements can be made to the kappa coefficient. For example, a weighted kappa (Cohen, 1968) can be used when the researcher considers some mistakes to be more important than others. This type of kappa weights disagreements differently, depending on how serious the researcher considers a particular error to be. Modified versions of the simple kappa coefficient have also been derived to assess agreement among any number of observers (Fleiss, 1971; Krippendorff, 2013; Uebersax, 1982) and for use with ordinal-, interval-, and ratio-level data (Krippendorff, 2013).

A very useful parametric alternative to the use of percentage agreement in general, and kappa in particular, to assess interobserver agreement is to use a generalizability theory approach (R. L. Brennan, 2001; Cronbach, Gleser, Nanda, & Rajaratmam, 1972; Shavelson & Webb, 1991) to decompose the various errors of measurement into their appropriate components. Shavelson and Webb (1991), in particular, offer a very clearly written overview for nonmathematicians of the theory and methods of this approach.

Examples From Published Research

Beach, E. K., Maloney, B. H., Plocica, A. R., Sherry, S. E., Weaver, M., Luthringer, L., & Utz, S. (1992). The spouse: A factor in recovery after acute myocardial infarction. *Heart & Lung: The Journal of Critical Care, 21,* 30–38.

Capio, C. M., Sit, C. H. P., & Abernethy, B. (2011). Fundamental movement skills testing in children with cerebral palsy. *Disability & Rehabilitation, 33*(25/26), 2519–2528. doi: 10.3109/09638288.2011.577502

THE POINT BISERIAL CORRELATION

The phi, Cramér, and kappa coefficients are suitable for assessing the strength of association in categorical data. There may be occasions, however, when researchers are interested in assessing the strength of relationship between one variable that is at the interval or ratio level of measurement and a second variable that is either dichotomous or at the ordinal level of measurement (e.g., gender vs. depression scores or one scale item vs. the total scale score). The point biserial correlation is used to examine strength of association in the first instance (dichotomous vs. interval/ratio data), and the biserial correlation is used in the second instance (ordinal vs. interval data). In this section, we will examine the point biserial correlation in greater detail; the biserial correlation will be briefly addressed when examining the Spearman rho correlation coefficient.

An Appropriate Research Question for the Point Biserial Correlation

The point biserial correlation has been used in a number of health care research projects. Damrosch and Perry (1989) used the point biserial correlation in their analysis of patterns of adjustment, frequency of chronic sorrow, and coping behaviors of parents of children with Down syndrome. Burnette, Ramundo, Stevenson, and Beeson (2009) also used the point biserial correlation in their evaluation of a web-based asynchronous pediatric emergency medicine learning tool for residents and medical students. Eskander et al. (2012) used the same point biserial correlation to examine the association between preoperative spinal cord rotation and postoperative C5 nerve palsy. Another common use of the point biserial correlation is to compare an individual's performance on a single item (e.g., yes, no) with his or her total score on a particular test. Renzaho and Polonsky (2012), for example, used the statistic for that purpose to develop and evaluate a knowledge questionnaire about blood donation in African migrant communities in Australia.

In our hypothetical study, a number of possible research questions could be answered using the point biserial correlation. For example, suppose we were interested in examining the strength of association between the average number of sleep environment interruptions experienced by a hospitalized child during the course of a staff-initiated intervention and his or her distress at Day 2 postintervention. A research question that could be answered using this statistic would be as follows:

> What is the strength of association between a hospitalized child's average number of sleep environment interruptions during the course of a staff-initiated intervention and his or her distress (not distressed, distressed) at Day 2 post intervention?

Null and Alternative Hypotheses

Table 9.7 presents null and alternative hypotheses that were generated from our research question and that could be answered using a point biserial correlation. The data set that we will be using is hospitalized children with cancer-30 cases.sav (study.sagepub.com/pett2e). Note that the variable of distress at Day 2 is nominal (0 = not distressed,

Table 9.7 Example of Null and Alternative Hypotheses Suitable for a Point Biserial Correlation Coefficient

Null Hypothesis
H_0: There is no association between the variables of the average number of environmental sleep disturbances during a staff-initiated intervention and his or her distress (not distressed, distressed) at Day 2 following the intervention.
Alternative Hypothesis
H_a: There is an association between the variables of the average number of environmental sleep disturbances during a staff-initiated intervention and his or her distress (not distressed, distressed) at Day 2 following the intervention.

1 = distressed) and that the average number of sleep environment disturbances during the intervention is at the interval level of measurement (range: 0–12), with higher values indicating more sleep environment disturbances.

Overview of the Procedure

The point biserial correlation is a special case of a parametric statistic, the Pearson product-moment correlation. Although there may be some disagreement in the statistics literature as to whether the point biserial correlation is a parametric or nonparametric statistic, it is considered by some writers (Daniel, 1990) to be nonparametric because one of the variables being assessed is dichotomous.

Calculation of the point biserial correlation, r_{pb}, is rather straightforward and is merely a simplified version of the Pearson *r*:

$$r_{pb} = \sqrt{\frac{n_1 n_0}{N}} \left(\frac{(\bar{x}_1 - \bar{x}_0)}{\sqrt{\Sigma (x - \bar{x})^2}} \right)$$

where

N = total sample size,

n_0 = the number of cases when the value of the dichotomous variable = 0,

n_1 = the number of cases when the value of the dichotomous variable = 1,

$\bar{x}_0$ = mean of the continuous variable when the dichotomous variable = 0,

$\bar{x}_1$ = mean of the continuous variable when the dichotomous variable = 1,

x = individual observations for entire group, and

$\bar{x}$ = the mean for the entire group.

The value of the point biserial correlation coefficient can range between −1 and +1, with higher absolute values indicating a greater strength of relationship. The point biserial correlation is tested in a manner similar to that for the Pearson *r*. The null hypothesis of no relationship between the dichotomous and continuous variables will be rejected if the obtained value of the correlation coefficient exceeds a critical value with $df = N - 2$ at a prestated alpha level (e.g., .05) or, alternatively, if the resulting *p* value is less than the prestated alpha.

Because of the close relationship of r_{pb} to the Pearson *r*, the strength of association for r_{pb} can be evaluated using the criteria for r^2 (Table 7.7) (Hinkle et al., 2003). That is, values of r_{pb}^2 above .81 indicate an extremely strong relationship, .49 to .80 a strong relationship, .25 to .48 a moderate relationship, .09 to .24 a low relationship, and .00 to .08 a weak relationship.

Critical Assumptions of the Point Biserial Correlation

The point biserial correlation has a number of assumptions that are associated with both nonparametric and parametric statistics.

1. *The randomly selected observations are paired, with one variable being dichotomous and the other at the interval/ratio level.*
2. *The dichotomous (Y) variable has mutually exclusive groups whose values have been coded 0 and 1.*
3. *The continuous (X) variable is distributed normally overall and within each level of the dichotomous variable.*
4. *The continuous (X) variable has equal variances across each level of the dichotomous variables.*

Note that all four of these assumptions are similar to those of the parametric independent (or Student's) *t* test. The difference in the two tests is that whereas the independent *t* test is a test of differences in the means of two groups, the point biserial correlation is a measure of association between two variables. Moreover, whereas the independent variable for the *t* test *must* be dichotomous, there is no such restriction for the point biserial correlation. Either the independent or dependent variable may be dichotomous.

In our hypothetical study, the dependent variable, distress, is dichotomous, and the independent variable, average number of sleep environment disturbances, is at the interval level. Using the *Analyze . . . Descriptive Statistics . . . Explore* dialog box in SPSS for Windows can generate the plots and K-S statistics to determine whether we meet the assumption of normality of distribution for the continuous variable across both levels of the dichotomous variable (see Chapter 3 for details).

Homogeneity of variance could also be assessed in SPSS for Windows by opening the *Analyze . . . Compare Means . . . Independent-Samples T Test* dialog box in the menu. The *grouping variable* is the dichotomous variable (e.g., *Distress_T2*), and the test variable is the continuous variable (e.g., *Sleep_Environment_Interruptions*). The resulting independent t test also provides information about *Levene's test for equality of variances,* which is a test of homogeneity of variance. The null hypothesis of equal variances will be rejected if the generated p value of Levene's test is less than our alpha (e.g., $\alpha = .05$). For this test, we do not want to reject H_0 because that would imply that the variances are not equal.

Computer-Generated Output

Figure 9.7 presents the descriptive statistics, the syntax commands, and computer-generated output for the point biserial correlation obtained in SPSS for Windows. The data set that we will be using is hospitalized children with cancer-30 cases.sav (study.sagepub .com/pett2e) Descriptive statistics can be obtained by opening *Analyze . . . Descriptive Statistics . . .* and clicking on either *Frequencies . . . Descriptives . . .* or *Explore.* SPSS for Windows does not produce a point biserial correlation directly. Because this statistic is a special case of the Pearson correlation coefficient, it is possible to obtain the point biserial correlation by opening the *Analyze . . . Correlate . . . Bivariate* dialog box, identifying both the nominal- and interval-level variables of interest (i.e., *Sleep_Environment_Interruptions* and *Distress_T2*), and selecting the *Pearson* correlation coefficient.

Figure 9.7 indicates that the point biserial correlation coefficient generated from SPSS for Windows is +.490 ($p = .006$) (1). This value could also have been obtained directly from the formula for the point biserial correlation:

$$r_{pb} = \sqrt{\frac{n_1 n_0}{N}} \left(\frac{(\bar{x}_1 - \bar{x}_0)}{\sqrt{\Sigma (x - \bar{x})^2}} \right)$$

The descriptive statistics in Figure 9.7 provide us with the following information concerning sample sizes, group means, and the total variance for the continuous variable.

$N = 30$,

$n_0 = 14$ (the number of cases in the intervention group for which distress = 0),

$n_1 = 16$ (the number of cases in the control group for which distress = 1),

$$s^2_{sleep\ interruptions} = \frac{\Sigma\left(X - \bar{X}\right)^2}{(N-1)} = 7.633$$

$$\Sigma(X - \bar{X})^2 = (N-1)s^2 = (30-1)(7.633) = 221.357$$

$\bar{X}_0 = 6.1429$ (the mean value of number of environmental interruptions for the group for which distress = 0), and

$\bar{X}_1 = 8.8125$ (the mean value of number of environmental interruptions for the group for which distress = 1).

Figure 9.7 Descriptive statistics, syntax, and computer-generated output in SPSS for Windows (v. 22–23) for the point biserial correlation.

Descriptives

	distress_t2 distress immediately post-intervention			Statistic	Std. Error
Sleep_Environment_Interruptions average number of sleep environmental interruptions per night during intervention	.00 not distressed	Mean		6.1429	.71757
		95% Confidence Interval for Mean	Lower Bound	4.5926	
			Upper Bound	7.6931	
		5% Trimmed Mean		6.2143	
		Median		6.0000	
		Variance		7.209	
		Std. Deviation		2.68492	
		Minimum		.00	
		Maximum		11.00	
		Range		11.00	
		Interquartile Range		1.50	
		Skewness		-.734	.597
		Kurtosis		1.709	1.154
	1.00 distressed	Mean		8.8125	.55692
		95% Confidence Interval for Mean	Lower Bound	7.6255	
			Upper Bound	9.9995	
		5% Trimmed Mean		8.8472	
		Median		9.0000	
		Variance		4.963	
		Std. Deviation		2.22767	
		Minimum		5.00	
		Maximum		12.00	
		Range		7.00	
		Interquartile Range		3.50	
		Skewness		-.352	.564
		Kurtosis		-.662	1.091

Descriptive Statistics

	N	Minimum	Maximum	Mean	Std. Deviation	Variance
Sleep_Environment_Interruptions average number of sleep environmental interruptions per night during intervention	30	.00	12.00	7.5667	2.76285	7.633
distress_t2 distress immediately post-intervention	30	.00	1.00	.5333	.50742	.257
Valid N (listwise)	30					

```
***Data set : Hospitalized children with cancer-30 cases.sav***

CORRELATIONS
 /VARIABLES=distress_t2 Sleep_Environment_Interruptions
 /PRINT=TWOTAIL NOSIG
 /MISSING=PAIRWISE.
```

Correlations

		distress_t2 distress immediately post-intervention	Sleep_Environment_Interruptions average number of sleep environmental interruptions per night during intervention
distress_t2 distress immediately post-intervention	Pearson Correlation	1	(1) .490**
	Sig. (2-tailed)		.006
	N	30	30
Sleep_Environment_Interruptions average number of sleep environmental interruptions per night during intervention	Pearson Correlation	.490**	1
	Sig. (2-tailed)	.006	
	N	30	30

**. Correlation is significant at the 0.01 level (2-tailed).

Now it is possible to generate the value for the point biserial correlation:

$$r_{pb} = \sqrt{\frac{n_1 n_0}{N}} \left(\frac{(\bar{x}_1 - \bar{x}_0)}{\sqrt{\Sigma (x - \bar{x})^2}} \right)$$

$$\sqrt{\frac{(16)(14)}{30}} \left(\frac{(8.8125 - 6.1429)}{\sqrt{(221.357)}} \right) = (2.7325)(0.1794) = +0.49$$

Is the value of the point biserial correlation, +.49, sufficiently large to reject the null hypothesis of no relationship between the variables of number of sleep environment interruptions and children's distress? We can determine this in one of two ways: by calculating a *t* statistic based on the point biserial correlation or by evaluating the *p* value that is presented in the printout.

Calculating a *t* statistic based on the point biserial correlation.

To determine the significance of r_{pb}, if N is sufficiently large (e.g., $N > 25$), a *t* statistic can be obtained:

$$t = r_{pb} \sqrt{\frac{N-2}{1 - r_{pb}^2}} = 0.49 \sqrt{\frac{30-2}{1 - 0.49^2}} = (0.49)(6.07) = 2.97$$

This *t* statistic is distributed as a *t* distribution with $df = N - 2$ or, in our case, $30 - 2 = 28$. We will reject the null hypothesis of no association between the variables distress and number of sleep environment interruptions if and only if our calculated *t* (2.97) is larger than the critical value at our prestated level of alpha (e.g., $\alpha = .05$).

Table A.3 in Appendix A presents the critical values of the *t* distribution at various one- and two-tailed levels of alpha. For a two-tailed $\alpha = .05$, that critical value is ±2.048. Since +2.97 is larger than +2.048, we will reject the null hypothesis and conclude that there is an association between the variables distress and number of sleep environment interruptions. That is, those children who experienced more sleep environment interruptions during the intervention were also more likely to be distressed at Day 2.

Evaluating the *p* value presented in the printout.

Since we are presented with a *p*-value, not a *t statistic,* in the computer printout from SPSS for Windows (v. 22–23) (Figure 9.7), we will need to interpret this *p* value instead ($p = .006$ (1)). In this case, we will reject the null hypothesis if the generated *p* value is less than our predetermined two-tailed alpha (e.g., $\alpha = .05$). Because .006 is less than .05, we will reject the null hypothesis of no association and conclude that there is a statistically significant relationship between number of sleep environmental interruptions and children's distress.

If our research hypothesis had been directional, we would either have chosen a one-tailed test of significance (e.g., 1.701, Table A.3, Appendix A) or have divided the resulting *p* value from Figure 9.7 in half and compared it to our one-tailed α level. The positive correlation that we have obtained suggests that the distress group assigned the value of 1 (distressed at Day 2) had a greater average number of sleep environmental disruptions during the intervention than the distressed group assigned the value of 0 (nondistressed at Day 2). According to our guidelines regarding strength of association, the relationship between average number of sleep environmental disruptions and distress is moderate because $r^2_{pb} = (.49)^2 = .24$.

Internet Resources for Generating the Point Biserial Correlation

The point biserial correlation can be calculated using a number of free Internet resources. One such currently available user-friendly Internet site is vassarstats.net/pbcorr.html. The instructions are clearly presented and easily followed. That is, using a spreadsheet such as the Excel file, hospitalized children with cancer.xlsx, we are requested to copy and paste the values for the continuous variable (e.g., *Number of environmental interruptions*) when the dichotomous variable (e.g., *Distress at Day 2*) = 0. Next we copy and paste the values of the same continuous variable when the dichotomous variables = 1. By clicking on *Calculate . . .*, we are presented with the output presented in Figure 9.8.

The results presented in Figure 9.8 confirm our previous findings (e.g., $r_{pb} = +.49$, $t = 2.98$, two-tailed $p = .006$).

Figure 9.8 Internet-generated output for the point biserial correlation.

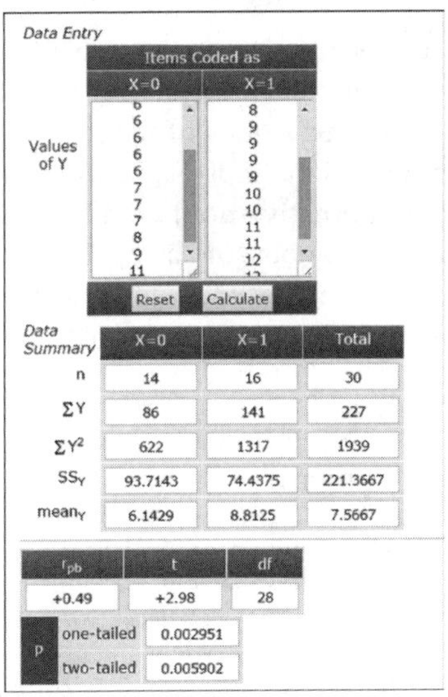

Presentation of Results

Although the point biserial correlation could be presented in a table similar to Table 9.10, it is probably best suited to presentation in the text if there is only one biserial correlation to report.

> A point biserial correlation was undertaken to evaluate the strength of association between the continuous variable, average number of sleep environment disturbances during the intervention, and the nominal level variable, distress at Day 2 postintervention. The results of this analysis (r_{pb} = +.49, p = .006) indicate that, although those who were distressed at Day 2 had experienced a statistically significantly higher number of nocturnal sleep interruptions during the intervention than those who were not distressed, the relationship between distress and number of environmental sleep interruptions was moderate with a shared variance of 23%.

Advantages, Limitations, and Alternatives to the Point Biserial Correlation

The point biserial correlation is used to examine the strength of relationship between a nominal-level and a variable that is at least interval level of measurement. It would be an especially useful statistic, therefore, when the researcher has found a significant difference between two groups (e.g., intervention vs. control) and wants to know how strong the relationship is between this nominal-level independent variable and a continuous dependent variable. Neither the *t* test nor any of its nonparametric alternatives (e.g., the Mann-Whitney test) can provide this information except as a report of effect size.

A disadvantage to this statistic is that it must meet the parametric assumption of a normally distributed continuous variable. The categorical variable of interest must also be dichotomous, with assigned values of 0 and 1.

As indicated, the point biserial correlation is a special case of the Pearson product-moment correlation. An alternative nonparametric measure for ascertaining strength of association between a dichotomous and a continuous variable was suggested by Freeman (1965). This statistic has been found to have a distribution very similar to the Mann-Whitney *U* statistic (Buck & Finner, 1985; Daniel, 1990) but is not currently available in SPSS for Windows.

Examples From Published Research

Burnette, K., Ramundo, M., Stevenson, M., & Beeson, M. S. (2009). Evaluation of a Web-based asynchronous pediatric emergency medicine learning tool for residents and medical students. *Academic Emergency Medicine, 16*(12), S46–S50. doi: 10.1111/j.1553-2712.2009.00598.x

Damrosch, S. P., & Perry, L. A. (1989). Self-reported adjustment, chronic sorrow, and coping of parents of children with Down syndrome. *Nursing Research, 38,* 25–30.

Eskander, M. S., Balsis, S. M., Balinger, C., Howard, C. M., Lewing, N. W., Eskander, J. P., . . . Jenis, L. G. (2012). The association between preoperative spinal cord rotation and postoperative c5 nerve palsy. *Journal of Bone & Joint Surgery, American Volume, 94*(17), 1605–1609.

Renzaho, A. M. N., & Polonsky, M. J. (2012). Examining demographic and socio-economic correlates of accurate knowledge about blood donation among African migrants in Australia. *Transfusion Medicine (Oxford, England), 22*(5), 321–331. doi: 10.1111/j.1365-3148.2012.01175.x

THE SPEARMAN RANK-ORDER CORRELATION COEFFICIENT

The Spearman rank-order correlation coefficient (also known as *Spearman's rho* or r_s) (Spearman, 1904) is one of the best-known and frequently used nonparametric statistics in health care research. A brief search of the PsycINFO, CINAHL, and MEDLINE databases for the years 2000–2014, for example, yielded more than 1,300 research articles published in academic journals that had reported the use of Spearman's rho. This statistic is most often used to examine the relationship between two ordinal-level variables. It is also a very suitable alternative to its parametric alternative, the Pearson product-moment correlation coefficient, when for various reasons the data do not meet that test's assumptions.

An Appropriate Research Question for the Spearman Rank-Order Correlation Coefficient

Numerous studies have used Spearman's rho to evaluate the degree of association between the rankings of two continuous variables. For example, Roy, Forrester, Macko, and Krebs (2013) used a Spearman rank-order correlation coefficient to examine the relationship between changes in passive ankle stiffness and gait function in persons with chronic stroke. In addition to their use of kappa, Capio et al. (2011) used the Spearman rho to assess the relationship between product-oriented and process-oriented measures of fundamental movement skills among children with cerebral palsy. Tomarken et al. (2008) used that same correlation coefficient to examine factors associated with complicated grief predeath in caregivers of cancer patients.

In our hypothetical study, we might be interested in examining the relationship between the 30 children's postintervention anxiety scores and parents' initial evaluations of their children's posthospital adjustment. The anxiety scores were measured on a 7-point Likert-type scale (1 = *not at all anxious,* 7 = *very anxious*) and thus were at the ordinal level of measurement. Although the posthospital adjustment scores were at the interval level of measurement, with a range of 63 to 93, they were not normally distributed, a requirement of the parametric Pearson product-moment correlation. A research question that could be answered using the Spearman rank-order correlation coefficient is as follows:

> To what extent is there a negative relationship between children's postintervention anxiety scores and parents' perceptions of their children's immediate posthospital adjustment?

Null and Alternative Hypotheses

An example of null and alternative hypotheses that are based on our research question that would be suitable for a Spearman rank-order correlation coefficient is presented in Table 9.8. Because our research question is directional, the alternative hypothesis is also directional.

Overview of the Procedure

Like the point biserial correlation coefficient, Spearman's rho is a special case of the Pearson *r*. For Spearman's rho, however, a Pearson correlation coefficient is obtained for the rankings of the observations, not their actual scores.

To compute r_s, the observations for each of the *X* and *Y* variables are ranked for each subject from lowest (rank = 1) to highest (rank = *N*). Tied observations are assigned the average rank that would have been assigned without ties. For example, if three observations on one variable were tied for third position and would have occupied positions 3, 4, and 5, they would all receive the rank of 4 (i.e., [3 + 4 + 5]/3 = 4). Next, for each subject, the difference between his or her rank on the *X* and *Y* variables, d_p, is obtained, squared, and summed across all subjects. If there are no ties, the Spearman rho correlation coefficient can be obtained using the following formula:

$$r_s = 1 - \frac{6\sum_{i=1}^{N} d_i^2}{N^3 - N}$$

where

d_i = the difference in the ranks on the two paired variables, *X* and *Y*, for a particular subject, and

N = the number of pairs of observations.

Table 9.8 Example of Null and Alternative Hypotheses Suitable for a Spearman Rank-Order Correlation Coefficient

Null Hypothesis
H_0: There is no association between children's postintervention anxiety and their parents' perceptions of their children's immediate posthospital adjustment.
Alternative Hypothesis
H_a: There is a negative association between children's postintervention anxiety and their parents' perceptions of their children's immediate posthospital adjustment.

This formula does not adjust for ties. Ties appear to have a minimal effect on the value of r_s provided there are few ties or the number of ties within a group of ties is small. The following formula for r_i adjusts for ties (Daniel, 1990; Siegel & Castellan, 1988):

$$r_s = \frac{(N^3 - N) \; - \; 6 \sum d_i^2 - (T_x + T_y)/2}{\sqrt{(N^3 - N)^2 [T_x + T_y)(N^3 - N)] + T_x T_y}}$$

The values for d_i and N are the same as for the formula presented previously. The correction factors for tied ranks, T_x and T_y, are obtained using the following formula (Siegel & Castellan, 1988):

$$T_x = \sum_{i-1}^{g} (t_i^3 - t_i)$$

where

T_x = the correction factor for the x variable,

T_y = the correction factor for the y variable,

g = the number of groupings of different tied ranks, and

t_i = the number of tied ranks in the ith grouping.

With these formulas, we could calculate Spearman's rho for the children's postintervention anxiety and immediate posthospital adjustment scores by hand using the raw data presented in Table 9.9. Because there are so many ties for both the independent and dependent variables, it will be necessary to use the Spearman rho formula that corrects for ties; therefore, we need to compute not only the sum of d^2 (the sum of the squared differences in the rankings of the X and Y variables) (Table 9.9, (1)) but also T_x and T_y. It is relatively easy to obtain the number of ties (T_x) for the anxiety variable using the anxiety variable from Table 9.9, column 3(2):

$$\begin{aligned} T_x = \sum_{i=1}^{g} (t_i^3 - t_i) &= (4^3 - 4) + (7^3 - 7) + (11^3 - 11) + (6^3 - 6) + (2^3 - 2) \\ &= 60 + 336 + 1320 + 210 + 6 = 1932 \end{aligned}$$

The number of ties for the adjustment variable, T_y, is a bit more cumbersome to calculate since we must first list out the rankings for the adjustment variable listed in column 4 (3) (e.g., 1, 4.5, 4.5, 7, 7, 7, 9, 11, 11, 11, 13, 14, 15, 16.5, 16, 5, 19.5, 19.5, 19.5, 19.5, 22, 23.5, 25.5, 25.5, 27.5, 27.5, 29.5, 29.5) in order to calculate T_y:

$$\begin{aligned} T_y = \sum_{i=1}^{g} (t_i^3 - t_i) &= \left(2^3 - 2\right) + \left(2^3 - 2\right) + \left(3^3 - 3\right) + \left(2^3 - 2\right) + \left(4^3 - 4\right) \\ &\quad + \left(2^3 - 2\right) + \left(2^3 - 2\right) + \left(2^3 - 2\right) + \left(2^3 - 2\right) \\ &= 7\left(2^3 - 2\right) + 2\left(3^3 - 3\right) + \left(4^3 - 4\right) = 150 \end{aligned}$$

Table 9.9 Raw Data for Spearman Rho and Kendall's Tau-b Calculations

Anxiety	*Calculations for the Spearman Rho Correlation*					*Calculations for Kendall's tau*		
	Posthospital Adjustment	*Rankings*		*Difference*		*# Natural Order Pairs Concordant*	*# Reverse Order Pairs Discordant*	*# Ties*
(X) ④	*(Y)* ⑤	R_x ②	R_y ③	*d*	d^2	*(C)* ⑥	*(D)* ⑦	*(T)* ⑧
3	76	2.5	11	–8.5	72.25	16	9	1
3	76	2.5	11	–8.5	72.25	16	9	1
3	85	2.5	19.5	–17	289	9	15	2
3	85	2.5	19.5	–17	289	9	15	2
4	75	8	9	–1	1	11	8	0
4	85	8	19.5	–11.5	132.25	5	14	0
4	85	8	19.5	–11.5	132.25	5	14	0
4	89	8	23.5	–15.5	240.25	4	15	0
4	89	8	23.5	–15.5	240.25	4	15	0
4	90	8	25.5	–17.5	306.25	4	15	0
4	90	8	25.5	–17.5	306.25	4	15	0
5	62	17	1	16	256	8	0	0
5	67	17	7	10	100	4	4	0
5	67	17	7	10	100	4	4	0
5	67	17	7	10	100	2	4	0
5	79	17	14	3	9	2	6	0
5	82	17	15	2	4	2	6	0
5	83	17	16.5	0.5	0.25	1	6	1
5	92	17	27.5	–10.5	110.25	0	8	0
5	92	17	27.5	–10.5	110.25	0	8	0
5	93	17	29.5	–12.5	156.25	0	8	0
5	93	17	29.5	–12.5	156.25	0	8	0
6	78	25.5	4.5	21	441	0	2	0

Table 9.9 (Continued)

	Calculations for the Spearman Rho Correlation					*Calculations for Kendall's tau*		
Anxiety	*Posthospital Adjustment*	*Rankings*		*Difference*		*# Natural Order Pairs Concordant*	*# Reverse Order Pairs Discordant*	*# Ties*
(X) ④	*(Y)* ⑤	R_x ②	R_y ③	*d*	d^2	*(C)* ⑥	*(D)* ⑦	*(T)* ⑧
6	76	25.5	4.5	21	441	0	2	0
6	66	25.5	11	14.5	210.25	0	2	0
6	66	25.5	13	12.5	156.25	0	2	0
6	83	25.5	16.5	9	81	0	2	0
6	86	25.5	22	3.5	12.25	0	2	0
7	65	29.5	2.5	27	729	0	0	0
7	65	29.5	2.5	27	729	0	0	0
TOTAL				①	5,983	112	218	7

Given these values for T_x (1,932) and T_y (150), it is now possible to calculate r_s:

$$r_s = \frac{(N^3 - N^2) - 6\sum d_i^2 - (T_x + T_y)/2}{\sqrt{(N^3 - N^2 - [(T_x + T_y)(N^3 - N)] + T_x T_y}} \infty$$

$$= \frac{(30^3 - 30) - 6(5983) - (1932 + 150)/2}{\sqrt{(30^3 - 30)^2 - [(1932 + 150)(30^3 - 30)] + (1932)(150)}}$$

$$= \frac{-9969}{25913.69} = -.385.$$

There are two ways to determine significance of r_s. As with the point biserial correlation, if N is sufficiently large (e.g., $N > 25$), a t statistic can be calculated. Alternatively, one can examine the Spearman rank order correlation coefficient directly by comparing it to an expected value. The following formula is used to obtain the t statistic:

$$t = r_s \sqrt{\frac{N - 2}{1 - r_s^2}}$$

$$= -.385 \sqrt{\frac{30 - 2}{1 - (-.385)^2}} = -2.207$$

This t statistic is approximately distributed as a Student's t with $df = N - 2$, where N is the number of pairs. The null hypothesis that $r_s = 0$ will be rejected if the obtained value of the t statistic is greater than the absolute critical value at the prestated one- or two-tailed α (e.g., $\alpha = .05$) and $df = (N - 2)$ (provided, of course, for one-tailed tests that the t value is in the predicted direction).

Because the research hypothesis in our hypothetical study is directional in the negative direction and $\alpha = .05$, we will compare our calculated t value with a critical one-tailed t value with $df = 28$. We will reject the null hypothesis if the actual t value we obtained, −2.207, is *smaller* than our critical value. It is *smaller* because we are predicting an inverse or negative relationship between anxiety and adjustment and because only then will our actual t statistic fall within the one-tailed region of rejection of the t distribution.

Table A.3 in Appendix A presents the one- and two-tailed critical values for the t statistic at various levels of alpha. From this table, we can see that the one-tailed critical value for this t distribution at $df = 28$ is 1.70. Because we are predicting an inverse or negative relationship between anxiety and adjustment, we need to make that critical value negative. As a result, −1.70 is larger than our calculated value, −2.205. We can, therefore, reject the null hypothesis and determine that, indeed, there is a statistically significant negative association between children's postintervention anxiety and their posthospital adjustment scores. That is, those children who had higher postintervention anxiety scores were assessed by their parents to have lower immediate posthospital adjustment.

For smaller N (e.g., when the number of pairs is ≤ 30), one can use Table A.4 in Appendix A to obtain the critical values of r_s at set levels of alpha. Given that we have 30 pairs of observations, a one-tailed $\alpha = .05$, and an alternative hypothesis that predicts a negative relationship between postintervention anxiety and post-hospital adjustment, we will reject the null hypothesis of no association if our obtained r_s is *smaller* than the negative critical value of −.3059. Since our actual r_s (−.385) is less than our critical value (−.3059), we will again reject the null hypothesis of no association and conclude that there is an inverse relationship between postintervention anxiety and postintervention adjustment.

Critical Assumptions of the Spearman Rank-Order Correlation Coefficient

1. *The two randomly selected variables, X and Y, are continuous variables with at least an ordinal level of measurement.*
2. *The two variables, X and Y, are paired observations.*

The data from our hypothetical study partially meet these assumptions. The two variables, children's anxiety and mothers' assessments of posthospital adjustment, are paired observations that are at least at the ordinal level of measurement. The data were not, however, drawn from a random sample. Although the children were randomly assigned to intervention and usual care, they were originally obtained from a sample of convenience.

Computer Commands

Figure 9.9 presents the SPSS for Windows dialog box for the Spearman rho. This dialog box was opened by highlighting *Analyze . . . Correlate . . . Bivariate . . .* in the menus and selecting the *Spearman rho* statistic. Because we are undertaking a directional test, the *one-tailed* significance level was chosen.

Computer-Generated Output

Figure 9.10 presents the SPSS for Windows syntax commands and computer printout for Spearman's rho. Note that although we used the same dialog box that would be used to generate the Pearson *r*, the syntax commands have indicated that we are using a nonparametric correlation coefficient (2).

Figure 9.10 also presents the 2 × 2 correlation matrix for the Spearman's rho. Notice that on the diagonal, we are presented with 1's (the correlation of the variable with itself). On the off-diagonal, we are given the correlation coefficient, one-tailed *p* value, and

Figure 9.9 Computer commands for generating the Spearman rho correlation coefficient in SPSS for Windows (v. 22–23).

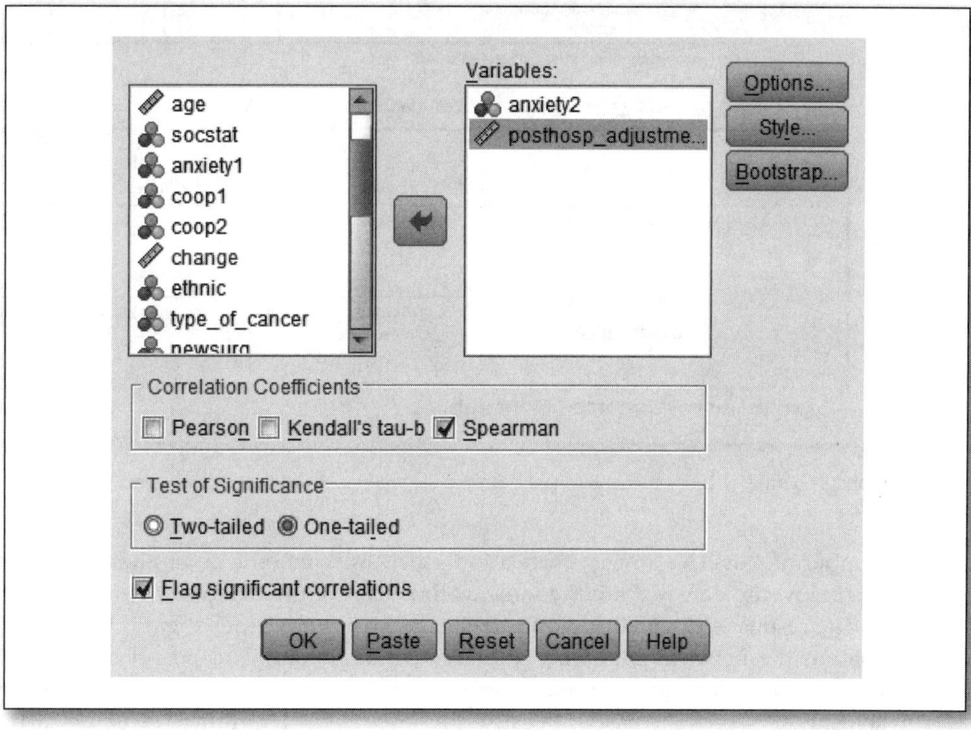

Figure 9.10 SPSS for Windows (v. 22–23) computer-generated output for the Spearman rho rank-order correlation coefficient and Kendall's tau coefficient.

```
***Data set: hospitalized children with cancer-30 cases. sav

NONPAR CORR (2)
 /VARIABLES=anxiety2 posthosp_adjustment
 /PRINT=SPEARMAN ONETAIL NOSIG
 /MISSING=PAIRWISE.
```

Correlations

			anxiety2 post-intervention anxiety	posthosp_adjustment parent's assessment of child's adjustment upon discharge
Spearman's rho	anxiety2 post-intervention anxiety	Correlation Coefficient	1.000	-.385*
		Sig. (1-tailed)	.	.018
		N	30	30
	posthosp_adjustment parent's assessment of child's adjustment upon discharge	Correlation Coefficient	(3) -.385*	1.000
		Sig. (1-tailed)	.018	.
		N	30	30

*. Correlation is significant at the 0.05 level (1-tailed). (4)

Correlations

			anxiety2 post-test anxiety	posthosp posthospital adjustment
Kendall's tau_b	anxiety2 post-test anxiety	Correlation Coefficient	1.000	(9) -.283*
		Sig. (1-tailed)	.	(10) .024
		N	30	30
	posthosp posthospital adjustment	Correlation Coefficient	-.283*	1.000
		Sig. (1-tailed)	.024	.
		N	30	30

*. Correlation is significant at the 0.05 level (1-tailed).

number of pairs (*N*). Since a correlation matrix is symmetric about the diagonal, the values below the diagonal are the same as those above the diagonal.

The results of this analysis indicate that, as we found earlier, there is indeed a negative relationship between children's postintervention anxiety and post-hospital adjustment, $r_s = -.385$. That is, as children's postintervention anxiety decreased, their posthospital adjustment scores increased. Because the one-tailed significance level, $p = .018$ (3), is less than our preset one-tailed $\alpha = .05$, we can reject the null hypothesis and conclude that this inverse relationship is significant.

Notice that the output indicates that the "correlation is significant at the .05 level (1-tailed)" (4). That statement is only true *if* we have predicted in the right direction. Suppose we had predicted an inverse relationship between anxiety and adjustment but, in reality, the actual r_s was +.385, not −.385. The computer, in its ignorance, would have still indicated that the correlation was significant when, in fact, we could not have rejected the null hypothesis. So, bottom line, do not believe all that you are presented with in an output without having first checked to see if the results were in the direction predicted.

Determining the strength of the relationship of r_s.

There is some discussion in the literature (Daniel, 1990; Strahan, 1982) as to whether r_s^2 can be used to assess the strength of relationship, because Spearman's rho addresses ranks and not actual values. Strahan (1982) argues that r_s^2 is a good estimator of r^2 because, under the circumstances of a normal distribution, the magnitude of r_s is quite close to that of the Pearson *r*. He suggests, therefore, that r_s^2 is a reasonable nonparametric estimate of the percentage of variance in the dependent variable that can be explained by the independent variable.

In our hypothetical example, $r_s^2 = (-.385)^2 = .1482$, which would suggest that approximately 14.82% of the variance in the children's posthospital adjustment scores is shared with their postintervention anxiety scores. According to the r^2 values presented in Table 7.6, this relationship is, at best, weak.

Internet Resources for Generating the Spearman Rank-Order Correlation Coefficient

Several currently available free-access resources can generate a Spearman rank-order correlation coefficient. One useful resource is www.vassarstats.net. Once you have gained access to the website, click on *Correlation & Regression*, *Rank Order Correlation*. When the page opens, you will be asked to enter the number of paired items (e.g., 30 pairs of anxiety and adjustment data). Data entry can be in the form of the raw data or its ranks, or the data can be imported via a spreadsheet such as an Excel file (e.g., hospitalized children with cancer-30 cases.xlsx). The instructions were easy to follow.

Figure 9.11 presents a screenshot of the output for the Spearman rho, the *t* statistic, and one- and two-tailed *p* values that were generated from this website. The values of r_s (−.3847), the *t* statistic (−2.21), and the *p* value (.018) were similar to those that we obtained when generating the statistic by hand and when running the data in SPSS for Windows.

Presentation of Results

Table 9.10 is an example of a suitable presentation of the results of the Spearman rho correlation coefficient. Because the upcoming Kendall's tau also used parents' evaluations of children's posthospital adjustment as a dependent variable, this statistic is also presented. The results of the Spearman rho analysis could also be presented in the text as follows:

Figure 9.11 Screenshot of output obtained for the Spearman rank-order correlation.

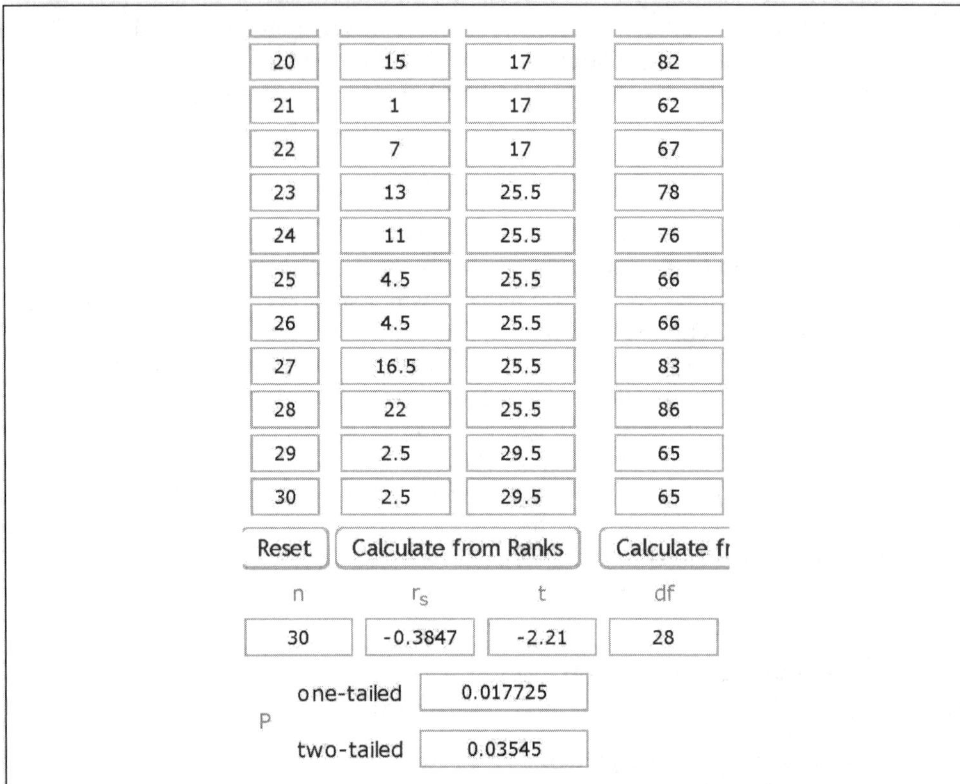

SOURCE: VassarStats.net (Richard Lowrey, author).

Table 9.10 Results of Tests of Association for Spearman's Rho and Kendall's Tau Correlations

	Posthospital Adjustment	
	r	*p*
Children's postintervention anxiety		
Spearman rho	−.38	.018
Kendall's tau	−.28	.024

The Spearman rank-order correlation coefficient was used to examine the extent to which children's postintervention anxiety scores were negatively associated with parents' evaluations of children's posthospital adjustment. The results of this analysis ($r_s = -.385$, $p = .018$) indicated that children with greater postintervention anxiety were evaluated by their parents to have poorer posthospital adjustment. The strength of this relationship ($r_s^2 = .148$) was weak in that only 14.8% of the variance in the children's posthospital adjustment scores could be explained by postintervention anxiety.

Advantages, Limitations, and Alternatives to the Spearman Rank-Order Correlation Coefficient

The Spearman rho correlation coefficient is an extremely useful, easily calculated statistic that can be used when the assumptions of the parametric Pearson correlation coefficient have not been met sufficiently. When the assumptions underlying the Pearson *r* have been met, Spearman's rho is 91% as efficient as the Pearson *r* in rejecting the null hypothesis (Daniel, 1990; Siegel & Castellan, 1988). This means that if a correlation between two continuous variables really exists in a population that has a bivariate normal distribution, Spearman's rho will detect that relationship in 100 cases with the same significance as the Pearson *r* does in 91 cases (Siegel & Castellan, 1988).

Another advantage is that Spearman's rho closely approximates the numerical size of the Pearson *r*, and its squared value is considered by some researchers to be a close nonparametric approximation of the coefficient of determination, r^2. A disadvantage of Spearman's rho is that it requires a larger sample size than does Kendall's tau to approximate a normal distribution and also does not have the same relationship to a partial correlation coefficient as does Kendall's tau.

The Pearson product-moment correlation coefficient (Pearson *r*) is the parametric equivalent to the Spearman rho rank-order correlation coefficient. A nonparametric alternative to Spearman's rho is Kendall's tau coefficient. This statistic will be discussed in the next section.

Examples From Published Research

Capio, C. M., Sit, C. H. P., & Abernethy, B. (2011). Fundamental movement skills testing in children with cerebral palsy. *Disability & Rehabilitation, 33*(25/26), 2519–2528. doi: 10.3109/09638288.2011.577502

Roy, A., Forrester, L. W., Macko, R. F., & Krebs, H. I. (2013). Changes in passive ankle stiffness and its effects on gait function in people with chronic stroke. *Journal of Rehabilitation Research & Development, 50*(4), 555–571. doi: 10.1682/JRRD.2011.10.0206

Tomarken, A., Holland, J., Schachter, S., Vanderwerker, L., Zuckerman, E., Nelson, C., . . . Prigerson, H. (2008). Factors of complicated grief pre-death in caregivers of cancer patients. *Psycho-Oncology, 17*(2), 105–111.

KENDALL'S TAU COEFFICIENT

Kendall's tau coefficient was developed by Kendall (1938) as an alternative measure of association to Spearman's rho. It has been described as a measure of discrepancy or discordance between two continuous variables (Daniel, 1990; Siegel & Castellan, 1988). This coefficient is represented in research reports by various symbols (e.g., τ, T, or t) and also has been referred to as the Kendall rank-order correlation coefficient (Siegel & Castellan, 1988). In this text, the statistic will be referred to as *Kendall's tau* (τ).

An Appropriate Research Question for Kendall's Tau Coefficient

Kendall's tau coefficient may be used under the same conditions as Spearman's rho; that is, it can be used to examine the degree of association or dependence between two continuous variables. For example, in addition to Spearman's rho, Ruff, Riechers Ii, Wang, Piero, and Ruff (2012) used Kendall's tau to evaluate the relationship between improved posttraumatic stress, disorder severity, sleep, and symptomatic improvement among veterans with mild traumatic brain injury. Bursztein Lipsicas et al. (2013) also used this coefficient to examine the gender distribution of suicide attempts among immigrant groups in European countries. Gini and Pozzoli (2013) used the same coefficient in their meta-analysis of bullied children and their psychosomatic problems.

Because of its similarity to the Spearman rho coefficient, a research question similar to that posed in our hypothetical study for the Spearman rho will be used for Kendall's tau so that we can compare the results of these two nonparametric measures of association:

> To what extent is there a negative relationship between children's postintervention anxiety scores and parents' perceptions of their children's posthospital adjustment?

Null and Alternative Hypotheses

The null and alternative hypotheses for Kendall's tau are similar to those of Spearman's rho (Table 9.8). In our hypothetical study, for example, the null hypothesis for the above-stated research question would state that there is no relationship between children's postintervention anxiety scores and parents' perceptions of their children's posthospital adjustment. The alternative or research hypothesis would postulate an inverse or negative relationship between the two variables: Children with higher postintervention anxiety will have poorer posthospital adjustment. Because the alternative hypothesis is directional, this is a one-tailed test.

Overview of the Procedure

Like Spearman's rho, Kendall's tau is based on the ranking of data that are at least ordinal level of measurement. Under most conditions, the values of this coefficient range between −1 and −1, with the value of −1 suggesting a perfect inverse relationship between two continuous variables, 0 the lack of a relationship, and +1 a perfect direct relationship. Because of the differences in the way the two statistics are calculated, however, there are often discrepancies in their calculated values.

To calculate Kendall's tau, the original values for variable *X* are first ranked in ascending order from lowest to highest (Daniel, 1990). These ascending values are considered to be in *natural order*. In Table 9.9, the Anxiety variable (*X*) is ranked from 3 to 7 (4). Next, the values of variable *Y* within each value of *X* are also ranked from lowest to highest. For example, in Table 9.9, the four values of the Adjustment variable (*Y*) have been ranked as 76, 76, 85, and 85 within the Anxiety score of 3 (5).

Each observation of *Y* is now compared to a *Y* value lying below it that does not share the same *X* value. For example, the value of 76 when $X = 3$ is compared to the values of 75, 85, 89, 90, and so on that do not have an Anxiety value equal to 3. This pair of *Y* values is said to be in *natural order* (*concordant*) if the *Y* value below is larger than the first *Y* value (e.g., 76 when *Anxiety* = *3* and 85 when *Anxiety* = *4*). The pair is in *reverse natural order* (*discordant*) if the *Y* value below is smaller than the *Y* value above (e.g., 76 for *Anxiety* = *3* and 75 for *Anxiety* = *4*). The pair of *Y* values is considered to be *tied* if they share the same value (e.g., 75 when *Anxiety* = *3* and 75 when *Anxiety* = *4*). The number of concordant, discordant, and tied *Y* pairs is obtained and summed across all values of *Y* to obtain the total number of *Y* pairs that are either in natural order (*C*) (6), in reverse order (*D*) (7), or tied (8).

From these data, a Kendall tau coefficient (tau-a) is calculated. If there are no tied *Y* pairs, the following formula is used:

$$\tau_a = \frac{C - D}{n(n-1)/2}$$

where

C = the number of *Y* pairs in natural order,

D = the number of *Y* pairs in reverse order,

n = the total number of paired (*X*, *Y*) observations, and

$n(n-1)/2 = \binom{n}{2}$ = the total number of possible pairs of observations.

If the majority of *Y* pairs are in natural order (i.e., they are concordant), the value of Kendall's tau will be positive (i.e., $C - D > 0$). A positive value implies that as the ranking of the *X* variable increases (or decreases), the ranking of the *Y* variable follows suit. If the majority of the *Y* pairs are in reverse order (i.e., they are discordant), the value of Kendall's tau will be negative (i.e., $C - D < 0$); that is, increased ranks of the *X* variable are associated with decreased ranks of the *Y* variable. If the numbers of concordant and discordant pairs are equal, the value of Kendall's tau will be 0, implying no association between the two variables.

If there are no ties, the value of this Kendall's tau ranges between +1 (a perfect positive relationship) and −1 (a perfect negative relationship). If there are ties, the range of possible values for this coefficient is smaller because the number of concordant and discordant pairs will always be smaller than the total number of pairs (concordant + discordant + ties). To alleviate this problem, Kendall developed a second coefficient (tau-b) that takes into account the number of tied X and Y observations:

$$\tau_b = \frac{C - D}{\sqrt{[n(n-1)/2] - T_x}\ \sqrt{[n(n-1)/2] - T_y}}$$

where

$T_x = \frac{1}{2}\sum t_x(t_x - 1)$,

$T_y = \frac{1}{2}\sum t_y(t_y - 1)$,

t_x = the number of X observations that are tied at a given rank, and

t_y = the number of Y observations that are tied at a given rank.

With the numbers of ties now being taken into account, the value of Kendall's tau-b can range from −1 to +1, with higher absolute values indicating a stronger degree of association between the two variables. The null hypothesis of no association between X and Y will be rejected if the calculated value of Kendall's tau (a or b) exceeds its critical value at a prespecified level of alpha. Alternatively, when presented with a computer printout, the null hypothesis will be rejected if the generated p value for Kendall's tau is less than alpha (e.g., $\alpha = .05$).

There are several ways to determine the critical value of Kendall's tau. Table A.6 in Appendix A presents the critical values of tau when the number of pairs of observations does not exceed $n = 20$. For larger samples ($n > 20$), Kendall's tau quickly becomes approximately normally distributed with a mean = 0 and a variance $(\sigma_\tau^2) = \dfrac{2(2N+5)}{9N(N-1)}$ (Abdi, 2007). Given these values, a z statistic can be generated that is approximately normally distributed with a mean of 0 and a variance of 1:

$$z = \frac{\tau}{\sigma_\tau} = \frac{\tau}{\sqrt{\dfrac{2(2N+5)}{9N(N-1)}}}$$

where

τ = the value of Kendall's tau,

σ_τ = the variance of tau, and

N = the number of pairs of observations.

The null hypothesis of no association between X and Y will be rejected if the absolute value of this calculated z statistic exceeds its absolute critical value (e.g., $|\pm 1.64|$) for a one-tailed $\alpha = .05$, provided that it is in the direction predicted. The two-tailed absolute value would be $|\pm 1.96|$ for a two-tailed $\alpha = .05$ (Table A.1, Appendix A).

Calculating Kendall's tau-b from actual *X* and *Y* values.

Table 9.9 presented the actual values for the anxiety (*X*) and posthospital adjustment (*Y*) scores for 30 children in our hypothetical study. From these data, we obtained the squared differences in ranks d_i^2 (1) so that we could calculate Spearman's rho. We can also use these data to calculate Kendall's tau.

To calculate Kendall's tau, the children's anxiety scores are first ranked in natural order from lowest ($X = 3$) to highest ($X = 7$) (4). The adjustment scores have also been ranked in natural order within each value of *X*. For example, for $X = 3$, the *Y* scores have been ranked 76, 76, 85, and 85 (5). The numbers of *Y* pairs *not included* in the particular *X* value that are in natural order, in reverse order, and tied are also presented. For $X = 3$ and $Y = 76$, for example, there were 16 concordant pairs (6), 9 discordant pairs (7), and 1 *Y* pair that shared the same value of 76 (8). Notice that the second value of $Y = 76$ when $X = 3$ is not counted as a tie because the pair share the same *X* value.

Because there are so many tied *X* and *Y* values in this hypothetical study, it will be necessary to use Kendall's tau-b. We will need to calculate the number of tied observations for both *X* and *Y*. For the *X* variable, *Anxiety,* we have 4 values of 3, 7 values of 4, 11 values of 5, and 6 values for 7. Therefore, according to our formula for the correction factor for ties, T_x,

$$\begin{aligned} T_x &= \frac{1}{2}\Sigma t_x(t_x - 1) \\ &= \frac{1}{2}[4(4-1) + 7(7-1) + 11(11-1) + 6(6-1) + 2(2-1)] \\ &= \frac{1}{2}[4(3) + 7(6) + 11)(10) + 6(5) + 2(1)] = \frac{1}{2}[196] = 98. \end{aligned}$$

T_y is calculated by listing all 30 values of *Y* in ascending order and counting the number of ties (t_y) for each *Y* value:

$$\begin{aligned} T_y &= \frac{1}{2}\Sigma t_y(t_y - 1) \\ &= \frac{1}{2}[(2(1) + 2(1) + 3(2) + 3(2) + 2(1) + 4(3) + 2(1) + 2(1) + 2(1) + 2(1)] = \frac{1}{2}(38) = 19. \end{aligned}$$

Now it is possible to calculate Kendall's tau-b for our hypothetical study:

$$\begin{aligned} \tau_b &= \frac{C - D}{\sqrt{[n(n-1)/2] - T_x}\ \sqrt{n(n-1)/2] - T_y}} \\ &= \frac{112 - 18}{\sqrt{[30(30-1)/2] - 98}\ \sqrt{[30(30-1)/2] - 19}} \\ &= \frac{-106}{\sqrt{337}\ \sqrt{416}} = -.2831. \end{aligned}$$

To determine whether the calculated tau value of $\tau_b = -.2831$ is sufficiently large to reject the null hypothesis of no association, we could either consult a table of critical values for Kendall's tau if $N \leq 20$ (e.g., Table A.6, Appendix A) or calculate the z statistic outlined previously.

Because we have 30 pairs of data, we would calculate the z statistic:

$$z = \frac{\tau}{\sigma_\tau} = \frac{\tau}{\sqrt{\frac{2(2N+5)}{9N(N-1)}}} = \frac{(-0.2831)}{\sqrt{\frac{2(2*30+5)}{9*30(30-1)}}} = \frac{(-0.2831)}{\sqrt{\frac{130}{7830}}} = -2.197$$

Our calculated z, −2.197, is less than the one-tailed critical value of z, −1.64, at $\alpha = .05$, and it is in the direction predicted. The conclusion to be drawn is that there is a significant negative relationship between children's postintervention anxiety and their posthospital adjustment.

Critical Assumptions of Kendall's Tau Coefficient

As for Spearman's rho, there are not many critical assumptions associated with the Kendall tau coefficient. They are as follows:

1. *The randomly selected data are sets of paired observations (X, Y) that have been collected from the same subjects.*
2. *The two continuous variables, X and Y, are measured on at least an ordinal scale.*

Except for the issue of random selection, both of these assumptions have been met in our hypothetical study. The two variables, postintervention anxiety and posthospital adjustment, are paired observations collected from a single set of subjects. These two variables are continuous, having at least an ordinal level of measurement.

Computer Commands

The computer commands in SPSS for Windows for Kendall's tau coefficient are similar to those for Spearman's rho (Figure 9.10). The dialog box for this statistic is opened by clicking on *Analyze . . . Correlate . . . Bivariate* in the menu, selecting the continuous variables to be analyzed (*Anxiety2* and *Posthosp*), and clicking on *Kendall's Tau-b*. Because our alternative hypothesis was directional, we also requested a one-tailed significance test.

Computer-Generated Output

Figure 9.10 presents not only the Spearman rho but also the computer-generated output for the Kendall tau-b coefficient obtained from SPSS for Windows. Note that, as indicated, the value for Kendall's tau-b, –.283, (9) is smaller in absolute value than that for the Spearman rho (–.385) and has a larger one-tailed p value: $p = .024$ for Kendall's tau-b (10) versus $p = .018$ for Spearman's rho (3). The conclusion regarding the null hypothesis is similar. Because this one-tailed p value, .024, is less than $\alpha = .05$, the null hypothesis will be rejected. The conclusion to be drawn is that, among the 30 children in our hypothetical study, there is an inverse relationship between postintervention anxiety and posthospital adjustment.

Internet Resources for Generating Kendall's Tau

Several currently available free-access resources can generate a Kendall's tau coefficient. One useful resource is http://www.wessa.net (Wessa, 2014). Once you have gained access to the website, click on *Descriptive Statistical Software . . . Kendall Rank Correlation . . .* and enter the values for your X variable (e.g., Anxiety, Table 9.9). Then enter the values for the Y variable (e.g., *posthospital adjustment*) that are associated with the X variable (Table 9.9). After you have (correctly) entered the data, click on *Compute. . . .* That will produce the output similar to that which is presented in Figure 9.12.

The value for Kendall's tau in Figure 9.12, –.283, is similar to that which we obtained when we calculated tau by hand and generated it in SPSS for Windows. The two-sided p value, however, is slightly different: .0502 versus 2*.024 = .048. The score, –106, and the denominator, 374.4, are similar to that which we obtained in our hand calculations, but it is not clear how the p value or the variance (of the score) was obtained. This would be no problem for our one-tailed test but would be somewhat questionable if we had a nondirectional (two-tailed) test since p (.0502) is larger than α (.05).

Figure 9.12 Internet-generated output for Kendall's tau coefficient.

Kendall tau Rank Correlation	
Kendall tau	-0.283102869987488
2-sided p-value	0.0502328351140022
Score	-106
Var(Score)	2875.83447265625
Denominator	374.422210693359

SOURCE: ©Wessa.Net 2002–2015 All rights reserved Free Statistics Software, Office for Research Development and Education, version 1.1.23-r7, Retrieved from http://www.wessa.net/

Presentation of Results

The presentation of the results for Kendall's tau-b is similar to that of the Spearman rho correlation (Table 9.10). A written summary of the analysis could also be presented in the text as follows:

> Kendall's tau-b coefficient was used to examine the extent to which children's postintervention anxiety scores were negatively associated with parents' evaluations of children's posthospital adjustment. The results of this analysis ($\tau_b = -.28$, one-tailed $p = .024$) indicate that children with greater postintervention anxiety were evaluated by their parents to have poorer posthospital adjustment.

Advantages, Limitations, and Alternatives to Kendall's Tau Coefficient

Kendall's tau-b is used in circumstances similar to those for Spearman's rho to evaluate the degree of association between two continuous variables. Like the Spearman rho, it is useful when the assumptions underlying the parametric correlation coefficient, the Pearson product-moment correlation, have not been met. It has the advantage of having its distribution approach a normal distribution more quickly than does the Spearman rho distribution.

Several statistics have been generated from the basic Kendall tau-b formula that have extended its usefulness beyond a mere test of association. For example, Kendall's coefficient of concordance, *W*, is used like the kappa coefficient to examine the degree of agreement among two or more raters concerning their rankings of objects or individuals (Daniel, 1990; Siegel & Castellan, 1988). Such a measure is especially useful for examining interrater reliability.

Unlike the Spearman rho, Kendall's tau-b can be generalized to a partial rank correlation coefficient that is very similar to the partial correlation coefficient obtained from the Pearson *r*. That is,

$$\tau_{xy,z} - \frac{\tau_{xy} - \tau_{xy}\tau_{yz}}{\sqrt{(1 - \tau_{xz}^2)(1 - \tau_{yz}^2)}}$$

This partial correlation coefficient examines the relationship between two variables, *X* and *Y*, while controlling for the effects of a third variable, *Z*. For example, in our hypothetical study, we might be interested in examining the relationship between the children's postintervention anxiety and posthospital adjustment, controlling for the effects of their preintervention anxiety. If we do not meet the assumptions of the parametric partial correlation coefficient using Pearson's *r*, we could use this nonparametric equivalent.

A disadvantage to Kendall's tau-b is the tediousness of calculating this statistic by hand, especially if the sample size is at all substantial. Fortunately, this is not a major consideration, given the availability of statistical computer packages.

The parametric equivalent to Kendall's tau coefficient is the Pearson product-moment correlation (*r*). A nonparametric alternative to Kendall's tau is the Spearman rho rank-order correlation coefficient. Although the Spearman rho appears to be the more commonly used nonparametric measure of association for continuous variables in the health care literature, both of these statistics have the same asymptotic efficiency (.912) compared to the Pearson *r* (Stuart, 1954). That is, given a bivariate normal distribution, both the Spearman rho and Kendall's tau will reject the null hypothesis with 100 cases, at a significance level similar to that of the Pearson *r* with 91 cases. This suggests that, in terms of power (i.e., the ability to correctly reject the null hypothesis), both of these statistics are nearly as powerful as the Pearson *r* given a normal distribution and can be more powerful than the Pearson *r* given a nonnormal bivariate distribution.

Examples From Published Research

Bursztein Lipsicas, C., Mäkinen, I. H., Wasserman, D., Apter, A., Kerkhof, A., Michel, K., . . . Schmidtke, A. (2013). Gender distribution of suicide attempts among immigrant groups in European countries—an international perspective. *European Journal of Public Health, 23*(2), 279–284. doi: 10.1093/eurpub/cks029

Gini, G., & Pozzoli, T. (2013). Bullied children and psychosomatic problems: A meta-analysis. *Pediatrics, 132*(4), 720–729. doi: 10.1542/peds.2013-0614

Ruff, R. L., Riechers Ii, R. G., Wang, X.-F., Piero, T., & Ruff, S. S. (2012). For veterans with mild traumatic brain injury, improved posttraumatic stress disorder severity and sleep correlated with symptomatic improvement. *Journal of Rehabilitation Research & Development, 49*(9), 1305–1320. doi: 10.1682/JRRD.2011.12.0251

Summary

In this chapter, we have examined six nonparametric measures of association between variables. Table 9.11 summarizes the statistics used and their expected levels of measurement. The phi, Cramér's *V*, and kappa coefficients are used when both the independent and dependent variables are categorical. The point biserial correlation coefficient is useful when one of the two variables is dichotomous and the other is interval, or ratio. When the independent and dependent variables are ordinal, interval, or ratio level of measurement, either Spearman's rho or Kendall's tau coefficient may be used. Three of these coefficients—the point biserial, phi, and Spearman's rho coefficients—are all special cases of a parametric statistic, the Pearson product-moment correlation coefficient (*r*).

There does not seem to be any definitive rule in the statistics literature as to which of the two rank-order coefficients, Spearman's rho or Kendall's tau, is preferred. It does appear from practice, however, that Spearman's rho is more commonly used in health care research. This coefficient does have the advantage of being closer in size to the Pearson *r* and, therefore, r_s^2 has sometimes been used as an estimate of the amount of variance in the dependent variable that is associated with the independent variable. On the other hand, Kendall's tau can produce a partial rank-order correlation coefficient that is useful when the assumptions of its parametric counterpart have not been met.

Table 9.11 Nonparametric Correlation Coefficients That Would Be Suitable With Variables of Specific Levels of Measurement

Variable 1		*Variable 2*		
		Nominal	*Ordinal*	*Interval/Ratio*
	Nominal	Phi (2 × 2) Contingency (r × c) Cramér *V* (r × c) Kappa		
	Ordinal	Rank biserial	Spearman's rho Kendall's tau	
	Interval/ratio	Point biserial	Spearman's rho Kendall's tau	Spearman's rho Kendall's tau

Regardless of the method chosen, the researcher should be cautioned about proper interpretation of measures of association. As Gibbons (1985) has aptly warned, a significant test of association (parametric or nonparametric) provides no evidence of a causal relationship between two variables. Such a significant association could, in fact, be the result of another set of variables as yet unidentified. The existence of such a significant association, therefore, is a necessary but not sufficient condition for inferring causality, and significant results should be interpreted with caution.

TEST YOUR KNOWLEDGE

1. Give an example from your area of research interest that would be suitable for the following nonparametric statistics (Note: in each instance, state the independent and dependent variables for your analysis and their levels of measurement):
   a. Phi coefficient
   b. Cramér's *V* coefficient
   c. Kappa coefficient
   d. Point biserial correlation
   e. Spearman rho rank-order correlation
   f. Kendall's tau
2. For each of the examples that you have provided in Question 1 above, please provide a null and alternative research hypothesis that could be used with the statistics you have listed.

3. Cramér's V versus phi:
   a. Under what conditions would you use the Cramér's V coefficient instead of the phi?
   b. When do these two coefficients have the same value?
   c. What are the general rules of thumb for assessing Cramér's V and phi?
4. Under what conditions would a researcher be inclined to use the point biserial correlation?
5. Why would a researcher decide to use a kappa coefficient instead of percent agreement when assessing the degree of agreement between two raters?
6. What are acceptable ranges of values for kappa?
7. Please give two similarities and two differences between the Spearman rho correlation coefficient and Kendall's tau coefficient.
8. What criteria would you use to assess the strength of a Spearman rho correlation?

COMPUTER EXERCISES

Using the data "hospitalized children with cancer-30 cases.sav", posted on the website study.sagepub.com/pett2e, please answer the following questions:

1. Assess the strength of association between group membership (staff-initiated intervention vs. usual care groups) and whether or not the hospitalized children are distressed prior to the intervention.
2. Assess the strength of the relationship between the children's social status position and the nurses' evaluation of their sleep quality at Day 2 of the intervention.
   a. What is the statistical test you will use to answer each of these tasks?
   b. What alpha level have you chosen?
   c. Please state the null and alternative hypotheses for each of these analyses.
   d. Undertake the analyses using a statistical computer package of your choice.
   e. Evaluate the strength of the relationship between the two variables listed in Questions 1 and 2.
   f. Summarize the results of your analyses of each of the tasks listed above.
   g. Choose an open access resource on the Internet to undertake your analyses as well. Do those results agree with your responses to f?

(Continued)

(Continued)

3. What is the relationship between the children's ages (in months) and their parents' assessment of the children's immediate posthospital adjustment?

   a. What are the independent and dependent variable(s) in this analysis, and what are their levels of measurement?
   b. What is the statistical test you will use to answer this research question?
   c. What alpha level have you chosen?
   d. Please state the null and alternative hypotheses for this research question.
   e. Undertake the analyses including post hoc tests using a statistical computer package of your choice.
   f. Summarize the results of your analysis, including the direction of the results.
   g. Choose an open access resource on the Internet to undertake your analyses as well. Do those results agree with your responses to f?

4. A researcher was interested in assessing the degree of agreement of two observers with regard to their assessment of 50 hospitalized children's distress (distressed, not distressed) prior to a staff-initiated intervention. This researcher obtained the following "confusion" matrix and wants to calculate both percentage agreement and a kappa coefficient.

Observer 1		*Observer 2*		
		Distressed	*Not Distressed*	*Total*
	Distressed	25	7	32
	Not Distressed	3	15	18
	Total	28	22	50

   a. Calculate the proportion of agreement between Observer 1 and Observer 2.
   b. Calculate the proportion of chance agreement between the two observers.
   c. Calculate kappa and evaluate its strength.
   d. Undertake the same analysis using a statistical software package of choice (e.g., SPSS for Windows). To what extent does your hand-calculated value for kappa agree with the results from your software package?
   e. Repeat the same analysis using a free Internet resource and compare your results.

Visit **study.sagepub.com/pett2e** to access SAS output, SPSS datasets, SAS datasets, and SAS examples.

CHAPTER 10

Logistic Regression

- The logic of logistic regression
- Odds ratios and relative risk
- Simple bivariate logistic regression
- Logistic regression with multiple independent variables

Consider this scenario: You are employed as a health care provider in a community clinic ("La Clinica") that provides comprehensive services to an underserved population of low-income adolescents living in an ethnically diverse metropolitan community. Among its many services is a culturally sensitive program for pregnant adolescents, the focus of which is to encourage the young women to participate more actively in their own care and to develop strong social support networks among their cohort. This particular program serves newly pregnant adolescents and follows them through to giving birth. It includes prenatal and primary care, prenatal education classes, and an array of comprehensive counseling services, including a smoking cessation program.

As part of its program evaluation strategy (and with institutional review board approval), La Clinica has elected to randomly assign approximately 100 pregnant adolescents upon enrollment to receive one of two models of care: a group-based service delivery model (*the intervention model*) or usual care with a single primary care provider (*the usual-care model*). La Clinica has hypothesized that provision of services through the intervention model will lead to greater improved health and pregnancy outcomes for the pregnant adolescents compared to those receiving services through a usual-care model.

Because of your expressed interest in team-oriented research, La Clinica is requesting your help in identifying those factors that best predict the odds of an adolescent mother giving birth to a normal-birthweight infant. You and your team of colleagues have identified four initial predictor variables that could have an impact on the odds that a teen mother would give birth to a normal-weight infant: (1) their participation in the group-based versus usual-care service delivery models, (2) the adolescents' smoking status, (3) the number of prenatal visits the adolescents had prior to giving birth, and (4) the perceived quality of their relationship with their parents. The challenge, however, is determining the best statistical test to analyze these data.

This scenario should not sound too foreign to you (although you might cringe at the thought of being responsible for the statistical analysis ☺). It often happens in health care research that we are interested in predicting the likelihood of a binary or dichotomous outcome, for example, having a normal-birthweight baby (yes, no) based on a set of predictors (e.g., type of intervention, mother's smoking status, her health, age, socioeconomic status, the number of prenatal visits, and prenatal complications). Depending on the level of measurement of the outcome variable, normal-birthweight baby, we would have two possible approaches to our statistical analysis. That is, if the outcome variable were interval or ratio (e.g., the actual weight of the baby in grams), we could consider using ordinary least squares (OLS) multiple linear regression to undertake the statistical analysis. If, however, the outcome variable were dichotomous (e.g., normal-birthweight baby vs. low-birthweight baby), multiple linear regression would not be an option since it assumes that the dependent variable is distributed normally. Our choice of statistical analysis, therefore, would be logistic regression.

In this chapter, we will examine logistic regression in greater detail. First, we will examine the "logic" of logistic regression and then review the meaning, calculation, and interpretation of an odds ratio and relative risk. Next we will undertake an examination of the assumptions and use of simple bivariate logistic regression. This will be followed by a discussion of the use of logistic regression with multiple independent variables.

It is not intended that this chapter provide a definitive discussion of the merits and machinations of logistic regression (LR). There are other fine textbooks that provide comprehensive analyses of this useful statistical tool (e.g., Allison, 2012; Garson, 2014; Hosmer, Lemeshow, & Sturdivant, 2013; Lomax & Hahs-Vaughn, 2012; Menard, 2010; Newcombe, 2012; Osborne, 2015; Pampel, 2000; Tabachnick & Fidell, 2013). The assumption is also made that you are somewhat familiar with OLS linear regression. For those who would like to refresh their knowledge of OLS multiple regression, the reader is referred to such textbooks as Field (2013), Kellar and Kelvin (2012), and Norman and Streiner (2008).

Some readers may wonder why logistic regression is being presented in a textbook on nonparametric statistics. Is logistic regression really a "nonparametric" technique? While there may be some question about this designation, logistic regression has been defined by some writers (e.g., Norman & Streiner, 2008; Osborne, 2015) as a nonparametric technique because it does not make assumptions about the distribution of the dependent variable. As indicated, logistic regression is most often used when the outcome of interest is a dichotomous nominal level variable coded "0" and "1." As you will soon see, it would not be appropriate to undertake an OLS regression (e.g., simple and multiple linear regression) because two major assumptions of this parametric statistic are that the dependent variable is distributed normally and that there is a linear relationship between the dependent variable and the interval- or ratio-level independent variables.

THE LOGIC OF LOGISTIC REGRESSION

The purpose of logistic regression is to examine the effects of a single or multiple independent variables on an outcome variable that is nominal level of measurement. Although this dependent variable can have more than two levels (and could also be an ordinal scale variable), most often it is dichotomous with the outcome of interest being assigned the value of "1" (e.g., having a given disease or giving birth to a normal-birthweight infant) and the alternative outcome coded "0" (e.g., not having the disease or having a low-weight infant). The predictor variable(s) can be of any level of measurement (nominal, ordinal, interval, or ratio).

Why Not Multiple Linear Regression?

Why should we use logistic regression in lieu of multiple linear regression? If the outcome variable were continuous, there would be no problem. We would choose multiple linear regression, provided we met the assumptions of this parametric technique. The problem with using multiple linear regression for a dichotomous dependent variable is that multiple linear regression uses an OLS solution to arrive at a regression equation. OLS assumes that the dependent or outcome variable is normally distributed. A nonordered nominal-level outcome variable will not be normally distributed. If the outcome variable is binary (i.e., dichotomous), its distribution will follow that of a binomial distribution.

Multiple linear regression also assumes a linear relationship between the independent and dependent variables. This is not achievable when the outcome variable is nominal level of measurement. According to our hypothetical scenario, we are interested in identifying those factors that would best predict whether or not an adolescent mother will give birth to a normal-birthweight infant. Our outcome variable, *normal-birthweight infant,* is dichotomous (0 = low-birthweight infant, 1 = normal-birthweight infant). As Figure 10.1 indicates, this outcome variable is necessarily bounded by 0 and 1. Any values that lie outside of that range are impossible values.

Figure 10.1 Illustration of the problems of using linear regression with a binary (dichotomous) outcome variable.

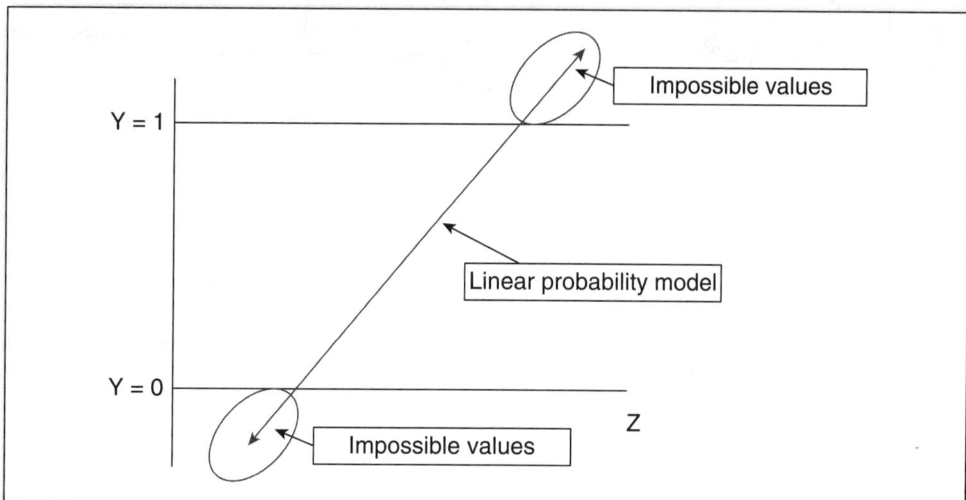

A distinct advantage to logistic regression is that it gives us information about how much more likely/unlikely it is for a given outcome to occur (e.g., an adolescent mother giving birth to a normal-birthweight child) given certain conditions (e.g., the intervention group the mother was randomly assigned to, mother being a smoker, the number of prenatal visits, and the perceived quality of her relationship with her parent(s)). These estimates are called *odds ratios.* Odds ratios represent the probability of an occurrence (e.g., having a normal-birthweight baby) given certain conditions (e.g., the intervention an adolescent mother received, her smoking status, number of prenatal visits, and the quality of her relationship with her parent(s)) over the probability of nonoccurrence (having a low-birthweight infant) given those same conditions.

Probabilities can range between 0 and 1, with larger values indicating greater probability of an occurrence. Probabilities also do not go in a straight line but rather take the form of an S-shaped curve such as that which is presented in Figure 10.2. This function is called the *logistic function* (Norman & Streiner, 2008). The challenge of logistic regression, therefore, is to arrive at some function of $P(Y = 1)$ (e.g., the probability of having a normal-birthweight infant) such that our prediction equation would model this S-shaped curve.

Obtaining the Logit Function

Arriving at a function that would model the S-shaped curve is not so difficult as it may first appear. We want to transform our OLS linear regression equation, $\hat{Y} = b_0 + b_1x_1 + b_2x_2 + \ldots + b_kx_k$, such that its values can range between 0 and 1. Afifi, May, and Clark

Figure 10.2 The S-shaped curve of the logistic function of a binary (dichotomous) outcome variable.

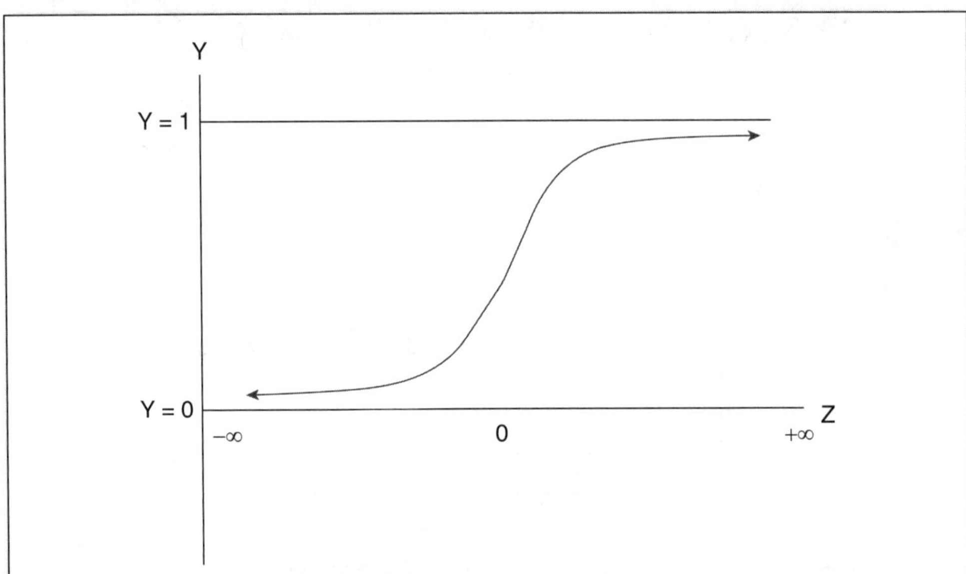

(2011) and Norman and Streiner (2008) present very clear approaches to obtaining such a function. Using our normal-birthweight example, if we were going to use OLS linear regression, we could write our regression equation as follows:

$$\hat{Y}_{\text{normal birthweight infant}} = b_0 + b_1(\text{treatment group}) + b_2(\text{smoking status}) + b_3(\text{number of prenatal visits}) + b_4(\text{quality of relationship with parents})$$

As indicated in Figure 10.1, the problem with this equation is that it is not bounded by 0 and 1. $\hat{Y}$ can have values that fall outside the restricted range. Therefore, we must seek an alternative solution. To do this, we will start with probabilities. That is, using the definition for a conditional probability, let

$$Y = Pr\left(\textit{normal birthweight infant}\,(NBW)\,\textit{given our regression equation},\ \hat{Y}\right)$$

$$= \Pr(\text{NBW} \mid \hat{Y}) = 1 \big/ \left(1 + e^{-\hat{Y}}\right)$$

where

"|" = the phrase "given," and

e = the constant, 2.71828.

This equation must lie between 0 and 1 because it is a probability (Afifi et al., 2011). Also, when $\hat{Y} = -\infty$, Y approaches the value of 0 since $e^{-(-\infty)}$ is a very large number and $1/(1 + e^{-(-\infty)}) \to 0$. When $\hat{Y} = +\infty$, $1/(1 + e^{-(+\infty)}) \to 1$, since $e^{-(+\infty)}$ is a very small number. When $\hat{Y} = 0$, $1/(1 + e^{-0}) = 1/(1 + 1) = 0.5$. This transformation is called the *logistic transformation* (Norman & Streiner, 2008).

The problem with this transformation is that our regression equation, $\hat{Y}$, is an exponent of *e*, the constant, making it difficult to interpret. For that reason, we will rearrange the equation *Y* to create a more direct expression for $\hat{Y}$. With a few algebraic manipulations we can achieve this.

$$Y = 1 \big/ \left(1 + e^{-\hat{Y}}\right)$$

By cross multiplying, we arrive at the following equation:

$$Y\left(1 + e^{-\hat{Y}}\right) = 1$$

Then, by dividing both sides by *Y*, we obtain

$$\left(1 + e^{-\hat{Y}}\right) = \frac{1}{Y}$$

Subtracting 1 from both sides and cleaning up the equation, we arrive at

$$e^{-\hat{Y}} = \frac{1}{Y} - 1 = \frac{1-Y}{Y}$$

Now we will take the natural log (ln) of both sides of the equation:

$$\ln\left(e^{-\hat{Y}}\right) = \ln\frac{1-Y}{Y}$$

Recall from algebra that the $\ln(e^a) = a$. It follows, therefore, that $\ln(e^{-\hat{Y}}) = -\hat{Y}$ and we obtain the following formula:

$$-\hat{Y} = \ln\left(\frac{1-Y}{Y}\right)$$

Then, multiplying both sides by –1, we arrive at the following equation for $-\hat{Y}$:

$$\hat{Y} = -\ln\left(\frac{1-Y}{Y}\right)$$

Again, from algebra, $-\ln(c/d) = \ln(d/c)$; therefore $-\ln\left(\frac{1-Y}{Y}\right) = \ln\left(\frac{Y}{1-Y}\right)$ and the above formula can be simplified:

$$\hat{Y} = \ln\left(\frac{Y}{1-Y}\right)$$

This last equation is known as the *logit function* of $\hat{Y}$ (Afifi et al., 2011; Norman & Streiner, 2008) and can be rewritten as follows:

$$logit\left(\hat{Y}\right) = \ln\left(\frac{Y}{1-Y}\right) = b_0 + b_1X_1 + b_2X_2 + \ldots b_kX_k$$

In the case of our normal-birthweight example,

$$logit\left(\hat{Y}\right) = b_0 + b_1\left(treatment\ group\right) + b_2\left(smoking\ status\right) +$$

$$b_3\left(number\ of\ prenatal\ visits\right) + b_4\left(quality\ of\ relationship\ with\ parents\right)$$

This logit function represents the "log of the odds," [Ln(Odds)], where "Odds" represents the probability that $Y = 1$ given the independent variables in our equation over the probability that $Y = 0$, given those same variables in the equation. In our example, it is the log of the odds of having a normal-birthweight baby given the treatment group the adolescent mother was assigned to, her current smoking status, the number of prenatal visits, and the quality of her relationship with her parent(s) over the probability that the adolescent will have a low-birthweight baby given those same independent variables.

Maximum likelihood estimation.

How do we obtain this logit function? Prior to the advent of powerful and easily accessible computers, obtaining a solution to the logit function was computationally challenging. Thanks to readily available statistical computer packages, we can direct the computer to undergo a series of iterations to arrive at the best solution that will maximize the likelihood of detecting the observed outcome given the respondents' scores on the predictor variables. The approach used to obtain this "best solution" is called *maximum likelihood estimation* (*MLE*) (Lomax & Hahs-Vaughn, 2012; Norman & Streiner, 2008; Osborne, 2015; Stoltzfus, 2011).

MLE starts with an initial estimation of the logistic regression coefficients (i.e., the parameters) given the patterns in the sample data, arrives at a preliminary solution, and then compares this outcome to a given criterion. If the criterion has not been met, MLE will continue these iterations (and comparisons) until either a final estimation is reached that meets the set criterion or the computer is unable to achieve a solution and terminates the analysis (Osborne, 2015). We will illustrate this process when we undertake a logistic regression analysis in SPSS for Windows (v. 22–23). First, let us first review what is meant by an odds ratio and relative risk and what type of information these statistics provide us.

THE ODDS RATIO AND RELATIVE RISK

An advantage to logistic regression is that it provides us with information about how much more likely/unlikely it is for the outcome to be present given certain circumstances. This is called an *odds ratio* (OR). These ORs approximate what is known as relative risk, particularly if the condition being studied is rare. An OR represents the change in odds of an outcome of interest (e.g., giving birth to a normal-birthweight child) given a one-unit increase in the independent variable (e.g., usual care vs. group-based intervention) while controlling for other variables in the model. When the independent variable is dichotomous (e.g., type of intervention), the OR compares the group that equals "0" (e.g., the usual-care group) to the group that equals "1" (e.g., the group-based intervention). These odds ratios can range from 0 to $+\infty$ and can be interpreted as follows:

OR < 1: The exposure is associated with lower odds of the outcome.

OR = 1: The exposure has no effect on the odds of the outcome.

OR > 1: The exposure is associated with greater odds of the outcome.

Relative risk (RR) is often used in cohort studies. A cohort design is one in which one or more groups of individuals (aka *cohorts*) are followed prospectively to evaluate whether exposure to a particular treatment or lifestyle choice affects the risk of a particular outcome (Sedgwick, 2013). Relative risk is the ratio of the probability of an event occurring (e.g., an adolescent mother having a normal-birthweight infant) in the exposed group (e.g., the group-based intervention group) compared to a nonexposed group (e.g., the usual-care group). Let's take a look at how relative risk and the odds ratio are calculated by starting with a relatively simple example:

> What are the odds of having a normal-birthweight infant given that the adolescent mother received the group-based intervention compared to those adolescent mothers who received usual care?

Table 10.1 presents a contingency table that was generated in SPSS for Windows (v. 22–23) (*Analyze . . . Descriptive statistics . . . Crosstabs*) that compared *group_assignment* (the row variable) to *normal_birthweight_baby* (the column variable).

Calculating relative risk.

To calculate relative risk (RR) from Table 10.1, we would use the following formula:

$$RR = \frac{Pr_{event\ when\ exposed}}{Pr_{event\ when\ not\ exposed}}$$

$$= \frac{Pr(NBW \mid adolescent\ mother\ is\ in\ the\ intervention\ group)}{Pr(NBW \mid adolescent\ mother\ is\ in\ the\ traditional\ services\ group)}$$

$$= \frac{A/(A+B)}{C/(C+D)} = \frac{41/50}{30/50} = \frac{.82}{.50} = 1.64$$

Table 10.1 Comparison of the Numbers of Low- and Normal-Birthweight Babies by Usual-Care vs Group-Based Intervention

Group_assignment group assignment-group-based delivery model (intervention) vs traditional care-single primary care provider (control) * normal_birthweight_baby How much did child weigh at birth? Crosstabulation

Count

		normal_birthweight_baby How much did child weigh at birth?		
		.00 less than 2500 gr	1.00 2500 gr or more	Total
Group_assignment group assignment-group-based delivery model (intervention) vs traditional care-single primary care provider (control)	.00 traditional care-single primary care provider U	D 20	C 30	50
	1.00 intervention-group-based delivery model G	B 9	A 41	50
Total		29	71	100

How do we interpret this relative risk?

> The risk (probability) of an adolescent mother in the intervention group having a normal-birthweight infant was 1.64 times higher than the risk (probability) for an adolescent mother in the usual-care group.

The word *risk* sounds strange when referring to something as positive as having a normal-birthweight baby. Keep in mind, however, that *risk* implies the probability of an outcome whether positive or negative.

Obtaining a confidence interval for relative risk.

As was pointed out in Chapter 7, a 95% confidence interval defines a range of values such that the population parameter of interest (in this case, relative risk) will fall within this range in 95% of samples (Field, 2009). This means that if we were to resample the population 100 times, the "true" value in the population for relative risk would lie between the two values 95 out of 100 times. These confidence intervals are built around the value for relative risk that was calculated based on our sample. In our example, we could state the following: "There is a 95% probability that the true population relative risk for having a normal-birthweight baby given that the mother was in the intervention versus usual-care group falls between _____ and _____."

The confidence interval (CI) for relative risk (RR) is easily calculated given a simple 2 × 2 table of frequencies such as Table 10.1 (Morris & Gardner, 1988). We can obtain a 100(1 – α)% CI for the RR by first calculating the standard error (SE) for the log of RR, ln(RR), finding the CI for ln(RR), and then converting that CI back into a CI for RR by raising the CI for ln(RR) to the base e. For example, given the RR that we obtained above (RR = 1.64), using the data presented in Table 10.1, and assuming that we would like a 95% CI (i.e., α = .05), we obtain the following:

$$100(1-\alpha)\%\,\text{CI for ln (RR)} = \text{ln (RR)} \pm Z_{\alpha/2}[\text{SE(lnRR)}]$$

$$95\%\,\text{CI for RR} = \ln(1.64) \pm 1.96\,[\text{SE}(\ln(1.64))]$$

where

$$\text{Ln}\left(1.64\right) = 0.4947$$

$$\text{SE}\left(\text{lnRR}\right) = \sqrt{\frac{1}{A} - \frac{1}{A+B} + \frac{1}{C} - \frac{1}{C+D}}$$

$$= \sqrt{\frac{1}{41} - \frac{1}{41+9} + \frac{1}{30} - \frac{1}{30+20}} = \sqrt{\frac{1}{41} - \frac{1}{50} + \frac{1}{30} - \frac{1}{50}}$$

$$= \sqrt{0.0244 - 0.02 + 0.0333 - 0.02} = \sqrt{0.0177} = 0.1332$$

Given this information, we can now calculate the 95% CI for ln(RR):

$$95\%\text{CI for } \ln(\text{RR}) = .4947 \pm 1.96[1.332]$$

$$= 0.4947 \pm 0.2611 = 0.2336,\ 0.7558$$

To obtain the 95% CI for the RR, we would raise these two values to their exponential:

$$e^{0.2336} = 1.26$$

$$e^{0.7558} = 2.13$$

Our 95% confidence interval for our relative risk, therefore, is 1.26 – 2.13. This 95% CI for RR could be interpreted as follows:

> There is a 95% probability that the true population relative risk for having a normal-birthweight baby given that the adolescent mother participated in the group intervention (compared to the usual care) lies between 1.26 and 2.13.

Notice that this confidence interval does not contain "1.0". If the CI did contain "1", we would not be able to reject the null hypothesis of no statistically significant difference in risk between the two groups (i.e., RR = 1). Our conclusion, therefore, is that our relative risk is statistically significant at $p \leq .05$.

Calculating an odds ratio.

An odds ratio (OR) is calculated slightly differently from relative risk. That is, ORs represent the odds of an event occurring given one condition over the odds of that same event given the alternative condition. The general formula for conditional probabilities ("D given E") is as follows:

> Pr(D | E) = (#D occurrences contained in category E) divided by the total occurrences in category E.

For example, from Table 10.1, the probability of a normal-birthweight infant (NBW) given the adolescent mother receives the group-based delivery model (G) would be as follows:

$$\Pr(\text{NBW} \mid \text{G}) = \text{A} / (\text{A} + \text{B}) = 41 / 50 = 0.82$$

Similarly, from Table 10.1, the probability of a low-birthweight infant (LBW) given the adolescent mother receives the group-based delivery model (G) would be

$$\Pr(\text{LBW} \mid \text{G}) = \text{B} / (\text{A} + \text{B}) = 9 / 50 = 0.18$$

We can also use the data from Table 10.1 to calculate the probability of an NBW given the adolescent mother receives the usual-care model (U):

$$\Pr(\text{NBW} \mid \text{U}) = \text{C} / (\text{C} + \text{D}) = 30 / 50 = 0.60$$

The probability of an LBW given the adolescent mother is in the usual group (U) would be obtained as follows:

$$\Pr(\text{LBW} \mid \text{U}) = \text{D} / (\text{C} + \text{D}) = 20 / 50 = 0.40$$

These probabilities enable us to obtain the odds of a normal-birthweight infant given the adolescent mother receives the group-based intervention:

$$\text{Odds}(\text{NBW} \mid \text{Group intervention}) = \left(\frac{\Pr(\text{occurrence})}{\Pr(\text{nonoccurrence})} \right) = \frac{\Pr(\text{NBW} \mid \text{G})}{\Pr(\text{LBW} \mid \text{G})} = \frac{0.82}{0.18}$$
$$= 4.56$$

The odds of a normal-birthweight infant given that the adolescent mother receives usual care would be

$$\text{Odds}(\text{NBW} \mid \text{usual care}) = \left(\frac{\Pr(\text{occurrence})}{\Pr(\text{nonoccurrence})} \right) = \frac{\Pr(\text{NBW} \mid \text{U})}{\Pr(\text{LBW} \mid \text{U})} = \frac{0.60}{0.40} = 1.50$$

The OR, then, would be a comparison of the two odds:

$$\frac{\text{Odds of normal-birthweight infant when receiving the group intervention}}{\text{Odds of normal-birthweight infant when receiving usual care}} = \frac{4.56}{1.50}$$
$$= 3.04$$

This OR could be interpreted as follows:

> The odds of having a normal-birthweight infant given that the adolescent mother received the group-based intervention are 3.04 times higher than for those adolescent mothers who received usual care.

Notice that this odds ratio, 3.04, is considerably higher than the relative risk ratio (1.64). Osborne (2015) and Sedgwick (2014) point out that odds ratios tend to overestimate relative risk, especially when the outcome (e.g., having a normal-birthweight baby) is relatively common (e.g., it occurs in more than 5%–10% of the population). As a result, the OR will overestimate the effect of the "treatment" on the outcome measure. In this situation, Osborne (2015) suggests reporting the RR rather than OR. Sedgwick (2014) also indicates that the OR will be greater than the RR if the RR is greater than 1.0 and less than the RR otherwise. Norman and Streiner (2008) suggest that as the prevalence of a condition increases, the OR not only becomes larger than the RR but also sets an upper bound for the RR (p. 163). Newcombe (2012) presents an excellent in-depth discussion of the relative merits of relative risk and odds ratios.

Obtaining a confidence interval for the odds ratio.

The odds ratio is like any other point estimate: It is a single estimate of the population odds ratio. Since we rarely, if ever, know what the true population parameter is, this single estimate of the odds ratio in the population may not be particularly accurate. Therefore, as with any other point estimate (e.g., the mean, median, correlation, relative risk), confidence intervals that give us an estimate of the range of possible values for the OR should also be reported.

Typically, you will see either 90% or 95% confidence intervals for the odds ratio reported in the clinical research literature. These confidence intervals have a common form:

$$100(1-\alpha)\%\ \text{confidence interval} = \text{statistic} \pm z_{\alpha/2}(SE_{\text{statistic}})$$

where

α = the two-tailed Type I error you have set (e.g., .10 or .05);

$z_{\alpha/2}$ = the two-tailed value of the standard normal distribution, z, for the α you have set (e.g., $z_{\alpha/2} = 1.96$ if $\alpha = .05$ or $z_{\alpha/2} = 1.64$ if $\alpha = .10$); and

$SE_{\text{statistic}}$ = the standard error of the statistic we are interested in (e.g., the odds ratio).

Most statistical packages provide the confidence interval (CI) for the OR. To give you a sense of how these CIs are obtained, we will calculate the 95% CI for the OR (3.04) that we obtained for our data presented in Table 10.1. Bland and Altman (2000) and Morris and Gardner (1988) present a relatively straightforward method for estimating a confidence interval for the OR, using what is known as the "logit method" (Breslow & Day, 1980; Morris & Gardner, 1988).

Since the values for an OR are limited at the lower end of its distribution (it cannot be a negative value), the OR distribution is necessarily skewed. As we saw in an earlier discussion, the log of the OR (i.e., the logit) can take on any value and approximates a normal distribution. We can also estimate the standard error (SE) of this ln(OR). For a 2 × 2 table such as that presented in Table 10.1, the SE(ln OR) is estimated by taking the square root of the reciprocals of the four frequencies, *A* to *D:*

$$SE(\ln OR) = \sqrt{\left(\frac{1}{A} + \frac{1}{B} + \frac{1}{C} + \frac{1}{D}\right)}$$

From Table 10.1, we can insert the values *A* to *D* to obtain SE(ln OR):

$$SE(\ln OR) = \sqrt{\left(\frac{1}{41} + \frac{1}{9} + \frac{1}{30} + \frac{1}{20}\right)} = \sqrt{0.2188} = 0.4678$$

The 95% CI for ln(OR) is given as follows (Morris & Gardner, 1988):

$$95\%CI(\ln OR) = \ln(OR) \pm 1.96(SE(\ln OR))$$

In our example, we need to calculate the natural log of our OR (3.04) and then plug that value into the above formula along with the SE(ln OR) (.4678).

$$\ln(OR) = \ln(3.04) = 1.112$$

$$95\%\ CI(\ln OR) = 1.112 \pm 1.96(0.4678) = 1.112 \pm 0.9169 = 0.1951, 2.0289$$

By raising these two limits (.1951, 2.0289) to their exponential, we obtain the 95% CI for the OR:

$$95\%\ \text{CI}\left(\text{OR}\right) = e^{0.1951}, e^{2.0289} = 1.21, 7.60$$

Interpreting the confidence interval for the odds ratio.

We now have the two limits for our OR: 1.21 and 7.60. We can interpret this CI as follows: Controlling for other variables in the model, there is a 95% probability that the true population odds ratio for having a normal-birthweight baby given that the mother was in the intervention compared to the usual care group lies between 1.21 and 7.60.

Because we do not have any other variables in our model, we could omit the statement, *controlling for other variables in the model*. However, if we do have additional predictors in our model, we need to make certain that the statement is included since, as previously indicated, odds ratios change depending on the variables included in the model.

Notice that the confidence interval for the relative risk (1.26–2.13) is much tighter than that of the odds ratio for the same data (1.21–7.60), although both are statistically significant at $p \le .05$ since neither CI contains 1.0. The tighter confidence interval for the relative risk would suggest that the 95% CI for relative risk is more accurate than that of the odds ratio.

A word of caution with regard to the 95% CI for the OR: When one of the cells (e.g., A, B, C, or D) is equal to 0, the estimated SE(ln OR) cannot be calculated since 1/0 is in error and any value close to 0 in the denominator approaches infinity. Should that occur, an exact approach rather than the asymptotic approach for obtaining SE(lnOR) needs to be used. Shan and Wang (2014) illustrate the use of an approach developed by Buehler (1957) to obtaining exact confidence intervals. Unfortunately, this approach is not available in SPSS for Windows (v. 22–23).

SIMPLE BIVARIATE LOGISTIC REGRESSION

Simple bivariate logistic regression (LR) is used to evaluate the outcome of a dichotomous dependent variable based on the effects of a single independent variable. The outcome of interest should be coded "1" and its alternative coded "0." The predictor variable can be any level of measurement. However, as noted, interpretation of an odds ratio is easier when continuous data (e.g., number of cigarettes smoked/day) have been collapsed into discrete categories (e.g., 0 = nonsmoker, 1 = up to 10/day, 2 = 11–20 cigarettes/day, 3 = greater than a pack/day).

In our simple LR example, both the outcome (normal-birthweight baby) and predictor (type of treatment) variables are dichotomous and coded 0 and 1. Using an online resource or a statistical computer package, we can generate a 2 × 2 table similar to Table 10.1 in which the data represent frequencies, not scores. ORs can also be obtained.

Since simple LR is the easiest LR form to understand and interpret, we will start with this approach. We will use the example, the effects of the type of intervention (usual care vs. a group-based intervention) on the adolescent mother's birth outcome (normal- vs. low-birthweight infant). Then, after "mastering" the interpretation of logistic regression with a single independent variable, we will proceed with a multivariate logistic regression in which there are two or more independent variables.

An Appropriate Research Question for Simple Bivariate Logistic Regression

Like OLS multiple regression, LR attempts to answer two basic questions: (1) How well does our generated logistic regression model fit our actual data? (2) To what extent do each of the independent variables add to the fit of the model? These two questions necessitate separate assessments in multiple LR. With simple bivariate LR, in which there is only one independent variable in the model, these two questions can be answered simultaneously.

A number of examples in the health care literature demonstrate the versatility and use of simple bivariate logistic regression. This approach is often accompanied by the use of multiple logistic regression to determine the best set of predictors of a binary outcome variable. For example, Goffman, Madden, Harrison, Merkatz, and Chazotte (2007) used both simple and multivariate logistic regression in their assessment of predictors of maternal mortality and near-miss maternal morbidity. Niemeier, Marwitz, Lesher, Walker, and Bushnik (2007) used a similar approach to evaluate gender differences in executive functions following traumatic brain injury. Zhong et al. (2014) also used these statistics in their population-based retrospective cohort study of barriers to immediate breast reconstruction in the Canadian universal health care system.

The hypothetical example that was given earlier in this chapter will be used to illustrate the approach to evaluating output generated for a simple bivariate logistic regression. For example, we are interested in assessing the effect of the intervention (group based vs. usual care) on the ultimate birthweight of the child. An appropriate research question that could be asked, therefore, would be as follows:

> What are the odds of having a normal-birthweight infant given that the adolescent mother received the group-based intervention compared to those adolescent mothers who received usual care?

Null and Alternative Hypotheses

Table 10.2 presents examples of null and alternative hypotheses generated from the research question outlined above that could be analyzed using simple logistic regression. Notice that, in our example, the alternative hypothesis is nondirectional. We could have predicted a direction; we could have said that the odds of having a normal-birthweight infant given that the adolescent was in the group-based intervention was greater than that of the usual-care group.

Critical Assumptions and Conditions for Binary Logistic Regression

Because logistic regression is a nonparametric technique, it does not have assumptions regarding the distribution of its outcome variable (Osborne, 2015). That does not

Table 10.2 Example of Null and Alternative Hypotheses Appropriate for Use With a Simple Logistic Regression

Null Hypothesis
H_0: The odds of having a normal-birthweight infant given that the adolescent mother received the group-based intervention will be similar to that of adolescent mothers who received usual care. That is, the odds ratio (OR) =1.
Alternative Hypothesis
H_a: The odds of having a normal-birthweight infant given that the adolescent mother received the group-based intervention will be different from that of adolescent mothers who received usual care. That is, the odds ratio (OR) ≠1.

mean, however, that it is assumption-free. In addition to random selection (which rarely, if ever, occurs), a number of assumptions are applicable to both simple and multiple logistic regression when the dependent variable is binary (i.e., it is nominal level of measurement with two outcomes coded 0 and 1). These assumptions and conditions are summarized in Table 10.3. The following is a discussion of these issues in greater detail.

1. *The variables of interest have been measured without error.*

It is assumed that both the independent and dependent variables are measured without error, that we have reliable (and, hopefully, valid) measures for all of our variables of interest. Measurement error can occur in a variety of ways (e.g., researcher error, situational contaminants, issues related to the respondent, responses-set biases, and instrument clarity) (Pett, Lackey, & Sullivan, 2003). Osborne (2015) presents an excellent example of the

Table 10.3 Summary of Assumptions and Conditions of Logistic Regression

- The variables of interest have been measured without error.
- The dependent variable is dichotomous with its two levels coded "0" and "1."
- The independent variable(s) can be any level of measurement; if nominal with > 2 levels, they need to be dummy-coded.
- There is a sufficient ratio of cases to independent variables.
- There are sufficient responses in every given category.
- There is linearity of the logit with the continuous independent variables.
- The independent variables should have a significant impact on the dependent variable.
- Absence of multicollinearity.
- Absence of outliers.
- Independence of errors.

deleterious effects of an unreliable variable on logistic regression. As he points out, these effects are common to all statistical analyses: "Garbage in is Garbage out."

2. *The dependent variable is dichotomous with its two levels coded 0 and 1.*

Although the dependent variable needs to be dichotomous and coded 0 and 1, a continuous variable (e.g., the actual birthweight of the infant) could be collapsed into a dichotomous variable (e.g., normal- vs. low-birthweight infant). This assumption applies to both simple and multiple logistic regression. There are two additional forms of logistic regression: multinomial logistic regression (aka *polytomous logistic regression*) for unordered categories and ordered logistic regression. Because of the greater complexity of these two procedures, multinomial and ordinal logistic regression will not be addressed specifically in this chapter. Readers who are interested in exploring the use of these approaches are referred to Hosmer et al. (2013), Menard (2010), and Osborne (2015). It should be noted, therefore, that when referring to *logistic regression,* this chapter will deal only with logistic regression whose outcome variable is binary.

3. *The independent variable(s) can be any level of measurement.*

If the independent variable is nominal level of measurement with two categories (e.g., gender [male, female]), it needs to be coded 0 and 1 (e.g., 0 = male, 1 = female). If, however, the independent variable is a nonordered nominal-level variable with multiple levels (e.g., marital status), it needs to be collapsed into a maximum number (k – 1) of dummy variables where k = the number of categories. For example, if we had five categories for marital status (e.g., single, married, divorced/separated, widowed, and cohabiting), we could create a maximum of 5 –1 = 4 dummy variables, each of which was coded 0 for the absence of a trait and 1 for the presence of a trait. We could, for example, create a new variable, *Divorce,* for which 1 represented those persons who were divorced and 0 represented those persons who were not divorced. It is important to know which group has *not* been assigned a dummy variable (e.g., those persons who are single) because if all four of the newly created dummy variables are used simultaneously in a logistic regression analysis, then each of these dummy variables is essentially being compared to the group that has been "left out" (e.g., divorced vs. single) (Osborne, 2015).

Independent (aka *predictor*) variables that are ordinal (e.g., "stress" on a scale of 1–7), interval, or ratio can be used directly in logistic regression. Because odds ratios can be difficult to interpret if the independent variable's level of measurement is interval or ratio, researchers will often collapse interval/ratio data into a smaller set of ordered categories. Hosmer et al. (2013) suggest that, for continuous variables, collapsing data in multiples of 2, 5, or 10 may be the most meaningful and easily understood by the reader. Such collapsing needs to be undertaken carefully since disease outcomes may have different odds ratios depending on the collapsed level of the independent variable. For example, the odds of having coronary heart disease for a person aged 60 years may be very different from that of a person aged 80 years.

4. *There is a sufficient ratio of cases to independent variables.*

A number of problems can arise when there are not enough cases relative to the number of independent variables entered into the logistic regression equation (Tabachnick &

Fidell, 2013). Insufficient cases can result in extremely large parameter estimates and standard errors. We saw that earlier when calculating the SE(lnOR), cells with small or 0 cells raise havoc with our ability to estimate the standard error. As a result, the odds ratios (and confidence intervals) that are produced are inaccurate and often extremely high.

There is little consensus as to how large the sample size needs to be relative to the number of independent variables entered into an LR analysis. Some authors recommend at least 10 cases/independent variable (Norman & Streiner, 2008). In a simulation study of the number of events per variable in LR, Peduzzi, Concato, Kemper, Holford, and Feinstein (1996) conducted a Monte Carlo study to evaluate the number of events per variable needed for an LR analysis. The authors found few problems when the #cases/independent variable was > 10 but warned that fewer cases/independent variables could lead to significant problems (e.g., biased OR estimates and invalid tests of significance).

Determining sample size for LR is complex because the issue is not only the number of independent variables to be entered into the model but also the ratio of events to nonevents for the dependent variable. When there are a disproportionate number of cases to noncases (e.g., 90% to 10%), the required sample size will be larger than if the ratio of cases to noncases were more even (e.g., 50% to 50%). The following guidelines have been suggested when determining a minimum sample size for LR (http://www.medcalc.org/manual/logistic_regression.php):

If p = the *smallest* of the proportion of cases estimated in the population to be 0 or 1 for the dependent variable and k = the anticipated number of covariates (i.e., the number of independent variables), then minimum number of cases to include is

$$N = (10 * k) / p$$

In our normal-birthweight example, if we had four independent variables to include in our LR model (e.g., type of intervention, smoking status, number of prenatal visits, and quality of relationship with parents), and we knew that the proportion of normal-birthweight infants in the general adolescent mother population to be .60 (60%), then p = the smallest of the proportion of cases to be 0 or 1 (e.g., 1 − .60 = .40), and the minimum number of cases required would be

$$N = 10 * 4 / 0.40 = 100$$

We would then need 100 adolescent mothers to take part in our study . . . if this were the only analysis we planned to undertake. Since the sample size of 100 does not take into account dropouts or other forms of missing data, we would want to increase that size, perhaps by 25%. It has also been suggested that if the resulting number is less than 100, the sample size should be increased to at least 100 (Long, 1997).

While these estimates of sample size are useful, Osborne (2015) emphasizes the importance of reporting confidence intervals and of having large sample sizes, especially where there is a large discrepancy between cases and noncases. A statistical power analysis, using such programs as G*Power3 (Faul, Erdfelder, Buchner, & Lang, 2009; Faul, Erdfelder, Lang, & Buchner, 2007) or PASS-12 (Hintze, 2013) prior to undertaking the research will also help to determine an appropriate sample size for the given logistic regression analysis of interest.

5. *There are sufficient responses in every given category.*

There are several ways in which there might be insufficient responses in every given category. It could be, for example, that when creating a table that examines the distribution of responses of one nominal-level independent variable with regard to the dependent variable, we find that there is at least one cell that has a zero count. It could also be that, while there is no cell with zero counts, there are insufficient responses in a given category.

Logistic regression assumes that there will be no zero count cells for nominal-level independent variables. That means that one cell cannot contain all (or none) of persons within one of the outcomes of interest. If that were to occur, the two groups identified in the dependent variable would be perfectly separable because the odds of all the persons in a given cell would either be 0 or 1.0 (Lomax & Hahs-Vaughn, 2012). This would occur in our example if all the adolescent females who were nonsmokers gave birth to normal-birthweight babies. This condition would result in large standard errors, and the use of maximum likelihood estimates would be impossible (Tabachnick & Fidell, 2013).

Complete separation of groups can also occur when there are too many independent variables relative to the number of cases in one of the outcome categories (Hosmer et al., 2013; Tabachnick & Fidell, 2013). This is called *overfitting*. Overfitting is more difficult to detect in logistic regression because, unlike OLS linear regression, there is no form of adjusted R^2 that, when compared to unadjusted R^2, helps us to detect when the sample size is too small relative to the number of independent variables.

Because logistic regression uses both nominal-level independent and dependent variables, it is assumed that, for nominal-level independent variables, all expected frequencies are greater than 1 and no more than 20% of the expected frequencies should be less than 5. Note that these are *expected frequencies,* not actual frequencies. Lomax and Hahs-Vaughn (2012) offer several useful suggestions for addressing this problem (e.g., collapsing categories if the independent variable is nominal with more than two levels or adding a constant to each cell of the classification table). They also point out that if it is decided to retain the zero cell counts in a logistic regression analysis with multiple independent variables, the resulting higher standard errors and individual coefficients should be addressed as limitations.

6. *There is linearity of the logit with the continuous independent variables.*

Logistic regression assumes that there is a linear relationship between the logit transform (ln(odds)) and the continuous independent variables (Hosmer et al., 2013). There does not seem to be, however, an assumption regarding linear relationships among the independent variables (Tabachnick & Fidell, 2013). A number of suggested approaches (and solutions) can be used to assess and address the extent to which the continuous independent variables demonstrate sufficient linearity with the logit (Hosmer et al., 2013; Osborne, 2015). One solution, the Box-Tidwell approach (Box & Tidwell, 1962), will be illustrated when we undertake a multiple logistic regression analysis in SPSS for Windows.

7. *The independent variables should have a significant impact on the dependent variable.*

A goal of regression analysis, whether it is OLS linear regression or MLE logistic regression, is that of seeking a parsimonious model. That is, we would like to most accurately predict the outcome variable with the fewest number of independent variables. How, then, do we select the most appropriate variables to enter into our regression model?

The best place to start identifying the most meaningful independent variables is to generate a theoretical model from research and practice that best reflects the outcome variable of interest. While "fishing expeditions" are fun, they can easily result in statistically significant but clinically meaningless relationships between the predictor and outcome variables. Hosmer et al. (2013) outline a useful and systematic seven-step approach to purposefully selecting independent variables for a logistic regression analysis. These steps are summarized in Table 10.4. The interested reader will want to read the authors'

Table 10.4 A Suggested Systematic Approach to Selecting Meaningful Independent Variables for a Logistic Regression Analysis

Summary of Hosmer et al's (2013) seven-step process for selecting meaningful independent variables
1. Undertake a univariate analysis of the relationship of each independent variable (IV) to the dependent variable using chi square tests, *t*-tests, and point-biserial correlations; pay careful attention to cells with 0 frequencies; retain IVs whose $p < .25$.
2. Fit a multivariate model using all of the IVs from Step 1. Eliminate IVs that are not statistically significant per the Wald statistic. Compare the results obtained from the smaller model with the larger model. Make sure that the sample sizes are the same for both models.
3. Compare the estimated coefficients generated in the reduced model with those in the larger model. Look carefully at those coefficients that have changed > 20%; it means that one or more excluded IVs may be important. Continue the process of Steps 2 and 3 slowly and systematically until all important IVs are in the model.
4. Re-enter each nonsignificant IV from Step 1 one at a time into the model identified in Step 3. This will identify IVs that, while not statistically significant by themselves, may be important contributors to the model given other variables in the model.
5. Once a model has been determined in Step 4, examine the IVs closely; for continuous IVs, check for linearity with the logit.
6. Given the model selected in Step 5, check for interactions among the IVs in the model. To be included in the model, an interaction term should make both statistical ($p < \alpha$) and clinical sense.
7. Assess the adequacy and model fit of the final model.

SOURCE: Summarized from Hosmer, Lemeshow, and Sturdevant (2013), pp 90–93.

suggestions in depth (Hosmer et al., 2013, pp. 90–93). These suggestions are helpful guides to determining a final logistic regression model.

8. *Absence of multicollinearity.*

As with OLS multiple regression, an assumption of multiple logistic regression is that there is an absence of multicollinearity. *Multicollinearity* occurs when one or more independent variables (IVs) are highly correlated with each other. Correlations among IVs ≥ |.80| are of concern because they can produce large estimated standard errors and potentially nonsignificant coefficients (Tabachnick & Fidell, 2013). Multicollinearity can also occur when the multiple correlation between one IV and the remaining IVs is too high (e.g., ≥ .90). This can occur even when the individual correlations of the IVs with each other may not be especially high (Norman & Streiner, 2008).

One useful diagnostic to assess multicollinearity is the squared multiple correlation (SMC) of the IVs among themselves. That is, each IV serves as a dependent variable (DV), and the remaining IVs are regressed on that variable. SMCs and tolerance values (1 – SMC) then are obtained for each IV and evaluated. Low SMCs with corresponding high tolerance values are desired. Tabachnick and Fidell (2013) point out that tolerance values as low as .5 or .6 can be problematic.

Unlike OLS multiple regression, most statistical computer packages do not have collinearity diagnostics for logistic regression. These tests can be run, however, using OLS regression and the diagnostics evaluated. At the same time, we could examine the correlation matrix of the IVs to determine the extent to which the individual IVs are correlated with one another. Problematic IVs could then be dropped from the logistic regression analysis.

9. *Absence of outliers.*

Outliers occur in logistic regression when one or more cases are poorly predicted by the obtained model (Tabachnick & Fidell, 2013). That is, a case that is actually in one category of the outcome variable (e.g., an adolescent mother had given birth to a normal-birthweight child) is predicted, by our model, to have a strong probability of being in the other outcome category (e.g., giving birth to a low-birthweight child). This results in a poor fit of the model.

There are several ways that we can identify and evaluate these outliers. We can examine the classification table that is generated in the logistic regression analysis. We can also analyze the residuals. *Residuals* represent the difference between the actual outcome for a case and what we would have predicted given our generated logistic regression model. These residuals can be standardized with standardized residuals >|2.00| considered outliers. We will examine these outliers when we evaluate the residuals and also when we generate a multiple logistic regression solution in SPSS for Windows.

10. *Independence of errors.*

LR is not a repeated-measure design. Errors in prediction for an LR model have a binomial distribution that approximates normality with large samples. This assumes that individual responses are independent and are not influenced by the responses of others. Violating this assumption could result in underestimated standard errors, overestimated values of the test statistic, inaccurate confidence intervals, and, perhaps, rejecting the null hypothesis when in fact the null hypothesis is true (i.e., increased Type I error) (Lomax & Hahs-Vaughn, 2012). This could occur, for example, in a group treatment setting in which the group might have an influence on the responses of the participants. We might have this issue in our hypothetical study since the pregnant adolescents all came from the same community and may even be friends.

Steps for Interpreting a Logistic Regression Analysis

As indicated, in LR analysis we are seeking the answers to two questions:

1. How well does our overall LR model fit our data?

2. How well do our independent variables predict our outcome?

Answering these questions and interpreting the results of an LR analysis, whether simple or complex, is an iterative process. That is, we examine the fit of the model, evaluate the predictors, rerun the analyses, and repeat the process. This process can be a bit daunting because of the different kinds of statistics that are used to evaluate the LR process. Let us assume that, following the initial approach for selecting meaningful predictor variables suggested by Hosmer et al. (2013) (see Table 10.4), we have purposefully selected the independent variable(s) that we will include in our LR analysis. Next, we need to establish a coherent procedure for evaluating the results of the LR analysis.

Table 10.5 outlines an iterative procedure for analyzing and interpreting the results of an LR analysis, whether we are using simple or multivariate LR. These steps will be explained in more detail in the ensuing discussion. We will first approach these steps from the perspective of our simple LR analysis generated in SPSS for Windows using the data set, pregnant teen data for logistic regression-4 predictors.sav, that can be found on the SAGE website (study.sagepub.com/pett2e). Then we will repeat the same steps for our multiple LR analysis. For the interested reader, several excellent resources discuss these procedures in greater depth than can be outlined here. These include Hosmer et al. (2013), Osborne (2015), and Tabachnick and Fidell (2013).

Step 1. Undertake a logistic regression analysis using a statistical computer package or Internet resource. LR and ORs are easily generated in SPSS for Windows by clicking on *Analyze . . . Regression . . . Binary Logistic. . . .* The data set we will use is pregnant teen data for logistic regression-4 predictors.sav located on the SAGE website, study.sagepub.com/pett2e. These results are presented in Figure 10.3. The dependent variable (e.g., *normal_birthweight_baby*) is placed in the Dependent box (1) and the independent variable (group_ assignment) is placed in the Covariates list (Figure 10.3 (2)). Please note that independent variables are often referred to as *covariates* in logistic regression. By clicking on *Options* . . . , several statistics and plots, including classification plots, the Hosmer-Lemeshow goodness-of-fit test, residuals, correlations of estimates, iteration history, and the confidence interval for the odds ratio, exp(B), are offered (3). Predicted values, influence values, and residuals can also be saved

Table 10.5 Suggested Steps for Interpreting the Results of a Logistic Regression Analysis

Step	*Procedure*
1	Undertake a logistic regression analysis using a statistical computer package or Internet resource.
2	Evaluate the overall fit of the model. How well does the generated logistic regression model fit the data?
3	Examine the beta coefficients, their significance levels, odds ratios, and confidence intervals for the predictor variables.
4	Determine the extent to which the final model meets the assumptions for logistic regression.
5	Evaluate the effect size (e.g., Nagelkirke and Cox & Snell R^2).
6	Determine how successful a given model was in correctly classifying cases.
7	Analyze the residuals and leverage values.

for further analysis (4). We will ask for all of these statistics, plots, and saved values in order to obtain an understanding of what type of information each of these options provides. This will help us in completing Steps 2 to 7 of our LR analysis. Figure 10.3 also gives us the syntax commands that will generate the logistic regression output presented in Figure 10.4A–C (5).

The output for the simple bivariate LR analysis is presented in Figure 10.4A–C. The first output that we are given (Figure 10.4A) is the initial report of the variables included in the LR analysis. First we are presented with the Case Processing Summary (1). This summary indicates the number of cases that have been included in the analysis ($n = 100$ in our simple LR example) and any missing cases that we might have (missing = 0). We are also given information as to how the original values for our dependent variable (birthweight of the baby) will be coded by the computer (2). This output is important to examine because the computer, in its eternal wisdom, may decide to code the internal values for our dependent variable differently from our original coding scheme. That would mean that interpretation of the odds ratios would not be based on our original value (1) but rather its alternative (0). Figure 10.4A indicates that our original values (0,1) will have these same internal values as well (2).

Using an Internet resource to generate a simple logistic regression.

As of this writing, several Internet resources are available to generate a simple logistic regression. One in particular, http://vassarstats.net/logreg1.html, offers an easy-to-use calculator for obtaining an odds ratio. To use the program, however, we would need to specify the number of cases in each category of the predictor variable that are coded 0 or 1 for the outcome variable similar to that which was provided in Table 10.1. While we will not undertake this Internet analysis right now, you will get the opportunity to try out the program when completing the exercises at the conclusion of this chapter.

Figure 10.3 Generating a simple logistic regression analysis in SPSS for Windows.

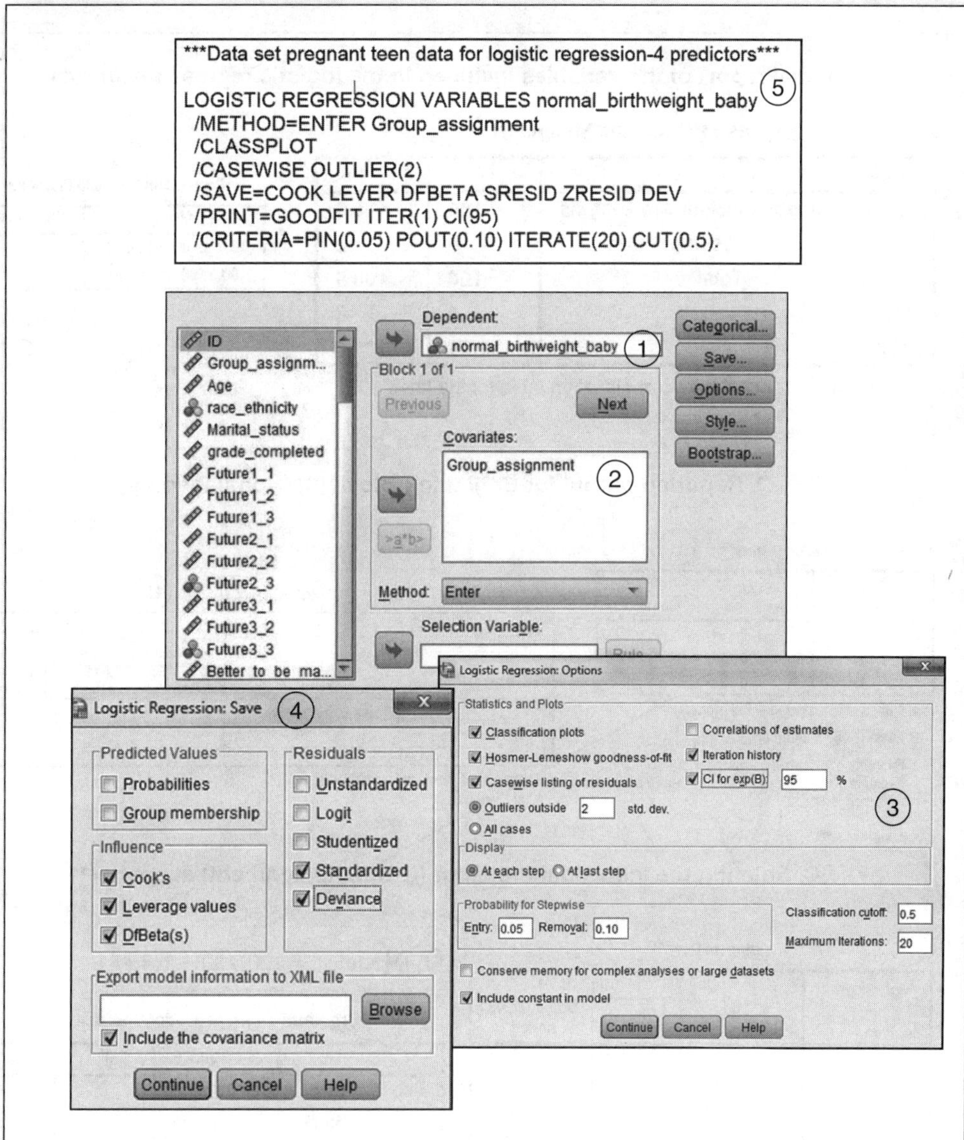

Step 2. Evaluate the overall fit of the model: How well does the generated LR model fit the data? As indicated earlier in this chapter, "likelihood" represents a probability. In this case, it is the probability that the observed values of the dependent variable can be predicted

Figure 10.4 Output for a simple bivariate logistic regression generated in SPSS for Windows (v. 22-23).

A. Initial report of the variables included in the logistic regression analysis

Case Processing Summary (1)

Unweighted Cases[a]		N	Percent
Selected Cases	Included in Analysis	100	100.0
	Missing Cases	0	.0
	Total	100	100.0
Unselected Cases		0	.0
Total		100	100.0

a. If weight is in effect, see classification table for the total number of cases.

Dependent Variable Encoding (2)

Original Value	Internal Value
.00 less than 2500 gr	0
1.00 2500 gr or more	1

B. Reported output for Beginning Block (0) (Constant only)

Iteration History[a,b,c] (3)

Iteration		-2 Log likelihood	Coefficients: Constant
Step 0	1	120.494	.840
	2	120.430	.895
	3	120.430	.895

a. Constant is included in the model.

b. Initial -2 Log Likelihood: 120.430

c. Estimation terminated at iteration number 3 because parameter estimates changed by less than .001.

Classification Table[a,b] (10)

Observed			Predicted: normal_birthweight_baby How much did child weight at birth? .00 less than 2500 gr	Predicted: normal_birthweight_baby How much did child weight at birth? 1.00 2500 gr or more	Percentage Correct
Step 0	normal_birthweight_baby How much did child weight at birth?	.00 less than 2500 gr	0	29	.0
		1.00 2500 gr or more	0	71	100.0
	Overall Percentage				71.0

a. Constant is included in the model.

b. The cut value is .500

C. Entering the Individual Predictor (Group Assignment) at Block (1)

Iteration History[a,b,c,d] (4)

Iteration		-2 Log likelihood	Coefficients: Constant	Coefficients: Group_assignment
Step 1	1	114.874	.400	.880
	2	114.442	.405	1.095
	3	114.441	.405	1.111
	4	114.441	.405	1.111

a. Method: Enter

b. Constant is included in the model.

c. Initial -2 Log Likelihood: 120.430

d. Estimation terminated at iteration number 4 because parameter estimates changed by less than .001.

(6) Model $\chi^2 = 120.430 - 114.441 = 5.99$

Omnibus Tests of Model Coefficients

		Chi-square	df	Sig.
Step 1	Step	(5) 5.990	1	(7) .014
	Block	5.990	1	.014
	Model	5.990	1	.014

Hosmer and Lemeshow Test (8)

Step	Chi-square	df	Sig.
1	.000	0	.

Model Summary (9)

Step	-2 Log likelihood	Cox & Snell R Square	Nagelkerke R Square
1	114.441[a]	.058	.083

a. Estimation terminated at iteration number 4 because parameter estimates changed by less than .001.

Classification Table[a] (11)

Observed			Predicted: normal_birthweight_baby How much did child weight at birth? .00 less than 2500 gr	Predicted: normal_birthweight_baby How much did child weight at birth? 1.00 2500 gr or more	Percentage Correct
Step 1	normal_birthweight_baby How much did child weight at birth?	.00 less than 2500 gr	0	29	.0
		1.00 2500 gr or more	0	71	100.0
	Overall Percentage				71.0

a. The cut value is .500

```
           Step number: 1

           Observed Groups and Predicted Probabilities

       80 +                                                                                                    +
          I                                                                                                    I
          I                                                                                                    I
F         I                                                                                                    I
R      60 +                                                                                                    +
E         I                                                                                                    I
Q         I                                                            2                    2                  I
U         I                                                            2                    2                  I
E      40 +                                                            2                    2                  +
N         I                                                            2                    2                  I
C         I                                                            2                    2                  I
Y         I                                                            2                    2                  I
       20 +                                                            1                    2                  +
          I                                                            1                    2                  I
          I                                                            1                    1                  I
          I                                                            1                    1                  I
Predicted ---------+---------+---------+---------+---------+---------+---------+---------+---------+----------
  Prob:   0        .1        .2        .3        .4        .5        .6        .7        .8        .9         1
  Group:  1111111111111111111111111111111111111111111111111122222222222222222222222222222222222222222222222222

          Predicted Probability is of Membership for 2500 gr or more
          The Cut Value is .50
          Symbols: 1 - less than 2500 gr
                   2 - 2500 gr or more
          Each Symbol Represents 5 Cases.
```

(12)

Casewise List[a]

a. The casewise plot is not produced because no outliers were found. (17)

Variables in the Equation (13)

		B	S.E.	Wald	df	Sig.	Exp(B)	95% C.I.for EXP(B) Lower	95% C.I.for EXP(B) Upper
Step 1[a]	Group_assignment	1.111	.468	5.639	1	(14) .018	(15) 3.037	1.214	7.597
	Constant	.405	.289	1.973	1	.160	1.500	(16)	

a. Variable(s) entered on step 1: Group_assignment.

from the observed values of the predictor variables (Garson, 2014). As with all probabilities, *likelihood* ranges from 0 to 1. Taking the log of this likelihood (LL) will result in values that range from 0 to $-\infty$ since the log of values less than 1 is negative. Multiplying LL by -2 will result in positive values for -2LL (0 to $+\infty$). This -2LL statistic is called the *likelihood ratio.* It is approximately distributed as a chi-square with degrees of freedom equal to the number of parameters included in the model. As the model improves, –LL becomes smaller in value.

LR uses MLE as its foundation to arrive at an LR solution. The goal is to maximize the LL that the obtained values of the outcome variable can be predicted from the observed values of the independent variables included in the model (Hosmer et al., 2013; Osborne, 2015). This computer-intensive iterative procedure begins with an initial "guestimate" of what the logit coefficient(s) or parameters should be. MLE then compares these estimates with a set criterion for what is "good." The resulting residuals are then retested, and an improved LL function is estimated. This procedure is repeated until the LL estimate does not change significantly given a set criterion. That would indicate that additional iterations will not improve the solution. It is the best that it can be. At this point, there is "convergence."

The iteration history that was generated for the null model with only the constant in Block (0) (3) and for the model that also included the group treatment variable in Block (1) (4) is presented in Figure 10.4B,C. In each instance we are given the values of –2 log likelihood (-2LL) and the estimated coefficients for the items entered into the model. The iterations for Step 0 with only the constant present terminated at iteration number 3 (-2LL = 120.430 (3)) because the parameter estimates changed by less than .001, the default value in SPSS for Windows. Similarly, the iterations for Block 1 with group assignment in the model terminated at Step 4 (-2LL = 114.441 (4)) for the same reason.

A number of different statistical approaches can help us to evaluate the overall fit of a generated model. These are called *goodness-of-fit statistics.* These statistics include the model chi-square (χ^2) test and the Hosmer-Lemeshow goodness-of-fit test. In addition, we can estimate the approximate strength of our generated model and can use a classification table to assess the extent to which our generated model can successfully predict the actual values of our outcome variable. In this section, we will examine each of the goodness-of-fit indices and interpret the output that is generated in SPSS for Windows.

Model chi-square (χ^2).

The likelihood ratio is used to test the goodness of fit of a given set of LR models. For example, we can compare how well our model fits compared to a null model that contains only a constant. Or, we can examine what happens when we add an additional independent variable to our reduced model. Regardless of the comparisons, the models being compared need to be nested. That is, all parameters that are contained in the smaller model need to be included in the larger model.

The *model chi-square (χ^2) test* compares the –2LL for a full model (one that contains all of the independent variables of interest) with the –2LL of an initial or null model (which contains only the constant)—that is, model $\chi^2 = (-2LL_{\text{smaller model}}) - (-2LL_{\text{bigger model}})$. The null hypothesis states that, with the exception of the constant, all of the LR coefficients = 0. We will reject this null hypothesis if the difference between the -2LL's (also a χ^2 statistic) is statistically significant at our set level of alpha (e.g., $\alpha = .05$). The degrees of freedom (*df*) for this χ^2 is the difference between the *df* for the bigger and smaller models. Should this χ^2 be statistically significant, we would conclude that our full model is a better predictor of our outcome variable than the null model: At least one of the LR coefficients for our predictor variables is not equal to 0.

With more than one predictor in our model, a statistically significant model χ^2 test does not mean that *all* of the predictor variables are statistically significant. For that we would need to evaluate the statistical significance of each of the independent predictors.

Figure 10.4C presents the model chi-square (χ^2) test that was generated from our commands presented in Figure 10.3. The value of this χ^2 is 5.990 with $df = 1$ (5). It is the difference between the –2LL for the model with only the constant ($-2LL_0 = 120.440$) and –2LL for the model with group assignment added ($-2LL_1 = 114.441$) (6):

$$\text{Model}\,\chi^2 = (-2LL_0) - (-2LL_1) = 120.440 - 114.411 = 5.99$$

The degrees of freedom (*df*) for this model χ^2 is $2 - 1 = 1$ since there were 2 *df*s for the "full" model and 1 *df* for the null model with only the constant. We will reject the null hypothesis that the full model is no better than the null model since our *p* value of .014 (7) is less than $\alpha = .05$. Alternatively, from Appendix A, Table A.2, we can determine that the critical value for a χ^2 with $df = 1$ is 3.841. Since our actual χ^2 (5.99) is greater than the critical value of the χ^2 (3.841), we can reject the null hypothesis and conclude that our "full" model with group assignment added is statistically significantly better than our "null" model that contained only the constant.

Notice that the χ^2 values for the "Step," the "Block," and the "Model" in Block = 1 are exactly the same ($\chi^2 = 5.990$) (6). The reason for this is that there was only one predictor variable, group assignment, entered into our model; therefore, the "step," "block," and "model" are the same. Later, when we undertake a logistic regression analysis with multiple predictor variables, these values will most likely be different from one another.

Hosmer-Lemeshow goodness-of-fit test.

A second goodness-of-fit statistic that is routinely available in statistical computer packages is the Hosmer-Lemeshow goodness-of-fit test (Hosmer & Lemeshow, 1980; Hosmer et al., 2013; Lemeshow & Hosmer, 1982). It is used when one or more of the predictor variables have more than two levels. Several authors (Garson, 2014; Osborne, 2015) have indicated that they prefer this test to the model χ^2 and classification tables when evaluating model fit because it is more robust, especially for models with continuous variables and studies with small samples. Because our predictor variable, group assignment, is dichotomous, this test will not yield meaningful results for our simple logistic regression but will be meaningful when we undertake a multiple logistic regression with at least one continuous predictor variable.

To obtain the Hosmer-Lemeshow goodness-of-fit test, respondents are first listed in order of their predicted probabilities based on the generated LR model and then divided into 10 groups or *deciles* according to these predicted probabilities. For example, respondents with predicted probabilities ≤ .10 would be in the first group, while those with predicted probabilities > .9 would be in the 10th group. Next, the participants are further separated into two groups reflecting their actual position on the outcome variable (e.g., 1 = having a normal-birthweight baby, 0 = low-birthweight baby). From these data, a 10 × 2 contingency table is generated that reflects the observed frequencies in each cell. Expected frequencies are also obtained for the 20 cells (expected frequency = [row total][column total]/*N*). From these data, a χ^2 statistic with $df = 8$ (df = #deciles – 2 = 10 – 2 = 8) is obtained. The null hypothesis states that the model fits the data. The alternative hypothesis states that the model does not fit the data.

Unlike the model χ^2 test, a nonsignificant χ^2 is desirable with the Hosmer-Lemeshow test. That would indicate that, for those persons whose value on the outcome variable = 0 (i.e., in our example, they had a low-birthweight baby), their estimated probabilities would be located among the lower deciles (e.g., .1, .2). For those whose outcome variable = 1 (i.e., they had a normal-birthweight baby), their estimated probabilities would cluster in the higher deciles (e.g., .8, .9). That would mean that the observed frequencies for each cell were similar to the expected values, thus resulting in a nonsignificant χ^2. If the model does not fit the data, then the probabilities for the respondents in both categories will be distributed across all of the deciles. The observed frequencies in the cells would not match the expected frequencies, resulting in a statistically significant χ^2 and a poor model fit.

As indicated, the value for our Hosmer and Lemeshow test reported in Figure 10.4C (8) has produced meaningless results (chi-square = 0) since our predictor variable, group assignment, is dichotomous and, therefore, could not be separated into meaningful deciles.

R^2 values.

The coefficient of determination, R^2, in OLS multiple linear regression represents the proportion of variance in the dependent variable that can be predicted by the independent or predictor variables in the model. Its values range between 0 and 1.0, with higher values indicating a greater proportion of variance in the dependent variable that can be explained by the independent variable(s) in the model. These R^2 values help us to evaluate the strength or effect size of a given model and to compare it to other models that are not necessarily nested but that share the same dependent variable.

Because LR is dealing with an outcome variable that is nominal level, it does not have a true analog to the R^2 in multiple linear regression in which the outcome variable is continuous. Several approximations to R^2 (sometimes called *pseudo-*R^2) have been suggested (Menard, 2000). Three of these, which can be obtained in SPSS for Windows, are the Cox and Snell (1989), Nagelkerke (1991), and McFadden (1974) pseudo-R^2 measures. SPSS reports the Cox and Snell and Nagelkerke measures for binary logistic regression and the McFadden measure for multinomial logistic regression. Each of these measures appears to have challenges, and as a result, there is no consensus as to which approach is preferred. To help you to understand the output that you obtain from these measures, the differences among the three measures will be briefly addressed.

The Cox and Snell R^2 can be obtained by the following formula (Allison, 2012, 2013; Menard, 2000):

$$R^2_{C\&S} = 1 - \left(L_0 / L_M \right)^{2/n}$$

where

L_0 = likelihood function for the null model with only the constant,

L_M = likelihood function for the model containing the predictors being evaluated, and

n = sample size.

The problem with the Cox and Snell R^2 is that its upper bound is less than 1.0. According to Allison (2013), the upper bound for the Cox and Snell R^2 is $1 - L_0^{2/n}$, which can be much less than 1.0. Allison points out, for example, that when $p = .50$, the maximum that the Cox and Snell statistic can be is .75, and when $p = .90$, the upper bound is .48.

For that reason, Nagelkerke (1991) suggested dividing the Cox and Snell R^2 by its upper bound, thus creating an R^2 statistic that ranges between 0 and 1:

$$R^2_N = \frac{1 - \left(L_0 / L_M \right)^{2/n}}{1 - L_0^{2/n}}$$

The problem with this approach is that it lacks theoretical sense and can produce misleadingly high values (Allison, 2013). For this reason, Allison, for now, has recommended using the McFadden R^2 (McFadden, 1974). Its formula is given as follows:

$$R^2_{McF} = 1 - \ln(L_M) / \ln(L_0)$$

where $ln(x)$ represents the natural log of "x."

The McFadden R^2 is also known as the *likelihood ratio* R^2 (Menard, 2000). By simplifying the numerator and denominator of this R^2, we arrive at the following formula:

$$R^2_{McF} = R^2_L = Model\left(\chi^2\right) / -2LL_0$$

where the model χ^2 is the same as discussed above, and $-2LL_0$ is the -2 log-likelihood value for the null model with only the constant.

Allison (2013) argues that an advantage to the McFadden (likelihood ratio) approach is that it makes intuitive sense because it represents a proportional reduction in "error variance." This approach to R^2 is only available in SPSS for multinomial logistic regression, not the binary form. However, you will soon see that it is easily calculated by hand given the SPSS computer printout.

How would we interpret these R^2 estimates, and are they very useful in evaluating the overall strength of a model? Unlike the coefficient of determination obtained from OLS multiple linear regression, the pseudo-R^2 values that we obtain in logistic regression cannot be interpreted as a percentage of explained variance in the dependent variable. Rather, it has been suggested that we consider these R^2 values to be estimates of weak, moderate, or strong effect sizes (Garson, 2014).

Unfortunately, there do not appear to be any general guidelines for deciding on what constitutes a "weak," "moderate," or "strong" effect, especially when the three measures we have examined can produce different and, at times, dramatically conflicting results (Osborne, 2015). Certainly, the closer the R^2 value is to 0, the weaker the effect; the closer to 1.0, the stronger the effect. Garson (personal communication, October 18, 2014) suggests that, for Nagelkerke R^2, values of .09 to .29 could be considered to be "weak," .30 to .59 "moderate," and values ≥ .60 "strong". Similar criteria could also be applied to the McFadden/likelihood ratio R^2. An alternative approach is to use the same criteria that we would use to evaluate the strength of a correlation between two variables (r^2) (Hinkle, Wiersma, & Jurs, 2003). These are summarized in Table 10.6. These criteria suggest that values of 0 to .08 are weak, .09 to .24 low, .25 to .48 moderate, .49 to .80 strong, and .81 to 1.0 very strong. Regardless of the criteria we use, it is important to evaluate these measures carefully along with the other goodness-of-fit indices, including the classification tables.

The output for the Cox and Snell and Nagelkerke R^2 values (.058 and .083, respectively) are given to us in Figure 10.4C (9). Given the model χ^2 value of 5.99 and a $-2LL_0$ = 120.440 from Figure 10.4C (6), our McFadden/likelihood R^2 can be obtained as follows:

$$R^2_{McF} = R^2_L = \frac{Model\left(\chi^2\right)}{-2LL_0} = \frac{5.99}{120.440} = 0.0497$$

According to Table 10.6, all of these R^2 values (range: .0497–.083) demonstrate a weak effect. It is apparent, therefore, that despite its statistical significance (p = .014), our simple LR model that included only group assignment is a weak predictor of birthweight of the baby.

Classification tables.

An additional approach to evaluating goodness of fit of a given model is to examine the extent to which the model is successful in predicting a respondent's actual assignment

Table 10.6 Suggested Rule of Thumb for Interpreting Pseudo R^2 Values

Size of Pseudo R^2	*Effect size*
.81 – 1.00	Very strong
.49 – .80	Strong
.25 – .48	Moderate
.09 – .24	Low
.00 – .08	Weak

on the outcome variable. To do this, cases are assigned to either outcome of the dependent variable based on their computed probabilities generated from the logistic regression model. Typically, .50 is selected as the cutoff probability for assignment to one of the two values of the outcome variable, although, with justification, this default value can be changed. Cases with computed probabilities < .50 are assigned to the outcome whose value = 0 (e.g., in our example, 0 = low-birthweight babies). Cases with computed probabilities ≥ .50 are assigned to be in the outcome category whose value = 1 (e.g., 1 = normal-birthweight babies). The observed frequencies for both levels of the dependent variable are then compared to the assigned frequencies based on the computed probabilities derived from the logistic regression model, and the percentage of correct predictions is obtained.

There are two types of error in classifying cases: *false positives* and *false negatives*. A *false positive* (aka Type I error) occurs when, based on its computed probabilities, a case is assigned the value of 1 for the outcome variable when in fact the observed value = 0. A *false negative* (aka Type II error) occurs when, based on its computed probabilities, a case is assigned the predicted value of 0 for the outcome variable when, in reality, its observed value on the outcome variable = 1. In our example, we would have a *false positive* if we predicted that a child would be a normal-birthweight baby (1) when in fact it was of low birthweight (0). A *false negative* would have occurred if we had predicted that the baby would be low birthweight (0) when in fact it was of normal birthweight (1).

There are also two types of correct classification: *sensitivity* and *specificity*. *Sensitivity* represents the percentage of cases that were correctly classified as 1 on the outcome variable (e.g., normal-birthweight baby). *Specificity* is the percentage of cases that were correctly classified as a 0 on the outcome variable (e.g., low-birthweight baby).

Figure 10.4B presents the initial classification table for the null model with no predictor variables that was generated in SPSS for Windows (10). Given that this is a null model, these percentages are based merely on "guessing" that all of the observations would fall in the class of the outcome variable that had the largest sample size. Since, in our example, 71 of 100 cases were of normal birthweight, the computer "guesstimates" that all of the cases will fall in the normal-birthweight category. That means that, initially, the null model correctly predicted all of the cases whose outcome values = 1 (normal-birthweight babies ≥ 2,500 grams) with 100% sensitivity. However, it had 0 correct with regard to those babies who were of low birthweight (0% specificity). The overall % correct was 71.0% (71 correct/100 total n * 100 = 71.0%).

Next, the classification table is reconfigured once additional independent variable(s) have been entered into the logistic regression equation. We would then compare the classification table generated by the full model to that produced by the null model to determine the extent to which the additional predictor variable(s) improve the predictive ability of the model. The classification table in Figure 10.4C provides us with that information (11).

It appears that even with group assignment entered into the model (and setting our default probability cutoff at .50), we are not doing much better at predicting group membership than if we had guessed based on the group that had the largest sample size. That would mean that group assignment is not a very strong predictor of an adolescent mother having/not having a normal-birthweight infant. This outcome was supported by the weak R^2 values, .058 and .083, that we are presented with in Figure 10.4C (9).

The plot of the probability values in Figure 10.4C gives an indication as to why we have done so poorly in predicting low-birthweight babies based on their computed probabilities (12). Notice that all of the computed probabilities with group assignment in the model are either around .60 or .80. Since both of these predicted probabilities are greater than our cutoff value of .50, all of the cases would have been assigned to the normal-birthweight category (outcome variable = 1). Had we changed the default cutoff from .50 to .70, we would have changed the results of our classification table to something worse, in fact. As Osborne (2015) and Tabachnick and Fidell (2013) point out, the best way to improve the overall accuracy of classification is to find a better set of predictors.

So what do we make of all of this? While the model χ^2 indicated that we had a good model fit (model $\chi^2 = 5.99$, $p = .014$), other indicators of goodness of fit suggest that, while significant, the model is weak at best. This suggests that we may want to add additional predictors to our model. First, though, let's examine the individual statistics for our single predictor, group assignment, and interpret their meaning. With only one predictor, our interpretation will be relatively straightforward.

Step 3. Examine the beta coefficients, their significance levels, and odds ratios (and confidence interval) for each predictor variable. After examining the overall fit of the model, we will want to evaluate the generated coefficients for the independent variables to determine whether they are statistically significant contributors to the LR model. Given that for a simple LR, we only have one predictor, this will be an easy task. Two approaches can be taken when undertaking tests of the individual predictor variables. We could use either a Wald statistic or undertake a likelihood ratio test.

The Wald statistic.

The Wald statistic appears to be most often reported in the research literature, perhaps because it is easy to obtain, understand, and interpret. This statistic is calculated for each of the predictor variables in a proposed model; it is the default in SPSS for Windows. It can be obtained in one of two ways. Either it is treated as a *z statistic* or as a *chi square* (χ^2) *statistic* (Hosmer et al., 2013; Norman & Streiner, 2008; Tabachnick & Fidell, 2013). If it is treated as a *z statistic,* the Wald statistic is obtained by dividing the regression coefficient by its standard error (B/SE_B) and the results compared to a standard normal *z* distribution. Table A.1 in Appendix A presents the values for the cumulative distribution function (CDF) for the standard normal (*z*) distribution. If we have a nondirectional test and $\alpha = .05$, the critical value of the *z* statistic would be ±1.96 since that is where .025 lies to the right of +1.96 and left of −1.96. That is, the CDF for +1.96 is .975 (and 1 − .975 = .025); for −1.96, the CDF = .025.

A second approach, which is the default in SPSS for Windows, is to obtain a Wald statistic for each predictor by dividing the regression coefficient by its standard error and squaring the results:

$$\text{Wald statistic} = \left(\frac{B}{SE_B}\right)^2$$

This Wald statistic is distributed as a chi-square statistic (χ^2) with $df = 1$. We will reject the null hypothesis that the given independent variable is not a significant predictor in our model if the Wald statistic that we obtain is greater than a critical value for the Wald at our given level of α (e.g., .05) or if the p value we obtain is less than α. Using the χ^2 version of the Wald, we will reject the null hypothesis if and only if our actual Wald statistic is greater than the critical value of a χ^2 at our level of α with $df = 1$. Looking at a table of χ^2 values (e.g., Table A.2 in Appendix A), we can see that if $\alpha = .05$, then the critical value of a χ^2 with $df = 1$ is 3.841 or if $p < .05$.

Figure 10.4C presents the LR output for the Wald statistic for our group assignment variable that was generated in SPSS for Windows for the Wald statistic (13). In our example, besides the constant, we have only one predictor variable, group assignment. Therefore, we are given that variable's beta (B), standard error of beta (SE), the Wald statistic (Wald), degrees of freedom (*df*), *p* value (*Sig*), and odds ratio (Exp(B)). The beta we are presented with is 1.111 (standard error = .468). This results in a Wald statistic of 5.639. This was obtained as follows:

$$\text{Wald statistic} = \left(\frac{\text{B}}{\text{SE}_\text{B}}\right)^2 = \left(\frac{1.111}{0.468}\right)^2 = 5.636$$

The difference between this hand-calculated value, 5.636, and the computer-generated value, 5.639, can be attributed to round-off error. Since 5.636 (and 5.639) is greater than our critical χ^2 with $df = 1$ (3.841), we will reject the null hypothesis and conclude that there is an association between group assignment and subsequent birthweight of the child. This conclusion is supported by the fact that the generated *Sig* (the *p* value) for this analysis, .018 (Figure 10.4C (14)), is also less than our stated level of alpha ($\alpha = .05$).

Notice that, in Figure 10.4C, we are also given a Wald statistic for the constant. Hosmer et al. (2013) and Osborne (2015) point out that this constant is similar to the intercept in OLS regression. That is, the constant represents an estimate of the response when our predictor variable equals 0. In our example, it is the conditional odds of having normal-birthweight infant for persons assigned to the usual-care group (group assignment = 0). It is interesting that our constant is not statistically significant once the group assignment variable has entered the model.

Likelihood ratio test.

Despite the popularity of the Wald statistic, several authors have pointed out problems associated with these statistics (Hauck & Donner, 1977; Hosmer et al., 2013; Menard, 2002; Tabachnick & Fidell, 2013). Hauck and Donner (1977) found that, at times, the Wald statistic failed to reject the null hypothesis when the likelihood ratio test indicated the predictor variable was statistically significant. Menard (2010) concurred, indicating that large absolute values of the logistic regression coefficient tend to produce large values for its standard errors, increasing the likelihood of failing to reject the null hypothesis per the Wald test. For that reason, a likelihood ratio test may be a more reliable measure of the contribution of a given predictor variable to the LR model.

To generate a likelihood ratio test, a model χ^2 test is used to compare two models: one with and the other without the predictor variable of interest. Its purpose is to determine whether that predictor variable makes a statistically significant contribution to the improvement of a model's fit (Tabachnick & Fidell, 2013). A statistically significant model χ^2 would indicate that the predictor variable of interest improves the model fit.

A drawback to the likelihood ratio test is that it is labor and computer intensive and not readily available in all current statistical packages (Tabachnick & Fidell, 2013). That is, it requires evaluating each predictor variable independently for its unique contribution to the improvement of a model fit. Hosmer et al. (2013) indicate that they have not found large differences in the results of the Wald and likelihood tests. However, should there be discrepant results between the Wald and likelihood ratio statistics, the authors recommend that the results from the likelihood ratio test be reported.

In our simple logistic regression example with only one predictor variable (group assignment), our model χ^2 in Figure 10.4C (6) (5.99) indicates that, compared to the null model with only the constant present, group assignment is a statistically significant contributor to the improvement of model fit (p = .014 (7)). The Wald statistic for group assignment confirms that finding (p = .018 (14)).

Interpret the OR and its confidence interval.

As indicated earlier in this chapter, an OR represents the change in odds of an outcome of interest (e.g., giving birth to a normal-birthweight child) given a one-unit increase in the independent variable (e.g., 0 = usual care vs. 1 = group-based intervention) while controlling for other variables in the model. In SPSS for Windows, the OR is presented as an *Exp*(*B*) for each of the predictor variables entered into the LR model. Why *Exp*(*B*)? Despite the potential for confusion, *Exp*(*B*) is, in fact, the definition of the OR (OR = e^B).

Since we have only one predictor variable in our simple LR model, we have only one OR to interpret. Later in this chapter, we will see how we can not only interpret the ORs for several predictor variables but also evaluate which predictor variables make the greatest contribution to a given model.

The SPSS-generated OR for group assignment, 3.037, is presented in Figure 10.4C (15). This is the same value as that which we had hand-calculated earlier in this chapter. The 95% CI is also similar to our hand-calculated values: 1.214 and 7.597 (16).

There are several ways to interpret this OR and its 95% CI. First, we can interpret the OR and CI as we did earlier in this chapter:

> The odds of having a normal-birthweight infant given that the adolescent mother received the group-based intervention are 3.04 times higher than for those adolescent mothers who received usual care. Controlling for other variables in the model, there is a 95% probability that the true population odds ratio for having a normal-birthweight baby given that the mother was in the intervention compared to the usual-care group lies between 1.21 and 7.60.

Alternatively, the OR can be interpreted as a percentage (Hosmer et al., 2013). That is, with an OR = 3.04, we can say that there is a 204% [(3.04 – 1) * 100 = 204] increase in the odds of having a normal-birthweight infant (i.e., the outcome variable = 1) given that the adolescent mother took part in the group intervention (i.e., the predictor variable = 1) compared to the usual-care group (i.e., the predictor variable = 0).

Odds ratios are relatively easy to interpret when the predictor variable is dichotomous. As we will see when we examine multiple logistic regression, interpretation of the odds ratio becomes more cumbersome to interpret when the predictor variable is continuous. That is why you will often see continuous variables being collapsed into nominal- or ordinal-level data.

Step 4. Evaluate the extent to which the final model meets the assumptions for logistic regression. While LR is relatively free of assumptions and conditions, there are several steps that we need to take to determine the extent to which the adolescent data meet these assumptions and conditions. These were discussed in detail earlier in this chapter and summarized in Table 10.3.

For example, we would want to double-code our data and run descriptives on our variables of interest to be sure that the variables, group assignment and birth outcome, have been measured without error. Both our predictor and outcome variables are dichotomous; since there is only one predictor variable with 100 cases, we have a sufficient ratio of cases to independent variables. A single predictor variable also indicates that we do not have a problem with multicollinearity (i.e., high correlations among multiple predictor variables). The Crosstabs table presented in Table 10.1 indicates that we have sufficient cases in each category and, since our predictor variable, group assignment, is nominal level, we do not have an issue with linearity of the logit since that assumption applies to continuous predictor variables. Finally, the SPSS for Windows output (Figure 10.4C) has indicated that none of the residuals were found to be >|2.0|(17). *Independence of errors* could potentially be a problem. Although this was not a repeated-measures design, the pregnant adolescents came from the same neighborhood, some of whom were assigned to a group intervention. Therefore, there is the possibility that they influenced each other's responses.

Step 5. Undertake regression diagnostics. Once an LR model has been specified, it is important to undertake a series of regression diagnostics. These diagnostics, like those in OLS linear regression, help us to identify cases that are outliers. These are individual cases that either do not fit the specified model or are inappropriately influencing our results. Two diagnostic approaches are especially helpful: examination of the residuals and leverage values.

Statistical computer packages offer many, at times confusing, alternatives both with regard to residuals (e.g., unstandardized, logit, studentized, standardized, and deviance) and influence values (e.g., Cook's, leverage values, and Dbetas). To keep things relatively simple, we will focus on interpretation of the standardized and studentized residuals and leverage values (*Leverage* and *Cook's*). For the reader interested in exploring these and other values in greater depth, Hosmer et al. (2013), Menard (2010), Osborne (2015), and Sarkar, Midi, and Rana (2011) present excellent discussions of the meaning and interpretation of these and other residuals and leverage values.

Standardized and studentized residuals.

Residuals represent the difference between the predicted probability for a respondent based on our LR model and the actual value that the respondent had on the outcome variable. Suppose, for example, that one of the participating adolescents gave birth to a normal-weight infant (i.e., normal_birthweight = 1). Suppose, too, that, based on our model, the predicted probability for this adolescent giving birth to a normal-weight infant was .80. Then the difference between the actual outcome and the predicted probability would be 1 – .80 = .20. Thus, our predicted probability of having a normal-birthweight infant was off by .20. This is called a *residual*. The purpose of examining these residuals is to identify cases that either do not fit our model or appear to unduly influence the estimated parameters of our model.

Unstandardized residuals ($Y - \hat{Y}$) are limited in their interpretation; it is difficult to assess how "bad" the predicted probability is from the actual outcome on the outcome variable. To help evaluate these residuals, they can be standardized by adjusting them for their standard errors (Menard, 2010). These *standardized residuals* are sometimes referred to as *Pearson residuals* (Hosmer et al., 2013) or *normalized residuals* (Osborne, 2015). Residuals can also be *studentized*. *Studentized residuals* (aka *deviance residuals*) are residuals that have been divided by the standard deviation of the residuals, having first excluded a given case from the analysis (Osborne, 2015). They are an index of the extent to which a given case contributes to the lack of fit of a model (Osborne, 2015). They are useful for examining the leverage of a given case.

Residuals in LR are not expected to be normally distributed; it is assumed that these errors follow a binomial distribution (Menard, 2010). For larger sample sizes ($n \geq 30$), however, standardized residuals represent z scores with a mean = 0 and a standard deviation = 1. Values for standardized residuals that lie outside of a given value (e.g., $z \geq |3.0|$) are considered outliers (Osborne, 2015): They are cases that stand apart from the remainder of the data and do not fit our model very well. Similarly, studentized residuals also approximately follow a standard normal distribution for similar sample sizes. They are considered more stable than standardized residuals when the predicted probabilities approach the extremes (e.g., 0 or 1).

Upon request (see Figure 10.3), SPSS for Windows will indicate which cases have standardized residuals that are greater in absolute value than a prespecified cutoff. They can also be saved for further examination (Figure 10.3). From these data, we can identify which specific cases do not fit a specified model. These cases can then be checked for potential errors in coding and to try to determine why a particular case is an outlier. We can also assess the extent to which the χ^2 goodness-of-fit text would change as a result of deleting the outlier. We need to be careful, however, when deleting outliers. Not only does the LR model become less applicable to more diverse populations, but additional outliers may show up as a result of case deletion. Also, each time we run an LR model and save the residuals, a new version of the saved residuals (e.g., ZRE_1, ZRE_2, etc.) will appear at the end of the variable list. It can become very confusing as to which residuals apply to the model we are examining. For that reason, we will want to delete those unwanted versions of the saved residuals.

As indicated in Figure 10.4C (17), none of the standardized residuals generated from our simple LR model were found to be >|2.0|. That is not surprising since there is only one dichotomous predictor variable in the model. Later, when we examine an LR model with multiple predictor variables, we will revisit the interpretation of these standardized and studentized residuals.

Influence values.

Influence values represent those cases that are exerting an undue influence on the parameters of our model and, if removed, would result in a large change in those values (Belsley, Kuh, & Welsch, 2005; Menard, 2010). We will examine two such influence values: leverage and Cook's distance.

Leverage represents the importance of an observation to the fit of a given model (Hosmer et al., 2013; Sarkar et al., 2011). According to Osborne (2015), leverage values range from 0 to 1.0, where 0 indicates that a case has no influence on the LR parameters and 1.0 indicates that a case has a total influence on the model parameters. Osborne (2015) further suggests that leverage values greater than $3k/n$ (where k = the number of predictor variables in the model and n = the sample size) could serve as an indicator that a given case may be exerting undue influence on the model parameters. Menard (2010) proposes using the guidelines suggested by Belsley et al. (2005): Cases with leverage values > $(2(k)/n)$ are considered influential.

In our hypothetical example, $3k/n = (3 * 1)/100 = .03$ and $2(k)/n = 2(1)/100 = .02$. With only one dichotomous predictor variable, examining the leverage values for the 100 cases was not very helpful since the descriptive statistics indicated that all of the leverage values were the same: .02. As with residuals, these will be more useful when we run a logistic regression model with multiple predictors.

Cook's distance assesses the change in regression estimates and overall summary measures of fit as a result of removing a given case (or subjects with a particular covariance pattern) from the analysis (Garson, 2014; Hosmer et al., 2013; Menard, 2010). Standardizing Cook's distance produces yet another assessment of leverage: *Dbeta* (aka *DfBeta* in SPSS for Windows). Since DfBeta is standardized, values > |3.0| should be considered influential cases. There is a DfBeta value for each case for each predictor variable and constant. Hosmer et al. (2013) suggest graphing leverage values, Cook's distance, and DfBeta results against the estimated logistic probability values. The authors point out that these graphs are useful in visually identifying extreme values that lie outside a given cluster. We will not generate such graphs for our simple LR model since there is only one dichotomous predictor variable. However, we will briefly examine the Cook's and Dbeta coefficients when the LR model with multiple predictors is evaluated.

To summarize, a number of diagnostic assessments are available in statistical computer packages to help identify influential outliers in an LR analysis. Unfortunately, it may also be a bit bewildering to decide which of these many assessment tools we should use and how to interpret the generated results. Menard (2010) argues that, at the very minimum, we should pay close attention to values out of range for studentized residuals, leverage, and some form of Cook's distance (e.g., DfBeta). That will help us to identify potential errors and cases that are unduly influencing our results.

Presentation of the Results

The results of the statistical analysis of a simple logistic regression with only one variable could be presented in the form of a table similar to Table 10.7. Notice that the standardized beta coefficients were not presented in this table since there was only one predictor variable.

Table 10.7 Example of a Table of Results for a Simple Logistic Regression

Outcome Variable	*Predictor Variable*	*b*	*SE(b)*	*Wald*	*df*	p	*OR*	*95% CI (OR)*
Normal birthweight baby[a]	Treatment group[b]	1.11	0.47	5.64	1	0.018	3.64	1.21–7.60
	Constant	0.41	0.29	1.97	1	0.160	1.50	

NOTE: $R_L^2 = 0.0497$.

[a]Normal birthweight baby: 0 = low birthweight; 1 = normal birthweight.

[b]Treatment group: 0 = usual care; 1 = group-based intervention.

The results could also be presented in the text as follows:

> The results of the simple logistic regression analysis indicated that the intervention (usual-care vs. group-based intervention) was a statistically significant predictor of whether or not a pregnant adolescent would give birth to a normal-birthweight baby ($p = .018$). Adolescents who were randomly assigned to the group-based intervention were 3.64 times more likely to give birth to a normal-birthweight baby than adolescents in the usual-care group (95% CI: 1.21, 7.60). The strength of this relationship ($R_L^2 = .0497$) indicates that this was a weak effect.

Advantages, Limitations, and Alternatives to Simple Logistic Regression

Simple logistic regression is especially useful when a researcher is interested in obtaining an "unadjusted" odds ratio when there is only one predictor variable in the model. The drawback to simple logistic regression is that it tells us little about the contribution of that given predictor when additional predictor variables are entered into a logistic regression model. It also does not tell us which independent variable is most important in predicting our outcome variable.

For example, in our simple bivariate logistic regression analysis, we found that adolescent membership in a given intervention group was statistically significantly associated with having a normal-birthweight baby. But are there additional variables that may in fact have a stronger influence on adolescent birth outcomes (e.g., the number of prenatal visits, smoking status, and the quality of the adolescent's relationship with her parents)? Perhaps it is those variables that are more important than the intervention in predicting whether or not a pregnant adolescent will give birth to a normal-birthweight infant. To answer this question, we would need to turn to multiple logistic regression.

MULTIPLE LOGISTIC REGRESSION

Multiple LR is used when we have multiple independent variables and would like to examine their individual and collective influence on a dichotomous outcome variable. These independent or predictor variables can be of any level of measurement. If they are nominal level of measurement, they need to be dichotomous or have been recoded into dummy variables (see our earlier discussion about assumptions of LR, especially regarding the level of measurement of the predictor variables).

An Appropriate Research Question for Multivariate Logistic Regression

The model that we are testing in multivariate logistic regression is one that contains multiple independent variables:

$$logit\left(\hat{Y}\right) = b_0 + b_1\left(x_1\right) + b_2\left(x_2\right) + b_3\left(x_3\right) + \ldots + b_k\left(x_k\right)$$

The goal of this analysis is to determine how well our generated model fits our actual data and to determine the extent to which each of the independent variables adds to the fit of the model. Our ultimate goal is to correctly predict the outcome for individual cases.

There are many examples of the use of multivariate logistic regression in health care research. Lee-Lin et al. (2007) used multivariate logistic regression in an assessment of breast cancer beliefs and their influence on mammography screening practices among Chinese American immigrants. A similar approach was used by Mays et al. (2014) to examine the extent to which exposure to parental smoking affected adolescent smoking trajectories. Neuman et al. (2014) used multivariate logistic regression as well to examine predictors of readmissions among children previously hospitalized with pneumonia.

In our hypothetical example, we are interested in correctly predicting whether or not a pregnant adolescent will give birth to a normal-birthweight infant given the treatment group she was randomly assigned to, her smoking status, number of prenatal visits, and the quality of her relationship with her parent(s). The LR model we are examining, therefore, is the following:

$$logit\left(\hat{Y}\right) = b_0 + b_1\left(treatment\ group\right) + b_2\left(smoking\ status\right) + b_3\left(number\ of\ prenatal\ visits\right) + b_4\left(quality\ of\ relationship\ with\ parents\right)$$

An appropriate research question, given the model we have specified, could be as follows:

> To what extent do the following independent variables predict whether or not a pregnant adolescent will give birth to a normal-birthweight infant: the treatment group she was randomly assigned to, whether or not she is currently a smoker, the number of prenatal visits she had with her health care provider, and the quality of her relationship with her parents?

As we did with simple bivariate logistic regression, in answering this research question, we will address two separate but related issues:

1. How well does this overall LR model fit our data?
2. How well do our individual independent variables predict our outcome (e.g., birthweight of the child)?

The data set we will continue to use is pregnant teen data for logistic regression-4 predictors.sav that is posted on the SAGE website, study.sagepub.com/pett2e.

Methods of Entry in Logistic Regression

One of the first decisions to be made when undertaking a multivariate LR analysis is to determine the method that will be used to enter the predictor variables into the statistical analysis. This decision was easy in a simple bivariate LR analysis. Because there was only one predictor variable, we introduced the predictor variable into the model using the *Enter* command. With multivariate LR, the situation is a bit more complicated in that, as with OLS multiple regression, the choice of our method of entry for the predictor variables can affect the structure of our final model.

Our choice of approach to entry depends, in part, on whether we are testing a specified model, have generated hypotheses related to the order of importance of predictor variables, or are more interested in using an exploratory hypothesis-generating approach to model building. In the former examples (testing a specified model or predicting order of importance of predictor variables), the researcher takes control over the method of entry. In the latter example (a hypothesis-generating approach), the order of entry of predictor variables is controlled by the statistical software and is based on statistical significance.

User-specified approaches to entry.

User-specified methods of entry are preferred over software-specified entry. Using these methods, the researcher has control over how the predictor variables will be entered into the model. There are three basic approaches to variable entry if the researcher's goal is to test a specified model or predict the order of importance of a set of predictor variables: forced entry, hierarchical entry, and entering sets of predictor variables in blocks (Osborne, 2015).

Forced entry (aka *Enter* in SPSS for Windows) involves entering all of the predictor variables into the LR analysis simultaneously. Each predictor is then evaluated as if it had been entered last into the LR equation (Tabachnick & Fidell, 2013). While this approach is often used in LR analysis, it will retain predictor variables in the model that are not statistically significant.

Hierarchical entry involves entering each predictor variable step-by-step based on a prespecified theoretical model. The entering predictor variable is then evaluated for its contribution to the overall LR model fit by examining the change in the –2LL as a result of entering the predictor into the model. An advantage to this approach is that we can use the likelihood ratio test rather than the Wald statistic to evaluate the predictor variable's contribution to the model given the other variables in the model.

Entering predictor variables in blocks is similar to forced and hierarchical entry. Predictor variables are entered as prespecified blocks into the LR equation. This approach is especially useful if the researcher wants to examine the effect of a given set of variables on the outcome variable before evaluating the effects of other predictor variables in the model. For example, we may want to examine the effects of the group-based intervention on birthweight of the infant after having first controlled for a set of demographic variables (e.g., age of the adolescent, marital status, race/ethnicity). After creating dummy variables to represent the marital status and race/ethnicity variables, we could enter these variables first as a block and then, in the second step, enter the group assignment variable to assess the additional contribution of the intervention on birth outcomes having first controlled for the set of demographic variables in the first block. Osborne (2015) suggests that these blocks could also be used to assess dummy-coded variables as a single unit (e.g., those that represent marital status). We could also test a specific theoretical model of influence using these sets of blocks.

This approach is very useful in helping the researcher to determine the individual contributions of predictor variables to the logistic regression model. Osborne (2015) and Tabachnick and Fidell (2013) point out, however, that once the final set of predictor variables is in the model, it does not matter how they were entered (individually or in blocks). The model summary, classification table, individual statistics, and logistic regression equation will be the same because their parameters are estimated simultaneously controlling for all other variables in the model.

Software-determined entry.

A second approach to obtaining a logistic regression model is one that is based purely on statistical significance. In this case, the researcher is not testing a theoretical model but rather is focused on an exploratory hypothesis-generating analysis that is based solely on a computer algorithm. Predictor variables are entered (or removed) from an LR model based on their statistical, not theoretical, significance.

Two basic methods are used in software-determined entry: *stepwise forward* and *stepwise backward* solutions. Each uses set statistical criteria for entry or removal. Two commonly used criteria for both approaches are the likelihood ratio test and the Wald statistic.

A *stepwise forward* solution is one in which the predictor variables are initially examined for their statistically significant individual contributions to the LR model. The predictor variable with the most statistically significant contribution is entered first. The model is then reevaluated, and the next most statistically significant predictor variable given that the first variable is in the model is entered next. This process continues until the remaining predictor variables are no longer statistically significant at a preset level of alpha (e.g., $\alpha = .05$).

A *stepwise backward* solution is one in which all of the predictor variables are entered initially into the LR analysis. The nonsignificant predictor variables are then removed one by one based on their lack of statistical significance until only statistically significant predictor variables remain in the LR solution. The researcher can use either the significance of the likelihood ratio test or the Wald statistic to determine entry (or exit) of the predictor variables LR solution.

Regardless of approach, a method that is solely dependent on statistical significance is fraught with challenges. Critics liken this software-determined approach to going on a "fishing expedition." That is, while this approach has merit (e.g., nonsignificant predictors will not enter into the LR model), it also tends to produce unstable and less reproducible solutions. For example, age ($p = .04$) and years of schooling ($p = .043$) may both be statistically significant predictors of the birthweight of the baby, but, in the stepwise forward solution, age will enter first into the model because of its lower p value. Years of schooling could then be "bumped" from entry once age of the adolescent has entered into the model. Alternatively, future research may find that the p values of these two variables result in years of schooling coming in first, leading to different results and poor reproducibility. While this situation is less likely to occur with a stepwise backward LR approach, it still is a concern when researchers rely solely on software-determined entry criteria. These approaches tend to take advantage of random variations in the data and, as a result, produce results that are difficult to replicate in other samples.

While stepwise approaches offer the possibility of obtaining unexpected and often interesting findings, these results can also have occurred purely by chance. Osborne (2015) points out that this approach could be of value when the researcher's interest is in data mining of very large data sets; for smaller data sets, however, testing a clearly delineated theoretical model is preferable.

Computer-Generated Output for Multivariate Logistic Regression

Step 1. Undertake a logistic regression analysis using a statistical computer package or Internet resource. As was indicated earlier in this chapter, our first step is to undertake the LR analysis. In our hypothetical example, we are interested in four predictor variables (which, let us assume, were selected after a careful review of the literature) that have the potential for predicting whether or not a pregnant adolescent will give birth to a normal-birthweight infant: the intervention (usual care vs. a group-based intervention), number of prenatal visits, being a current smoker, and quality of the adolescent's relationship with her parent(s). While numerous other predictor variables could potentially predict birthweight outcomes (e.g., age of the adolescent, her delivery experience, income level, and drug- and alcohol-related experiences), we will focus on these four predictor variables to help us understand the process of LR. The data set that we will be using is the same as that which we used for the simple LR analysis: pregnant teen data for logistic regression-4 predictors.sav (study.sagepub.com/pett2e).

Because we do not have a clear idea which of these four predictor variables has the strongest effect on our LR equation, we will use the *Enter* approach to LR. That is, we will enter all of these variables simultaneously into the LR analysis. Heeding the advice of several authors (e.g., Garson, 2014; Menard, 2010; Osborne, 2015), we will also examine the likelihood ratio tests for the statistically significant variables after we have determined our model fit.

Figure 10.5 presents the SPSS for Windows (v. 22–23) syntax and SPSS for Windows commands for our multivariate LR. The dependent variable, *normal_birthweight_baby,*

Figure 10.5 Syntax and computer commands for a multivariate logistic regression analysis generated in SPSS for Windows (v. 22–23).

```
***Data set: Pregnant teen data for logistic regression-4 predictors.sav***

LOGISTIC REGRESSION VARIABLES normal_birthweight_baby
  /METHOD=ENTER Group_assignment quality_parental_relationship Prenatal_visits
    current_smoker
  /METHOD=ENTER Group_assignment
  /SAVE=PRED COOK LEVER DFBETA SRESID ZRESID DEV
  /CLASSPLOT
  /CASEWISE OUTLIER(2)
  /PRINT=GOODFIT CORR ITER(1) CI(95)
  /CRITERIA=PIN(0.05) POUT(0.10) ITERATE(20) CUT(0.5).
```

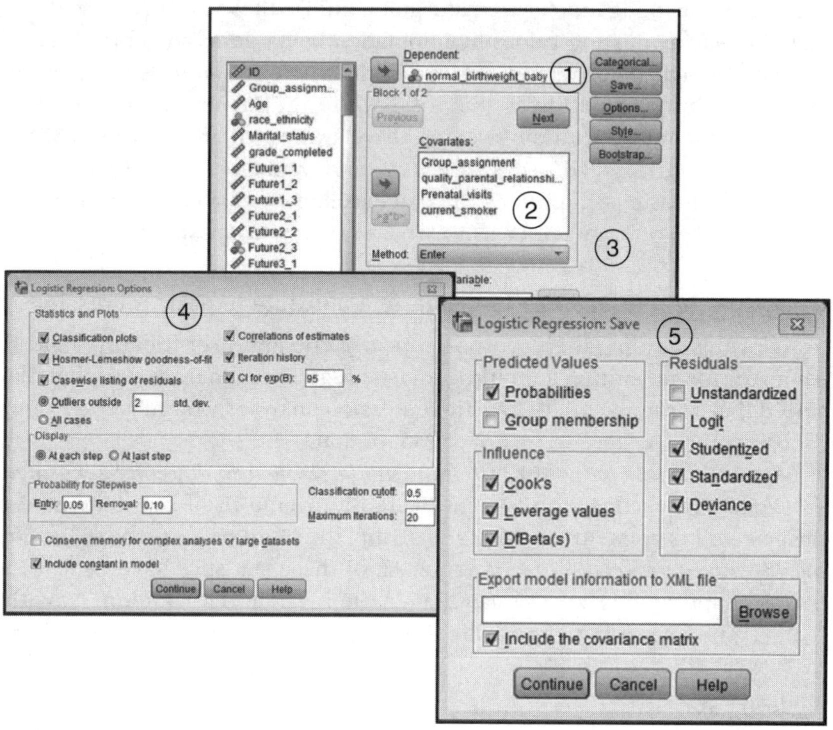

is dichotomous (0 = low-birthweight baby, 1 = normal-birthweight baby) and has been placed in the dependent list (1); the predictor variables are assigned to the *Covariates* list (2). Because we have elected to use the *Enter . . .* command (3), all of our predictor variables will be evaluated simultaneously for their contribution to our LR model.

By clicking on *Options . . .* we can choose among a set of statistics and plots (4). These include the classification plots, the Hosmer-Lemeshow goodness-of-fit test, case-wise listing of residuals, correlations of estimates, the iteration history, and the 95% confidence interval for the odds ratio. The classification cutoff has been set at the default (.50). The *Save . . .* function gives us the option of saving both the predicted values, influence values, and residuals (5). You will want to be conservative in what you save initially since these values are added to the end of the data file and can become a confusing array of extra variables.

Figure 10.6A–C presents the output that was generated from the SPSS for Windows computer commands presented in Figure 10.5. In Figure 10.6A, we are presented with the initial report of the numbers of cases included in the analysis and internal coding scheme for the outcome variable. Note that we have 17 missing cases (17.0%) out of a total of 100 respondents (1). This is a large amount of missing data that need to be examined in greater detail. Typically, we would want to review our questionnaires and data set to determine why these respondents have been excluded from the analysis. Are they missing at random, or is there something more systematic going on? Do these cases represent errors in coding? Would replacing missing values by imputation help address this problem?

Since LR in SPSS for Windows assumes that there are no missing values, it is important that we identify and address this loss. While the LR program itself does not offer a mechanism to address missing values, there are two programs within SPSS for Windows (*Analyze . . . Missing Values Analysis . . .* and *Transform . . . Missing Values . . .*) that can help address missing values. Several excellent resources (Osborne, 2015; Tabachnick & Fidell, 2013) offer guidance as to what to do about missing data.

Using an Internet resource to generate a multiple logistic regression.

As of this writing, there do not appear to be any user-friendly—and free—Internet resources for generating a multiple logistic regression analysis. For that reason, it is suggested that, for multivariate logistic regression analyses, you make use of proven statistical computer packages (e.g., SAS, SPSS, or Stata).

Step 2. Evaluate the overall fit of the model: How well does our generated LR model fit our data? The second step is to evaluate the overall fit of our generated model. To do this, we will examine the model χ^2 statistic, the Hosmer-Lemeshow goodness-of-fit test, the R^2 values, and classification table. All of these statistics have been described earlier in this chapter when we evaluated a simple bivariate LR solution. Now that we have a multivariate LR solution, hopefully this assessment will become even clearer.

Model χ^2 statistic.

The model χ^2 statistic (45.266) with $df = 4$ is presented in Figure 10.6C (2). Recall that the model χ^2 represents the difference between the –2LL for the beginning block of the

Figure 10.6 Computer-generated output for a multivariate logistic regression analysis generated in SPSS for Windows (v. 22–23).

A. Initial report of the variables included in the logistic regression analysis

Case Processing Summary

Unweighted Cases[a]		N	Percent
Selected Cases	Included in Analysis	83	83.0
	Missing Cases	(1) 17	17.0
	Total	100	100.0
Unselected Cases		0	.0
Total		100	100.0

a. If weight is in effect, see classification table for the total number of cases.

Dependent Variable Encoding

Original Value	Internal Value
.00 less than 2500 gr	0
1.00 2500 gr or more	1

B. Reported output for Beginning Block (0) (Constant only)

Iteration History[a,b,c]

Iteration		-2 Log likelihood	Coefficients: Constant
Step 0	1	104.730	.699
	2	104.713	.729
	3	(3) 104.713	.730

a. Constant is included in the model.

b. Initial -2 Log Likelihood: 104.713

c. Estimation terminated at iteration number 3 because parameter estimates changed by less than .001.

Classification Table[a,b] (9)

	Observed		Predicted: normal_birthweight_baby How much did child weight at birth? .00 less than 2500 gr	Predicted: normal_birthweight_baby How much did child weight at birth? 1.00 2500 gr or more	Percentage Correct
Step 0	normal_birthweight_baby How much did child weight at birth?	.00 less than 2500 gr	0	27	.0
		1.00 2500 gr or more	0	56	100.0
	Overall Percentage				67.5

a. Constant is included in the model.

b. The cut value is .500

C. Results after entering the individual predictors (Block 1, Method = Enter)

Iteration History[a,b,c,d]

Iteration		-2 Log likelihood	Coefficients: Constant	Group_assignment	quality_parental_relationship_interval	Prenatal_visits	current_smoker
Step 1	1	65.777	-4.549	.845	.104	.557	-.909
	2	60.080	-6.629	1.323	.147	.877	-1.359
	3	59.460	-7.561	1.548	.165	1.041	-1.572
	4	59.447	-7.718	1.586	.168	1.071	-1.609
	5	59.447	-7.722	1.587	.168	1.072	-1.610
	6	59.447	-7.722	1.587	.168	1.072	-1.610

a. Method: Enter

b. Constant is included in the model.

c. Initial -2 Log Likelihood: 104.713

d. Estimation terminated at iteration number 6 because parameter estimates changed by less than .001.

Omnibus Tests of Model Coefficients

		Chi-square	df	Sig.
Step 1	Step	45.266	4	.000
(2)	Block	45.266	4	.000
	Model	45.266	4	.000

(Continued)

Figure 10.6 (Continued)

Hosmer and Lemeshow Test

Step	Chi-square	df	Sig.
1	(5) 7.129	8	.523

Contingency Table for Hosmer and Lemeshow Test (6)

		normal_birthweight_baby How much did child weight at birth? = .00 less than 2500 gr		normal_birthweight_baby How much did child weight at birth? = 1.00 2500 gr or more		
		Observed	Expected	Observed	Expected	Total
Step 1	1	7	7.489	1	.511	8
	2	(7) 7	6.548	1	1.452	8
	3	3	5.122	5	2.878	8
	4	6	3.493	3	5.507	9
	5	2	1.714	6	6.286	8
	6	1	1.138	7	6.862	8
	7	1	.689	7	7.311	8
	8	0	.410	8	7.590	8
	9	0	.276	8	7.724	8
	10	0	.121	10	9.879	10

Model Summary

Step	-2 Log likelihood	Cox & Snell R Square	Nagelkerke R Square
1	(4) 59.447[a]	(8) .420	(8) .586

a. Estimation terminated at iteration number 6 because parameter estimates changed by less than .001.

Variables in the Equation

		(18) B	S.E.	(14) Wald	df	(15) Sig.	(16) Exp(B)	(17) 95% C.I.for EXP(B) Lower	Upper
Step 1[a]	Group_assignment	1.587	.694	5.238	1	.022	4.890	1.256	19.040
	quality_parental_relationship_interval	.168	.049	11.894	1	.001	1.183	1.075	1.302
	Prenatal_visits	1.072	.449	5.697	1	.017	2.922	1.211	7.046
	current_smoker	-1.610	.683	5.558	1	.018	.200	.052	.762
	Constant	-7.722	2.050	14.191	1	.000	.000		

a. Variable(s) entered on step 1: Group_assignment, quality_parental_relationship_interval, Prenatal_visits, current_smoker.

Classification Table[a] (10)

Observed			Predicted: normal_birthweight_baby How much did child weight at birth? .00 less than 2500 gr	1.00 2500 gr or more	Percentage Correct
Step 1	normal_birthweight_baby How much did child weight at birth?	.00 less than 2500 gr	18	9	66.7
		1.00 2500 gr or more	7	49	87.5
	Overall Percentage				80.7

a. The cut value is .500

```
          Step number: 1

          Observed Groups and Predicted Probabilities

                                                 (11)
       8 +                                                                                                    +
         I                                                                                                    I
         I                                                                                           (13)     I
F        I                                                                                                    I
R      6 +                                                                                               2  2 +
E        I                                                                                               2  2 I
Q        I              (12)                                                                             2  2 I
U        I                                                                                               2  2 I
E      4 +            2                                                                      2           2  22+
N        I            2                                                                      2           2  22I
C        I            1                                                                      2  2    2 2 22222I
Y        I            1                                                                      2  2    2 2 22222I
       2 +  1         1              12                 2                      2             2  2    222222222+
         I  1         1              12                 2                      2             2  2    222222222I
         I  1111 1    1 11 2 1      111    2  2   1     2 1   11   2     1   121 1   2222   12222112 222222222I
         I  1111 1    1 11 2 1      111    2  2   1     2 1   11   2     1   121 1   2222   12222112 222222222I
Predicted ---------+---------+---------+---------+---------+---------+---------+---------+---------+----------
  Prob:   0       .1        .2        .3        .4        .5        .6        .7        .8        .9         1
  Group:  1111111111111111111111111111111111111111111111111122222222222222222222222222222222222222222222222222

          Predicted Probability is of Membership for 2500 gr or more
          The Cut Value is .50
          Symbols: 1 - less than 2500 gr
                   2 - 2500 gr or more
          Each Symbol Represents .5 Cases.
```

Correlation Matrix

		Constant	Group_assignment	quality_parental_relationship_interval	Prenatal_visits	current_smoker
Step 1	Constant	1.000	-.260	-.842	-.499	.081
	Group_assignment	-.260	1.000	.053	.183	.009
	quality_parental_relationship_interval	-.842	.053	1.000	.028	-.185
	Prenatal_visits	-.499	.183	.028	1.000	-.155
	current_smoker	.081	.009	-.185	-.155	1.000

Casewise List[b]

Case	Selected Status[a]	Observed normal_birth weight_baby How much did child weight at birth?	Predicted	Predicted Group	Temporary Variable Resid	ZResid
19	S	1**	.886	2	-.886	-2.795
30	S	2**	.126	1	.874	2.637
51	S	1**	.878	2	-.878	-2.678

a. S = Selected, U = Unselected cases, and ** = Misclassified cases.

b. Cases with studentized residuals greater than 2.000 are listed.

LR analysis with only the constant (–2LL = 104.713 (3)) and –2LL for the model in which all of our predictor variables have been entered (–2LL = 59.447 (4)). Therefore, the model χ^2 = (104.713 – 59.447 = 45.266) (2). There are 4 degrees of freedom for this statistic because there are four predictor variables and one constant in the full model and $df = 5 - 1 = 4$.

A statistically significant value (in our case, $p = .000$) indicates that the "full" model is statistically significantly better than the "null" model with only the constant present. As we noted with the simple bivariate LR model, the step, block, and model χ^2 values are the same since we entered all four predictor variables simultaneously as a block into Step 1. Had we used a stepwise approach, these values would have been different from one another.

Hosmer-Lemeshow goodness-of-fit test.

The Hosmer-Lemeshow goodness-of-fit test (7.129) is also presented in Figure 10.6C (5). Recall that the null hypothesis for this statistic states that the model fits the data. For that reason, we do not want to reject the null hypothesis. Since the p value for this test ($p = .523$) is less than our prestated $\alpha = .05$, we will not reject the null hypothesis and conclude that our model fits the data.

The 10 × 2 contingency table from which the Hosmer-Lemeshow goodness-of-fit test was generated is also presented in Figure 10.6C (6). Each of the rows (1–10) represents deciles (e.g., 1 = .10, 2 = .20, 9 = .90, 10 = 1.00). The Hosmer-Lemeshow χ^2 statistic (7.129, $df = 10 - 2 = 8$) is obtained by subtracting the expected value for a given cell (*Exp*) from its observed (*Obs*) value, squaring this value, dividing by the expected value and then adding these resulting values across each cell:

$$\chi^2 = \Sigma\frac{(Obs - Exp)^2}{Exp} = \frac{(7.0 - 7.489)^2}{7.489} + \frac{(1.0 - 0.511)^2}{0.511} + \ldots + \frac{(0 - 0.121)^2}{0.121}$$

$$+ \frac{(10 - 9.879)^2}{9.879} = 7.129$$

Notice that the observed and expected values for each of the cells of this 10 × 2 contingency table for the Hosmer-Lemeshow test in Figure 10.6C (7) are rather similar, indicating that this χ^2 statistic is not likely to be statistically significant. Note also that the highest frequencies for low-birthweight babies (< 2,500 grams) are located in the lower deciles (e.g., .10–.40), while those for the normal-birthweight babies are located in the upper deciles (e.g., .50–1.00), again suggesting a "good" model fit.

R^2 values.

The Model Summary in Figure 10.6C reports that the Cox and Snell and Nagelkerke R^2 values are .420 and .586, respectively (8). Using the criteria suggested by Garson (personal communication, October 18, 2014), these would be considered "moderate" effects. According to the guidelines offered in Table 10.5, these effects would be considered "moderate to strong" effects.

As indicated when we examined a simple bivariate LR analysis, we could either report the results of these pseudo-R^2 values in our summary statement or calculate and report the McFadden (aka likelihood ratio) R^2:

$$R^2_{McF} = R^2_L = {Model(\chi^2)}\big/{-2LL_0} = 45.266\big/59.447 = .761$$

Both the Garson and Table 10.5 criteria indicate that this R^2 value (.761) is a "strong" effect size.

Classification tables.

In Figure 10.6A–C, we are also presented with two classification tables: one that assesses the model that contains only the constant (Figure 10.6A (9)), while the other evaluates the model containing all of the predictor variables (Figure 10.6C (10)). The null model that contained only the constant was assessed by assigning all of the pregnant adolescents to the outcome category that had the greatest sample size (those whose infants were of normal birthweight, $n = 56$). With only the constant in the model, the total overall percentage of correctly classified adolescents was 67.5%, with 0% of the adolescents with low-birthweight babies being correctly identified.

Figure 10.6C presents the classification table for the full model (10). Seventy-seven (18 + 49 = 67) of the 83 babies born to the adolescent mothers were correctly classified (80.7%). Nine babies were *false positives*. That is, based on our full model, they were assigned to the normal-birthweight group when in fact they were of low birthweight. Seven babies were *false negatives:* They were predicted to be of low birthweight when in fact they were of normal birthweight. Our *sensitivity value* (i.e., the percentage of cases correctly classified as a normal-birthweight baby) was 87.5% (.875 * 100 = 87.5%):

$$\textit{Sensitivity} = \frac{\textit{true positives}}{\textit{true positives} + \textit{false negatives}} = \frac{49}{49+7} = \frac{49}{56} = 0.875$$

Specificity was 66.7% (.667 * 100 = 66.7%):

$$\textit{Specificity} = \frac{\textit{true negatives}}{\textit{true negatives} + \textit{false positives}} = \frac{18}{18+9} = \frac{18}{27} = 0.667$$

It is apparent that the full model did a better job in correctly predicting normal-birthweight infants (87.5%) than low-birthweight babies (66.7%).

The plot of the probability values in Figure 10.6C (11) indicates visually where the errors in prediction have occurred. Recall that, based on the predetermined default cutoff value of .50, predicted probability values < .50 for the outcome variable (*normal_birth weight*) were assigned to the low-birthweight group (*normal_birthweight* = *0*); probability values ≥ .50 were assigned to the normal-birthweight group (*normal_birthweight* = *1*). Looking at the plot of these probability values, we can examine those cases that were at the extremes. For example, there were two cases in which, based on our full model, the babies were predicted to be in the low-birthweight group when, in fact, they were normal-birthweight babies (≥ 2,500 grams) (12). Similarly, there were seven cases at the extreme who, based on the probability values generated by the full model, were predicted to be in the normal-birthweight group when, in fact, the adolescent mothers had given birth to a low-birthweight baby (13).

To summarize the results of examining our overall model fit, with our four predictor variables, we have a good model fit. The model χ^2 is statistically significant (p < .001), indicating that our full model is superior to the null model. The Hosmer-Lemeshow test was not statistically significant (p = .523), indicating that, with the four predictor variables in the model, the full model fit the data. The calculated McFadden pseudo-R^2 (.761) demonstrated a strong effect. The classification table for the full model indicated that the overall percentage of correctly classified cases increased from 67.5% to 80.7%. However, the greatest percentage of correctly classified cases was with the normal-birthweight infants (87.5%) compared to the low-birthweight infants (66.7%). These results suggest that we would want to examine our data more closely to determine why our model did a better job of predicting normal-birthweight infants compared to low-birthweight infants. Now that we have examined the overall model fit, our next step is to examine the contribution of each of our predictor variables to the full model.

Step 3. Examine the beta coefficients, their significance levels, the odds ratios for each predictor variable, and their confidence intervals. Earlier in this chapter, we examined several approaches that can be used to assess the contributions of the predictor variables to the LR model. These included the Wald and likelihood ratio tests, as well as the odds ratios and their confidence intervals. Now that we have multiple predictor variables in our model, we will also examine the use of standardized beta coefficients to determine which predictor variables have the strongest impact on the outcome variable (normal-birthweight baby). We will also consider whether we should add interaction terms to our model.

Wald statistics.

The Wald statistics for the full model are presented in Figure 10.6C (14). You will recall from our earlier discussion that, in SPSS for Windows, these statistics are obtained using the following formula:

$$\text{Wald statistic} = \left(\frac{\text{B}}{\text{SE}_{\text{B}}}\right)^2$$

This Wald statistic is distributed as a χ^2 with $df = 1$. We will reject the null hypothesis that the predictor variable being examined is not a statistically significant contributor to our model if the p value we obtain (labelled *Sig* in SPSS for Windows) is less than our stated alpha level (e.g., $\alpha = .05$).

The p values for the Wald statistics that are presented in Figure 10.6C (15) indicate that all of the predictor variables that have been entered into our model are statistically significant with p values ranging from $p = .001$ (quality of the adolescent's relationship with her parents) to $p = .022$ (group assignment).

Likelihood ratio tests.

Likelihood ratio tests are generated by evaluating each predictor variable for its unique contribution to the improvement of the full model given the other independent variables in the LR equation. The LR model is calculated with and without the predictor variable of interest in the model, and the resulting model χ^2 values are compared. For our model with four predictors, we would need to run one analysis with the full model, run four separate LR analyses excluding one of the predictor variables, and then compare the results of the full model with that which excludes the predictor variable of interest. Assessing the difference between these two model χ^2 values represents the likelihood ratio test. It is a χ^2 with $df = 1$.

To obtain a full model in SPSS for Windows, go to *Analyze . . . Regression . . . Binary Logistic . . .* and then enter all the predictor variables of interest. After running that analysis and obtaining the model χ^2 value, repeat the process by removing one of the predictor variables from the model (e.g., group assignment) and comparing that resulting model χ^2 value with the full model.

Table 10.8 summarizes the results of these likelihood ratio tests. Unfortunately, in SPSS for Windows (v. 22–23), it is not possible to obtain the actual p values for the model χ^2 values for the differences. These can easily be obtained, however, by accessing an Internet χ^2 calculator (e.g., http://danielsoper.com/statcalc3/calc.aspx?id=11) and posting the generated model χ^2 difference value (e.g., 5.731) and its degrees of freedom (e.g., $df = 1$). This will return the p value for the model χ^2 difference (e.g., .016).

Table 10.8 Summary of the results for the likelihood ratio tests generated in SPSS for Windows

Full Model	*Excluded Predictor*	*Model χ^2 Full (df = 5)*	*Model χ^2 without predictor (df = 4)*	*Model χ^2 Difference (df = 1)*	p	*Wald*	p
Group assignment	Group assignment	45.266	39.531	5.731	.016	5.238	.022
Current smoker	Current smoker		39.254	6.012	.014	5.558	.018
# prenatal visits	# prenatal visits		36.822	8.444	.004	5.697	.017
Quality relationship with parent(s)	Quality relationship with parent(s)		27.040	18.226	.00002	11.894	.0006

Not surprisingly, since all of the Wald statistics were statistically significant, the resulting χ^2 difference values were also statistically significant at $\alpha < .05$. Notice, however, that in each instance, the model χ^2 difference values were all larger with lower p values than the Wald statistics, which are also χ^2 values with $df = 1$. Since the results of the Wald statistics and the likelihood ratio tests are somewhat discrepant, we might follow the suggestion of Hosmer et al. (2013) and report the likelihood ratio tests. In the literature, however, you will likely see the Wald statistic most often reported probably because of its ease of calculation.

Interpretation of the odds ratios and confidence intervals.

Returning to Figure 10.6C, we can now evaluate and interpret the ORs (16) and 95% CIs (17) for our predictor variables. These values ranged from .200 (95% CI: .052, .762) for current smoker to 4.890 (95% CI: 1.258, 19.040) for group assignment.

There are several issues that we need to address regarding the interpretation of these ORs and CIs. First, notice that there are OR values greater and less than 1.0. You will recall that OR values < 1.0 represent a *protective* effect: A decrease in exposure to the predictor variable increases the odds of obtaining a 1 on the dichotomous outcome variable. OR values > 1.0 indicate that the exposure increases the odds of obtaining a 1 on the outcome variable. OR values = 1 indicate that the predictor variable is not a statistically significant contributor to the LR model. It also means that the 95% CI will contain the value of 1.0 since we cannot reject the null hypothesis that the predictor is not a statistically significant contributor to the model. The value of OR = 1 could potentially be the true OR in the population.

Since the size of an odds ratio changes depending on what other predictor variables are in the model, we need to acknowledge their presence by adding the statement, *Controlling for other variables in the model. . . .* A similar statement also needs to be made when interpreting the confidence interval for the odds ratio.

We also need to be careful not to use the OR values as a determination of the importance of a given predictor variable unless all of the predictor variables are on the same scale of measurement. The reason for this is that the size of an OR depends, in part, on the scale of measurement of the predictor variable. For example, the OR for group assignment, a binary variable coded 0 and 1, was 4.890 (Wald p value = .022) (Figure 10.6C). In contrast, the OR for the quality of the adolescent's relationship with her parent(s) (a continuous variable, range: 20–50) was 1.183 (Wald p = .001) (Figure 10.6C). The OR interpretation for the group assignment variable is relatively straightforward:

> Controlling for the other variables in the model, pregnant adolescents who were in the group-based intervention group (group assignment =1) were 4.89 times more likely to give birth to a normal-birthweight infant than adolescents who were in the usual-care group (group assignment = 0).

In contrast, the OR interpretation for the predictor variable, quality of the adolescent's relationship with her parent(s), would be as follows:

> Controlling for the other variables in the model, for every 1-point increase in the adolescent's score on the relationship variable, there was a 1.183 times greater likelihood that she would give birth to a normal-birthweight infant compared to an adolescent with a 1-point lower score.

While an OR = 1.183 does not look particularly strong, it only reflects the odds of an occurrence given a 1-point increase in the predictor variable. As Menard (2010) has observed, ORs are least informative for continuous predictor variables. If, for example, we were to divide this predictor by 5 such that the range of our scale is now 4 to 10 rather than 20 to 50, the resulting odds ratio would increase substantially. That is one reason why researchers often choose to collapse continuous data into smaller categories so that the resulting OR is more easily interpretable. As part of the exercises at the end of this chapter, you will be asked to collapse the relationship data and compare the results.

Notice that the OR for current smoker is *protective* (OR = .200) (Figure 10.6C). Given that this is a nominal-level dichotomous predictor variable (0 = nonsmoker, 1 = smoker), the OR can be interpreted as follows:

> Controlling for the other variables in the model, adolescents who are smokers are 80% ([1 – .20 = .80] * 100 = 80%) less likely to have a normal-birthweight baby than adolescents who were nonsmokers.

An easier way to interpret this *protective effect* is to take the inverse of the OR (1/.20 = 5.0) and interpret this OR as follows:

> Controlling for the other variables in the model, the odds of an adolescent who was a nonsmoker giving birth to a normal-birthweight infant was five times greater than for an adolescent who was a smoker.

Table 10.9 summarizes the interpretation of the odds ratios and their confidence intervals for the four predictor variables in our model.

Table 10.9 Summary of Interpretation of Odds Ratios and 95% Confidence Intervals for the Full Model

Predictor variable	*Odds ratio (OR)*	*95% confidence interval (CI)*	*Interpretation: OR*	*Interpretation: 95% CI*
Group assignment (0 = usual care, 1 = group-based intervention)	4.89	1.26–19.04	Controlling for the other variables in the model, the odds of an adolescent in the group-based intervention giving birth to a normal birthweight baby is 4.89 times greater than an adolescent in the usual care group.	Controlling for the other variables in the model, there is a 95% probability that the true odds for the effect of group assigment on having a normal birthweight baby in the population lies between 1.26 and 19.04.
Quality relationship with parents (QRP) (range: 20–50)	1.18	1.08–1.30	Controlling for the other variables in the model, for every 1 point increase in the QRP variable there is a 1.18 (or 18%) increase in the odds of an adolescent giving birth to a normal birthweight infant.	Controlling for the other variables in the model, there is a 95% probability that the true odds for the effect of the quality of an adolescent's relationship with her parents on having a normal birth-weight baby in the population lies between 1.08 and 1.30.
# prenatal visits (1 = no visits, 2 = 1–3 visits, 3 = 4+ visits)	2.92	1.21–7.05	Controlling for the other variables in the model, adolescents who have more prenatal visits (e.g., 1–3 visits) are 2.92 times more likely to have a normal birthweight child than those adolescents who have had no prenatal visits.	Controlling for the other variables in the model, there is a 95% probability that the true odds for the effect of prenatal visits on having a normal birthweight infant in this pregnant adolescent population lies beteen 1.21 and 7.05.
Current smoker (0 = no, 1 = yes)	0.20	0.05–0.76	Controlling for the other variables in the model, adolescents who are non smokers are (1/0.20 = 5.0) 5.0 times more likely to have a normal birthweight child than adolescents who are smokers.	Controlling for the other variables in the model, there is a 95% probability that the true odds for the effect of smoking in this pregnant adolescent population lies between 1.32 (1/0.76 = 1.32) and 20.0 (1/0.05 = 20.0).

Standardized logistic regression beta coefficients.

In Figure 10.6C, we are presented with the unstandardized beta coefficients for the predictor variables in our full model (18). As with OLS multiple regression, the size of these unstandardized beta coefficients is influenced by the predictor variables' scale of measurement. The signs of these unstandardized coefficients (positive or negative) indicate whether an increase in the predictor value will increase (+) or decrease (–) the odds of obtaining a 1 on the outcome variable.

If all of the predictor variables were on the same scale of measurement, we could compare these unstandardized versions without any difficulty. Given a set of predictor variables that have diverse metrics, we would need to examine the standardized LR beta coefficients in order to determine which predictor variables have the strongest influence on our outcome variable, normal-birthweight baby. Unfortunately, we are not given these standardized beta coefficients in the logistic regression output generated by SPSS for Windows (v. 22–23). We will need to calculate them by hand.

While calculating standardized beta coefficients may sound daunting, it is not as difficult as it might seem. Menard (2010) offers an excellent chapter on approaches used to convert logistic regression coefficients into their standardized versions. He suggests that the following formula can be used to estimate a standardized beta coefficient (p. 89):

$$b^*_{yx} = (b_{yx})(s_x) / \sqrt{s^2_{logit(\hat{Y})} / R^2} = (b_{yx})(s_x)(R) / s_{logit(\hat{Y})}$$

where

b^*_{yx} = the estimated standardized beta coefficient for a predictor variable of interest,

b_{yx} = the unstandardized beta coefficient for that same predictor variable,

s_x = the standard deviation for the predictor variable of interest,

R = the simple correlation between the observed and predicted values for the outcome variable based on the LR model of interest, and

$s_{logit(\hat{Y})}$ = the standard deviation of the logit($\hat{Y}$).

Menard also outlines easy-to-follow steps (p. 89) that can be used to calculate a standardized beta coefficient for each of the predictor variables in a model. These are the steps that we will follow to obtain standardized beta coefficients for our four predictor variables.

First, we need to generate the unstandardized beta coefficients for the predictor variable included in our LR model of interest. As indicated, these unstandardized beta coefficients have been presented to us in Figure 10.6C. Then, using the results generated from our full model, we need to save the predicted values of Y (i.e., $\hat{Y}$). That is easily accomplished by requesting that the predicted values for the probabilities be saved (see Figure 10.5 (5)). These predicted values will show up at the end of the data file (*PRE_1*). Be sure that these are the latest predicted values since additional predicted values will appear each time the model is run.

Next, we need to calculate the zero-order correlation, *R,* between the predicted values of Y (*PRE_1*) and the actual values of Y. We can do this using the commands, *Analyze . . . Correlate . . . Bivariate . . .* and moving the two variables, *Pre_1* and *normal_birthweight,* into the *Variables* box (Figure 10.7 (1)). This command will generate the Pearson correlation (.682) between the predicted probabilities and the actual values of the outcome variable (e.g., normal-birthweight baby) that are presented in Figure 10.7 (2).

The next step is to compute a predicted value of the logit(Y) for each of our cases. We can approach this task in one of two ways. Using our unstandardized LR model, we could compute a logit score, logit(Y), for each of the cases. Recall that the formula for logit($\hat{Y}$) is

$$logit\left(\hat{Y}\right) = b_0 + b_1\left(x_1\right) + b_2\left(x_2\right) + b_3\left(x_3\right) + \ldots + b_k\left(x_k\right)$$

Based on our full model, our logit($\hat{Y}$) is

$$logit\left(\hat{Y}\right) = b_0 + b_1\left(treatment\ group\right) + b_2\left(current\ smoker\right) + b_3\left(number\ of\ prenatal\ visits\right) + b_4\left(quality\ of\ relationship\ with\ parents\right)$$

Given the output for the unstandardized regression coefficients presented to us in Figure 10.6C, we can generate the following equation:

$$logit\left(\hat{Y}\right) = -7.722 + 1.587\left(treatment\ group\right) + \left(-1.610\right)\left(current\ smoker\right) + 1.072\left(number\ of\ prenatal\ visits\right) + 0.168\left(quality\ of\ relationship\ with\ parents\right)$$

The *Transform . . . Compute . . .* command in SPSS for Windows (v. 22–23) opens a dialog box that allows us to create a new variable (*logit_Y_hat*) based on our generated ($\hat{Y}$) for our full model (Figure 10.7 (3)). By clicking on the *Paste . . .* command in that box, we can paste this compute statement into syntax, which could be saved for later use (Figure 10.7 (4)). Descriptives statistics could also be requested. This would result in the summary table of descriptive statistics presented in Figure 10.7 (5).

A second, somewhat easier approach to obtaining the predicted values of the logit(Y) is to use a second equation for the logit($\hat{Y}$) (Menard, 2010, p. 89):

$$logit\left(\hat{Y}\right) = ln\left[\hat{Y} / \left(1 - \hat{Y}\right)\right]$$

where $\hat{Y}$ = the predicted values for the outcome variable that were generated and saved for the LR model.

Using the *Transform . . . Compute . . .* commands we can calculate the values of logit($\hat{Y}$) for each of the cases (Figure 10.7 (6)) and run descriptive statistics. As you can see from the descriptive statistics output, the two formulae for the predicted values of logit($\hat{Y}$) generate similar, although not exact results (mean = 1.23, standard deviation = 2.24 (5)), the differences being attributed to round-off.

Figure 10.7 SPSS for Windows (v. 22–23) commands and output for generating predicted values of logit($\hat{Y}$).

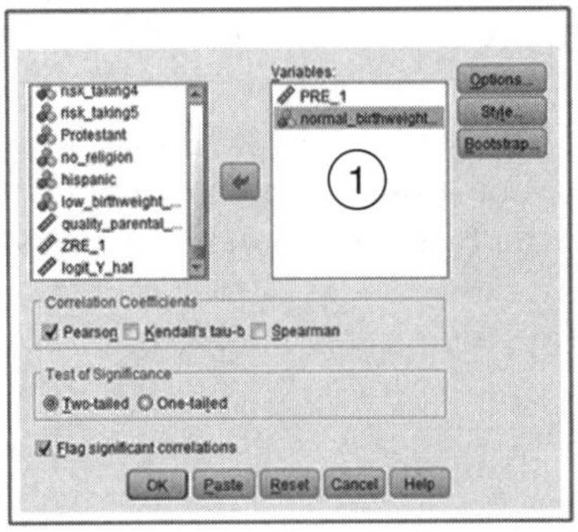

Correlations (2)

		PRE_1 Predicted probability	normal_birthweight_baby How much did child weight at birth?
PRE_1 Predicted probability	Pearson Correlation	1	.682**
	Sig. (2-tailed)		.000
	N	83	83
normal_birthweight_baby How much did child weight at birth?	Pearson Correlation	.682**	1
	Sig. (2-tailed)	.000	
	N	83	100

**. Correlation is significant at the 0.01 level (2-tailed).

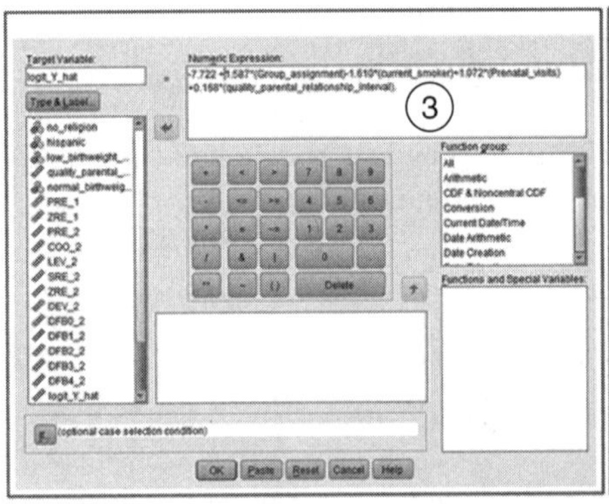

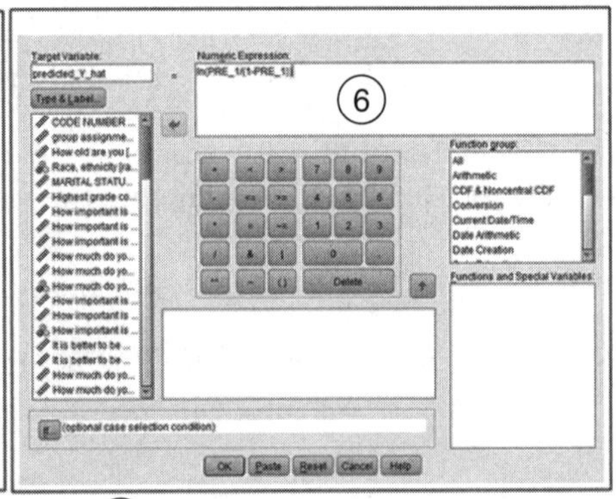

Descriptive Statistics (5)

	N	Minimum	Maximum	Mean	Std. Deviation
logit_Y_hat	83	-3.89	4.98	1.2278	2.24194
predicted_Y_hat	83	-3.89	4.99	1.2368	2.24329
Valid N (listwise)	83				

(4)

```
COMPUTE logit_Y_hat = -7.722+1.587*(Group_assignment) -1.610*(current_smoker)
+1.072*(Prenatal_visits)+ 0.168*(quality_parental_relationship_interval).

COMPUTE predicted_Y_hat = ln(PRE_1/(1-PRE_1)).

CORRELATIONS
 /VARIABLES=PRE_1 normal_birthweight_baby
 /PRINT=TWOTAIL NOSIG
 /MISSING=PAIRWISE.

DESCRIPTIVES VARIABLES=logit_Y_hat predicted_Y_hat
 /STATISTICS=MEAN STDDEV MIN MAX.

EXECUTE.
```

Next, we need to calculate the standard deviations for all of the predictor variables in the LR model. Menard (2010) cautions that these calculated values should be based only on the cases that were used to generate the LR model. Since we have 17 cases that were not included in the LR model, we will need to narrow down our analysis to 83 cases. We can easily achieve this in SPSS for Windows by going to *Data . . . Select cases . . . If condition is satisfied . . .* (Figure 10.8 (1)) and enter the limiting condition into the dialog box, for example, *NOT MISSING(logit_Y_hat)* (2). That will reduce our data set to only those 83 cases used to generate our LR model. Figure 10.8 presents the results of this analysis. Please note that, following this analysis, you want to be sure to change *Select cases . . .* back to the full data set (i.e., *Select all cases . . . all*) (3). The descriptive statistics, including their standard deviations for the variables that we have identified for the 83 cases included in our LR analysis, are also presented (4).

Now that we have all of the values needed to generate the standardized beta coefficients, our final task is to use the formula for b^*_{yx} to generate these values for each of the predictor variables in our LR model:

$$b^*_{yx} = \left(b_{yx}\right)\left(s_x\right)\left(R\right) / s_{logit(\hat{Y})}$$

$$b^*_{\text{group}} = \left(1.587\right)\left(0.503\right)\left(0.682\right) / 2.24 = 0.243$$

$$b^*_{\text{quality relationship}} = \left(0.168\right)\left(7.256\right)\left(0.682\right) / 2.24 = 0.371$$

$$b^*_{\text{prenatal visits}} = \left(1.072\right)\left(0.767\right)\left(0.682\right) / 2.24 = 0.250$$

$$b^*_{\text{current smoker}} = \left(-1.610\right)\left(0.490\right)\left(0.682\right) / 2.24 = -0.240$$

These standardized beta coefficients enable us to evaluate the relative importance of each predictor to the LR model. Their values range between −1.0 and +1.0; higher absolute values indicate a stronger relationship with the outcome variable. Examining the standardized betas for our four predictors, it is apparent that, controlling for the other variables in the model, the quality of the adolescent's relationship with her parent(s) was the strongest predictor of her giving birth to a normal-birthweight baby (b^* = .371). This is followed by number of prenatal visits (b^* = .250), group assignment (b^* = .243), and, finally, the adolescent's current smoking status (b^* = −.240). None of these standardized beta coefficients appear to be very strong predictors of our outcome variable, normal-birthweight baby.

Evaluating the impact of interaction effects on the full model.

From the analyses we have just undertaken, it looks as if our full LR model fits our data relatively well. What about the interaction effects among the predictor variables? Do they contribute to an improvement of our model? The following is a brief discussion of a suggested approach to creating, entering, and evaluating interaction effects among predictor variables. For an in-depth presentation regarding both interaction and curvilinear effects, the reader is referred to an excellent chapter in Osborne (2015): Chapter 8: "Logistic Regression With Multiple Independent Variables."

Figure 10.8 SPSS for Windows (v. 22–23) commands and output for generating standard deviations for the predictor variables (n = 83).

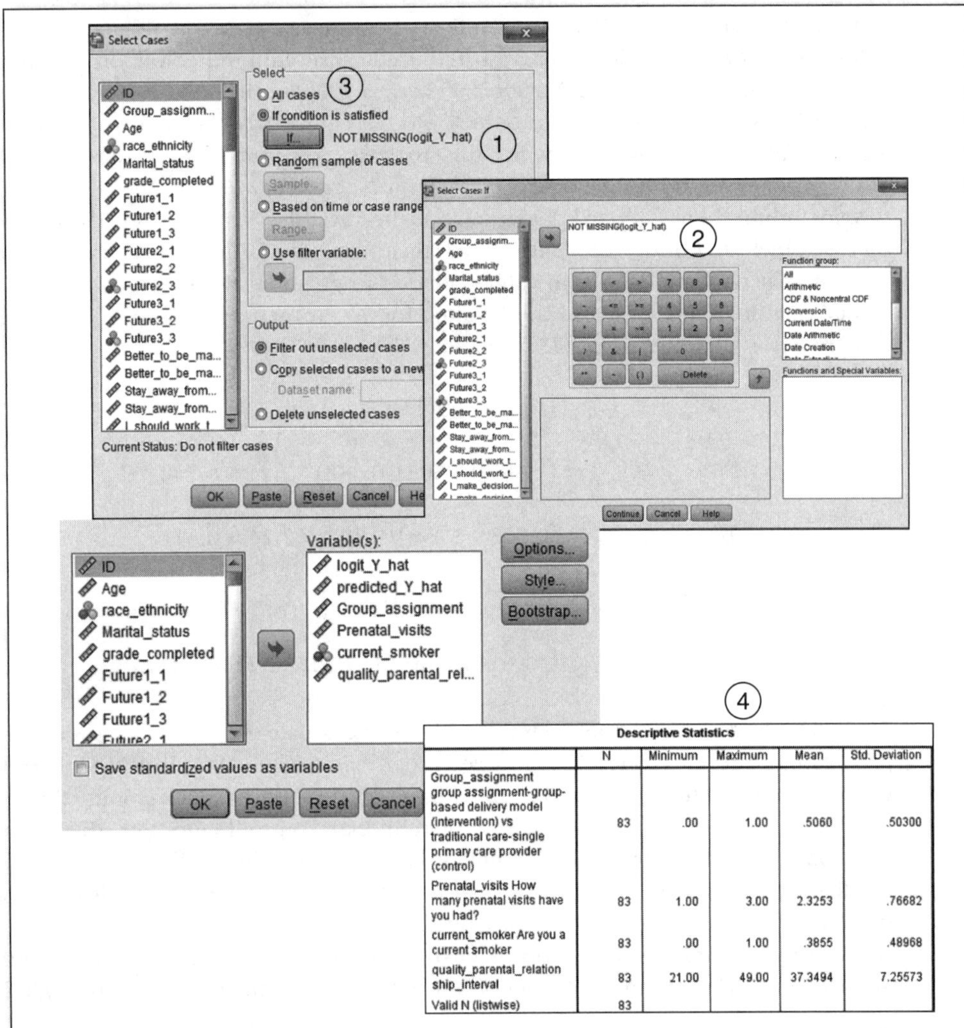

	N	Minimum	Maximum	Mean	Std. Deviation
Group_assignment group assignment-group-based delivery model (intervention) vs traditional care-single primary care provider (control)	83	.00	1.00	.5060	.50300
Prenatal_visits How many prenatal visits have you had?	83	1.00	3.00	2.3253	.76682
current_smoker Are you a current smoker	83	.00	1.00	.3855	.48968
quality_parental_relationship_interval	83	21.00	49.00	37.3494	7.25573
Valid N (listwise)	83				

Interaction effects refer to the interaction between two predictor variables. They represent the added effect of not only the simple effect of each predictor variable separately but also the two variables in combination. For example, we could determine whether there is a significant effect of adding the interaction between current smoking status and the number of prenatal visits, or the interaction between number of prenatal visits and the quality of the adolescent's relationship with her parent(s) on birthweight of the child.

To create an interaction effect, the two variables are multiplied by each other to create a third variable that represents the interaction between the two. When the two variables are dichotomous, this is easily achieved. When one or both predictor variables are continuous, the values for the continuous variables first need to be converted into z scores. This results in their values being "centered" at 0 (Osborne, 2015). Then their cross-products are obtained by multiplying the values of one "centered" variable by the other. Because these interactions are often highly correlated with the predictor variables they have been created from, Osborne (2015) suggests that interaction terms be entered in a separate step. If there are both statistically significant simple and interaction effects, Osborne recommends dropping the simple effects from the model.

Variables that represent the interaction of two or more variables can be obtained easily in SPSS for Windows. First, we will generate the z scores for the continuous predictor variables. By clicking on *Analyze . . . Descriptive statistics . . . Descriptives . . .* we can bring over our continuous variables of choice into the *Variables* box and then check the box that requests that the *standardized values be saved as variables* (Figure 10.9 ①). These standardized continuous variables are then saved at the end of the data file.

The next step is to create the interaction variables. In SPSS for Windows, this can be done by clicking on *Transform . . . Compute Variable . . .* and creating a new interaction variable (e.g., *Interaction_Zquality_parXgroup*) that is the cross-product of the standardized quality of relationship variable and group assignment (Figure 10.9 ②). It would be useful to *Paste . . .* this command into syntax so that additional interaction terms can be quickly created and used in future analyses. Figure 10.9 ③ presents the syntax commands that were generated by the *Transform . . . Compute . . .* statements. Notice that the dichotomous predictor variables were not standardized since they were already coded 0 and 1.

We are now ready to enter the simple predictor variables and their interactions into our model to determine which, if any, of our interaction terms were statistically significant contributors to the full LR model. Using the *Analyze . . . Regression . . . Binary logistic . . .* commands in SPSS for Windows, the four simple predictor variables were entered as a group in the first step using the *Enter . . . command* as presented in Figure 10.10 ①. Notice that the standardized versions of the continuous variables were used in this analysis. The interaction variables were then entered as a group in Step 2 ②. The syntax commands and results of the analysis are summarized in Figure 10.10.

As we would expect given our previous analyses, all of the simple predictor variables that were entered in Step 1 were statistically significant contributors to the full model ③. The model χ^2 value for this first step was also statistically significant (model χ^2 = 45.266, $df = 4$, $p = .000$ ④).

It is apparent, however, that none of the interaction terms that were added into the LR model in Step 2 were statistically significant contributors to the full model ⑤. This was also confirmed by the nonsignificant model χ^2 value for Step 2 (model $\chi^2 = 4.801$, $df = 5$, $p = .441$ ⑥). Not only were all of the interaction terms not statistically significant, but their presence in the model created havoc among the simple predictor variables. Notice that, with the interaction terms added in Step2, the *group assignment* variable is no longer statistically significant ($p = .056$). In addition, the 95% confidence interval went from 1.256 to 19.040 in Step 1 to .938 to 185.912 in Step 2 ⑦. This untenable 95% CI

Figure 10.9 SPSS for Windows (v. 22–23) commands and output for generating standardized scores and interaction terms for the continuous predictor variables in the LR model.

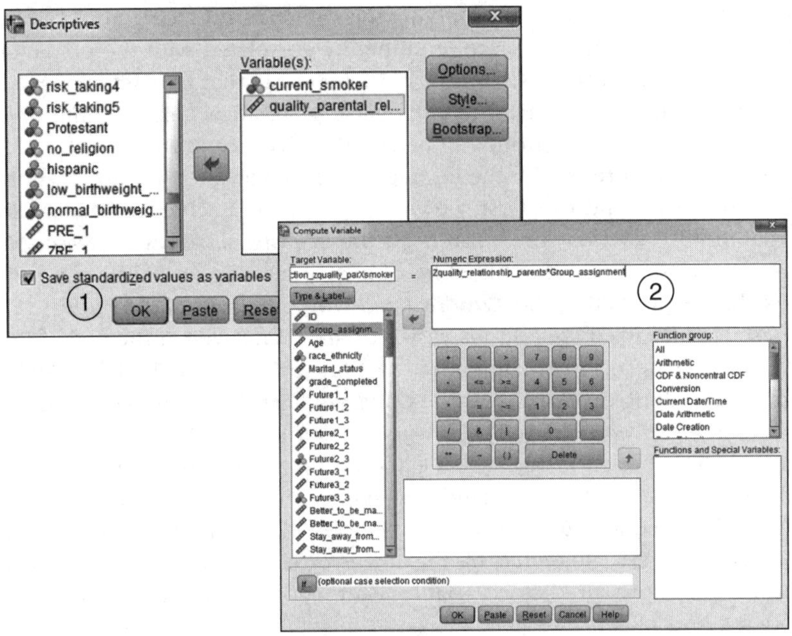


```
COMPUTE Interaction_Zquality_parXgroup = Zquality_relationship_parents*Group_assignment.
COMPUTE Interaction_group_x_smoker = Group_assignment*current_smoker.
COMPUTE Interaction_group_x_zprenatal_visits = Group_assignment*ZPrenatal_visits.
COMPUTE Interaction_zquality_parXsmoker = Zquality_relationship_parents*current_smoker.
COMPUTE Interaction_zquality_parXsmoker = Zquality_relationship_parents*zprenatal_visits.
COMPUTE Interaction_smoker_x_zprenatal_visits = current_smoker*zprenatal_visits.
EXECUTE.
```

3

value in Step 2 indicates that there is serious multicollinearity (i.e., overly strong intercorrelations) among the simple predictor variables and their interactions.

The conclusion to be drawn is that there is no benefit in adding interaction terms to our full model with four simple predictors. We can now move on to evaluating the extent to which this final model meets the assumptions for logistic regression.

Step 4. Evaluate the extent to which the final model meets the assumptions for logistic regression. Table 10.3 summarized the major assumptions and conditions of LR. Because the other assumptions were discussed in detail when examining simple LR, we will

Figure 10.10 SPSS for Windows (v. 22–23) commands and output for evaluating the contribution of the interaction terms to the LR model.

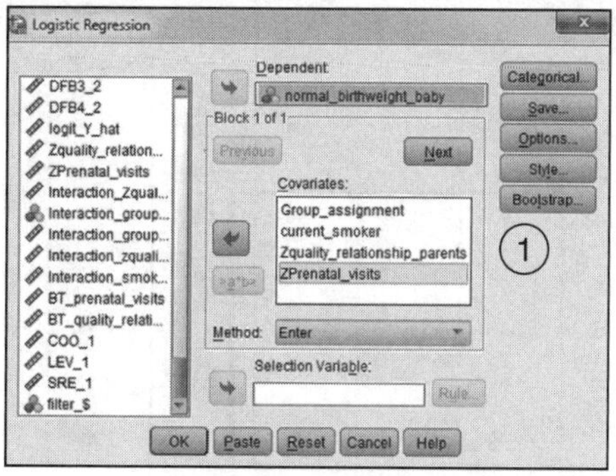

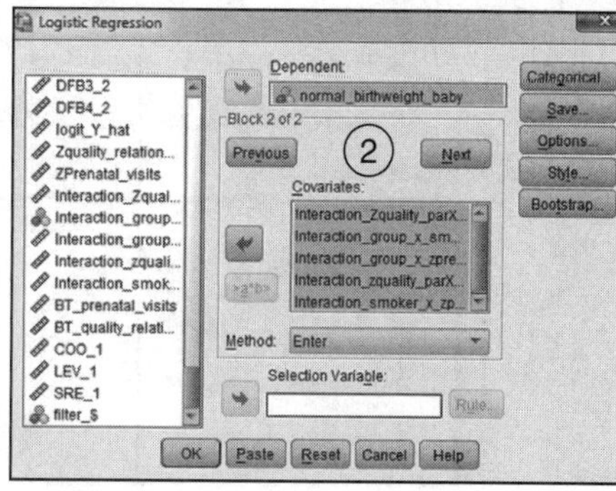

```
LOGISTIC REGRESSION VARIABLES normal_birthweight_baby
  /METHOD=ENTER Group_assignment current_smoker Zquality_relationship_parents ZPrenatal_visits
  /METHOD=ENTER Interaction_Zquality_parXgroup Interaction_group_x_smoker
    Interaction_group_x_zprenatal_visits Interaction_zquality_parXsmoker
    Interaction_smoker_x_zprenatal_visits
  /PRINT=GOODFIT ITER(1) CI(95)
  /CRITERIA=PIN(0.05) POUT(0.10) ITERATE(20) CUT(0.5).
```

Variables in the Equation

		B	S.E.	Wald	df	Sig.	Exp(B)	95% C.I.for EXP(B)	
								Lower	Upper
Step 1[a]	Group_assignment	1.587	.694	5.238	1	.022	4.890	1.256	19.040
	current_smoker	-1.610	.683	5.558	1	.018	.200	(7) .052	.762
(3)	Zquality_relationship_parents	1.236	.358	11.894	1	.001	3.442	1.705	6.950
	ZPrenatal_visits	.808	.339	5.697	1	.017	2.244	1.156	4.358
	Constant	1.034	.536	3.721	1	.054	2.811		

a. Variable(s) entered on step 1: Group_assignment, current_smoker, Zquality_relationship_parents, ZPrenatal_visits.

Omnibus Tests of Model Coefficients

		Chi-square	df	Sig.
Step 1	Step	45.266	4	.000
(4)	Block	45.266	4	.000
	Model	45.266	4	.000

Omnibus Tests of Model Coefficients

		Chi-square	df	Sig.
Step 1	Step	4.801	5	.441
(6)	Block	4.801	5	.441
	Model	50.067	9	.000

(Continued)

Figure 10.10 (Continued)

Variables in the Equation

		B	S.E.	Wald	df	Sig.	Exp(B)	95% C.I.for EXP(B) Lower	Upper
Step 1[a]	Group_assignment	2.583	1.351	3.657	1	.056	13.239	.938	186.912
	current_smoker	-1.734	.867	4.001	1	.045	.177	.032	.966
	Zquality_relationship_parents	.831	.434	3.658	1	.056	2.295	.980	5.378
	ZPrenatal_visits	.533	.490	1.184	1	.277	1.705	.652	4.455
	Interaction_Zquality_parXgroup	1.532	1.048	2.138	1	.144	4.627	.594	36.063
	Interaction_group_x_smoker	.781	1.902	.168	1	.682	2.183	.052	90.857
	Interaction_group_x_zprenatal_visits	1.146	.957	1.433	1	.231	3.145	.482	20.530
	Interaction_zquality_parXsmoker	.389	.381	1.042	1	.307	1.476	.699	3.114
	Interaction_smoker_x_zprenatal_visits	.561	.795	.498	1	.481	1.752	.369	8.330
	Constant	.894	.557	2.581	1	.108	2.445		

a. Variable(s) entered on step 1: Interaction_Zquality_parXgroup, Interaction_group_x_smoker, Interaction_group_x_zprenatal_visits, Interaction_zquality_parXsmoker, Interaction_smoker_x_zprenatal_visits.

(5) (7)

focus on two issues that have not been previously discussed: linearity of the logit and absence of multicollinearity. *Absence of outliers* will be addressed when we examine the residual diagnostics in the next section.

Linearity of the logit.

Linearity of the logit means that there is a linear relationship between the logit and each of the continuous predictor variables. We will use the Box-Tidwell transformation (Box & Tidwell, 1962) to assess this assumption. The Box-Tidwell transformation is obtained by multiplying each of the continuous variables (X_i) by its natural log ($\ln(X_i)$). Then, each transformation is entered into the LR equation along with the associated untransformed predictor variable to determine if the transformation is statistically significant. If a transformation is statistically significant, it is likely that we have violated the assumption of *linearity of the logit* (Hosmer et al., 2013; Menard, 2010). If that should happen, we would need to consider a curvilinear transformation of our continuous predictor variable. Hosmer et al. (2013), Menard (2010), and Osborne (2015) all provide excellent discussions of approaches to addressing curvilinear relationships among predictor variables in LR analyses.

We have two continuous predictor variables in our LR model: quality of the adolescent's relationship with her parent(s) and number of prenatal visits. Using the *Transform . . . Compute Variable . . .* command in SPSS for Windows, we will create two new variables, *BT_prenatal_visits* and *BT_quality_parental_relationship*. Figure 10.11 presents the dialog box (1) and syntax for creating these interaction variables (2). After creating these variables, we will repeat our LR analyses with the two Box-Tidwell transformations added to the analysis (3).

Figure 10.11 SPSS for Windows (v. 22–23) commands and output for generating Box-Tidwell transformations and evaluating the linearity of the logit.

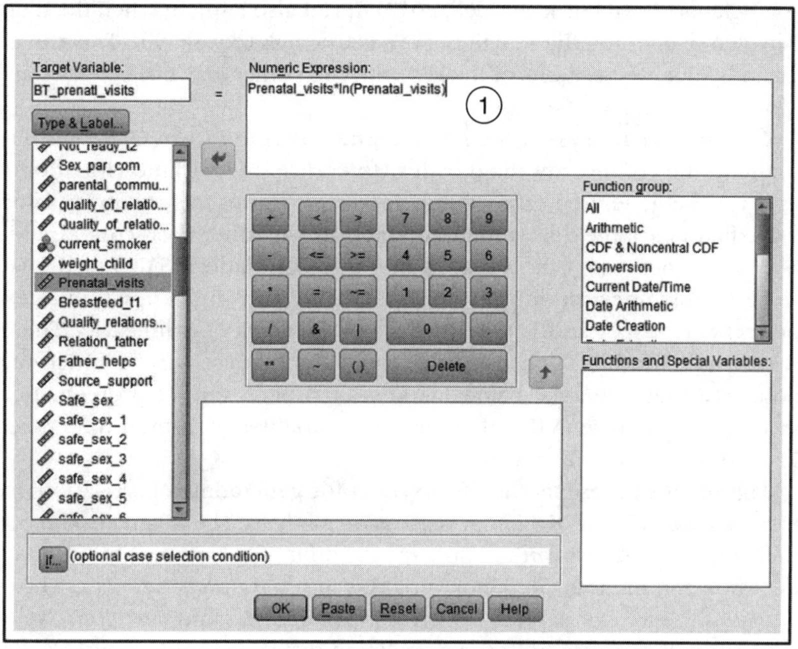


```
COMPUTE BT_prenatal_visits=prenatal_visits*ln(prenatal_visits).        (2)
COMPUTE BT_quality_relationship = quality_parental_relationship * ln(quality_parental_relationship).
EXECUTE.
```

Variables in the Equation

		B	S.E.	Wald	df	Sig.	Exp(B)	95% C.I.for EXP(B)	
								Lower	Upper
Step 1[a]	quality_parental_relationship	-.107	2.164	.002	1	.961	.899	.013	62.514
	Group_assignment	1.523	.710	4.607	1	.032	4.586	1.141	18.429
	Prenatal_visits	2.876	4.568	.396	1	.529	17.740	.002	137269.410
	current_smoker	-1.619	.692	5.471	1	.019	.198	.051	.769
(3)	BT_prenatal_visits	-1.083	2.718	.159	1	(4) .690	.339	.002	69.669
	BT_quality_relationship	.061	.476	.016	1	.899	1.062	.418	2.703
	Constant	-7.580	16.521	.211	1	.646	.001		

a. Variable(s) entered on step 1: BT_prenatal_visits, BT_quality_relationship.

It is evident that the two Box-Tidwell transformations for number of prenatal visits and quality of the adolescent's relationship with her parent(s) were not statistically significant (p = .690 and p = .699, respectively) (Figure 10.11 (4)). We can conclude, therefore, that we have met the assumption of linearity of the logit.

Multicollinearity.

You will recall that multicollinearity occurs when one or more independent variables (IVs) are highly correlated with each other. Correlations among IVs ≥ |.80| are of concern because they can produce large estimated standard errors and potentially nonsignificant coefficients (Tabachnick & Fidell, 2013). It can also happen when the multiple correlation between one IV and the remaining IVs is too high (e.g., ≥ .90). This can occur even when the individual correlations of the IVs with each other may not be especially high (Norman & Streiner, 2008).

One approach to assessing multicollinearity is to run an OLS multiple regression and evaluate the collinearity diagnostics (tolerance and variance inflation factor [VIF] values) for the generated OLS model. *Tolerance* represents the proportion of variance in a predictor variable that is not explained by the other predictor variables in the model (i.e., Tolerance = [1 – the squared multiple correlation (SMC) of the IVs among themselves]). Tolerance can range, therefore, between 0 and 1.0, with values of 0 indicating perfect collinearity and 1.0 indicating a perfect lack of collinearity. Therefore, low SMCs with corresponding high tolerance values are desired. Tabachnick and Fidell (2013) point out that tolerance values as low as .5 or .6 can be problematic. The VIF is the inverse of tolerance (VIF = 1/tolerance); variables with high tolerances will, per their inverse, have low VIF values.

Figure 10.12 presents the SPSS syntax for generating a correlation matrix and collinearity statistics in an OLS linear regression analysis. These can also be obtained by going to *Analyze . . . Regression . . . Linear . . .* adding the birthweight variable into the dependent box and the four predictor variables into the *Independents . . .* box. By clicking on *Statistics . . .* we can request *Collinearity diagnostics* and *descriptive statistics. . . .* These requests will generate both the correlation matrix and tolerance/VIF statistics.

When we examine the correlation matrix in Figure 10.12 for multicollinearity, we are only concerned with the predictor variables' correlations with each other, not with the outcome variable (*normal_birthweight_baby*). It is apparent that none of the predictor variables are highly correlated with one another. The strongest correlation was between quality of the adolescent's relationship with her parent(s) and the number of prenatal visits (r = .302 (1)). The tolerance and VIF collinearity statistics confirm the lack of multicollinearity with values for tolerance ranging from .888 to .955 (range for VIF: 1.047–1.126) (2), all within acceptable range.

Step 5. Undertake regression diagnostics. Our LR model with the four predictor variables (group assignment, current smoker, number of prenatal visits, and quality of the adolescent's relationship with her parent(s)) appears to be holding up reasonably well. There are no statistically significant interaction terms to be concerned about. We also appear to have met the major assumptions of logistic regression. The next and final step is to undertake the regression diagnostics to identify cases that do not seem to fit our model. Choosing the best approach to undertaking regression diagnostics is both an art and a science, and a number of textbooks and articles give much attention to the process. For the purposes of our discussion, we will use two diagnostic approaches to evaluating residuals and leverage values.

Figure 10.12 Syntax and output for the correlation matrix and collinearity diagnostics generated in SPSS for Windows (v. 22–23).

```
REGRESSION
 /DESCRIPTIVES MEAN STDDEV CORR SIG N
 /MISSING LISTWISE
 /STATISTICS COEFF OUTS R ANOVA COLLIN TOL
 /CRITERIA=PIN(.05) POUT(.10)
 /NOORIGIN
 /DEPENDENT normal_birthweight_baby
 /METHOD=ENTER quality_parental_relationship_interval Group_assignment
  current_smoker Prenatal_visits.
```

Correlations

		normal_birthweight_baby How much did child weight at birth?	quality_parental_relationship_interval	Group_assignment group assignment-group-based delivery model (intervention) vs traditional care-single primary care provider (control)	current_smoker Are you a current smoker	Prenatal_visits How many prenatal visits have you had?
Pearson Correlation	normal_birthweight_baby How much did child weight at birth?	1.000	.529	.343	-.348	.398
	quality_parental_relationship_interval	.529	1.000	.158	-.110	(1) .302
	Group_assignment group assignment-group-based delivery model (intervention) vs traditional care-single primary care provider (control)	.343	.158	1.000	-.158	.074
	current_smoker Are you a current smoker	-.348	-.110	-.158	1.000	-.143
	Prenatal_visits How many prenatal visits have you had?	.398	.302	.074	-.143	1.000

Coefficients[a]

Model		Unstandardized Coefficients		Standardized Coefficients			(2) Collinearity Statistics	
		B	Std. Error	Beta	t	Sig.	Tolerance	VIF
1	(Constant)	-.637	.223		-2.855	.006		
	quality_parental_relationship_interval	.026	.006	.399	4.526	.000	.888	1.126
	Group_assignment group assignment-group-based delivery model (intervention) vs traditional care-single primary care provider (control)	.211	.080	.226	2.651	.010	.955	1.047
	current_smoker Are you a current smoker	-.227	.082	-.236	-2.774	.007	.955	1.047
	Prenatal_visits How many prenatal visits have you had?	.139	.054	.227	2.583	.012	.897	1.115

a. Dependent Variable: normal_birthweight_baby How much did child weight at birth?

Residuals.

Figure 10.6A–C presented the casewise list of the three studentized residuals that were greater than |2.0|. This list is duplicated in Figure 10.13. The problematic cases were those adolescents whose information was posted on lines 19, 30, and 51 of the data set (1) with studentized residuals of –2.795, 2.637, and –2.678 (2). The three cases were misclassified because the adolescents were predicted to have given birth to a normal-birthweight infant when in fact they had a low-birthweight infant (Cases 19 and 52) or were predicted to have had a low-birthweight infant when, in reality, they had a normal-birthweight infant (Case 30). These are cases that should be closely examined to determine why they might have been misclassified. On the positive side, none of these residuals are > |3.0|.

Figure 10.13 SPSS for Windows (v. 22–23) residuals and influence diagnostics: studentized residuals > |2.0|, leverage values > .096, and plots of Cook's distance values.

Casewise List[b]

(1) Case	Selected Status[a]	Observed normal_birth weight_baby How much did child weight at birth?	Predicted	Predicted Group	Temporary Variable Resid	(2) ZResid
19	S	1**	.886	2	-.886	-2.795
30	S	2**	.126	1	.874	2.637
51	S	1**	.878	2	-.878	-2.678

a. S = Selected, U = Unselected cases, and ** = Misclassified cases.

b. Cases with studentized residuals greater than 2.000 are listed.

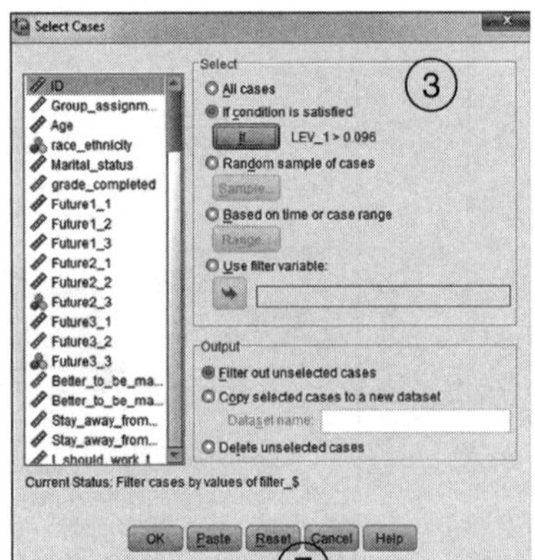

LEV_1 Leverage value

		Frequency	Percent	Valid Percent	Cumulative Percent
Valid	.09826	1	7.1	7.1	7.1
	.09976	1	7.1	7.1	14.3
	.10061	1	7.1	7.1	21.4
	.11129	2	14.3	14.3	35.7
	.11328	1	7.1	7.1	42.9
	.11386	1	7.1	7.1	50.0
	.12754	1	7.1	7.1	57.1
	.13734	1	7.1	7.1	64.3
(4)	.14530	1	7.1	7.1	71.4
	.14781	1	7.1	7.1	78.6
	.15821	1	7.1	7.1	85.7
	.16263	1	7.1	7.1	92.9
	.16891	1	7.1	7.1	100.0
	Total	14	100.0	100.0	

Case Summaries[a]

	ID CODE NUMBER OF QUESTIONNAIRE	LEV_1 Leverage value	COO_1 Analog of Cook's influence statistics	SRE_1 Standard residual
1 (8)	3366.00	.11129	.04940	-.86509
2	3349.00	.14781	.06218	-.84796
3	3540.00	.15821	.47184	-1.72728
4	3632.00	.16891	.07682	-.87841
5	6034.00	.14530	.19393	1.33459
6	4384.00	.11129	.31743	1.68569
7	3427.00	.11386	.02275	-.60663
8	1197.00	.10061	.22981	-1.57572
9	4349.00	.11328	.22180	-1.50675
10	3056.00	.13734	.18542	-1.33808
11	3477.00	.16263	.05652	.78108
12	3448.00	.09976	.02185	.63227
13	3463.00	.09826	.03410	.77705
14	3620.00	.12754	.25424	1.51986
Total N	14	14	14	14

a. Limited to first 100 cases.

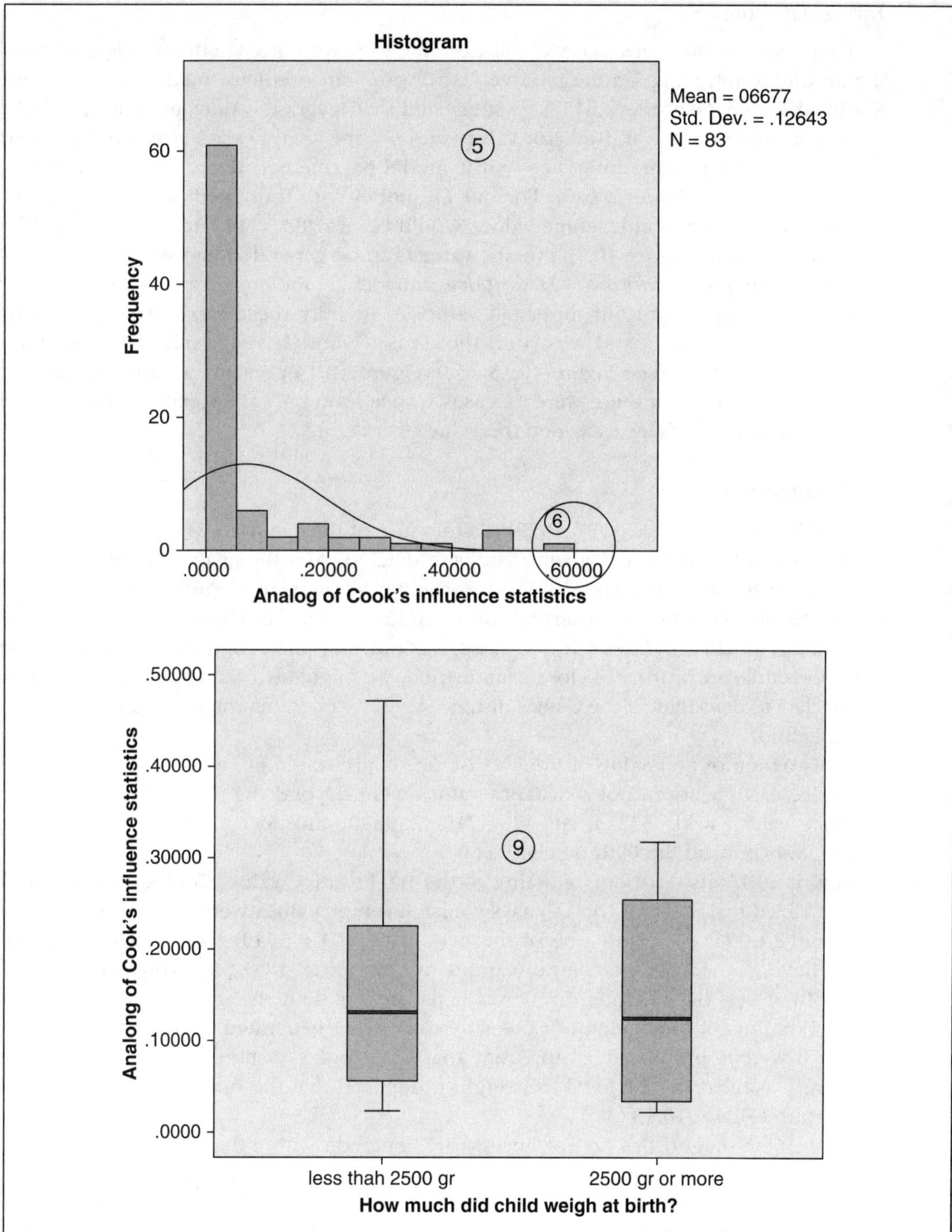
Histogram
Mean = 06677
Std. Dev. = .12643
N = 83
Frequency
60
40
20
0
.0000
.20000
.40000
.60000
Analog of Cook's influence statistics
5
6
Analong of Cook's influence statistics
.50000
.40000
.30000
.20000
.10000
.0000
less thah 2500 gr
2500 gr or more
How much did child weigh at birth?
9

Influence values.

There are two statistics that we will examine to determine whether cases are exerting an undue influence on the parameters for our four predictor model: leverage and Cook's distance. Osborne (2015) has suggested that leverage values greater than $3k/n$ (where k = the number of predictor values and n = the sample size) indicate that those cases are exerting undue influence on the model parameters. Menard (2010) prefers a more conservative value: $2(k)/n$. For our LR model with four predictor variables and 83 cases, the two critical leverage values would be 3(4)/83 = .144 and 2(4)/83 = .096.

As we saw from Figure 10.5, leverage values can be generated and saved to our data file. Then, using the *Analyze . . . Descriptive Statistics . . . Frequencies,* we can determine how many cases exceed our threshold value. To identify these cases, we could go to *Data . . . Select Cases . . .* and select only those cases whose leverage values exceeded the threshold (e.g., .096) (see Figure 10.13 (3)). Figure 10.13 presents a partial frequency table that indicates that there were 14 cases whose leverage values exceeded the cutoff value of .096, and 5 cases exceeded the value of .144 (4).

Cook's distance.

Cook's distance (Cook, 1977, 1979) is a measure of the extent to which the regression estimates would change if a given case were deleted from the analysis (Hosmer et al., 2013; Menard, 2010; Osborne, 2015). These values allow us to identify cases that either do not fit our model or are exerting undue influence on the parameters of the model (Hosmer et al., 2013). Cases whose values for Cook's distance lie outside of the 95th or 99th percentile are worthy of close examination. We might also want to examine subsets of our data to determine if the Cook's distance values were different, depending on group membership.

A histogram of an analog of Cook's distance is presented in Figure 10.13 (5). There were five cases whose Cook's distance values were beyond the 95th percentile. These distance values were .37224, .46647, .47184, .49890, and .55011. Only the last value, .55011, was beyond the 99th percentile (6).

Figure 10.13 also presents a listing of the ID, leverage value, Cook's distance, and standardized residuals for the 14 cases whose leverage values were outside the acceptable range (.096) (7). Only one of these 14 cases (ID = 3540) has a Cook's distance value beyond the 95th percentile (Cook's distance = .47184) (8). None of these 14 cases, however, have standardized residuals greater than the absolute value of 2.0. When boxplots of the analog of Cook's distance were generated for the low- and normal-birthweight groups, it is apparent that the Cook's distance values were more positively skewed for the low-birthweight group and that the outliers were located in that group (Figure 10.13 (9)).

Regression diagnostics do not necessarily conclude with a descriptive examination of residuals, leverage, and influence values. A number of additional diagnostics could be run on these values. Hosmer et al. (2013), Menard (2010), Osborne (2015), and Pregibon (1981) offer excellent advice regarding further approaches to analyzing residuals, leverage values, and influence statistics in logistic regression. In particular, the authors provide useful suggestions and examples for generating plots to identify outliers and influence values (e.g., a plot of Cook's distance against predicted values). While deleting cases with extreme residuals, leverage or influence values may be tempting; remember, though, that deleting extreme cases may—or may not—improve the generalizability of the model. They need to be examined closely to determine the reasons for their discrepancy.

Presentation of the Results

There are a number of different ways that researchers have used to summarize their findings with regard to an LR analysis. Table 10.10 presents one approach that could be used to present the findings obtained from an LR analysis with multiple predictor variables. In this example, the Wald statistic has been presented. If desired (and preferred by some researchers), the likelihood ratio test could be presented instead. Notice that both the unstandardized and standardized betas are presented. These results could also be summarized in the text as follows:

> A logistic regression analysis was conducted to determine the impact of the intervention (usual care vs. group-based intervention), number of prenatal visits, the quality of the pregnant adolescent's relationship with her parent(s), and her current smoking status on the birthweight of her infant (low vs. normal birthweight) (n = 83). Table 10.9 presents a summary of the results of this forced entry logistic regression analysis. A good model fit was obtained, as evidenced by a statistically significant model χ^2 value ($\chi^2 = 45.27$, $df = 4$, $p < .001$) and nonsignificant Hosmer-Lemeshow goodness-of-fit test ($\chi^2 = 7.13$, $df = 8$, $p = .52$).
>
> All four predictor variables (treatment group, number of prenatal visits, quality of the adolescent's relationship with her parent(s), and her current smoking status) were statistically significant ($p < .05$) predictors of whether or not she would give birth to a normal-birthweight baby. An examination of the standardized betas for these four predictors indicated that, controlling for the other variables in the model, the quality of the adolescent's relationship with her parent(s) was the strongest predictor of her giving birth to a normal-birthweight baby ($b^* = 0.371$, $p = .001$, OR = 1.18, 95% CI_{OR} = 1.08, 1.30). This was followed by number of prenatal visits ($b^* = .250$, $p = .017$, OR = 2.92, CI_{OR} = 1.21, 7.05), group assignment ($b^* = .243$, $p = .022$, OR = 4.89, CI_{OR} = 1.26, 19.0), and, finally, the adolescent's current smoking status ($b^* = -.240$, $p = .018$, OR = .20, CI_{OR} = .05, .76). After controlling for other variables in the model, those pregnant adolescents who were most likely to give birth to a normal-birthweight infant were those who had better relationships with their parent(s), had more prenatal visits, had been assigned to the group-based intervention, and were currently nonsmokers. While the overall effect of this model on birthweight of the infant was strong $\left(R_L^2 = .76\right)$, these variables' standardized beta coefficients indicated that, individually, these predictor variables had a low to moderate effect on strong predictors of our outcome variable.

Table 10.10 Suggested Summary Table Reporting the Results of the Logistic Regression Analysis (n = 83)

Outcome variable	*Predictor variables*	*Unstandardized coefficient (b)*	*SE (b)*	*Standardized coefficient (b*)*	*Wald*	df	p	*Odds Ratio (OR)*	*95% Confidence Interval (OR)*
Normal-birthweight baby[a]	Treatment group[b]	1.587	0.694	0.2327	5.238	1	.022	4.890	1.256–19.040
	# prenatal visits[c]	1.072	0.449	0.2370	5.697	1	.017	2.922	1.211–7.046
	Quality of relationship with parents[d]	0.168	0.049	0.3620	11.894	1	.001	1.183	1.075–1.302
	Current Smoker[e]	−1.610	0.683	−0.2333	5.558	1	.018	0.200	0.052–0.762
	Intercept	−7.722	2.050		14.191	1	.000	–	–

NOTE: $R_L^2 = 0.76$

[a]Normal-birthweight baby: 0 = low birthweight, 1 = normal birthweight.

[b]Treatment group: 0 = usual care, 1=group-based intervention.

[c]Number of prenatal visits: Range: 1 = no prenatal visits, 2 = 1–3 visits, 3 = ≥ 4 visits.

[d]Quality of relationship with parents: range: 20–50, higher scores indicate better relationship.

[e]Current smoker: 0 = no, 1 = yes.

Advantages, Limitations, and Alternatives to Binary Multiple Logistic Regression

Binary LR with multiple predictor variables is an extremely useful and increasingly popular statistical analysis technique. Given that it is relatively free of assumptions and can easily be undertaken in the most popular statistical packages, binary LR analyses have been undertaken in a variety of disciplines within a multitude of areas of interest.

While binary LR is relatively free of assumptions and conditions, this technique does assume that the outcome variable of interest is dichotomous, coded 0 and 1. Dependent variables that are continuous or have more than two levels need to be collapsed into a dichotomous outcome variable. Collapsing of data in this way may result in loss of sensitivity. In addition, this technique does not lend itself to repeated-measures designs.

One of the main drawbacks to binary LR is not that it is a limited technique; rather, as Menard has cogently observed, today's statistical software packages have not kept pace with the technique's increasing popularity. Unfortunately, Menard's wish in 2010 that his criticism of the software packages would be obsolete, all of the programs continue to have limitations regarding their LR packages with much needed room for improvement.

Alternatives to binary logistic regression.

There are several very useful alternatives to binary LR. When the outcome variable is continuous and normally distributed, OLS multiple regression is a good option. There are also more advanced options for binary LR. For example, multinomial and ordinal LR are useful techniques when the outcome variable has more than two non-ordered outcomes (multinomial LR) or has ordered categories (ordinal LR). Discriminant analysis is also an option when the predictor variables are continuous and the outcome variable is a nonordered categorical variable. Multilevel modeling is an excellent choice when data are nested within facilities (e.g., patients nested within hospital units) or have been collected across multiple time periods, especially when there is potential for missing data. Structural equation modeling is an excellent analytic tool when the researcher is interested in examining not only the direct but also the indirect effects of predictor variables on an outcome variable of interest. A number of excellent resources address these alternatives to binary logistic regression. These include (but are not limited to) Afifi et al. (2011), Allison (2012), Byrne (2010), Hosmer et al. (2013), Menard (2010), Osborne (2015), Stevens (2009), and Tabachnick and Fidell (2013).

Examples From Published Research

Goffman, D., Madden, R. C., Harrison, E. A., Merkatz, I. R., & Chazotte, C. (2007). Predictors of maternal mortality and near-miss maternal morbidity. *Journal of Perinatology, 27*(10), 597–601.

Lee-Lin, F., Menon, U., Pett, M., Nail, L., Lee, S., & Mooney, K. (2007). Breast cancer beliefs and mammography screening practices among Chinese American immigrants. *Journal of Obstetric, Gynecologic, & Neonatal Nursing, 36*(3), 212–221.

McFadden, D. (1974). Conditional logit analysis of qualitative choice behavior. In P. Zarembka (Ed.), *Conditional logit analysis of qualitative choice behavior* (pp. 105–142). New York, NY: Academic Press.

Neuman, M. I., Hall, M., Gay, J. C., Blaschke, A. J., Williams, D. J., Parikh, K., . . . Shah, S. S. (2014). Readmissions among children previously hospitalized with pneumonia. *Pediatrics, 134*(1), 100–109. doi: 10.1542/peds.2014-0331

Niemeier, J. P., Marwitz, J. H., Lesher, K., Walker, W. C., & Bushnik, T. (2007). Gender differences in executive functions following traumatic brain injury. *Neuropsychological Rehabilitation, 17*(3), 293–313.

Zhong, T., Fernandes, K. A., Saskin, R., Sutradhar, R., Platt, J., Beber, B. A., . . . Baxter, N. N. (2014). Barriers to immediate breast reconstruction in the Canadian universal health care system. *Journal of Clinical Oncology, 32*(20), 2133–2141. doi: 10.1200/JCO.2013.53.0774

TEST YOUR KNOWLEDGE

1. Give an example from your area of research interest that would be suitable for a simple and multiple logistic regression analysis using a binary outcome variable (Note: in each instance, state the independent and dependent variables for your analysis, their levels of measurement, and how you would code these variables).
2. For the two examples that you have provided in Question 1, please state the research questions that would be used with the logistic regression analyses that you have listed. Hint: there are two research questions that you would want to answer.
3. What is the difference between relative risk and odds ratios?
4. What are the assumptions and conditions underlying binary logistic regression, and how would you evaluate those assumptions?
5. Why would a researcher decide to use logistic regression given a binary outcome variable instead of ordinary least squares regression?
6. What are the main methods of entry for binary logistic regression, and what are their advantages and disadvantages?
7. Compare the differences between an unstandardized and standardized beta coefficient, indicating when each coefficient would be used.
8. What are the steps to undertaking a logistic regression analysis?
9. What statistics are used to evaluate overall model fit, and how would you interpret them?
10. What statistics are used to evaluate the contributions of the predictor variables to your model, and how would you interpret them?
11. What diagnostics would you use to evaluate the residuals and influence values?

COMPUTER EXERCISES

1. A team of researchers was interested in examining the impact of gender on anterior cruciate ligament (ACL) knee injuries among student athletes at a prestigious university in the intermountain West. A randomly selected group of 250 student athletes responded to their request regarding knee injuries experienced during the past 2 years. The following table presents the students' responses to an ACL injury (0 = no, 1 = yes), broken down by gender (0 = male, 1= female).

	Experienced an ACL injury?		
Gender	*Yes*	*No*	*Total*
Male	40	60	100
Female	80	70	150
Total	120	130	250

   a. What are the odds of experiencing an ACL knee injury given that a student was a female athlete compared to a male athlete? Calculate the odds ratio and 95% confidence interval for these data and interpret their values.
   b. What is the relative risk of a female having an ACL injury compared to that of a male athlete? Calculate the value for relative risk and its 95% confidence interval and interpret their values.
   c. Compare the results that you obtained for relative risk and the odds ratio.
   d. Input the data from the table into a suitable Internet resource (e.g., http://vassarstats.net/logreg1.html) and compare the results that you obtained in '*a.*' above.
   e. Repeat the process using the data (ACL injuries among University athletes.sav) posted on the SAGE website (study.sagepub.com/pett2e) and compare the results you obtained in '*a.*' and '*d.*'

2. A different team of researchers was interested in continuing their evaluation of the impact of various predictor variables on the likelihood that an adolescent mother would give birth to a low-birthweight infant (0 = normal birthweight, 1 = low birthweight). Based on a careful review of the literature (and excluding their intervention variable), they have selected seven predictor variables that they believe would have an impact on the birthweight of the child: age of the adolescent, number of prenatal visits, quality of the adolescent's relationship with her heath care provider, the quality of her relationship with her parent(s), her current smoking status, and the extent of her drug and alcohol use.
   a. Using the data set (pregnant teen data for logistic regression-4 predictors.sav) located on the SAGE website (study.sagepub.com/pett2e), undertake two logistic regression (LR)

(Continued)

(Continued)

analyses: (1) forced entry of all predictors simultaneously and (2) using a stepwise forward approach (e.g., likelihood ratio) (set $\alpha = .10$). Compare the two results. Which approach would you recommend these researchers use and why?

b. Using the model that you have recommended to the researchers, follow the procedures for undertaking an LR analysis outlined in this chapter to evaluate the overall model fit, including the pseudo-R^2 values as well as the contributions of the individual predictors to the model.

c. Interpret the odds ratios and 90% confidence intervals for the predictor variables in your model (remember that $\alpha = .10$).

d. Calculate the standardized beta coefficients for those same predictor variables and evaluate the variables' contributions to your model.

e. Examine the residuals and influence values for your model. Are there any cases that appear to be severe outliers? If so, how would you recommend the researchers handle these outliers?

f. Construct an LR table of findings similar to that presented in Table 10.10.

g. Summarize these results in paragraph form. Be sure to report the overall model fit as well as the direction and importance of the predictor variables to your model. Hint: you can use the example in the chapter as a model.

Visit **study.sagepub.com/pett2e** to access SAS output, SPSS datasets, SAS datasets, and SAS examples.

CHAPTER 11

Epilogue

These last 10 chapters have examined a variety of nonparametric statistics that can be used under a number of different conditions. We have examined nonparametric statistics that are useful for assessing shapes of distributions (Chapter 4), tests of repeated measures for two or more samples (Chapters 5 and 6), tests of differences between two or more independent groups (Chapters 7 and 8), measures of correlation between two variables (Chapter 9), and simple and multiple logistic regression (Chapter 10). The purpose of this final chapter is twofold: (1) to briefly summarize in table form the nonparametric statistics that have been examined in this textbook, the conditions under which they can be used, and their parametric counterparts and (2) to identify some promising nonparametric alternatives to commonly used higher level multivariate parametric techniques currently under development that hold promise both for the present and the future.

NONPARAMETRIC STATISTICAL PROCEDURES IDENTIFIED IN THIS TEXT

Table 11.1 provides a summary reference guide to the nonparametric statistical procedures reviewed in this text that are currently available in popular statistical computer packages. Although there are additional nonparametric statistics that are offered by computer packages, these particular statistics were selected for their practical applicability to problems in health care research. They are also some of the most commonly used nonparametric statistics in the field. The reader may find this guide helpful when trying to make informed decisions concerning the most suitable nonparametric statistic to use given his or her data and purpose. The table also provides information as to which chapter the reader could turn to for further information concerning the nonparametric statistic of interest. For example, if you have an ordinal level outcome variable (e.g., level of pain measured on a Likert-type scale) and wanted to undertake a test of association with a predictor variable that was nominal level with multiple levels (e.g., type of cancer), you could consider using the median, Kruskal-Wallis, or two-way analysis of variance (ANOVA) by ranks tests that are found in Chapter 9. If, on the other hand, you are examining changes in pain levels for a single sample across multiple time periods, a Friedman test (Chapter 6) might be an appropriate choice (Table 11.1).

Table 11.1 Summary of the Nonparametric Statistical Tests Reviewed in This Text

	Single Sample	*Related Samples*		*Independent Samples*			
		# Measures		*# Levels*			
	"Goodness of Fit"	*2*	*> 2*	*2*	*> 2*	*Tests of Association*	*Logistic Regression*
Chapter Location	*4*	*5*	*6*	*7*	*8*	*9*	*10*
Dependent Variable							
Nominal	Binomial[a]; chi-square goodness of fit	McNemar	Cochran's *Q*	Fisher's exact[a]; chi-square	Chi-square; Mantel-Haenszel	Phi[a]; Cramér's V; kappa; point biserial	Simple, bivariate logistic regression
Ordinal/interval/ratio	Kolmogorov-Smirnov one- and two-sample tests	Sign; Wilcoxon signed ranks	Friedman	Median[b]; Mann-Whitney *U*	Median; Kruskal-Wallis; two-way ANOVA by ranks	Spearman's rho; Kendall's tau	

[a]Requires dichotomous outcome variable.

[b]See Chapter 8 for description.

For those readers who are trying to decide between a parametric and a nonparametric test, Table 11.2 outlines some nonparametric alternatives to particular parametric tests. A nonparametric Spearman rho correlation coefficient, for example, is a good alternative to the parametric Pearson product moment correlation. Two nonparametric alternatives to the independent *t* test are the median and the Mann-Whitney *U* tests.

Obviously, some nonparametric tests do not have parametric alternatives because the variables being evaluated are at the nominal level of measurement (e.g., the chi-square tests, the phi, and the Cramér coefficient). In other instances (e.g., structural equation modeling), there are presently no suitable nonparametric alternatives to the parametric tests available in the more commonly used statistical computer packages. You will soon see in this next section, however, that nonparametric alternatives to other multivariate parametric statistics (e.g., analysis of covariance [ANCOVA] and repeated-measures ANOVA using ranked data) are being developed; hopefully, they will soon be offered in the more popular statistical computer packages (e.g., Stata, SAS and SPSS).

Table 11.2 Parametric Tests and Their Nonparametric Alternatives

Type of Problem		*Parametric Test*	*Nonparametric Alternative*
Repeated measures			
	2 time periods	Paired *t* test	Sign Wilcoxon signed ranks
	> 2 time periods	Repeated measures ANOVA ($1 \times c$)	Friedman
Independent samples			
1 IV	2 groups	Independent *t* test	Median Mann-Whitney *U*
1 IV	> 2 groups	One-way ANOVA	Median Kruskal-Wallis
> 1 IV	> 2 groups	Two-way ANOVA	Two-way ANOVA by ranks
Measures of association			
		Pearson *r*	Spearman's rho Kendall's tau Point biserial
Regression			
1 IV		Simple linear regression	Simple binary logistic regression[a]
> 1 IV		Multiple linear regression	Multiple logistic regression[a] Ordinal logistic regression[b] Multinomial logistic regression[c]

NOTE: ANOVA = analysis of variance; IV = independent variable.

[a]Requires a dichotomous outcome variable.

[b]Requires an ordered nominal-level outcome variable.

[c]Requires a nonordered nominal-level outcome variable with more than two levels.

When faced with data that do not meet the sometimes strict assumptions of multivariate statistical analyses, researchers can seek out simpler solutions. It may be possible to transform the dependent variable to achieve a more nearly normal distribution (see Chapter 3 for details). It might also be feasible to dichotomize the dependent variable and to consider using logistic regression in place of multiple regression. For repeated-measures ANOVA and ANCOVA, it might be advantageous to create change scores (e.g., Change = Time2 – Time1) and to undertake Kruskal-Wallis tests on these change scores. A serious disadvantage to change scores, however, is that they focus on *change,* not on scores that have been adjusted for the effects of a covariate. The results from these analyses could be subject to different outcomes and interpretations.

As has been emphasized throughout this text, it is extremely important that researchers be aware of the assumptions underlying the parametric or nonparametric test being considered and to assess the extent to which their data meet those assumptions. All of the chapters presented in this textbook have tried to provide you with the tools to undertake a responsible evaluation of a test's assumptions. No statistical test is powerful if its assumptions have been seriously violated. It is, therefore, the researcher's ethical responsibility to ensure that tests of such assumptions have been carefully undertaken and reported.

SOME PROMISING NONPARAMETRIC STATISTICS

A number of nonparametric alternatives to higher level parametric techniques (e.g., survival and event history modeling, as well as longitudinal and time-series data analysis) that are extremely useful in health sciences research have been developed, some of which are available in the commonly used statistical computer packages (Biswas, 2008; Brunner, Domhof, & Langer, 2002; Hosmer & Lemeshow, 1999; Kleinbaum, 1996; Korosteleva, 2014; MacKenzie & Peng, 2014). As Akritas and Politis (2003) have observed, with the development of affordable high-speed computers, such nonparametric techniques for use with time-to-event analyses, function smoothing, bootstrapping, data mining, and "bagging, subagging and bragging" (Bŭhlmann, 2003) have become practically available. For example, nonparametric estimators of time-to-event analyses—for example, the Kaplan-Meier estimator of the survival function (Kaplan & Meier, 1958), the log-rank test of comparing two survival functions, and the Cox proportional hazards model—are now available in both SPSS for Windows and SAS (Korosteleva, 2014). Bootstrapping methods (Davison & Hinkley, 2006; Mooney & Duval, 1993) to obtain standard errors on samples from populations with unknown or nonnormal distributions are increasing in popularity because of their availability in easy-to-use programs (e.g., AMOS) (Byrne, 2010). Similarly, kernel density estimation methods for smoothing (Dubnicka, 2011; Gijbels, 2003; Horová, Koláček, & Zelinka, 2012) and expanded permutation tests (Edgington & Onghena, 2007; Good, 2005; Lehmann & Romano, 2005) are increasingly being used in health care research.

Despite these developments, however, there still remain major *lacunae,* or holes, in the availability of these nonparametric alternatives in the more commonly used statistical computer packages, especially with regard to the more complex research designs. As Menard (2010) has suggested, these statistical computer packages have not all kept pace with the interesting developments in nonparametric statistics. For example, although the Friedman test is a useful alternative when there are multiple observations taken from a single sample, there are a few nonparametric alternatives available for multivariate analysis of variance (MANOVA) (Finch, 2005) and repeated-measures designs with multiple independent variables and time periods (Brunner et al., 2002). Akritas and Brunner (2003), in their review article on recent developments related to nonparametric models for ANOVA and ANCOVA, pointed out a number of nonparametric approaches that are being developed that could be viable alternatives to ANOVA, MANOVA, and ANCOVA. Bathke and Brunner (2003) also consider a nonparametric analog to the parametric ANCOVA that is based on rank methods for use with Likert-type dependent variables. The authors also offer a SAS macro on their website (www.ams.med.uni-goettingen.de) that enables researchers to undertake this analysis. On that same website, they also provide detailed information on the use of this macro.

Another interesting development is the work of Noguchi, Gel, Brunner, and Konietschke (2012) and the working group from the Department of Medical Statistics at the University of Göttingen in Germany. These authors offer a software package developed in R entitled **nparLD** ("*nonparametric longitudinal data*"), the purpose of which is to provide a user-friendly statistical package that enables researchers to use rank-based approaches to the analysis of longitudinal data. The authors report that the package offers nonparametric approaches for the most frequently used factorial designs and is freely available from the Comprehensive R Archive Network (http://CRAN.R-project.org/package=nparLD). There are also detailed help files, instructions, and examples that accompany the program. An advantage to the use of these rank-based methods for longitudinal analyses is that the approach is not restricted to the analysis of data measured on a continuous scale but can also be used with ordered categorical, dichotomous, and heavily skewed data (Konietschke, Bathke, Hothorn, & Brunner, 2010; Noguchi et al., 2012).

Multiple logistic regression and its nonparametric relatives (ordinal and multinomial logistic regression) for ordered and nonordered nominal-level outcome variables with more than two levels offer useful alternatives to multiple linear regression. In the area of diagnostics, Brunner and Zapf (2014) provide an overview of nonparametric receiver operating characteristic (ROC) curve methods that could be used in the analysis of diagnostic trials. Martinez-Camblor, Carleos, and Corral (2011) also suggest the use of a nonparametric approach to comparing multiple independent ROC curves. In a slightly different context, McKean and Hettmansperger (2011) present robust nonparametric statistical methods that can be used not only in the univariate but also with the multivariate situation.

Unfortunately, these nonparametric alternatives, while promising, still need to be translated into practical computer applications that can be understood and used by nonstatisticians. Clinical researchers also need to gain a stronger familiarity with the workings of the less user-friendly statistical computer packages. Until both occur, the theoretical development of nonparametric statistics will continue to supersede the practical development of computer applications that would facilitate the introduction of these nonparametric statistics into health care research. When they are available, nonparametric statistics offer a feasible and potentially powerful alternative to the more restrictive parametric tests. As statistical computer packages catch up with theoretical developments in nonparametric statistics, researchers in the health sciences and other disciplines can look forward to ever-expanding tools with which to reach informed decisions about research evidence.

Appendix: Statistical Tables

Table A.1A-B Table of Values for the Cumulative Distribution Function (CDF) for the Standard Normal Distribution

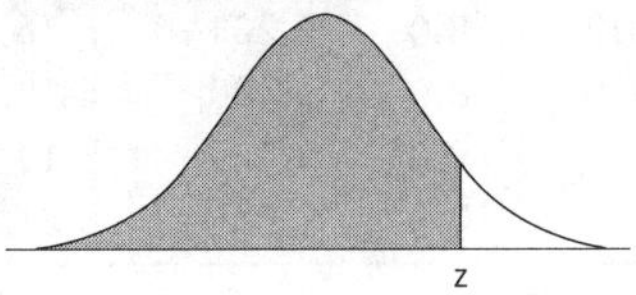

A. Cumulative Distribution Function (CDF) for the Standard Normal Distribution From -∞ to Z

Z	0.00	0.01	0.02	0.03	0.04	0.05	0.06	0.07	0.08	0.09
0.0	0.5000	0.5040	0.5080	0.5120	0.5160	0.5199	0.5239	0.5279	0.5319	0.5359
0.1	0.5398	0.5438	0.5478	0.5517	0.5557	0.5596	0.5636	0.5675	0.5714	0.5753
0.2	0.5793	0.5832	0.5871	0.5910	0.5948	0.5987	0.6026	0.6064	0.6103	0.6141
0.3	0.6179	0.6217	0.6255	0.6293	0.6331	0.6368	0.6406	0.6443	0.6480	0.6517
0.4	0.6554	0.6591	0.6628	0.6664	0.6700	0.6736	0.6772	0.6808	0.6844	0.6879
0.5	0.6915	0.6950	0.6985	0.7019	0.7054	0.7088	0.7123	0.7157	0.7190	0.7224
0.6	0.7257	0.7291	0.7324	0.7357	0.7389	0.7422	0.7454	0.7486	0.7517	0.7549
0.7	0.7580	0.7611	0.7642	0.7673	0.7704	0.7734	0.7764	0.7794	0.7823	0.7852
0.8	0.7881	0.7910	0.7939	0.7967	0.7995	0.8023	0.8051	0.8078	0.8106	0.8133
0.9	0.8159	0.8186	0.8212	0.8238	0.8264	0.8289	0.8315	0.8340	0.8365	0.8389
1.0	0.8413	0.8438	0.8461	0.8485	0.8508	0.8531	0.8554	0.8577	0.8599	0.8621
1.1	0.8643	0.8665	0.8686	0.8708	0.8729	0.8749	0.8770	0.8790	0.8810	0.8830
1.2	0.8849	0.8869	0.8888	0.8907	0.8925	0.8944	0.8962	0.8980	0.8997	0.9015
1.3	0.9032	0.9049	0.9066	0.9082	0.9099	0.9115	0.9131	0.9147	0.9162	0.9177
1.4	0.9192	0.9207	0.9222	0.9236	0.9251	0.9265	0.9279	0.9292	0.9306	0.9319
1.5	0.9332	0.9345	0.9357	0.9370	0.9382	0.9394	0.9406	0.9418	0.9429	0.9441
1.6	0.9452	0.9463	0.9474	0.9484	0.9495	0.9505	0.9515	0.9525	0.9535	0.9545
1.7	0.9554	0.9564	0.9573	0.9582	0.9591	0.9599	0.9608	0.9616	0.9625	0.9633
1.8	0.9641	0.9649	0.9656	0.9664	0.9671	0.9678	0.9686	0.9693	0.9699	0.9706
1.9	0.9713	0.9719	0.9726	0.9732	0.9738	0.9744	0.9750	0.9756	0.9761	0.9767
2.0	0.9772	0.9778	0.9783	0.9788	0.9793	0.9798	0.9803	0.9808	0.9812	0.9817
2.1	0.9821	0.9826	0.9830	0.9834	0.9838	0.9842	0.9846	0.9850	0.9854	0.9857
2.2	0.9861	0.9864	0.9868	0.9871	0.9875	0.9878	0.9881	0.9884	0.9887	0.9890
2.3	0.9893	0.9896	0.9898	0.9901	0.9904	0.9906	0.9909	0.9911	0.9913	0.9916
2.4	0.9918	0.9920	0.9922	0.9925	0.9927	0.9929	0.9931	0.9932	0.9934	0.9936
2.5	0.9938	0.9940	0.9941	0.9943	0.9945	0.9946	0.9948	0.9949	0.9951	0.9952
2.6	0.9953	0.9955	0.9956	0.9957	0.9959	0.9960	0.9961	0.9962	0.9963	0.9964
2.7	0.9965	0.9966	0.9967	0.9968	0.9969	0.9970	0.9971	0.9972	0.9973	0.9974
2.8	0.9974	0.9975	0.9976	0.9977	0.9977	0.9978	0.9979	0.9979	0.9980	0.9981
2.9	0.9981	0.9982	0.9982	0.9983	0.9984	0.9984	0.9985	0.9985	0.9986	0.9986
3.0	0.9987	0.9987	0.9987	0.9988	0.9988	0.9989	0.9989	0.9989	0.9990	0.9990

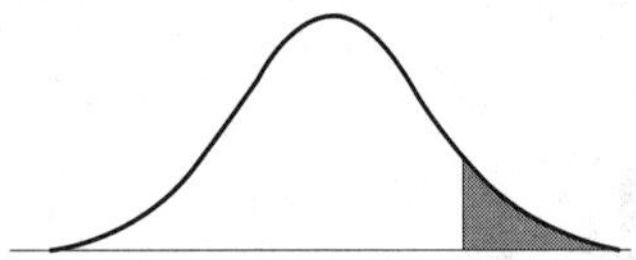

z

B. Far Right Tail Probabilities

Z	P{Z to ∞ }	Z	P{Z to ∞}	Z	P{Z to ∞}	Z	P{Z to ∞}	
2.0	0.02275	3.0	0.001350	4.0	0.00003167	5.0	2.867	E-7
2.1	0.01786	3.1	0.0009676	4.1	0.00002066	5.5	1.899	E-8
2.2	0.01390	3.2	0.0006871	4.2	0.00001335	6.0	9.866	E-10
2.3	0.01072	3.3	0.0004834	4.3	0.00000854	6.5	4.016	E-11
2.4	0.00820	3.4	0.0003369	4.4	0.000005413	7.0	1.280	E-12
2.5	0.00621	3.5	0.0002326	4.5	0.000003398	7.5	3.191	E-14
2.6	0.004661	3.6	0.0001591	4.6	0.000002112	8.0	6.221	E-16
2.7	0.003467	3.7	0.0001078	4.7	0.000001300	8.5	9.480	E-18
2.8	0.002555	3.8	0.00007235	4.8	7.933 E-7	9.0	1.129	E-19
2.9	0.001866	3.9	0.00004810	4.9	4.792 E-7	9.5	1.049	E-21

SOURCE: These tables are public domain and are available at http://www.math.unb.ca/~knight/utility/NormTble.htm. They were produced by APL programs written by the author, Dr. William Knight and are reproduced with his permission.

Table A.2 Critical Points of the Chi Square Distribution

Critical Points of the Chi Square Distribution

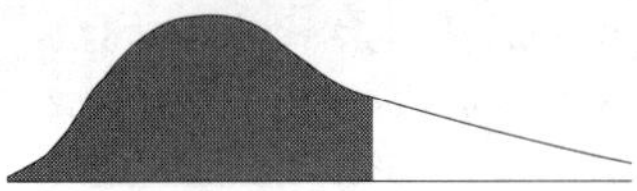

D. F.	Cumulative probability												
	0.005	*0.010*	*0.025*	*0.05*	*0.10*	*0.25*	*0.50*	*0.75*	*0.90*	*0.95*	*0.975*	*0.99*	*0.995*
1	0.39E-4	0.00016	0.00098	0.0039	0.0158	0.102	0.455	1.32	2.71	3.84	5.02	6.63	7.88
2	0.0100	0.0201	0.0506	0.103	0.211	0.575	1.39	2.77	4.61	5.99	7.38	9.21	10.6
3	0.0717	0.115	0.216	0.352	0.584	1.21	2.37	4.11	6.25	7.81	9.35	11.3	12.8
4	0.207	0.297	0.484	0.711	1.06	1.92	3.36	5.39	7.78	9.49	11.1	13.3	14.9
5	0.412	0.554	0.831	1.15	1.61	2.67	4.35	6.63	9.24	11.1	12.8	15.1	16.7
6	0.676	0.872	1.24	1.64	2.20	3.45	5.35	7.84	10.6	12.6	14.4	16.8	18.5
7	0.989	1.24	1.69	2.17	2.83	4.25	6.35	9.04	12.0	14.1	16.0	18.5	20.3
8	1.34	1.65	2.18	2.73	3.49	5.07	7.34	10.2	13.4	15.5	17.5	20.1	22.0
9	1.73	2.09	2.70	3.33	4.17	5.9	8.34	11.4	14.7	16.9	19.0	21.7	23.6
10	2.16	2.56	3.25	3.94	4.87	6.74	9.34	12.5	16.0	18.3	20.5	23.2	25.2
11	2.60	3.05	3.82	4.57	5.58	7.58	10.3	13.7	17.3	19.7	21.9	24.7	26.8
12	3.07	3.57	4.40	5.23	6.30	8.44	11.3	14.8	18.5	21.0	23.3	26.2	28.3
13	3.57	4.11	5.01	5.89	7.04	9.3	12.3	16.0	19.8	22.4	24.7	27.7	29.8
14	4.07	4.66	5.63	6.57	7.79	10.2	13.3	17.1	21.1	23.7	26.1	29.1	31.3
15	4.60	5.23	6.26	7.26	8.55	11.0	14.3	18.2	22.3	25.0	27.5	30.6	32.8
16	5.14	5.81	6.91	7.96	9.31	11.9	15.3	19.4	23.5	26.3	28.8	32.0	34.3
17	5.70	6.41	7.56	8.67	10.1	12.8	16.3	20.5	24.8	27.6	30.2	33.4	35.7
18	6.26	7.01	8.23	9.39	10.9	13.7	17.3	21.6	26.0	28.9	31.5	34.8	37.2
19	6.84	7.63	8.91	10.1	11.7	14.6	18.3	22.7	27.2	30.1	32.9	36.2	38.6
20	7.43	8.26	9.59	10.9	12.4	15.5	19.3	23.8	28.4	31.4	34.2	37.6	40.0
21	8.03	8.90	10.3	11.6	13.2	16.3	20.3	24.9	29.6	32.7	35.5	38.9	41.4
22	8.64	9.54	11.0	12.3	14.0	17.2	21.3	26.0	30.8	33.9	36.8	40.3	42.8
23	9.26	10.2	11.7	13.1	14.8	18.1	22.3	27.1	32.0	35.2	38.1	41.6	44.2
24	9.89	10.9	12.4	13.8	15.7	19.0	23.3	28.2	33.2	36.4	39.4	43.0	45.6
25	10.5	11.5	13.1	14.6	16.5	19.9	24.3	29.3	34.4	37.7	40.6	44.3	46.9
26	11.2	12.2	13.8	15.4	17.3	20.8	25.3	30.4	35.6	38.9	41.9	45.6	48.3
27	11.8	12.9	14.6	16.2	18.1	21.7	26.3	31.5	36.7	40.1	43.2	47.0	49.6
28	12.5	13.6	15.3	16.9	18.9	22.7	27.3	32.6	37.9	41.3	44.5	48.3	51.0
29	13.1	14.3	16.0	17.7	19.8	23.6	28.3	33.7	39.1	42.6	45.7	49.6	52.3
30	13.8	15.0	16.8	18.5	20.6	24.5	29.3	34.8	40.3	43.8	47.0	50.9	53.7
31	14.5	15.7	17.5	19.3	21.4	25.4	30.3	35.9	41.4	45.0	48.2	52.2	55.0
32	15.1	16.4	18.3	20.1	22.3	26.3	31.3	37.0	42.6	46.2	49.5	53.5	56.3
33	15.8	17.1	19.0	20.9	23.1	27.2	32.3	38.1	43.7	47.4	50.7	54.8	57.6

34	16.5	17.8	19.8	21.7	24.0	28.1	33.3	39.1	44.9	48.6	52.0	56.1	59.0
35	17.2	18.5	20.6	22.5	24.8	29.1	34.3	40.2	46.1	49.8	53.2	57.3	60.3
36	17.9	19.2	21.3	23.3	25.6	30.0	35.3	41.3	47.2	51.0	54.4	58.6	61.6
37	18.6	20.0	22.1	24.1	26.5	30.9	36.3	42.4	48.4	52.2	55.7	59.9	62.9
38	19.3	20.7	22.9	24.9	27.3	31.8	37.3	43.5	49.5	53.4	56.9	61.2	64.2
39	20.0	21.4	23.7	25.7	28.2	32.7	38.3	44.5	50.7	54.6	58.1	62.4	65.5
40	20.7	22.2	24.4	26.5	29.1	33.7	39.3	45.6	51.8	55.8	59.3	63.7	66.8
41	21.4	22.9	25.2	27.3	29.9	34.6	40.3	46.7	52.9	56.9	60.6	65.0	68.1
42	22.1	23.7	26.0	28.1	30.8	35.5	41.3	47.8	54.1	58.1	61.8	66.2	69.3
43	22.9	24.4	26.8	29.0	31.6	36.4	42.3	48.8	55.2	59.3	63.0	67.5	70.6
44	23.6	25.1	27.6	29.8	32.5	37.4	43.3	49.9	56.4	60.5	64.2	68.7	71.9
45	24.3	25.9	28.4	30.6	33.4	38.3	44.3	51.0	57.5	61.7	65.4	70.0	73.2
	0.005	**0.010**	**0.025**	**0.05**	**0.10**	**0.25**	**0.50**	**0.75**	**0.90**	**0.95**	**0.975**	**0.99**	**0.995**

This public table is in the public domain. It was produced using APL programs written by the author, William Knight / Univ. of New Brunswick/Canada

Table A.3 *t* Table

cum. prob	$t_{.50}$	$t_{.75}$	$t_{.80}$	$t_{.85}$	$t_{.90}$	$t_{.95}$	$t_{.975}$	$t_{.99}$	$t_{.995}$	$t_{.999}$	$t_{.9995}$
one-tail	*0.50*	*0.25*	*0.20*	*0.15*	*0.10*	*0.05*	*0.025*	*0.01*	*0.005*	*0.001*	*0.0005*
two-tails	*1.00*	*0.50*	*0.40*	*0.30*	*0.20*	*0.10*	*0.05*	*0.02*	*0.01*	*0.002*	*0.001*
df											
1	0.000	1.000	1.376	1.963	3.078	6.314	12.71	31.82	63.66	318.31	636.62
2	0.000	0.816	1.061	1.386	1.886	2.920	4.303	6.965	9.925	22.327	31.599
3	0.000	0.765	0.978	1.250	1.638	2.353	3.182	4.541	5.841	10.215	12.924
4	0.000	0.741	0.941	1.190	1.533	2.132	2.776	3.747	4.604	7.173	8.610
5	0.000	0.727	0.920	1.156	1.476	2.015	2.571	3.365	4.032	5.893	6.869
6	0.000	0.718	0.906	1.134	1.440	1.943	2.447	3.143	3.707	5.208	5.959
7	0.000	0.711	0.896	1.119	1.415	1.895	2.365	2.998	3.499	4.785	5.408
8	0.000	0.706	0.889	1.108	1.397	1.860	2.306	2.896	3.355	4.501	5.041
9	0.000	0.703	0.883	1.100	1.383	1.833	2.262	2.821	3.250	4.297	4.781
10	0.000	0.700	0.879	1.093	1.372	1.812	2.228	2.764	3.169	4.144	4.587
11	0.000	0.697	0.876	1.088	1.363	1.796	2.201	2.718	3.106	4.025	4.437
12	0.000	0.695	0.873	1.083	1.356	1.782	2.179	2.681	3.055	3.930	4.318
13	0.000	0.694	0.870	1.079	1.350	1.771	2.160	2.650	3.012	3.852	4.221
14	0.000	0.692	0.868	1.076	1.345	1.761	2.145	2.624	2.977	3.787	4.140
15	0.000	0.691	0.866	1.074	1.341	1.753	2.131	2.602	2.947	3.733	4.073
16	0.000	0.690	0.865	1.071	1.337	1.746	2.120	2.583	2.921	3.686	4.015
17	0.000	0.689	0.863	1.069	1.333	1.740	2.110	2.567	2.898	3.646	3.965
18	0.000	0.688	0.862	1.067	1.330	1.734	2.101	2.552	2.878	3.610	3.922
19	0.000	0.688	0.861	1.066	1.328	1.729	2.093	2.539	2.861	3.579	3.883
20	0.000	0.687	0.860	1.064	1.325	1.725	2.086	2.528	2.845	3.552	3.850
21	0.000	0.686	0.859	1.063	1.323	1.721	2.080	2.518	2.831	3.527	3.819
22	0.000	0.686	0.858	1.061	1.321	1.717	2.074	2.508	2.819	3.505	3.792
23	0.000	0.685	0.858	1.060	1.319	1.714	2.069	2.500	2.807	3.485	3.768
24	0.000	0.685	0.857	1.059	1.318	1.711	2.064	2.492	2.797	3.467	3.745
25	0.000	0.684	0.856	1.058	1.316	1.708	2.060	2.485	2.787	3.450	3.725
26	0.000	0.684	0.856	1.058	1.315	1.706	2.056	2.479	2.779	3.435	3.707
27	0.000	0.684	0.855	1.057	1.314	1.703	2.052	2.473	2.771	3.421	3.690
28	0.000	0.683	0.855	1.056	1.313	1.701	2.048	2.467	2.763	3.408	3.674
29	0.000	0.683	0.854	1.055	1.311	1.699	2.045	2.462	2.756	3.396	3.659
30	0.000	0.683	0.854	1.055	1.310	1.697	2.042	2.457	2.750	3.385	3.646
40	0.000	0.681	0.851	1.050	1.303	1.684	2.021	2.423	2.704	3.307	3.551
60	0.000	0.679	0.848	1.045	1.296	1.671	2.000	2.390	2.660	3.232	3.460
80	0.000	0.678	0.846	1.043	1.292	1.664	1.990	2.374	2.639	3.195	3.416
100	0.000	0.677	0.845	1.042	1.290	1.660	1.984	2.364	2.626	3.174	3.390
1000	0.000	0.675	0.842	1.037	1.282	1.646	1.962	2.330	2.581	3.098	3.300
z	0.000	0.674	0.842	1.036	1.282	1.645	1.960	2.326	2.576	3.090	3.291
	0%	50%	60%	70%	80%	90%	95%	98%	99%	99.8%	99.9%
	Confidence Level										

Table A.4-A

Critical Values for the Wilcoxon/Mann-Whitney Test (U)
2-tailed (non-directional) α=.10;
1-tailed (directional) α=.05

n_1 \ n_2	1	2	3	4	5	6	7	8	9	10	11	12	13	14	15	16	17	18	19	20
1	-	-	-	-	-	-	-	-	-	-	-	-	-	-	-	-	-	-	0	0
2	-	-	-	-	0	0	0	1	1	1	1	2	2	2	3	3	3	4	4	4
3	-	-	0	0	1	2	2	3	3	4	5	5	6	7	7	8	9	9	10	11
4	-	-	0	1	2	3	4	5	6	7	8	9	10	11	12	14	15	16	17	18
5	-	0	1	2	4	5	6	8	9	11	12	13	15	16	18	19	20	22	23	25
6	-	0	2	3	5	7	8	10	12	14	16	17	19	21	23	25	26	28	30	32
7	-	0	2	4	6	8	11	13	15	17	19	21	24	26	28	30	33	35	37	39
8	-	1	3	5	8	10	13	15	18	20	23	26	28	31	33	36	39	41	44	47
9	-	1	3	6	9	12	15	18	21	24	27	30	33	36	39	42	45	48	51	54
10	-	1	4	7	11	14	17	20	24	27	31	34	37	41	44	48	51	55	58	62
11	-	1	5	8	12	16	19	23	27	31	34	38	42	48	50	54	57	61	65	69
12	-	2	5	9	13	17	21	26	30	34	38	42	47	51	55	60	64	68	72	77
13	-	2	6	10	15	19	24	28	33	37	42	47	51	56	61	65	70	75	80	84
14	-	2	7	11	16	21	26	31	36	41	45	51	56	61	66	71	77	82	87	92
15	-	3	7	12	18	23	28	33	39	44	50	55	61	65	72	77	83	88	94	100
16	-	3	8	14	19	25	30	36	42	48	54	60	65	71	77	83	89	95	101	107
17	-	3	9	15	20	26	33	39	45	51	57	64	70	77	83	89	96	102	109	115
18	-	4	9	18	22	28	35	41	48	55	61	68	75	82	88	95	102	109	116	123
19	0	4	10	17	23	30	37	44	51	58	65	72	80	87	94	101	109	116	123	130
20	0	4	11	18	25	32	39	47	54	62	69	77	84	92	100	107	115	123	130	138

Table A.4-B 2-tailed (non-directional) α=.05; 1-tailed (directional) α=.025

	n_2																			
n_1	1	2	3	4	5	6	7	8	9	10	11	12	13	14	15	16	17	18	19	20
1	-	-	-	-	-	-	-	-	-	-	-	-	-	-	-	-	-	-	-	-
2	-	-	-	-	-	-	-	0	0	0	0	1	1	1	1	1	2	2	2	2
3	-	-	-	-	0	1	1	2	2	3	3	4	4	5	5	6	6	7	7	8
4	-	-	-	0	1	2	3	4	4	5	6	7	8	9	10	11	11	12	13	13
5	-	-	0	1	2	3	5	6	7	8	9	11	12	13	14	15	17	18	19	20
6	-	-	1	2	3	5	6	8	10	11	13	14	16	17	19	21	22	24	25	27
7	-	-	1	3	5	6	8	10	12	14	16	18	20	22	24	26	28	30	32	34
8	-	0	2	4	6	8	10	13	15	17	19	22	24	26	29	31	34	36	38	41
9	-	0	2	4	7	10	12	15	17	21	23	26	28	31	34	37	39	42	45	48
10	-	0	3	5	8	11	14	17	20	23	26	29	33	36	39	42	45	48	52	55
11	-	0	3	6	9	13	16	19	23	26	30	33	37	40	44	47	51	55	58	62
12	-	1	4	7	11	14	18	22	26	29	33	37	41	45	49	53	57	61	65	69
13	-	1	4	8	12	16	20	24	28	33	37	41	45	50	54	59	63	67	72	76
14	-	1	5	9	13	17	22	26	31	36	40	45	50	55	59	64	67	74	78	83
15	-	1	5	10	14	19	24	29	34	39	44	49	54	59	64	70	75	80	85	90
16	-	1	6	11	15	21	26	31	37	42	47	53	59	64	70	75	81	86	92	98
17	-	2	6	11	17	22	28	34	39	45	51	57	63	67	75	81	87	93	99	105
18	-	2	7	12	18	24	30	36	42	48	55	61	67	74	80	86	93	99	106	112
19	-	2	7	13	19	25	32	38	45	52	58	65	72	78	85	92	99	106	113	119
20	-	2	8	14	20	27	34	41	48	55	62	69	76	83	90	98	105	112	119	127

Table A.4-C 2-tailed (non-directional) α=.01; 1-tailed (Directional) α=.005

n_1 \ n_2	1	2	3	4	5	6	7	8	9	10	11	12	13	14	15	16	17	18	19	20
1	-	-	-	-	-	-	-	-	-	-	-	-	-	-	-	-	-	-	-	-
2	-	-	-	-	-	-	-	-	-	-	-	-	-	-	-	-	-	-	0	0
3	-	-	-	-	-	-	-	-	0	0	0	1	1	1	2	2	2	2	3	3
4	-	-	-	-	-	0	0	1	1	2	2	3	3	4	5	5	6	6	7	8
5	-	-	-	-	0	1	1	2	3	4	5	6	7	7	8	9	10	11	12	13
6	-	-	-	0	1	2	3	4	5	6	7	9	10	11	12	13	15	16	17	18
7	-	-	-	0	1	3	4	6	7	9	10	12	13	15	16	18	19	21	22	24
8	-	-	-	1	2	4	6	7	9	11	13	15	17	18	20	22	24	26	28	30
9	-	-	0	1	3	5	7	9	11	13	16	18	20	22	24	27	29	31	33	36
10	-	-	0	2	4	6	9	11	13	16	18	21	24	26	29	31	34	37	39	42
11	-	-	0	2	5	7	10	13	16	18	21	24	27	30	33	36	39	42	45	46
12	-	-	1	3	6	9	12	15	18	21	24	27	31	34	37	41	44	47	51	54
13	-	-	1	3	7	10	13	17	20	24	27	31	34	38	42	45	49	53	56	60
14	-	-	1	4	7	11	15	18	22	26	30	34	38	42	46	50	54	58	63	67
15	-	-	2	5	8	12	16	20	24	29	33	37	42	46	51	55	60	64	69	73
16	-	-	2	5	9	13	18	22	27	31	36	41	45	50	55	60	65	70	74	79
17	-	-	2	6	10	15	19	24	29	34	39	44	49	54	60	65	70	75	81	86
18	-	-	2	6	11	16	21	26	31	37	42	47	53	58	64	70	75	81	87	92
19	-	0	3	7	12	17	22	28	33	39	45	51	56	63	69	74	81	87	93	99
20	-	0	3	8	13	18	24	30	36	42	46	54	60	67	73	79	86	92	99	105

References

Abdi, H. (2007). The Kendall rank correlation coefficient. In N. J. Salkind (Ed.), *Encyclopedia of measurement and statistics* (pp. 508–510). Thousand Oaks, CA: Sage.

Ackerman, I. N., Ademi, Z., Osborne, R. H., & Liew, D. (2013). Comparison of health-related quality of life, work status, and health care utilization and costs according to hip and knee joint disease severity: A national Australian study. *Physical Therapy, 93*(7), 889–899. doi: 10.2522/ptj.20120423

Afifi, A., May, S., & Clark, V. A. (2011). *Practical multivariate analysis.* Boca Raton, FL: CRC Press.

Agresti, A. (2003). Dealing with discreteness: Making 'exact' confidence intervals for proportions, differences of proportions and odds ratios more exact. *Statistical Methods in Medical Research, 12,* 3-21.

Agresti, A. (2013). *Categorical data analysis.* Chicago: John Wiley and Sons.

Agresti, A., & Coull, B. A. (1998). Approximate is better than "exact" for interval estimation of binomial proportions. *The American Statistician, 52*(2), 119–126. doi: 10.1080/00031305.1998.10480550

Agresti, A., & Liu, I. (2001). Strategies for modeling a categorical variable allowing multiple category choices. *Sociological Methods & Research, 29*(4), 403–434. doi: 10.1177/0049124101029004001

Akritas, M. G. (1990). The rank transform method in some two-factor designs. *Journal of the American Statistical Association, 85*(409), 73–78.

Akritas, M. G. (2011). Nonparametric models for ANOVA and ANCOVA designs. In M. Lovric (Ed.), *International encyclopedia of statistical science* (pp. 964–968). Berlin, Germany: Springer.

Akritas, M. G., & Arnold, S. F. (1994). Fully nonparametric hypotheses for factorial designs I: Multivariate repeated measures designs. *Journal of the American Statistical Association, 89,* 336–343.

Akritas, M. G., Arnold, S. F., & Brunner, E. (1997). Nonparametric hypothesis and rank statistics for unbalanced factorial designs. *Journal of the American Statistical Association, 92*(437), 258–265.

Akritas, M. G., & Brunner, E. (2003). Nonparametric models for ANOVA and ANCOVA: A review. In In M. G. Akritas & Politis, D. N. (Eds.), *Recent advances and trends in nonparametric statistics* (pp. 79–91). Amsterdam: JAI.

Akritas, M. G., & Politis, D. N. (2003). *Recent advances and trends in nonparametric statistics.* Amsterdam: Elsevier.

Akritas, M. G., Stavropoulos, A., & Caroni, C. (2009). Asymptotic theory of weighted F-statistics based on ranks. *Journal of Nonparametric Statistics, 21,* 177–191.

Allison, P. D. (2012). *Logistic regression using SAS: Theory and application.* Cary, NC: SAS Institute.

Allison, P. D. (2013). What's the best R-squared for logistic regression? http://www.statisticalhorizons.com/r2logistic

Altman, D. G. (1990). *Practical statistics for medical research.* Boca Raton, FL: CRC Press.

Altman, D. G. (1991). Statistics in medical journals: Developments in the 1980s. *Statistics in Medicine, 10*(12), 1897.

Altman, D. G. (1994). The scandal of poor medical research. *British Medical Journal, 308*(6924), 283.

Altman, D. G. (2000). Statistics in medical journals: Some recent trends. *Statistics in Medicine, 19*(23), 3275–3289.

Anders, M. E., & Evans, D. P. (2010). Comparison of PubMed and Google Scholar literature searches. *Respiratory Care, 55*(5), 578–583.

Armitage, P. (1955). Tests for linear trends in proportions and frequencies. *Biometrics, 11,* 375–386. doi: 10.2307/3001775

Armitage, P., Berry, G., & Matthews, J. N. S. (2008). *Statistical methods in medical research.* New York: John Wiley.

Armstrong, G. D. (1981). Parametric statistics and ordinal data: A pervasive misconception. *Nursing Research, 30*(1), 60–62.

Bakeman, R., & Gottman, J. M. (1997). *Observing interaction: An introduction to sequential analysis* (2nd ed.). Cambridge, UK: Cambridge University Press.

Balanda, K. P., & MacGillivray, H. (1988). Kurtosis: A critical review. *The American Statistician, 42*(2), 111–119.

Barfield, J. P., & Malone, L. A. (2013). Perceived exercise benefits and barriers among power wheelchair soccer players. *Journal of Rehabilitation Research & Development, 50*(2), 231–238. doi: 10.1682/JRRD.2011.12.0234

Barnard, G. A. (1945). A new test for 2 × 2 tables. *Nature, 156,* 177, 183.

Basta, T., Shacham, E., & Reece, M. (2008). Psychological distress and engagement in HIV-related services among individuals seeking mental health care. *AIDS Care, 20*(8), 969–976.

Bathke, A., & Brunner, E. (2003). A nonparametric alternative to analysis of covariance. In M. G. Akritas & D. M. Brunner (Eds.), *Recent advances and trends in nonparametric statistics.* Amsterdam: Elsevier.

Beach, E. K., Maloney, B. H., Plocica, A. R., Sherry, S. E., Weaver, M., Luthringer, L., & Utz, S. (1992). The spouse: A factor in recovery after acute myocardial infarction. *Heart & Lung: The Journal of Critical Care, 21,* 30–38.

Belsley, D. A., Kuh, E., & Welsch, R. E. (2005). *Regression diagnostics: Identifying influential data and sources of collinearity* (Vol. 571). New York: John Wiley.

Bennett, B. M., & Underwood, R. E. (1970). On McNemar's test for the 2 × 2 table and its power function. *Biometrics, 6,* 339–343.

Benyamini, Y., Gerber, Y., Molshatzki, N., Goldbourt, U., & Drory, Y. (2014). Recovery of self-rated health as a predictor of recurrent ischemic events after first myocardial infarction: A 13-year follow-up. *Health Psychology, 33*(4), 317–325. doi: 10.1037/a0031371

Berry, J. G., Poduri, A., Bonkowsky, J. L., Zhou, J., Graham, D. A., Welch, C., . . . Srivastava, R. (2012). Trends in resource utilization by children with neurological impairment in the United States inpatient health care system: A repeat cross-sectional study. *PLoS Medicine, 9*(1), e1001158. doi: 10.1371/journal.pmed.1001158

Berry, K. J., & Mielke, P. W. (1987). Exact chi-square and Fisher's exact probability test for 3 by 2 cross-classification tables. *Educational and Psychological Measurement, 47*(3), 631–636. doi: 10.1177/001316448704700312

Bewick, V., Cheek, L., & Ball, J. (2004). Statistics review 10: Further nonparametric methods. *Critical Care, 8*(3), 196–199.

Bhambhani, Y., Mactavish, J., Warren, S., Thompson, W. R., Webborn, A., Bressan, E., . . . Vanlandewijck, Y. (2010). Boosting in athletes with high-level spinal cord injury: Knowledge, incidence and attitudes of athletes in paralympic sport. *Disability & Rehabilitation, 32*(26), 2172–2190. doi: 10.3109/09638288.2010.505678

Bilder, C., & Loughin, T. (2004). Testing for marginal independence between two categorical variables with multiple responses. *Biometrics, 60*(1), 241–248.

Biswas, A. (2008). *Statistical advances in the biomedical sciences: Clinical trials, epidemiology, survival analysis and bioinformatics.* Hoboken, NJ: John Wiley.

Blair, R. C., & Higgins, J. J. (1985). Comparison of the power of the paired samples t-test to that of Wilcoxon's signed ranks test under various population shapes. *Psychological Bulletin, 97,* 119–128.

Blair, R. C., Sawilowsky, S. S., & Higgins, J. J. (1987). Limitations of the rank transform statistic in tests for interactions. *Communications in Statistics-Simulation and Computation, 16*(4), 1133–1145.

Bland, J. M., & Altman, D. G. (2000). The odds ratio. *British Medical Journal, 320,* 1468.

Bontempi, J. B., Mugno, R., Bulmer, S. M., Danvers, K., & Vancour, M. L. (2009). Exploring gender differences in the relationship between HIV/STD testing and condom use among undergraduate college students. *American Journal of Health Education, 40*(2), 97–105.

Bowring, A. L., Peeters, A., Freak-Poli, R., Lim, M. S., Gouillou, M., & Hellard, M. (2012). Measuring the accuracy of self-reported height and weight in a community-based sample of young people. *BMC Medical Research Methodology, 12,* 175–175.

Box, G. E. P., & Tidwell, P. W. (1962). Transformation of the independent variables. *Technometrics, 4,* 531–550.

Brennan, R. L. (2001). *Generalizability theory.* New York: Springer-Verlag.

Brennan, R. L., & Prediger, D. J. (1981). Coefficient kappa: Some uses, misuses, and alternatives. *Educational and Psychological Measurement, 41,* 678–699.

Breslow, N. E., & Day, N. E. (1980). *Statistical methods in cancer research: Vol. 1. The analysis of case-control studies* (Vol. 1). Lyons, France: International Agency for Research on Cancer.

Brown, L. D., Cai, T. T., & DasGupta, A. (2001). Interval estimation for a binomial proportion. *Statistical Science, 16,* 101–117.

Brunner, E., Domhof, S., & Langer, F. (2002). *Nonparametric analysis of longitudinal data in factorial experiments.* New York: John Wiley.

Brunner, E., & Zapf, A. (2014). Nonparametric ROC analysis for diagnostic trials. In N. Balakrishnan (Ed.), *Methods and applications of statistics in clinical trials* (pp. 483–495), New York: John Wiley.

Buck, J. L., & Finner, S. L. (1985). A still further note on Freeman's measure of association. *Psychometrika, 50,* 365–366.

Buehler, R. J. (1957, December 1). confidence intervals for the product of two binomial parameters. *Journal of the American Statistical Association, 52*(280), 482–493.

Bŭhlmann, P. (2003). Bagging, subagging and bragging for improving some prediction algorithms. In M. G. Akritas & D. N. Politis (Eds.), *Recent advances and trends in nonparametric statistics* (pp. 19–34). Amsterdam: Elsevier.

Burnette, K., Ramundo, M., Stevenson, M., & Beeson, M. S. (2009). Evaluation of a web-based asynchronous pediatric emergency medicine learning tool for residents and medical students. *Academic Emergency Medicine, 16*(12), S46–S50. doi: 10.1111/j.1553-2712.2009.00598.x

Butar, F., & Park, J.-W. (2008). Permutation tests for comparing two populations. *Journal of Mathematical Sciences & Mathematics Education, 3*(2), 19–30.

Byrne, B. M. (2010). *Structural equation modeling with AMOS: Basic concepts, applications, and programming* (2nd ed.). New York: Routledge.

Cai, J., & Zeng, D. (2004). Sample size/power calculation for case-cohort studies. *Biometrics, 60*(4), 1015–1024.

Camilli, G. (1990). The test of homogeneity for 2 × 2 contingency tables: A review of and some personal opinions on the controversy. *Psychological Bulletin, 108*(1), 135–145.

Campbell, I. (2007). Chi-squared and Fisher-Irwin tests of two-by-two tables with small sample recommendations. *Statistics in Medicine, 26,* 3661–3765.

Canto, J. G., Shlipak, M. G., Rogers, W. J., Malmgren, J. A., Frederick, P. D., Lambrew, C. T., . . . Kiefe, C. I. (2000). Prevalence, clinical characteristics, and mortality among patients with myocardial infarction presenting without chest pain. *Journal of the American Medical Association, 283*(24), 3223–3229.

Cao, H., Lake, D. E., Griffin, M. P., & Moorman, J. R. (2004). Increased nonstationarity of neonatal heart rate before the clinical diagnosis of sepsis. *Annals of Biomedical Engineering, 32*(2), 233–244.

Capio, C. M., Sit, C. H. P., & Abernethy, B. (2011). Fundamental movement skills testing in children with cerebral palsy. *Disability & Rehabilitation, 33*(25/26), 2519–2528. doi: 10.3109/09638288.2011.577502

Carifio, J., & Perla, R. (2008). Resolving the 50-year debate around using and misusing Likert scales. *Medical Education, 42*(12), 1150–1152. doi: 10.1111/j.1365-2923.2008.03172.x

Cerulli, C., Talbot, N. L., Tang, W., & Chaudron, L. H. (2011). Co-occurring intimate partner violence and mental health diagnoses in perinatal women. *Journal of Women's Health, 20*(12), 1797–1803. doi: 10.1089/jwh.2010.2201

Charan, J., & Biswas, T. (2013). How to calculate sample size for different study designs in medical research? *Indian Journal of Psychological Medicine, 35*(2), 121.

Chumbler, N. R., Huanguang, J., Phipps, M. S., Xinli, L., Ordin, D., Williams, L. S., . . . Bravata, D. M. (2013). Postdischarge quality of care: Do age disparities exist among Department of Veterans Affairs ischemic stroke patients? *Journal of Rehabilitation Research & Development, 50*(2), 263–272. doi: 10.1682/JRRD.2011.08.0145

Closas, P., Coma, E., & Méndez, L. (2012). Sequential detection of influenza epidemics by the Kolmogorov-Smirnov test. *BMC Medical Informatics and Decision Making, 12,* 112. doi: 10.1186/1472-6947-12-112

Cochran, W. G. (1952). The χ^2 test of goodness of fit. *Annals of Mathematical Statistics, 25,* 315–345.

Cochran, W. G. (1954). Some methods for strengthening the common χ^2 tests. *Biometrics, 10,* 417–451.

Cohen, J. (1960). A coefficient of agreement for nominal scales. *Educational and Psychological Measurement, 20,* 37–46.

Cohen, J. (1968). Weighted kappa: Nominal scale agreement with provision for scaled disagreement or partial credit. *Psychological Bulletin, 70,* 213–220.

Collado, V., Faulks, D., Nicolas, E., & Hennequin, M. (2013). Conscious sedation procedures using intravenous midazolam for dental care in patients with different cognitive profiles: A prospective study of effectiveness and safety. *PLoS ONE, 8*(8), e71240.

Collingridge, D. S. (2013). A primer on quantitized data analysis and permutation testing. *Journal of Mixed Methods Research, 7*(1), 79–95.

Conover, W. J. (1999). *Practical nonparametric statistics* (3rd ed.). New York: John Wiley.

Conover, W. J., & Iman, R. L. (1976). On some alternative procedures using ranks for the analysis of experimental designs. *Communications in Statistics, A5*(14), 1349–1368.

Conover, W. J., & Iman, R. L. (1981). Rank transformations as a bridge between parametric and nonparametric statistics. *American Statistician, 35*(3), 124–129.

Conover, W. J., & Iman, R. L. (1982). Analysis of covariance using the rank transformation. *Biometrics, 38*(3), 715–724.

Cook, R. D. (1977). Detection of influential outliers in linear regression. *Technometrics, 19,* 15–18.

Cook, R. D. (1979). Influential observations in linear regression. *Journal of the American Statistical Association, 74,* 169–174.

Cox, D. R., & Snell, E. J. (1989). *Analysis of binary data* (2nd ed.). New York: Chapman & Hall.

Cramér, H. (1946). *Mathematical models of statistics*. Princeton, NJ: Princeton University Press.

Cronbach, L. J., Gleser, G. C., Nanda, H., & Rajaratmam, N. (1972). *The dependability of behavioral measurements: Theory of generalizability of scores and profiles*. New York: John Wiley.

Curtis, D. A., & Marascuilo, L. A. (1992). Point estimates and confidence intervals for the parameters of the two-sample and matched-pair combined tests for ranks and normal scores. *Journal of Experimental Education, 60*(3), 243–269. doi: 10.1080/00220973.1992.9943879

Damrosch, S. P., & Perry, L. A. (1989). Self-reported adjustment, chronic sorrow, and coping of parents of children with Down syndrome. *Nursing Research, 38,* 25–30.

Daniel, W. W. (2000). *Applied nonparametric statistics* (2nd ed.). Pacific Grove, CA: Duxbury.

Davison, A. C., & Hinkley, D. V. (2006). *Bootstrap methods and their application*. Cambridge, England: Cambridge University Press.

DeCarlo, L. T. (1997). On the meaning and use of kurtosis. *Psychological Methods, 2*(3), 292–307. doi: 10.1037/1082-989X.2.3.292

Delyzer, T. L., & Yazdani, A. (2013). Characterizing the lateral slope of the aging female eyebrow. *Canadian Journal of Plastic Surgery, 21*(3), 173–177.

Demir, S. G., & Erdil, F. (2013). Effectiveness of home monitoring according to the Model of Living in hip replacement surgery patients. *Journal of Clinical Nursing, 22*(9/10), 1226–1241. doi: 10.1111/jocn.12255

Dexter, F. (1994). Analysis of statistical tests to compare doses of analgesics among groups. *Anesthesiology, 81,* 610–615.

Donlan, W., & Lee, J. (2010). Coraje, nervios, and susto: Culture-bound syndromes and mental health among Mexican migrants in the United States. *Advances in Mental Health, 9*(3), 288–302.

Dubnicka, S. R. (2011). Kernel density estimation with missing data: Misspecifying the missing data mechanism. In J. L. Rosenberger, T. P. Hettmansperger, D. R. Hunter, D. S. P. Richards, & J. L. Rosenberger (Eds.), *Nonparametric statistics and mixture models: A Festschrift in honor of Thomas P. Hettmansperger.* Singapore: World Scientific.

Dunn, O. J. (1964). Multiple comparisons using rank sums. *Technometrics, 6*(3), 241–252.

Eaves, R. C., & Milner, B. (1993). The criterion-related validity of the Childhood Autism Rating Scale and the Autism Behavior Checklist. *Journal of Abnormal Child Psychology, 21,* 481–491.

Edgington, E., & Onghena, P. (2007). *Randomization tests.* Boca Raton, FL: CRC Press.

Elizondo-Montemayor, L., Gutierrez, N. G., Moreno, D. M., Martínez, U., Tamargo, D., & Treviño, M. (2013). School-based individualised lifestyle intervention decreases obesity and the metabolic syndrome in Mexican children. *Journal of Human Nutrition & Dietetics, 26,* 82–89. doi: 10.1111/jhn.12070

Eskander, M. S., Balsis, S. M., Balinger, C., Howard, C. M., Lewing, N. W., Eskander, J. P., . . . Jenis, L. G. (2012). The association between preoperative spinal cord rotation and postoperative c5 nerve palsy. *Journal of Bone & Joint Surgery, American Volume, 94*(17), 1605–1609.

Evans, S., Ferrando, S., Carr, C., & Haglin, D. (2011). Mindfulness-based stress reduction (MBSR) and distress in a community-based sample. *Clinical Psychology & Psychotherapy, 18*(6), 553–558. doi: 10.1002/cpp.727

Fagerland, M. (2012). *t*-Tests, non-parametric tests, and large studies—a paradox of statistical practice? *BMC Medical Research Methodology, 12*(1), 78.

Fagerland, M., & Sandvik, L. (2009). The Wilcoxon-Mann-Whitney test under scrutiny. *Statistics in Medicine, 28,* 1487–1497.

Fallin, A., Johnson, A. O., Riker, C., Cohen, E., Rayens, M. K., & Hahn, E. J. (2013). An intervention to increase compliance with a tobacco-free university policy. *American Journal of Health Promotion, 27*(3), 162–169. doi: 10.4278/ajhp.110707-QUAN-275

Faul, F., Erdfelder, E., Buchner, A., & Lang, A. (2009). Statistical power analyses using G*Power 3.1: Tests for correlation and regression analyses. *Behavior Research Methods, 41*(4), 1149–1160.

Faul, F., Erdfelder, E., Lang, A., & Buchner, A. (2007). G* Power 3: A flexible statistical power analysis program for the social, behavioral, and biomedical sciences. *Behavior Research Methods, 39*(2), 175–191.

Feuer, E. J., & Kessler, L. G. (1989). Test statistic and sample size for a two-sample McNemar test. *Biometrics, 45*(2), 629–636.

Feuerman, M., & Miller, A. R. (2008). Relationships between statistical measures of agreement: Sensitivity, specificity and kappa. *Journal of Evaluation in Clinical Practice, 14*(5), 930–933. doi: 10.1111/j.1365-2753.2008.00984.x

Field, A. (2009). *Discovering statistics using SPSS* (3rd ed.). Thousand Oaks, CA: Sage.

Field, A. (2013). *Discovering statistics using IBM SPSS statistics.* Los Angeles, CA: Sage.

Finch, H. (2005). Performance of nonparametric and parametric MANOVA test statistics. *Methodology, 1*(1), 27–38.

Fisher, R. A. (1935). *The design of experiments.* New York: Hafner.

Fleiss, J. L. (1971). Measuring nominal scale agreement among many raters. *Psychological Bulletin, 76,* 378–382.

Fleiss, J. L., Cohen, J., & Everitt, B. S. (1969). Large sample standard errors of kappa and weighted kappa. *Psychological Bulletin, 72,* 323–327.

Freelon, D. (2010). ReCal: Intercoder reliability calculation as a web service. *International Journal of Internet Science, 5*(1), 20–33.

Freeman, G., & Halton, J. (1951). Note on an exact treatment of contingency, goodness of fit and other problems of significance. *Biometrika, 38*(1/2), 141–149.

Freeman, L. C. (1965). *Elementary applied statistics: For students in behavioral science.* New York: John Wiley.

Freidlin, B., & Gastwirth, J. L. (2000). Should the median test be retired from general use? *The American Statistician, 54*(3), 161–164.

Fromm, R. E., Levine, R. L., & Pepe, P. E. (1992). Circadian variation in the time of request for helicopter transport of cardiac patients. *Annals of Emergency Medicine, 23,* 75–80.

Gaddis, G. M., & Gaddis, M. L. (1994). Non-normality of distribution of Glasgow Coma Scores and Revised Trauma Scores. *Annals of Emergency Medicine, 23,* 75–80.

Gaither, N., & Glorfeld, L. (1983). An evaluation of the use of tests of significance in organizational behavior research. *Academy of Management Review, 10,* 787–793.

Gaither, N., & Glorfeld, L. (1985). An evaluation of the use of tests of significance in organizational behavior research. *Academy of Management Review, 10*(4), 787–793. doi: 10.2307/258046

Garrett, N. A., Alesci, N. L., Schultz, M. M., Foldes, S. S., Magnan, S. J., & Manley, M. W. (2004). The relationship of stage of change for smoking cessation to stage of change for fruit and vegetable consumption and physical activity in a health plan population. *American Journal of Health Promotion, 19*(2), 118–127.

Garson, G. D. (2014). *Logistic regression: Binary & multinomial.* Asheboro, NC: Statistical Publishing Associates.

Gibbons, J. D. (1985). *Nonparametric methods for quantitative analysis.* Columbus OH: American Sciences Press.

Gibbons, J. D., & Chakraborti, S. (1991). Comparisons of the Mann-Whitney, Student's t, and alternate t tests for means of normal distributions. *Journal of Experimental Education, 59,* 258–267.

Gijbels, I. (2003). Inference for nonsmooth regression curves and surfaces using kernel-based methods. In M. G. Akritas & D. N. Politis (Eds.), *Recent advances and trends in nonparametric statistics* (pp. 183–202). Amsterdam: Elsevier.

Gini, G., & Pozzoli, T. (2013). Bullied children and psychosomatic problems: A meta-analysis. *Pediatrics, 132*(4), 720–729. doi: 10.1542/peds.2013-0614

Glazer, W. M., Morgenstern, H., & Doucette, J. (1994). Race and tardive dyskinesia among outpatients at a CMHC. *Hospital and Community Psychiatry, 45,* 38–42.

Goffman, D., Madden, R. C., Harrison, E. A., Merkatz, I. R., & Chazotte, C. (2007). Predictors of maternal mortality and near-miss maternal morbidity. *Journal of Perinatology, 27*(10), 597–601.

Good, P. I. (1995). *Permutation tests: A practical guide to resampling methods for testing hypothesis.* New York: Springer.

Good, P. I. (2005). *Permutation, parametric and bootstrap tests of hypotheses* (3rd ed.). New York: Springer.

Goodman, L. A. (1954). Kolmogorov-Smirnov tests for psychological research. *Psychological Bulletin, 51,* 160–168.

Graves, K. D., Carter, C. L., Anderson, E. S., & Winett, R. A. (2003). Quality of life pilot intervention for breast cancer patients: Use of social cognitive theory. *Palliative & Supportive Care, 1*(2), 121–134.

Green, S. B. (1981). A comparison of three indexes of agreement between observers: Proportion of agreement, G-Index, and kappa. *Educational and Psychological Measurement, 41,* 1069–1072.

Guadagnolo, B. A., Cina, K., Koop, D., Brunette, D., & Petereit, D. G. (2011). A pre-post survey analysis of satisfaction with health care and medical mistrust after patient navigation for American Indian cancer patients. *Journal of Health Care for the Poor and Underserved, 22*(4), 1331–1343. doi: 10.1353/hpu.2011.0115

Haberman, S. J. (1984). The analysis of residuals in cross-classified tables. *Biometrics, 29,* 205–220.

Hair, J. F., Black, W., Babin, C., Anderson, R. E., & Tatham, R. L. (2010). *Multivariate data analysis* (7th ed.). Englewood Cliffs, NJ: Prentice Hall.

Hair, J. F., Jr., Anderson, R. E., Tatham, R. L., & Black, W. C. (1995). *Multivariate data analysis: With readings* (3rd ed.). New York: Macmillan.

Han, L. (2009). SouthEast SAS Users Group. Calculating the point estimate and confidence interval of Hodges-Lehmann's median using SAS software: SESUG 2008: The Proceedings of the SouthEast SAS Users Group, St Pete Beach, FL, 2008. http://analytics.ncsu.edu/sesug/2008/ST-154.pdf

Harwell, M. R. (1988). Choosing between parametric and nonparametric tests. *Journal of Counseling & Development, 67*(1), 35–38. doi: 10.1002/j.1556-6676.1988.tb02007.x

Hauck, W. N., & Donner, A. (1977). Wald's test as applied to hypotheses in logit analysis. *Journal of the American Statistical Association, 72,* 851–853.

Hayes, A. F., & Krippendorff, K. (2007). Answering the call for a standard reliability measure for coding data. *Communication Methods and Measures, 1,* 77–89.

Hayes, L., Quine, S., & Bush, J. (1994). Attitude change amongst nursing students towards Australian Aborigines. *International Journal of Nursing Studies, 31*(1), 67–76.

Hays, W. (1994). *Statistics* (5th ed.). Belmont, CA: Wadsworth/Cengage Learning.

Hempton, C., Dow, B., Cortes-Simonet, E. N., Ellis, K., Koch, S., LoGiudice, D., . . . Ames, D. (2011). Contrasting perceptions of health professionals and older people in Australia: What constitutes elder abuse? *International Journal of Geriatric Psychiatry, 26*(5), 466–472. doi: 10.1002/gps.2549

Herman, T., Giladi, N., & Hausdorff, J. M. (2011). Properties of the 'timed up and go' test: More than meets the eye. *Gerontology, 57*(3), 203–210. doi: 10.1159/000314963

Hettmansperger, T. P. (1984). *Statistical inference based on ranks.* New York: John Wiley.

Higgins, J., & Green, S. (Eds.). (2011). *Cochrane handbook for systematic reviews of interventions* (5.1.0 ed.). www.cochrane-handbook.org

Higgins, J., Thompson, S. G., Deeks, J. J., & Altman, D. G. (2003). Measuring inconsistency in meta-analyses. *British Medical Journal, 327*(7414), 557–560.

Hinds, P. S., Hockenberry, M., Rai, S. N., Zhang, L., Razzouk, B. I., McCarthy, K., . . . Rodriguez-Galindo, C. (2007). Nocturnal awakenings, sleep environment interruptions, and fatigue in hospitalized children with cancer. *Oncology Nursing Forum, 34*(2), 393–402. doi: 10.1188/07.ONF.393-402

Hinds, P. S., & Hockenberry-Eaton, M. (2001). Developing a research program on fatigue in children and adolescents diagnosed with cancer. *Journal of Pediatric Oncology Nursing, 18*(2, Suppl. 1), 3–12.

Hinkelman, K., & Kempthorne, O. (2007). Factorial experiments: Basic ideas. In K. Hinkelman & O. Kempthorne (Eds.), *Design and analysis of experiments* (pp. 419–495). New York: John Wiley.

Hinkle, D. E., Wiersma, W., & Jurs, S. G. (2003). *Applied statistics for the behavioral sciences.* Boston, MA: Houghton Mifflin.

Hintze, J. (2013). *PASS 12.* Kaysville, UT: NCSS, LLC. www.ncss.com

Hirji, K. F., Tan, S.-J., & Elashoff, R. M. (1991). A quasi-exact test for comparing two binomial proportions. *Statistics in Medicine, 10*(7), 1137–1153. doi: 10.1002/sim.4780100713

Hockenberry, M. J., Hinds, P. S., Barrera, P., Bryant, R., Adams-McNeill, J., Hooke, C., . . . Manteuffel, B. (2003). Three instruments to assess fatigue in children with cancer: The child, parent and staff perspectives. *Journal of Pain and Symptom Management, 25*(4), 319–328.

Hodges, J. L., & Lehmann, E. L. (1963). Estimates of location based on rank tests. *Annals of Mathematical Statistics, 34,* 598–611.

Holland, B. S., & Copenhaver, M. D. (1988). Improved Bonferroni-type multiple testing procedures. *Psychological Bulletin, 104*(1), 145.

Horová, I., Koláček, J., & Zelinka, J. (2012). *Kernel smoothing in MATLAB: Theory and practice of kernel smoothing.* Singapore: World Scientific Publishing.

Horton, N. J., & Switzer, S. S. (2005). Statistical methods in the journal. *New England Journal of Med, 353*(18), 1977–1979.

Hosmer, D. W., & Lemeshow, S. (1980). Goodness of fit tests for the multiple logistic regression model. *Communications in Statistics—Theory and Methods, 9*(10), 1043–1069.

Hosmer, D. W., & Lemeshow, S. (1999). *Applied survival analysis.* New York: John Wiley.

Hosmer, D. W., Lemeshow, S., & Sturdivant, R. X. (2013). *Applied logistic regression.* http://utah.eblib.com/patron/FullRecord.aspx?p=1138225

Howell, D. C. (2011). *Statistical methods for psychology.* Belmont, CA: Cengage Learning.

Huebner, R. A., Johnson, K., Bennett, C. M., & Schneck, C. (2003). Community participation and quality of life outcomes after adult traumatic brain injury. *American Journal of Occupational Therapy, 57*(2), 177–185. doi: 10.5014/ajot.57.2.177

IBM. (2012). *IBM SPSS Statistics for Windows* (Version 21.0). Armonk, NY: Author.

IBM® SPSS® (2015). *IBM® SPSS® SamplePower* (v.3.0.1) Chicago: IBM SPSS, Inc.

Jagsi, R., Motomura, A. R., Amarnath, S., Jankovic, A., Sheets, N., & Ubel, P. A. (2009). Under-representation of women in high-impact published clinical cancer research. *Cancer, 115*(14), 3293–3301. doi: 10.1002/cncr.24366

Jamieson, S. (2004). Likert scales: How to (ab)use them. *Medical Education, 38*(12), 1217–1218. doi: 10.1111/j.1365-2929.2004.02012.x

Jenkins, S. J., Fuqua, D. R., & Froehle, T. C. (1984). A critical examination of use of non-parametric statistics in the *Journal of Counseling Psychology. Perceptual and Motor Skills, 59*(1), 31–35. doi: 10.2466/pms.1984.59.1.31

Jin, Z., Yu, D., Zhang, L., Meng, H., Lu, J., Gao, Q., . . . He, J. (2010). A retrospective survey of research design and statistical analyses in selected Chinese medical journals in 1998 and 2008. *PLoS ONE, 5*(5), e10822. doi: 10.1371/journal.pone.0010822

Johnson, A. F. (1985). Beneath the technological fix: Outliers and probability statements. *Journal of Chronic Diseases, 38*(11), 957–961.

Jooste, P. L., Weight, M. J., & Lombard, C. J. (2000). Short-term effectiveness of mandatory iodization of table salt, at an elevated iodine concentration, on the iodine and goiter status of schoolchildren with endemic goiter. *American Journal of Clinical Nutrition, 71*(1), 75–80.

Kaartinen, M., Puura, K., Mäkelä, T., Rannisto, M., Lemponen, R., Helminen, M., . . . Hietanen, J. (2012). Autonomic arousal to direct gaze correlates with social impairments among children with ASD. *Journal of Autism & Developmental Disorders, 42*(9), 1917–1927. doi: 10.1007/s10803-011-1435-2

Kabaila, P., & Lloyd, C. J. (2000). Profile upper confidence limits from discrete data. *Australian and New Zealand Journal of Statistics, 39,* 193-204.

Kallenberg, W. C. M., Oosterhoff, J., & Schriever, B. F. (1985). The number of classes in chi-squared goodness-of-fit tests. *Journal of the American Statistical Association, 80,* 959–968.

Kallert, T. W., Glöckner, M., & Schützwohl, M. (2008). Involuntary vs. voluntary hospital admission: A systematic literature review on outcome diversity. *European Archives of Psychiatry and Clinical Neuroscience, 258*(4), 195–209.

Kaplan, E. L., & Meier, P. (1958). Nonparametric estimation from incomplete observations. *Journal of the American Statistical Association, 53,* 457–481.

Kasiulevičius, V., Šapoka, V., & Filipavičiūtė, R. (2006). Sample size calculation in epidemiological studies. *Gerantologija, 7*(4), 225–231.

Katerndahl, D. A. (1990). Comparison of panic symptom sequences and pathophysiologic models. *Journal of Behavior Therapy and Experimental Psychiatry, 21,* 101–111.

Katz, N., & Sachs, D. (1991). Meaning ascribed to major professional concepts: A comparison of occupational therapy students and practitioners in the United States and Israel. *American Journal of Occupational Therapy, 45*(2), 137–145.

Kellar, S. P., & Kelvin, E. A. (2012). *Munro's statistical methods for health care research.* Philadelphia, PA: Wolters Kluwer Health/Lippincott Williams & Wilkins.

Kendall, M. G. (1938). A new measure of rank correlation. *Biometrika, 30,* 81–93.

King, D. J., Gotch, F. M., & Larsson-Sciard, E. L. (2001). T-cell re-population in HIV-infected children on highly active anti-retroviral therapy (HAART). *Clinical and Experimental Immunology, 125*(3), 447–454.

Kleinbaum, D. G. (1996). *Survival analysis: A self-learning text.* New York: Springer-Verlag.

Klosky, J. L., Foster, R. H., Li, Z., Peasant, C., Howell, C. R., Mertens, A. C., . . . Ness, K. K. (2013). Risky sexual behavior in adolescent survivors of childhood cancer: A report from the Childhood Cancer Survivor Study. *Health Psychology, 33,* 868–877. doi: 10.1037/hea0000044

Knapp, T. R. (1990). Treating ordinal scales as interval scales: An attempt to resolve the controversy. *Nursing Research, 39*(2), 121–123.

Koeslag, J. H., Schach, S. R., & Melzer, C. W. (1987). A reappraisal of the use of the phi coefficient in multiple choice examinations. *Medical Education, 21,* 46–52.

Konietschke, F., Bathke, A., Hothorn, L., & Brunner, E. (2010). Testing and estimation of purely nonparametric effects in repeated measures designs. *Computational Statistics and Data Analysis, 54,* 1895–1905.

Korosteleva, O. (2014). *Nonparametric methods in statistics with SAS applications.* Boca Raton, FL: CRC Press.

Kothari, C. L., Zielinski, R., James, A., Charoth, R. M., & Sweezy Ldel, C. (2014). Improved birth weight for Black infants: Outcomes of a Healthy Start program. *American Journal of Public Health, 104*(Suppl. 1), S96–S104. doi: 10.2105/AJPH.2013.301359

Krippendorff, K. (2013). *Content analysis: An introduction to its methodology* (3rd ed.). Thousand Oaks, CA: Sage.

Kruskal, W. H. (1988). Miracles and statistics: The casual assumption of independence. *Journal of the American Statistical Association, 83*(404), 929–940.

Kruskal, W. H. (1952). A nonparametric test for the several sample problem. *Annals of Mathematical Statistics, 23*(4), 525–540.

Kruskal, W. H., & Wallis, W. A. (1952). Use of ranks in one-criterion variance analysis. *Journal of the American Statistical Association, 47*, 583–621.

Kydd, A., Touhy, T., Newman, D., Fagerberg, I., & Engstrom, G. (2014). Attitudes towards caring for older people in Scotland, Sweden and the United States. *Nursing Older People, 26*(2), 33–40. doi: 10.7748/nop2014.02.26.2.33.e547

Kyrgiou, M., Koliopoulos, G., Martin-Hirsch, P., Arbyn, M., Prendiville, W., & Paraskevaidis, E. (2006). Obstetric outcomes after conservative treatment for intraepithelial or early invasive cervical lesions: Systematic review and meta-analysis. *Lancet, 367*(9509), 489–498.

Landis, J. R., & Koch, G. G. (1977). The measurement of observer agreement for categorical data. *Biometrica, 33*, 159–174.

Lee-Lin, F., Menon, U., Pett, M., Nail, L., Lee, S., & Mooney, K. (2007). Breast cancer beliefs and mammography screening practices among Chinese American immigrants. *Journal of Obstetric, Gynecologic, & Neonatal Nursing, 36*(3), 212–221.

Lehman, R. S. (1991). *Statistics and research design in the behavioral sciences.* Belmont, CA: Wadsworth/Thomson Learning.

Lehmann, E. L. (2006). *Nonparametrics: Statistical methods based on ranks.* New York: Springer-Verlag.

Lehmann, E. L., & Romano, J. P. (2005). *Testing statistical hypotheses* (3rd ed.). New York: Springer.

Lemeshow, S., & Hosmer, D. W. (1982). A review of goodness of fit statistics for use in the development of logistic regression models. *American Journal of Epidemiology, 115*(1), 92–106.

Lennon, O., Carey, A., Gaffney, N., Stephenson, J., & Blake, C. (2008). A pilot randomized controlled trial to evaluate the benefit of the cardiac rehabilitation paradigm for the non-acute ischaemic stroke population. *Clinical Rehabilitation, 22*(2), 125–133. doi: 10.1177/0269215507081580

Libsicas, C.B., Mäkinen, I. H., Wasserman, D., Apter, A., Kerkhof, A., Michel, K., Renberg, E.S., van Heeringen, K. Värnik, A. & Schmidtke, A. (2013). Gender distribution of suicide attempts among immigrant groups in European countries—an international perspective. *European Journal of Public Health, 23*(2), 279–284. doi: 10.1093/eurpub/cks029

Lilliefors, H. W. (1967). On the Kolmogorov-Smirnov test for normality with mean and variance unknown. *Journal of the American Statistical Association, 62*, 399–402.

Lloyd, C. J. (2007). Exact one-sided confidence limits for the difference between two correlated proportions. *Statistics in Medicine, 26*, 3369–3384.

Lloyd, C. J. (2013). Accurate confidence limits for stratified clinical trials. *Statistics in Medicine, 32*, 3415–3413.

Loerakker, S., Huisman, E. S., Glatz, J. F., Baaijens, F. P. T., Oomens, C. W. J., & Bader, D. L. (2012). Plasma variations of biomarkers for muscle damage in male nondisabled and spinal cord injured subjects. *Journal of Rehabilitation Research & Development, 49*(4), 361–372. doi: 10.1682/JRRD.2011.06.0100

Lomax, R. G., & Hahs-Vaughn, D. L. (2012). *Statistical concepts: A second course* (4th ed.). New York: Routledge/Taylor & Francis Group.

Long, J. S. (1997). *Regression models for categorical and limited dependent variables.* Thousand Oaks, CA: Sage.

Ludbrook, J., & Dudley, H. (1994). Issues in biomedical statistics: Analysing 2 × 2 tables of frequencies. *Australian and New Zealand Journal of Surgery, 64*(11), 780–787.

MacKenzie, G., & Peng, D. (Eds.). (2014). *Statistical modelling in biostatistics and bioinformatics.* New York: Springer.

Mann, H. B., & Whitney, D. R. (1947). On a test of whether one of two random variables is stochastically larger than the other. *Annals of Mathematical Statistics, 18*(1), 50–60.

Mansell, J. L., Tierney, R. T., Higgins, M., McDevitt, J., Toone, N., & Glutting, J. (2010). Concussive signs and symptoms following head impacts in collegiate athletes. *Brain Injury, 24*(9), 1070–1074. doi: 10.3109/02699052.2010.494589

Mantel, N. (1963). Chi-square tests with one degree of freedom; extensions of the Mantel-Haenszel Procedure. *Journal of the American Statistical Association, 58*(303), 690–700. doi: 10.1080/01621459.1963.10500879

Mantel, N., & Haenszel, W. (1959). Statistical aspects of the analysis of data from retrospective studies of disease. *Journal of the National Cancer Institute, 22,* 719–748.

Martinez-Camblor, P., Carleos, C., & Corral, N. (2011). Powerful nonparametric statistics to compare *k* independent ROC curves. *Journal of Applied Statistics, 38*(7), 1317–1332. doi: 10.1080/02664763.2010.498504

Mays, D., Gilman, S. E., Rende, R., Luta, G., Tercyak, K. P., & Niaura, R. S. (2014). Parental smoking exposure and adolescent smoking trajectories. *Pediatrics, 133*(6), 983–991. doi: 10.1542/peds.2013-3003

McCain, G. C. (1992). Facilitating inactive awake states in preterm infants: A study of three interventions. *Nursing Research, 40,* 359–363.

McFadden, D. (1974). Conditional logit analysis of qualitative choice behavior. In P. Zarembka (Ed.), *Conditional logit analysis of qualitative choice behavior* (pp. 105–142). New York: Academic Press.

McIntosh, C. G., Tonkin, S. L., & Gunn, A. J. (2013). Randomized controlled trial of a car safety seat insert to reduce hypoxia in term infants. *Pediatrics, 132*(2), 326–331. doi: 10.1542/peds.2013-0127

McKean, J., & Hettmansperger, T. P. (2011). *Robust nonparametric statistical methods.* Boca Raton, FL: CRC Press.

McNemar, Q. (1969). *Psychological statistics* (4th ed.). New York: John Wiley.

Meiser-Stedman, R., Smith, P., Glucksman, E., Yule, W., & Dalgleish, T. (2007). Parent and child agreement for acute stress disorder, post-traumatic stress disorder and other psychopathology in a prospective study of children and adolescents exposed to single-event trauma. *Journal of Abnormal Child Psychology, 35*(2), 191–201.

Menard, S. (2000). Coefficients of determination for multiple logistic regression analysis. *The American Statistician, 54,* 17–24.

Menard, S. (2002). *Applied logistic regression analysis.* Thousand Oaks, CA: Sage.

Menard, S. (2010). *Logistic regression: From introductory to advanced concepts and applications.* Thousand Oaks, CA: Sage.

Merrill, R. M., Lindsay, C. A., Shields, E. C., & Stoddard, J. (2007). Have the focus and sophistication of research in health education changed? *Health Education & Behavior, 34*(1), 10–25. doi: 10.1177/1090198106288564

Mier, N., Tanguma, J., Millard, A. V., Villarreal, E. K., Alen, M., & Ory, M. G. (2011). A pilot walking program for Mexican-American women living in colonias at the border. *American Journal of Health Promotion, 25*(3), 172–175. doi: 10.4278/ajhp.090325-ARB-115

Miletic, D., Sekulic, D., & Ostojic, L. (2007). Body physique and prior training experience as determinants of SEFIP score for university dancers. *Medical Problems of Performing Artists, 22*(3), 110–115.

Mooney, C. Z., & Duval, R. (1993). *Bootstrapping: A nonparametric approach to statistical inference.* Newbury Park, CA: Sage.

Morris, J. A., & Gardner, M. J. (1988). Calculating confidence intervals for relative risks (odds ratios) and standardised ratios and rates. *British Medical Journal, 296,* 1313–1316.

Myers, J. L., DCecco, J. V., White, J. B., & Borden, V. M. (1982). Repeated measurements of dichotomous variables: Q and F tests. *Psychological Bulletin, 92,* 517–525. doi: 10.1037/0033-2909.92.2.517

Nagelkerke, N. J. D. (1991). A note on a general definition of the coefficient of determination. *Biometrika, 78,* 691–692.

Neave, H. R., & Worthington, P. L. (1988). *Distribution-free tests.* London, UK: Routledge.

Neter, J., Wasserman, W., & Whitmore, G. (1993). *Applied statistics.* Englewood Cliffs, NJ: Prentice Hall.

Neuman, M. I., Hall, M., Gay, J. C., Blaschke, A. J., Williams, D. J., Parikh, K., . . . Shah, S. S. (2014). Readmissions among children previously hospitalized with pneumonia. *Pediatrics, 134*(1), 100–109. doi: 10.1542/peds.2014-0331

Newcombe, R. G. (2006). Confidence intervals for an effect size measure based on the Mann-Whitney statistic. Part 2: Asymptotic methods and evaluation. *Statistics in Medicine, 25*(4), 559–573.

Newcombe, R. G. (2012). *Confidence intervals for proportions and related measures of effect size.* Boca Raton, FL: CRC Press.

Newson, R. (2006). Confidence intervals for rank statistics: Somers' D and extensions. *Stata Journal, 6*(3), 309.

Newson, R. (2007, September). *Robust confidence intervals for Hodges–Lehmann median difference.* Paper presented at the 2007 UK Stata Users Group meeting, London, England. http://ideas.repec.org/p/boc/usug07/01.html

Ng, K., Scott, J. B., Drake, B. F., Chan, A. T., Hollis, B. W., Chandler, P. D., . . . Fuchs, C. S. (2014). Dose response to vitamin D supplementation in African Americans: Results of a 4-arm, randomized, placebo-controlled trial. *American Journal of Clinical Nutrition, 99*(3), 587–598. doi: 10.3945/ajcn.113.067777

Niemeier, J. P., Marwitz, J. H., Lesher, K., Walker, W. C., & Bushnik, T. (2007). Gender differences in executive functions following traumatic brain injury. *Neuropsychological Rehabilitation, 17*(3), 293–313.

Noguchi, K., Gel, Y. R., Brunner, E., & Konietschke, F. (2012). nparLD: An R software package for the nonparametric analysis of longitudinal data in factorial experiments. *Journal of Statistical Software, 50*(12), 1–23.

Nokes, N. R., & Tucker, L. A. (2012). Changes in hip bone mineral density and objectively measured physical activity in middle-aged women: A 6-year prospective study. *American Journal of Health Promotion, 26*(6), 341–347. doi: 10.4278/ajhp.100622-QUAN-208

Norman, G. (2010). Likert scales, levels of measurement and the "laws" of statistics. *Advances in Health Sciences Education, 15*(5), 625–632. doi: 10.1007/s10459-010-9222-y

Norman, G. R., & Streiner, D. L. (2008). *Biostatistics: The bare essentials.* Shelton, CT: People's Medical Publishing House.

Nunnally, J. C., & Bernstein, I. (1994). *Psychometric theory.* New York: McGraw-Hill.

Osborne, J. W. (2015). *Best practices in logistic regression.* Thousand Oaks, CA: Sage.

Overall, J. E., & Hornick, C. W. (1982). An evaluation of power and sample-size requirements for the continuity-corrected Fisher Exact test. *Perceptual and Motor Skills, 54*(1), 83–86. doi: 10.2466/pms.1982.54.1.83

Pampel, F. C. (2000). *Logistic regression: A primer.* Thousand Oaks, CA: Sage.

Park, H. M. (2008). *Univariate analysis and normality test using SAS, Stata, and SPSS.* Bloomington: University Information Technology Services, Indiana University.

Pastore, L. M., Morris, W. L., & Karns, L. B. (2008). Emotional reaction to fragile X premutation carrier tests among infertile women. *Journal of Genetic Counseling, 17*(1), 84–91. doi: 10.1007/s10897-007-9129-9

Patil, K. D. (1975). Cochran's Q test: Exact distribution. *Journal of the American Statistical Association, 70,* 186–189.

Pedhazur, E., & Schmelkin, L. (1991). *Measurement, design, and analysis: An integrated analysis.* Hillsdale, NJ: Lawrence Erlbaum.

Peduzzi, P., Concato, J., Kemper, E., Holford, T. R., & Feinstein, A. R. (1996). A simulation study of the number of events per variable in logistic regression analysis. *Journal of Clinical Epidemiology, 49*(12), 1373–1379.

Pell, G. (2005). Use and misuse of Likert scales. *Medical Education, 39*(9), 970. doi: 10.1111/j.1365-2929.2005.02237.x

Pett, M. A., Lackey, N. R., & Sullivan, J. J. (2003). *Making sense of factor analysis: The use of factor analysis for instrument development in health care research*. Thousand Oaks, CA: Sage.

Pett, M. A., & Sehy, Y. (1996). *The use and potential for misuse of parametric statistics in nursing research*. Salt Lake City: University of Utah College of Nursing.

Philip, P. A., Ayyangar, R., Vanderbilt, J., & Gaebler-Spira, D. J. (1994). Rehabilitation outcomes in children after treatment of primary brain tumor. *Archives of Physical Medicine and Rehabilitation, 75*, 36–39.

Preacher, K. J. (2001). Calculation for the chi-square test: An interactive calculation tool for chi-square tests of goodness of fit and independence [Computer software]. http://quantpsy.org

Pregibon, D. (1981). Logistic regression diagnostics. *Annals of Statistics, 9*, 705–724.

Price, J. W. (2013). Creatinine normalization of workplace urine drug tests: Does it make a difference? *Journal of Addiction Medicine, 7*(2), 129–132. doi: 10.1097/ADM.0b013e318283698c

Puri, M. L., & Sen, P. K. (1985). *Nonparametric methods in general linear models*. New York: John Wiley.

Quade, D. (1979). Using weighted rankings in the analysis of complete blocks with additive block effects. *Journal of the American Statistical Association, 74*(367), 680–683. doi: 10.2307/2286991

Qualls, M., Pallin, D. J., & Schuur, J. D. (2010). Parametric versus nonparametric statistical tests: The length of stay example. *Academic Emergency Medicine, 17*(10), 1113–1121. doi: 10.1111/j.1553-2712.2010.00874.x

Ratner, P. (1995). Indicators of exposure to wife abuse. *Canadian Journal of Nursing Research, 27*(1), 31.

Reed, J. A., Price, A. E., Grost, L., & Mantinan, K. (2012). Demographic characteristics and physical activity behaviors in sixteen Michigan parks. *Journal of Community Health: The Publication for Health Promotion and Disease Prevention, 37*(2), 507–512. doi: 10.1007/s10900-011-9471-6

Rentinck, I. C. M., Gorter, J. W., Ketelaar, M., Lindeman, E., & Jongmans, M. J. (2009). Perceptions of family participation among parents of children with cerebral palsy followed from infancy to toddler hood. *Disability & Rehabilitation, 31*(22), 1828–1834. doi: 10.1080/09638280902822286

Renzaho, A. M. N., & Polonsky, M. J. (2012). Examining demographic and socio-economic correlates of accurate knowledge about blood donation among African migrants in Australia. *Transfusion Medicine (Oxford, England), 22*(5), 321–331. doi: 10.1111/j.1365-3148.2012.01175.x

Rigby, A. S. (2000). Statistical methods in epidemiology: V. Towards an understanding of the kappa coefficient. *Disability & Rehabilitation, 22*(8), 339–344.

Robichaud-Ekstrand, S. (1991). Shower versus sink bath: Evaluation of heart rate, blood pressure, and subjective response of the patient with myocardial infarction. *Heart & Lung: The Journal of Critical Care, 20*, 375–382.

Robinson, J. G., Wang, S., Smith, B. J., & Jacobson, T. A. (2009). Meta-analysis of the relationship between non-high-density lipoprotein cholesterol reduction and coronary heart disease risk. *Journal of the American College of Cardiology, 53*(4), 316–322.

Robl, J., Jewell, T., & Kanotra, S. (2012). The effect of parental involvement on problematic social behaviors among school-age children in Kentucky. *Maternal & Child Health Journal, 16*, 287–297. doi: 10.1007/s10995-012-1187-4

Rosen, M. G., Debanne, S. M., Thompson, K., & Dickinson, J. C. (1992). Abnormal labor and infant brain damage. *Obstetrics and Gynecology, 80*(6), 961–965.

Rothman, K. J., Greenland, S., & Lash, T. L. (2008). *Modern epidemiology.* Philadelphia, PA: Lippincott Williams & Wilkins.

Roy, A., Forrester, L. W., Macko, R. F., & Krebs, H. I. (2013). Changes in passive ankle stiffness and its effects on gait function in people with chronic stroke. *Journal of Rehabilitation Research & Development, 50*(4), 555–571. doi: 10.1682/JRRD.2011.10.0206

Ruff, R. L., Riechers Ii, R. G., Wang, X.-F., Piero, T., & Ruff, S. S. (2012). For veterans with mild traumatic brain injury, improved posttraumatic stress disorder severity and sleep correlated with symptomatic improvement. *Journal of Rehabilitation Research & Development, 49*(9), 1305–1320. doi: 10.1682/JRRD.2011.12.0251

Ruttimann, U. E., & Pollack, M. M. (1991). Objective assessment of changing mortality risks in pediatric intensive care unit patients. *Critical Care Medicine, 19*(4), 474–483.

Salkind, N. J. (2010). *Statistics for people who (think they) hate statistics* (4th ed.). Thousand Oaks, CA: Sage.

Salkind, N. J. (2012). *Statistics for people who (think they) hate statistics: Excel 2010 edition.* Los Angeles, CA: Sage.

Sarkar, S. K., Midi, H., & Rana, S. (2011). Detection of outliers and influential observations in binary logistic regression: An empirical study. *Journal of Applied Sciences, 11,* 26–35.

Sawilowsky, S. (1990). Nonparametric tests of interaction in experimental design. *Review of Educational Research, 60,* 91–126.

Schrager, S. M., Wong, C. F., Weiss, G., & Kipke, M. D. (2011). Human immunodeficiency virus testing and risk behaviors among men who have sex with men in Los Angeles County. *American Journal of Health Promotion, 25*(4), 244–247. doi: 10.4278/ajhp.090203-ARB-43

Scott, W. (1955). Reliability of content analysis: The case of nominal scale coding. *Public Opinion Quarterly, 19*(3), 321–325.

Sedgwick, P. (2013). Case-control studies: Measures of risk. *British Medical Journal, 346,* f1185–f1185. doi: 10.1136/bmj.f1185

Sedgwick, P. (2014). Relative risks versus odds ratios. *British Medical Journal, 348,* 1407.

Shan, G., Ma, C., Hutson, A. D., & Wilding, G. F. (2012). An efficient and exact approach for detecting trends with binary endpoints. *Statistics in Medicine, 31,* 155–164.

Shan, G., & Wang, W. (2013). ExactCIdiff: An R package for computing exact confidence intervals for the difference of two proportions. *R Journal, 5,* 63–67.

Shan, G., & Wang, W. (2014). Exact one-sided confidence limits for Cohen's kappa as a measurement of agreement. *Statistical Methods in Medical Research, 0*(0), 1–17.

Shavelson, R. J., & Webb, N. M. (1991). *Generalizability theory: A primer.* Newbury Park, CA: Sage.

Sheskin, D. J. (2003). *Handbook of parametric and nonparametric statistical procedures.* Boca Raton, FL: CRC Press.

Siegel, S., & Castellan, N. J. (1988). *Nonparametric statistics for the behavioral sciences.* New York: McGraw-Hill.

Siegler, J. C., Rehman, S., Bhumireddy, G. P., Abdula, R., Klem, I., Brener, S. J., . . . Heitner, J. F. (2011). The accuracy of the electrocardiogram during exercise stress test based on heart size. *PLoS ONE, 6*(8), e23044. doi: 10.1371/journal.pone.0023044

Sim, J., & Wright, C. C. (2005). The kappa statistic in reliability studies: Use, interpretation, and sample size requirements. *Physical Therapy, 85*(3), 257–268.

Singer, B. (1979). Distribution-free methods for non-parametric problems: A classified and selected bibliography. *British Journal of Mathematical and Statistical Psychology, 32*(1), 1–60. doi: 10.1111/j.2044-8317.1979.tb00750.x

Slakter, M. J. (1965). A comparison of the Pearson chi-square and Kolmogorov goodness-of-fit test with respect to validity. *Journal of the American Statistical Association, 60,* 854–858.

Smirnov, N. V. (1939). Estimate of deviation between empirical distribution functions in two independent samples. *Bulletin Moscow University, 2*(2), 3–16.

Snoey, E., Housset, B., Guyon, P., ElHaddad, S., Valty, J., & Hericord, P. (1994). Analysis of emergency department interpretation of electrocardiograms. *Journal of Accident & Emergency Medicine, 11*(3), 149–153.

Spearman, C. (1904). The proof and measurement of association between two things. *American Journal of Psychology, 15,* 72–101.

Sprent, P., & Smeeton, N. C. (2001). *Applied nonparametric statistical methods* (3rd ed.). Boca Raton, FL: Chapman & Hall/CRC.

Stevens, J. (2009). *Applied multivariate statistics for the social sciences* (5th ed.). New York: Taylor & Francis.

Stevens, J. P. (2013). *Intermediate statistics: A modern approach.* New York: Routledge Academic.

Stevens, S. (1951). Mathematics, measurements and psychophysics. In S. S. Stevens (Ed.), *Handbook of experimental psychology* (pp. 1–49). New York: John Wiley.

Stevens, S. (1968). Measurement, statistics, and the schemapiric view. *Science, 161*(3844), 849–856.

Stevens, S. S. (1946). On the theory of scales of measurement. *Science, 103,* 677–680. doi: 10.1126/science.103.2684.677

Stoltzfus, J. C. (2011). Logistic regression: A brief primer. *Academic Emergency Medicine, 18*(10), 1099–1104. doi: 10.1111/j.1553-2712.2011.01185.x

Stone, R. A., Huffman, J., Istwan, N., Desch, C., Rhea, D., Stanziano, G., & Joy, S. (2011). Pregnancy outcomes following bariatric surgery. *Journal of Women's Health, 20*(9), 1363–1366. doi: 10.1089/jwh.2010.2714

Stork, C. M., Brown, K. M., Reilly, T. H., Secreti, L., & Brown, L. H. (2006). Emergency department treatment of viral gastritis using intravenous ondansetron or dexamethasone in children. *Academic Emergency Medicine, 13*(10), 1027–1033.

Strahan, R. F. (1982). Assessing magnitude of effect from rank-order correlation coefficients. *Educational and Psychological Measurement, 42,* 763–765.

Stroman, G. A., Stewart, W. C., Golnik, K. C., Curé, J. K., & Olinger, R. E. (1995). Magnetic resonance imaging in patients with low-tension glaucoma. *Archives of Ophthalmology, 113*(2), 168–172. doi: 10.1001/archopht.1995.01100020050027

Stuart, A. (1954). The efficiencies of tests of randomness against normal regression. *Journal of the American Statistical Association, 51,* 285–287.

Tabachnick, B. G., & Fidell, L. S. (2013). *Using multivariate statistics* (6th ed.). Boston, MA: Pearson.

Theodorsson-Norheim, E. (1987). Friedman and Quade tests: BASIC computer program to perform nonparametric two-way analysis of variance and multiple comparisons on ranks of several related samples. *Computers in Biology and Medicine, 17*(2), 85–99. doi: http://dx.doi.org/10.1016/0010-4825(87)90003-5

Thompson, G. L. (1991). A note on the rank transform for interactions. *Biometrica, 78,* 697–701.

Thompson, G. L., & Ammann, L. P. (1989). Efficiencies of the rank-transform in two-way models with no interaction. *Journal of the American Statistical Association, 84,* 325–330.

Thornbury, J. M. (1992). Cognitive performance on Piagetian tasks by Alzheimer's disease patients. *Research in Nursing & Health, 15*(1), 11–18. doi: 10.1002/nur.4770150104

Tomarken, A., Holland, J., Schachter, S., Vanderwerker, L., Zuckerman, E., Nelson, C., . . . Prigerson, H. (2008). Factors of complicated grief pre-death in caregivers of cancer patients. *Psycho-Oncology, 17*(2), 105–111.

Toothaker, L. E., & Newman, D. A. (1994). Nonparametric competitors to the two-way ANOVA. *Journal of Educational and Behavioral Statistics, 19*(3), 237–273.

Uebersax, J. S. (1982). A generalized kappa coefficient. *Educational and Psychological Measurement, 42,* 181–183.

Van den Broeck, C., Himpens, E., Vanhaesebrouck, P., Calders, P., & Oostra, A. (2008). Influence of gestational age on the type of brain injury and neuromotor outcome in high-risk neonates. *European Journal of Pediatrics, 167*(9), 1005–1009.

Vereecken, C., Covents, M., & Maes, L. (2010). Comparison of a food frequency questionnaire with an online dietary assessment tool for assessing preschool children's dietary intake. *Journal of Human Nutrition and Dietetics, 23*(5), 502–510. doi: 10.1111/j.1365-277X.2009.01038.x

Walsh, J. E. (1946). On the power function of the sign test for slippage of means. *Annals of Mathematical Statistics, 17*(3), 358–362.

Wang, H., & Akritas, M. G. (2004). Rank tests for ANOVA with large number of factor levels. *Journal of Nonparametric Statistics, 16*(3–4), 563–589.

Wang, W. (2006). Smallest confidence intervals for one binomial proportion. *Journal of Statistical Planning and Inference, 136,* 4293–4306.

Wang, W. (2010). On construction of the smallest one-sided confidence interval for the difference of two proportions. *The Annals of Statistics, 38, 1227-1243.*

Waninge, A., Evenhuis, I. J., van Wijck, R., & van der Schans, C. P. (2011). Feasibility and reliability of two different walking tests in people with severe intellectual and sensory disabilities. *Journal of Applied Research in Intellectual Disabilities, 24*(6), 518–527. doi: 10.1111/j.1468-3148.2011.00632.x

Waninge, A., van der Weide, W., Evenhuis, I. J., van Wijck, R., & van der Schans, C. P. (2009). Feasibility and reliability of body composition measurements in adults with severe intellectual and sensory disabilities. *Journal of Intellectual Disability Research, 53*(4), 377–388. doi: 10.1111/j.1365-2788.2009.01153.x

Warner, R. M. (2012). *Applied statistics: From bivariate through multivariate techniques* (2nd ed.). Los Angeles, CA: Sage.

Wessa, P. (2014). Free Statistics software. 1.1.23-r7. http://www.wessa.net

Whellan, D. J., Droogan, C. J., Fitzpatrick, J., Adams, S., McCarey, M. M., Andrel, J., . . . Keith, S. (2012). Change in intrathoracic impedance measures during acute decompensated heart failure admission: Results from the Diagnostic Data for Discharge in Heart Failure Patients (3D-HF) pilot study. *Journal of Cardiac Failure, 18*(2), 107–112.

Wilcox, R. R. (1992). Comparing the medians of dependent groups. *British Journal of Mathematical and Statistical Psychology, 45,* 151–162.

Wilcoxon, F. (1945). Individual comparisons by ranking methods. *Biometrics Bulletin, 1*(6), 80–83.

Williams, J. G., Allison, C., Scott, F. J., Bolton, P. F., Baron-Cohen, S., Matthews, F. E., & Brayne, C. (2008). The Childhood Autism Spectrum Test (CAST): Sex differences. *Journal of Autism & Developmental Disorders, 38*(9), 1731–1739.

Yates, F. (1934). Contingency tables involving small numbers and the χ^2 test. *Journal of the Royal Statistical Society, 1,* 217–235.

Yim, K. H., Nahm, F. S., Han, K. A., & Park, S. Y. (2010). Analysis of statistical methods and errors in the articles published in the *Korean Journal of Pain. Korean Journal of Pain, 23*(1), 35–41.

Zahniser, S. C., Gupta, S. C., Kendrick, J. S., Lee, N. C., & Spirtas, R. (1994). Tubal pregnancy and cigarette smoking: Is there an association? *Journal of Women's Health, 3*(5), 329–336.

Zhang, Y., Lee, E. T., Cowan, L. D., Fabsitz, R. R., & Howard, B. V. (2011). Coffee consumption and the incidence of Type 2 diabetes in men and women with normal glucose tolerance: The Strong Heart Study. *Nutrition, Metabolism, and Cardiovascular Diseases, 21*(6), 418–423.

Zhong, T., Fernandes, K. A., Saskin, R., Sutradhar, R., Platt, J., Beber, B. A., . . . Baxter, N. N. (2014). Barriers to immediate breast reconstruction in the Canadian universal health care system. *Journal of Clinical Oncology, 32*(20), 2133–2141.

Zhou, X. H., & Dinh, P. (2005). Nonparametric confidence intervals for the one- and two-sample problems. *Biostatistics, 6*(2), 187–200.

Zimmerman, D. W. (2012). A note on consistency of non-parametric rank tests and related rank transformations. *British Journal of Mathematical and Statistical Psychology, 65*(1), 122–144. doi: 10.1111/j.2044-8317.2011.02017.x

Zimmerman, D. W., & Zumbo, B. D. (1993). Relative power of the Wilcoxon test, the Friedman test, and repeated-measures ANOVA on ranks. *Journal of Experimental Education, 62*(1), 75–86.

Author Index

Abernathy, B., 282, 292, 311
Ackerman, I. N., 178, 197
Adams, S., 110
Ademi, Z., 178, 197
Afifi, A., 326-327, 328, 393
Agresti, A., 54, 56, 59, 400, 401
Akritas, M. G., 252, 253, 265
Alen, M., 120
Alesci, N. L., 280
Allison, C., 235
Allison, P. D., 324, 351, 393
Altman, D. G., 5, 125, 219, 334
Amarnath, S., 61
Ames, D., 280
Ammann, L. P., 253
Anders, M. E., 177
Anderson, E. S., 101, 110
Anderson, R. E., 37
Andrel, J., 110
Antozzi, C., 280
Apter, A., 319
Arbyn, M., 134
Armitage, P., 219, 220
Armstrong, G. D., 19
Arnold, S. F., 252
Artbuthnot, J. 3
Ayyangar, R., 135

Babin, C., 37
Bakeman, R., 281, 283, 285, 286
Balanda, K. P., 25
Balinger, C., 300
Balis, S. M., 300
Ball, J., 237
Barfield, J. P., 236, 251
Barnard, G. A., 163
Baron-Cohen, S., 235
Basta, T., 276, 280
Bathke, A., 401
Baxter, N. N., 395
Beach, E. K., 282, 292
Beber, B. A., 395
Becker, P. T., 197
Beeson, M. S., 293, 300
Belsley, D. A., 359
Bennett, B., 61
Bennett, B. M., 92
Benyamini, Y., 236, 251
Bernstein, I., 20
Berry, G., 219
Berry, J. G., 218, 219, 225
Berry, K. J., 163
Bewick, V., 237
Bhambhani, Y, 153, 163
Bhumireddy, G. P., 177
Biswas, A., 400
Biswas, T., 221
Black, R. L., 37
Blair, R. C., 119, 253
Blake, C., 111, 120
Bland, R. C., 334
Blaschke, A. J., 395
Bolton, P. F., 235
Bonkowsky, J. L., 218, 225
Bontempi, J. B., 153, 164
Borden, V. M., 134
Bowring, A. L., 111
Box, G. E. P., 340, 384-385
Brand, F. N., 75
Brayne, C., 235
Brener, S. J., 177
Brennan, P. F., 281
Brennan, R. L., 292
Breslow, N. E., 334
Bressan, E., 163
Brouwer, B., 251
Brown, K. M., 202, 218
Brown, L. D., 53, 54, 56, 59
Brown, L. H., 202, 218
Brunette, D., 111, 120

Brunner, E., 252, 253, 400, 401
Buchner, A., 11, 43, 339
Buck, J. L., 300
Buehler, R. J., 335
Bühlmann, P., 400
Bulmer, S. M., 153, 164
Burnette, K., 293, 300
Bursztein Lipsicas, C., 312, 319
Bush, J., 111, 120
Bushnik, T., 336, 395
Butar, F., 197
Byrne, B. M., 393, 400

Cai, J., 221
Cai, T. T., 53
Calders, P., 276, 280
Camilli, G., 163
Campbell, I., 175
Campbell, J. P., 87
Canto, J. G., 226, 235
Cao, H., 83, 87
Capio, C., 282, 292, 301
Capio, C. M., 311
Carey, A., 111, 120
Carifio, J., 19
Carleos, C., 401
Caroni, C., 252
Carr, 11, 111
Carter, C. L., 101, 110
Castellan, N. J., 8, 13-14, 43, 79, 82, 88, 92, 94, 110, 125, 126, 127, 134, 149, 155, 156, 170-171, 175, 196, 211, 226, 237, 238, 277, 278, 285, 303, 311, 312, 318
Cerulli, C., 153, 164
Chakraborti, S., 196
Chan, A. T., 251
Chandler, P. D., 251
Chaplin, D., 120
Charan, J., 221
Charoth, R. M., 202, 218, 225
Chaudron, L. H., 153, 165
Chazotte, C., 336, 394
Cheek, L., 237
Chumbler, N. R., 236
Cina, K., 111, 120
Clark, V. A., 326-327
Closas, P., 77, 83
Cochran, W. G., 61, 175
Cohen, E., 197
Cohen, J., 281, 285, 292
Collado, V., 153, 164
Collingridge, D., 197
Collins, J. V., 235
Coma, E., 83
Confalonieri, P., 280
Conover, W. J., 31, 76, 78, 85, 101, 137, 138, 143, 144, 149, 155, 177, 183, 196, 225, 237, 252, 253, 255, 261-262, 265
Cook, R. D., 390-391
Cornelio, F., 280
Corral, N., 401
Cortes-Simonet, E. N., 280
Coull, B. A., 54
Covents, M., 111
Cowan, L. D., 219, 225
Cox, D. R., 350
Cramér, H., 173-174, 276-280
Cronbach, L. J., 292
Cunningham, M. D., 120
Curé, J. K., 111

D'Agnostino, R. B., 75
Dalgleish, T., 270, 276
Damrosch, S. P., 293, 300
Daniel, W. W., 52, 75, 78, 83, 114, 158, 251, 277, 294, 300, 303, 309, 311, 312, 313, 318
Danvers, K., 153, 164
DasGupta, A., 53
Davison, A. C., 400
Day, N. E., 334
DCecco, J. V., 134
Debanne, S. M., 83
DeCarlo, L. T., 25
Deeks, J. J., 125
Deitz, J., 120
Delyzer, T. L., 178
Demir, S. G., 92, 101
DeMoivre, 3
Dexter, E., 251
Dickinson, J. C., 77, 83
Dinh, P., 183
Disbrow, D., 60
Domhof, S., 400
Donlan, W., 270, 275
Donner, A., 355
Doucette, J., 219, 225

Dow, B., 280
Drake, B. F., 251
Droogan, C. J., 110
Drory, Y., 236, 251
Dubnicka, S. R., 400
Dudley, H., 175
Dunn, O. J., 242-247
Duval, R., 400

Eaves, R. C., 270, 275
Edgington, E., 400
Elashoff, R. M., 163
ElHaddad, E., 101
Elizondo-Montemayor, L., 92, 101
Ellis, K., 280
Engstrom, G., 236, 251
Erdfelder, E., 11, 43, 339
Erdil, F., 92, 101
Eskander, J. P., 300
Eskander, M .S., 293, 300
Evans, D. P., 177
Evans, S., 111
Evenhuis, I. J., 111
Everitt, B. S., 285

Fabsitz, R. R., 219, 225
Fagerberg, I., 236, 251
Fagerland, M., 5, 177, 196
Fallin, A., 178, 197
Faul, F., 11, 43, 339
Faulks, D., 153, 164
Feinstein, A. R., 339
Fernandes, K. A., 395
Ferrando, S., 111
Feuer, E. J., 92, 100
Feurerman, M., 281
Fidell, L. S., 37, 38, 39, 44, 252, 324, 338-339, 340, 342, 343, 355, 356, 362, 363, 386, 393
Field, A., 183, 191, 255, 324, 331
Filipavičiūtė, R., 221
Finch, H., 401
Finner, S. L., 300
Fisher, R. A., 197
Fitzpatrick, J., 110
Fleiss, 71, 285, 286, 292
Foldes, S. S., 280
Forrester, L. W., 301, 311
Frederick, P. D., 235
Freelon, D., 290
Freeman, G., 163
Freeman, L. C., 300
Freidlin, B., 235
Froehle, T. C., 5
Fromm, R. E., 77, 83
Fuchs, C. S., 251
Fuqua, D. R., 5

Gaddis, G. M., 61, 75
Gaddis, M. L., 61, 75
Gaebler-Spira, D. J., 135
Gaffney, N., 111, 120
Gaither, N., 4, 5
Gardner, M. J., 331, 334
Garrett, N. A., 276, 280
Garson, G. D., 324, 348, 352, 359, 365
Gastwirth, J. L., 235
Gatty, C. M., 76
Gay, J. C., 395
Gel, Y. R., 401
Gerber, Y., 236, 251
Gibbons, J. D., 68, 196, 251
Gijbels, I., 400
Giladi, N., 77, 83
Gini, G., 312, 319
Glazer, W. M., 219, 225
Gleser, G. C., 292
Glöckner, M., 270, 275
Glorfeld, L., 4, 5
Glucksman, E., 270, 276
Glutting, J., 275
Godersky, J. C., 164
Goetz, A. M., 164
Goffman, D., 336, 394
Goldbourt, U., 236, 251
Golnik, K. C., 111
Good, P. I., 197, 400
Goodman, L. A., 82
Gorter, J. W., 124, 134
Gotch, F. M., 84, 87
Gottman, J. M., 281, 283, 285, 286
Graff-Radford, N. R., 164
Graham, D. A., 218, 225
Gratton, M. C., 87
Graves, K. D., 101, 110
Green, S., 125

Green, S. B., 281
Greenland, S., 219
Griffin, M. P., 83, 87
Grost, L., 48, 61, 76
Grunwald, P., 197
Guadagnolo, B. A., 111, 120
Gunn, A. J., 178, 197
Gupta, S. C., 61, 76
Gutierrez, N. G., 101
Guyon, P., 101

Haberman, S. J., 171
Haenszel, 219
Haglin, D., 111
Hahn, E. J., 197
Hahs-Vaughn, D. L., 329, 340, 343
Hair, J. F., 37, 38
Halton, J., 163
Han, K. A., 5
Han, L., 117
Harrison, E. A., 394
Harsham, J., 60
Harwell, M. R., 12
Hauck, N. W., 355
Hausdorff, J. M., 77, 83
Hayes, A. F., 290
Hayes, L., 75, 111, 120
Hays, W., 52, 53, 54, 68, 75, 156, 161, 276
Heitner, J. F., 177
Hempton, C., 276, 280
Hennequin, M., 153, 164
Hericord, P., 101
Herman, T., 83
Hettmansperger, T. P., 148, 196, 401
Higgins, J., 125
Higgins, J. J., 119, 253
Higgins, M., 275
Himpens, E., 276, 280
Hinds, P. S., 7, 20
Hinkelman, K., 123
Hinkle, D. E., 8, 170-171, 173, 211, 255, 272, 275, 276, 295
Hinkley, D. V., 400
Hintze, J., 11, 43, 60, 339
Hirji, K. F., 163
Hockenberry, M., 20
Hockenberry-Eaton, M., 20
Hodges, J. L., 117, 183
Holford, T. R., 339
Holland, J., 311
Hollis, B. W., 251
Hornick, C. W., 163
Horová, I., 400
Horton, N. J., 5
Hosmer, D. W., 324, 338, 340, 341, 342, 343, 348, 349-350, 355, 356, 357, 358, 359, 373, 391, 393, 400
Hothorn, L., 401
Housset, B., 101
Howard, B. V., 219, 225
Howard, C. M., 300
Howell, D. C., 67
Huebner, R. A., 61
Hutson, A. D., 59

Iman, R. L., 252, 253, 255, 261-262, 265

Jacobson, T. A., 125, 135
Jaffe, K. M., 120
Jagsi, J., 48
Jagsi, R., 61
James, A., 202, 218, 225
Jamieson, S., 19
Jankovic, A., 61
Jeffrey, P. K., 235
Jenis, L. G., 300
Jenkins, S. J., 5
Jewell, T., 164, 177
Jin, Z., 5
Johnson, A. F., 38
Johnson, A. O., 197
Johnson, K., 61
Jones, M. P., 164
Jongmans, M. J., 124, 134
Jooste, P. L., 226, 235
Jurs, S. G., 8, 170-171, 272

Kaartinen, M., 135
Kabaila, P., 59
Kallenberg, W. C. M., 75
Kallert, T. W., 270, 275
Kanotra, S., 164, 177
Kaplan, E. L., 400
Karns, L. B., 153
Kase, C. S., 75
Kasiulevi☒ius, V., 221

Katerndahl, D. A., 77, 83
Kay, A. B., 235
Keith, S., 110
Kellar, S. P., 8, 25, 26, 191, 324
Keller, J. H., 60
Kelly-Hayes, M., 75
Kelvin, E. A., 25, 26, 191, 324
Kemper, E., 339
Kempthorne, O., 123
Kendall, M. G., 311-319
Kendrick, J. S., 61, 76
Kerkhof, A., 319
Kessler, L. G., 92, 100
Ketelaar, M., 124, 134
Kiefe, C. I., 235
King, D. J., 84, 87
Kipke, M. D., 124, 135
Kleinbaum, D. G., 400
Klem, I., 177
Klosky, J. L., 153
Knapp, T. R., 19, 20
Koch, G. G., 286
Koch, S., 280
Koeslag, J. H., 270
Koláček, J., 400
Koliopoulos, G., 134
Kolmogorov, 39, 83
Konietschke, F., 401
Koop, D., 111, 120
Korosteleva, O., 400
Kothari, C. L., 202, 218, 225
Koval, 281
Krebs, H. I., 301, 311
Krippendorff, K., 281, 286, 290, 292
Kruskal, W. H., 37, 236
Kuh, E., 359
Kydd, A., 236, 251
Kyrgiou, M, 125, 134

Lackey, N. R., 337
Lake, D. E., 83, 87
Lambrew, C. T., 235
Landis, J. R., 286
Lang, A., 11, 43, 339
Langer, F., 400
Larsson-Sciard, E. L., 84, 87
Lash, T. L., 219
Lee, E. T., 219, 225
Lee, J., 270, 275
Lee, N. C., 61, 76
Lee, S., 394
Lee-Lin, F., 361, 394
Lehman, R. S., 25
Lehmann, E. L., 117, 119, 183, 400
Lemeshow, S., 349-350, 400
Lennon, O., 111, 120
Leonardi, M., 280
Lesher, K., 395
Levine, R. L., 77, 83
Lewing, N. W., 300
Liew, D., 178, 197
Lilliefors, H. W., 82
Lindeman, E., 124, 134
Linsay, C. A., 5
Lloyd, C. J., 59
Loerakker, S., 135
LoGiudice, D., 280
Lomax, R. G., 329, 340, 343
Lombard, C. J., 226, 235
Long, J. S., 339
Lowry, R., 163
Ludbrook, J., 175
Luthringer, L., 292

Ma, C., 59
MacGillivray, H., 25
MacKenzie, G., 400
Macko, R. F., 301, 311
Mactavish, J., 163
Madden, R. C., 336, 394
Maes, L., 111
Maggi, L., 280
Magnan, S. J., 280
Mäkinen, I. H., 319
Malmgren, J. A., 235
Malone, L. A., 236, 251
Maloney, B. H., 292
Manley, M. W., 280
Mansell, J. L., 270, 275
Mantegazza, R., 280
Mantel, N., 218
Mantinan, K., 48, 61, 76
Marascuilo, L. A., 183
Martínez, U., 101
Martinez-Camblor, P., 401
Martin-Hirsch, P., 134

Marwitz, J. H., 395
Matthews, F. E., 219, 235
May, S., 326-327
Mays, D., 361
McCain, G. C., 135
McCarey, M. M., 110
McDevitt, J., 275
McFadden, D., 350, 351, 395
McGuirck, J. M., 75
McIntosh, C. G., 178, 197
McKean, J., 401
McMurdo, M. E., 197
McNemar, Q., 153
Meier, P., 400
Meiser-Stedman, R., 270, 276
Melzer, C. W., 270
Menard, S., 338, 350, 351, 355, 357, 358, 359, 365, 376, 379, 391, 393, 400-401
Méndez, L., 77, 83
Menon, U., 394
Merkatz, I. R., 336, 394
Merrill, R. M., 5
Michel, K., 319
Midi, H., 357
Mielke, P. W., 163
Mier, N., 111, 120
Miletic, D., 101, 110
Millard, A. V., 120
Miller, A. R., 281
Milner, B., 270, 275
Molshatzki, N, 236, 251
Mooney, C. Z., 400
Mooney, K., 394
Moorman, J., 197
Moorman, J. R., 83, 87
Moreno, D. M., 101
Morgenstern, H., 219, 225
Morris, W. L., 153, 331, 334
Motomura, A. R., 61
Muder, R. R., 164
Mungo, R., 153, 164
Myers, J. L., 134

Nagelkerke, N. J., 350, 351
Nahm, F. S., 5
Nail, L., 394
Nanda, H., 292
Neave, H. R., 251
Nelson, C., 311
Nelson, F. C., 235
Neter, J., 10, 23, 25, 43, 75, 76, 77, 177
Neuman, M. I., 361, 395
Newcombe, R. G., 194, 333
Newman, D., 236, 251
Newman, D. A., 252, 253, 265
Newson, R., 117, 183
Ng, K., 236, 251
Nicolas, E., 153, 164
Niemeier, J. P., 395
Noguchi, K., 401
Nokes, N. R., 218, 219, 225
Norman, G., 19
Norman, G. R., 324, 326, 327, 328, 329, 333, 342, 386
Novack, C. M., 120
Nunnally, J. C., 20

Olinger, R. E., 111
Onghena, P., 400
Oosterhoff, J., 75
Oostra, A., 276, 280
Ory, M. G., 120
Osborne, J. W., 324, 329, 333, 336, 337, 338, 339, 343, 348, 352, 355, 357, 358, 359, 362, 363, 365, 381, 391, 393
Osborne, R. H., 178, 197
Ostojic, L., 101, 110
Overall, J. E., 163

Packer, T. L., 251
Pallin, D. J., 5
Pampel, F. C., 324
Paraskevaidis, E., 134
Parikh, K., 395
Park, H. M., 23, 25, 197
Park, S. Y., 5
Pastore, L. M., 153
Pearson, Karl, 3
Pedhazur, E., 19, 20, 38
Peduzzi, P., 339
Pell, G., 19
Peng, D., 400
Pepe, P. E., 83
Perla, R., 19
Perry, L. A., 293, 300

Petereit, D. G., 111, 120
Philip, P. A., 135
Piero, T., 312, 319
Platt, J., 395
Plocica, A. R., 292
Poduri, A., 218, 225
Politis, D. N., 400
Pollack, M. M., 61
Polonsky, M. J., 293, 301
Pousti, T. J., 120
Pozzoli, T., 312, 319
Preacher, K. J., 67
Prediger, D. J., 281
Pregibon, D., 391
Prendiville, W., 134
Price, A. E., 48, 61, 76
Price, J. W., 92, 101
Puri, M. L., 252, 253, 255, 261, 262

Quade, D., 149
Qualls, M., 5
Quine, S., 111, 120

Raggi, A., 280
Rajaratmam, N., 292
Ramundo, M., 293, 300
Rana, S., 357
Ratner, P., 61
Raynes, M. K., 197
Reading, James, 27-28
Reece, M., 276, 280
Reed, J. A., 48, 61, 76
Rehman, S., 177
Reilly, T. H., 202, 218
Rennie, L. M., 197
Rentinck, I. C. M., 124, 134
Renzaho, A. M., 293, 301
Riechers Ii, R. G., 312, 319
Rigby, A. S., 281
Riker, C., 197
Robichaud-Ekstrand, S., 44
Robinson, J. G., 125, 135
Robl, J., 164, 177
Rogers, W. J., 235
Romano, J. P., 400
Rosen, M. G., 77, 83
Rothman, K. J., 219, 220
Roy, A., 301, 311
Ruff, R. L., 312, 319
Ruff, S. S., 312
Ruff, S.S., 319
Ruttimann, U. E., 61

Salkind, N. J., 25, 191
Salls, J. S., 76
Salomone, J. A., 87
Sandvik, L., 177, 196
Šapoka, V., 221
Sarkar, S. K., 357, 359
Saskin, R., 395
Sauriol, A., 251
Sawilowsky, S., 265
Sawilowsky, S. S., 253
Schach, S. R., 270
Schachter, S., 311
Schmelkin, L., 19, 20, 38
Schmidtke, A., 319
Schneck, C., 61
Schrager, S. M., 124, 135
Schriever, B. F., 75
Schultz, M. M., 280
Schützwohl, M., 270, 275
Schuur, J. D., 5
Scott, F. J., 235
Scott, J. B., 251
Scott, W., 290
Secreti, L., 202, 218
Sedgwick, P., 329, 333
Sehy, Y., 44
Sekulic, D., 101, 110
Sen, P. K., 252, 253, 255, 261, 262
Shacham, E., 276, 280
Shah, S. S., 395
Shan, G., 59, 335
Shavelson, R. J., 292
Sheets, N., 61
Sherry, S. E., 292
Sheskin, 03, 255
Shields, E. C., 5
Shlipak, M. G., 235
Siegel, S., 8, 13-14, 43, 79, 82, 88, 92, 94, 110, 125, 126, 127, 134, 149, 155, 156, 170-171, 175, 196, 211, 226, 237, 238, 277, 278, 285, 303, 311, 312, 318
Siegler, J. C., 164, 177
Sills, J H., 120

Silverman, L. N., 76
Sim, 05, 281, 286
Singer, B., 3
Sit, C. H . P., 282, 292, 311
Slakter, 65, 82
Smeeton, N. C, 78, 183, 235, 236
Smirnov, N. V., 83
Smith, B. J., 125, 135
Smith, P., 270, 276
Snell, E. J., 350
Snoey, E., 93, 101
Spirtas, R., 61, 76
Sprent, P., 78, 183, 235
Squier, C., 164
Srivastava, R., 218, 225
Stavropoulos, A., 252
Stephenson, J., 111, 120
Stevens, J., 37, 393
Stevens, J. P., 255
Stevens, S., 19, 20
Stevenson, M., 293, 300
Stewart, W. C., 111
Stoddard, J., 5
Stoltzfus, J. C., 329
Stone, R. A., 153
Stork, C. M., 202, 218
Strahan, R. F., 309
Streiner, D. L., 324, 326, 327, 328, 329, 333, 342, 386
Stroman, G. A., 111
Stuart, A., 319
Stuhr, S., 197
Sullivan, J. J., 337
Sudtrahar, R., 395
Sweezy Ldel, C., 218, 225
Switzer, S. S., 5

Tabachnick, D. G., 37, 38, 39, 44, 252, 324, 338-339, 340, 342, 343, 355, 356, 362, 363, 386, 393
Talbot, N. L., 153, 164
Tamargo, D., 101
Tan, S.-J., 163
Tang, W., 153, 164
Tanguma, J., 120
Tatham, R. L., 37
Theodorsson-Norheim, E., 149
Thompson, G. L., 253, 265
Thompson, K., 77, 83
Thompson, S. G., 125
Thompson, W. R., 163
Thornbury, J. M., 84, 87
Tidwell, 62, 340, 384-385
Tierney, R. T., 275
Tomarken, A., 311
Tonkin, S. L., 178, 197
Toone, N., 275
Toothacker, L. E., 252, 253, 265
Touhy, T., 236, 251
Treviño, M., 101
Tucker, L. A., 218, 219, 225

Ubel, P. A., 61
Uebersax, J. S., 292
Underwood, R. E., 92
Utz, S., 292

Valty, J., 101
Vancour, M. L., 153, 164
Van den Broeck, C., 276, 280
Vanderbilt, J., 135
van der Schans, C. P., 111
van der Weide, W., 111
Vanderwerker, L., 311
Vanhaesebrouck, P., 276, 280
Vanlandewijck, Y, 163
van Wijck, R., 111
Vereecken, C., 111
Villareal, E. K., 120

Waffarn, F., 120
Wagener, M. M., 164
Wald, 354-355
Walker, W. C., 395
Wallis, W. A., 236
Walsh, J. E., 110
Wang, H., 265
Wang, S., 125, 135
Wang, W., 59, 335
Wang, X.-F., 312, 319
Waninge, A., 111
Warden, M. J., 120
Wardlaw, A. J., 235
Warner, R. M., 8, 10
Warren, S., 163
Wasserman, D., 319

Wasserman, W., 10, 23, 177
Watson, W. A., 87
Weaver, M., 292
Webb, N. M., 292
Webborn, A., 163
Weight, M. J., 226, 235
Weiss, G., 124, 135
Welch, C., 218, 225
Welsch, R. E., 359
Wessa, P., 317
Whellan, D. J., 101-102, 110
White, J. B., 134
Whitmore, G., 10, 23, 177
Wiersma, W., 8, 170-171, 272
Wilcox, R. R., 119
Wilcoxon, R. R., 111
Wilding, G. F., 59
Williams, D. J., 395
Williams, J. G., 235
Winett, R. A., 101, 110
Wolf, P. A., 75
Wong, C. F., 124, 135
Worthington, P. L., 251
Wright, C. C., 281, 286

Yates, F., 66-67
Yazdani, A., 178
Yim, K. H., 5
Yule, W., 270, 276

Zahniser, S. C., 61, 76
Zapf, A., 401
Zelinka, J., 400
Zeng, D., 221
Zhang, Y., 219, 225
Zhong, T., 336, 395
Zhou, J., 218, 225
Zhou, X. H., 183
Zielinski, R., 202, 218, 225
Zimmerman, D. W., 149, 196, 197
Zuckerman, E., 311
Zumbo, B. D., 149, 196

Subject Index

Academic Emergency Medicine, 218, 300
Advances in Mental Health, 275
Agreement, kappa coefficient and, 282. *See also* Kappa coefficient
Agresti-Coull interval, 54
Aids Care, 280
Alpha:
  null hypothesis and, 11
  setting, 10
  significant level, 9
Alternative hypothesis:
  binomial tests, 48
  chi-square tests and, 62, 165, 203
  Cochran's *Q* test and, 125-126
  Cramér's *V* coefficient, 277
  Fisher's exact test, 153-154
  Friedman test and, 136
  kappa coefficient, 282-283
  Kendall's tau coefficient, 312
  Kolmogorov-Smirnov one-sample test and, 77-78
  Kolmogorov-Smirnov two-sample test and, 84
  Kruskal-Wallis one-way ANOVA by rank, 236, 237 (fig.)
  Mantel-Haenszel chi-square test for trends, 220
  McNemar test and, 93-94
  Median test, 226-227
  phi coefficient, 270-271
  point biserial correlation, 293-294
  sign test and, 102
  simple bivariate regression, 336, 337 (tab.)
  Spearman rank-order correlation coefficient, 302
  two-way ANOVA by ranks, 253-254
  Wilcoxon-Mann-Whitney *U* test, 178-179
  Wilcoxon signed-rank test and, 112
American Journal of Clinical Nutrition, 235, 251
American Journal of Health Education, 164
American Journal of Health Promotion, 197, 218, 225, 280
American Journal of Infection Control, 164
American Journal of Occupational Therapy, 76
American Journal of Public Health, 218, 225
American Review of Respiratory Disease, 235
AMOS (computer program), 400
Analysis of covariance. *See* ANCOVA
Analysis of logistic regression, 343-349
Analysis of variance. *See* ANOVA
ANCOVA, 44
  alternatives to, 401
  error rate and, 13
Annals of Biomedical Engineering, 87
Annals of Emergency Medicine, 75, 83, 87
ANOVA:
  alternatives to, 401
  error rates and, 12-13
  two-way, 44
  two-way ANOVA by ranks. *See* Two-way ANOVA by ranks
Archives of Physical Medicine and Rehabilitation, 197, 120, 251
Association, determine strength of, chi-square test and, 210
Assumptions:
  parametric tests and, 2
  report assessment of and violation of, 44
  See also Critical assumptions

Bayesian interval, 56
Beta coefficients, standardized logistic regression, 376-379
Beta error, 11

Binary logistic regression, alternatives to, 393
Binomial probability calculator, 51
Binomial tests, 47-61
- advantages/limitations & alternatives to, 59-60
- confidence intervals for, 52-54
- critical assumptions of, 56-57
- examples from published research, 60-61
- output, computer-generated, 57-59
- overview of, 49-51
- presentation of results, 59
- research question for, 48
- sample size for, 60
- SPSS for Windows, commands, 54-56
- *z* approximation to, 51-52

BMC Medical Informatics and Decision Making, 83
Bonferroni adjustment, 133
Bonferroni correction, 125
Bonferroni's inequity, 133
Boxplots:
- figure, 35
- univariate outliers, assess with, 36-37

Box-Tidwell approach, 340
Box-Tidwell transformation, 384-385
Brain Injury, 275

Calculators:
- binomial probability, 51
- chi-square, 65-67, 217
- chi-square test for *K* independent samples, 205
- distress data, 155-156
- intensity of fatigue data, Wilcoxon-Mann-Whitney *U* test and, 180-183
- Kendall's tau coefficient from *X* and *Y* values, 315-316
- K-W test for diagnosis/awakenings, 238-241
- McNemar test, 99-100
- statistical, 50, 51 (fig.)

Cancer (research journal), 61
Cardiff University, 194
Categorical data, 4
Cell influence, examine residuals, chi-square test for *K* independent samples and, 211
Childhood Autism Spectrum Test (CAST), 226
Childhood Fatigue Scale (CFS), 20
Chi-square statistic, 354-355
Chi-square test, for two independent samples, 164-177
- advantages/limitations & alternatives for, 175-176
- analyzing residuals, 171
- contingency coefficient, Cramérs *V* and, 173-174
- critical assumptions for, 167-168
- determine strength of association between two variables, 172-174
- distress data, calculating for, 166-167
- examples from research, 177
- Internet resources for generating, 174-175
- null/alternative hypotheses, 165
- output, computer-generated, 168-171
- overview, 165-166
- phi coefficient and, 172-173
- presentation of results, 175
- research question, 164-165
- SPSS for windows commands, 168

Chi-square test, goodness-of-fit, 61-76
- advantages/limitations, alternatives to, 73-75
- collapse cells, eliminate minimum size violations, 72
- critical assumptions of, 67-69
- determining value of, using Internet, 65-67
- examples from research, 75-76
- null/alternative hypotheses and, 62
- output, computer-generated, 69-72
- overview of, 62-63
- presentation of results, 72-73
- research question for, 61
- SPSS for Windows, commands, 69
- table, interpreting, 63-65

Chi-square test for *K* independent samples, 202-218
- advantages/limitations & alternatives to, 217-218
- association, determine strength of, 210
- cell influences, examine residuals, 211
- computer commands, 206-207

contingency table, partitioning, 211-213
critical assumptions of, 205-206
examples from research, 218
Internet resources for generating, 213-217
null/alternative hypotheses, 203
output, computer-generated, 207-210
overview, 203-205
research question, 202-203
results, presentation of, 217
SPSS for Windows, 206-213
subtables, analyze partitioned, 213
CI. *See* Confidence interval
CINAHL database, 178, 236, 253, 301
Classification tables, 352-354
Clinical and Experimental Immunology, 87
Clinical Rehabilitation, 120
Cochran's *Q* test, 124-135
advantages/limitations & alternatives to, 134
critical assumptions of, 128-129
examples from research, 134-135
Internet resources to determine, 133
null/alternative hypotheses and, 125-126
output, computer-generated, 129-130
overview of, 126-128
presentation of results, 133-134
research question for, 124-125
SPSS for Windows, commands, 129-130
Coefficient of determination (R^2), 350-352
Cohen's kappa. *See* Kappa coefficient
Cohorts, 329
Comprehensive R Archive Network, 401
Computer-generated output. *See* SPSS software
Computer programs, statistical testing, 11, 43
Conditional logit analysis of qualitative choice behavior (McFadden), 395
Confidence intervals:
interpret, for odds ratio, 335
odds ratio, 333-335
relative risk, 331-332
Wilcoxon-Mann-Whitney *U* test and, 190-193
Wilcoxon-Mann-Whitney *U* test and, 183-185
Confidence intervals, binomial tests and, 52-54
Conover-Iman rank transformation, 261-262
Contingency table, partitioning, chi-square test for *K* independent samples and, 211-213
Contingency coefficient Cramér's *V* and, 173-174
Continuous probability distribution, 76
Cook's distance, 359, 390-391
Cook's leverage values, 357
Correlations, Mantel-Haenszel chi-square test for trends and, 222-224
Cox and Snell R^2, 350-351
Cox proportional hazards model, 400
Cramér's *V* coefficient, 173-174, 210, 276-280
advantages/limitations & alternatives to, 280
computer commands, 278
critical assumptions, 278
examples of research, 280
null/alternative hypotheses, 277
output, computer-generated, 278-279
overview, 277-278
research question, 276
results, presentation of, 279-280
SPSS for Windows, 278-279
Critical assumptions:
binomial tests, 56-57
chi-square tests, 67-69, 167-168, 205-206
Cochran's *Q* test, 128-129
Cramér's *V* coefficient, 278
Fisher's exact test, 156-158
Friedman test, 139
kappa coefficient, 287
Kendall's tau coefficient, 316
Kolmogorov-Smirnov one-sample test, 78-79
Kruskal-Wallis one-way ANOVA by rank, 241
Mantel-Haenszel chi-square test for trends, 221-222
McNemar test, 95-96
median test, 229
nonparametric tests and, 3-4
phi coefficient, 272
point biserial correlation, 295-296
sign test, 104
simple bivariate regression, 336-343

Spearman rank-order correlation coefficient, 306
two-way ANOVA by ranks, 255
Wilcoxon-Mann-Whitney *U* test, 185-186
Wilcoxon signed-rank test, 113-114
Cumulative Binomial Probability Calculator, 50, 51 (fig.)
Cumulative distributions, 77

DanielSoper.com, website, 50, 156, 174-175, 213
Data:
categorical, 4
characteristics of levels of measurement. *See also* Levels of measurement, 17-21
dichotomous. *See* Cochran's *Q* test
distress, for Chi-square test, for two independent samples, 166-167
distress, for Fisher's exact test, 155-156
intensity of fatigue, Wilcoxon-Mann-Whitney *U* test and, 180-183
parametric tests and (box), 2
transformation considerations, 38-39
Data transformations, 252. *See also* Transformation
Dbeta coefficient, 359
Deciles, 349-350
Decisions, in hypothesis testing (box), 9
Dependent variables, parametric tests and (box), 2
Detrended normal probability plot, 28-31
Deviance residuals, 358-359
DfBeta coefficient, 359
Dichotomous data. *See* Cochran's *Q* test
Dichotomous variables, 47
continuous probability, 76
McNemar test and, 92
Differences, among groups, 242-249
Disability & Rehabilitation, 134, 164, 292, 311
Discriminant analysis, 393
Distress data:
chi-square test, for two independent samples, 166-167
Fisher's exact test, 155-156
Distribution:
assessing shape of, Wilcoxon-Mann-Whitney *U* test, 187
exponential, 76
independent/dependent variables and, 235
Poisson, 76
theoretical cumulative, 77
uniform, 77
z approximation to binomial, 51-52
Distribution, normality of, 21-35
comparison of forms of (fig.), 24
dependent variable by subgroups, 33-35
kurtosis, 25-26
normal/detrended normal probability plots, 28-31
probability plot, examples, 31
shape of, 26-31
skewness, 22-25
statistical tests, normality, 31-33
Distribution-free tests, 2-3
Dummy-coded variables, 363
Dunn multiple comparisons procedure, 242-247

EPI Stat, 133
EpiTools, 221
Equidistant intervals, 19
Errors:
beta, 11
false positives/false negatives, 353
logistic regression and, 342-343
types, 10
See also Type I error; Type II error
European Archives of Psychiatry and Clinical Neuroscience, 275
European Journal of Pediatrics, 280
European Journal of Public Health, 319
Excel, Microsoft, 108, 194, 290
Expected frequencies, 340
Eyeball test, 27-28

False negatives, 353, 371
False positives, 353, 370-371
Fisher's coefficient, 25
Fisher's exact test, 100
advantages/limitations & alternatives to, 162-163
calculate distress data for, 155-156
critical assumptions of, 156-158
examples from research, 163-164
Internet resources for generating, 161-162

null/alternative hypotheses, 153-154
output, computer-generated, 158-161
overview, 154-155
parametric/nonparametric alternatives to, 163
presentation of results, 162-163
research question for, 153
SPSS for Windows, commands, 158
Fleiss's kappa, 290
Forced-entry, 362-363
Fragile X permutation test, 153
Freeman-Halton extension, Fisher's exact test, 163
Frequency:
data, 4
expected, 340
preintervention (fig.), 27
Friedman test, 44, 135-149, 401
advantages/limitations & alternatives to, 147-148
critical assumptions of, 139
null/alternative hypotheses, 136
output, computer-generated, 140-143
overview of, 136-139
parametric/nonparametric alternatives to, 148-149
post hoc comparisons, differences in rank and, 143-145
presentation of results, 146-147
research question for, 135
SPSS for Windows, commands, 139-140
F statistics, 252
F test, 125

Gerontology, 83
Gibbons, 85, 320
Glasgow Coma Score (GCS), 61
Goodness-of-fit statistics, 348
Goodness-of-fit tests:
binomial, 47-61. *See also* Binomial tests
chi-square. *See also* Chi-square tests, 61-76
classification tables for, 352-354
Hosmer-Lemeshow, 343, 348, 349-350, 369-370. *See also* Hosmer-Lemeshow goodness-of-fit
Kolmogorov-Smirnov one sample, 76-83. *See also* Kolmogorov-Smirnov one sample
Kolmogorov-Smirnov two-sample test. *See also* Kolmogorov-Smirnov two-sample test, 83-88
Google Scholar, 3, 164
G*Power 3 (software), 11, 43, 339
Grand median, 227
Grouping variable, 185-186
Groups:
differences among, 242-249
Hosmer-Lemeshow test, 349-350
nonparametric tests for (fig.), 266

Health care research, nonparametric tests and, 4-6
Health Psychology, 251
Heart & Lung: The Journal of Critical Care, 292
Heterogeneity, 125
Hierarchical entry, logistic regression, 363
Hodges-Lehmann confidence interval:
Wilcoxon-Mann-Whitney U test, 183
Wilcoxon signed-rank test, 117
Hodges-Lehmann estimator, 183, 185, 190
Homogeneity of variance, 39-42, 125
Homoscedasticity, parametric tests and (box), 2
Hosmer-Lemeshow goodness-of-fit test, 343, 348, 349-350
Hospital and Community Psychiatry, 225
Hypotheses, parametric tests and (box), 2. *See also* Alternative hypothesis; Null hypothesis

IBM registered trade mark, 43
Independence of errors, 357
Independent samples, chi-square test for *K*. *See* Chi-square test for *K* independent samples
Influence values, 359, 390
Intensity of fatigue data, Wilcoxon-Mann-Whitney *U* test and, 180-183
Interaction effects, impact on full model, 379-384
International Journal of Geriatric Psychiatry, 280
International Journal of Nursing Studies, 120
Internet resources for:
chi-square test for *K* independent samples, 213-217
Cochran's *Q* test, 133

determine outcome of McNemar test using, 99-100
chi-square test, for two independent samples, 174-175
Fisher's exact test, 161-162
free, x
Friedman test, 146
kappa coefficient, 290
Kruskal-Wallis one-way ANOVA by rank, 249
Mantel-Haenszel chi-square test for trends, 224
Median test, 234
multiple logistic regression, 366
phi coefficient, 274-275
point biserial correlation, 299
sign test, 106-108
Simple bivariate regression, 344-348
simple logistic regression, generate, 344-348
Spearman rank-order correlation coefficient, 309
two-way ANOVA by ranks, 262-264
Wilcoxon-Mann-Whitney *U* test, 194
Wilcoxon signed-ranks test, 118-119
See also Websites
Interobserver agreement, 281
Interpreting logistic regression analysis, 343-359
classification tables, 352-354
Hosmer-Lemeshow goodness-of-fit test, 349-350
influence values, 359
Internet resources for generating, 344-348
likelihood ratio test, 355-356
model chi-square, 348-349
odds ratio and confidence level, 356-357
R^2, 350-352
standardized/studentized residuals, 358-359
Wald statistic, 354-355
Interval levels of measurement, 19-20

Jeffrey's estimate, 56, 59
Journal of Abnormal Child Psychology, 275, 276
Journal of Accident & Emergency Medicine, 101
Journal of Addiction Medicine, 101
Journal of American Health Promotion, 120
Journal of Autism & Developmental Disorders, 235
Journal of Behavior Therapy and Experimental Psychiatry, 83
Journal of Bone & Joint Surgery, American Volume 94, 301
Journal of Cardiac Failure, 110
Journal of Clinical Nursing, 101
Journal of Clinical Oncology, 395
Journal of Community Health: The Publication for Health Promotion and Disease Prevention, 61, 76
Journal of Health Care for the Poor and Underserved, 120
Journal of Health Promotion, 135
Journal of Human Nutrition & Dietetics, 101
Journal of Obstetric, Gynecologic, & Neonatal Nursing, 394
Journal of Perinatology, 120, 394
Journal of Rehabilitation Research & Development, 251, 311, 319
Journal of the American College of Cardiology, 135
Journal of the American Diet Association, 60
Journal of the American Medical Association, 235
Journal of Women's Health, 76, 165

Kappa coefficient, 281-292
advantages/limitations & alternatives to, 292-
assessing, 285-287
critical assumptions, 287
examples from research, 292
null/alternative hypotheses, 282-283
output, computer-generated, 287-290
overview, 283-284
research question, 282
results, presentation of, 290-291
SPSS for Windows, 287-290
Kendall's coefficient of concordance (W), 149
Kendall's tau coefficient, 312-319

advantages/limitations & alternatives to, 318-319
calculating, from *X* and *Y* values, 315-316
computer commands, 316
critical assumptions, 316
examples from research, 319
Internet resources, for calculating, 317
null/alternative hypotheses, 312
output, computer-generated, 316-317
overview, 312-316
research question, 312
results, presentation of, 318
SPSS for Windows and, 316-317
Kernel density estimation, 400
Kolmogorov-Smirnov (K-S) Lilliefors statistics, 31-33, 35
Kolmogorov-Smirnov one-sample test, 76-83
advantages/limitations & alternatives to, 82
critical assumptions of, 78-79
examples, 83
null/alternative hypotheses, 77-78
output, computer-generated, 80-82
overview of, 78
presentation of results, 82
research question for, 77
SPSS for Windows, commands, 79-80
Kolmogorov-Smirnov two-sample test, 83-88
advantages/limitation & alternatives to, 88
critical assumptions of, 85
examples from published research, 88
null/alternative hypotheses, 84
overview of, 84-85
presentation of results, 88
SPSS computer commands, 85-86
Krippendorff's alpha, 290
Kruskal-Wallis one-way ANOVA by rank, 235-251
advantages/limitations & alternatives to, 250-251
calculate for diagnosis/awakenings, 238-241
computer commands, 241-242
critical assumptions, 241
Dunn multiple comparisons procedure, 242-247
examples from research, 251
group differences, 242-249
Holms step-down procedure for post hoc comparisons, 247-249
internet resources for generating, 249
null/alternative hypotheses, 236, 237 (fig.)
output, computer-generated, 242
overview, 236-241
pairwise comparisons, 246-247
research question for, 236
results, presentation of, 249-250
SPSS for Windows, 241-249
Kruskal-Wallis test, 225
K sample, 149
Kurtosis, 25-26
K-W. *See* Kruskal-Wallis one-way ANOVA by rank

Lancet, 134
Leptokurtic, 25
Leptokurtic distributions, 38-39
Levels of measurement:
best type of, 21
characteristics of (tab.), 18
interval, 19-20
nominal, 17-18
ordinal, 18-19
ratio, 20-21
Levene's test, 39, 261, 296
Leverage values, 357
Likelihood ratio, 56, 348
Likelihood ratio R^2, 351
Likelihood ratio test, 355-356, 372-373
Likert-type scale, 4
Linearity of the logit, 384-385
Logic, of logistic regression, 324-325
Logistic function, 326
Logistic regression, 61
interpreting analysis, 343-349
logic of, 324-325
logit function and, 326-328
maximum likelihood estimation, 329
multinominal, 338
multiple, 361-394. *See also* Multiple logistic regression
multiple linear *v.*, 325-326
odds ratio & relative risk, 329-335. *See also* Relative risk; Odds ratio

polytomous, 338
simple bivariate, 335-361. *See also* Simple bivariate regression,
Logistic transformation, 327
Logit function, logistic regression and, 326-328, 328
Log of the odds, 328
LR. *See* Logistic regression

Mahalanobis distance, 37
Mann-Whitney tests, 5, 83, 88
pairwise comparisons, 247, 248 (fig.)
See also Wilcoxon-Mann-Whitney
Mann-Whitney *U* tests, 398
MANOVA, 44, 401
Mantel-Haenszel chi-square test for trends, 218-225
advantages/limitations & alternatives to, 225
computer commands, 222
critical assumptions of, 221-222
examples from research, 225
Internet resources for generating, 224
null/alternative hypotheses, 220
overview, 220-221
research question, 219
results, presentation of, 224
SPSS for Windows, 222-224
Maternal & Child Health Journal, 177
Maximum likelihood estimation, logistic regression, 329, 341, 348
McFadden R^2, 351
McNemar test, 92-101
advantages/limitations & alternatives to, 100-101
critical assumptions of, 95-96
examples from published research, 101
null/alternative hypotheses, 93-94
outcomes, determine using website, 99-100
output, computer-generated, 96-99
overview of, 94-95
presentation of results, 100
research question for, 92-93
SPSS for Windows, commands, 96
Measurement, levels of. *See* Levels of measurement
Medcalc.org, website, 133
Median test, 225-235
advantages/limitations & alternatives to, 234-235
calculating, for T2 data, 228-229
computer commands, 230
critical assumptions, 229
data interpretation, cautions, 232-233
examples from research, 235
Internet resources for, 234
null/alternative hypothesis, 226-227
output, computer-generated, 230-233
overview, 227-229
research question for, 226
results, presentation of, 234
SPSS for Windows, 230-233
Medical Problems of Performing Artists, 110
MEDLINE database, 301
Medline database, 178, 236, 253
Mesokurtic, 25
Methods of entry, in logistic regression, 362-364
predictor variables, entering in blocks, 363
software-determined entry, 363-364
user-specific entry, 362-363
M-H test. *See* Mantel-Haenszel chi-square test for trends
Minimum sample size, 42-43
MLE. *See* Maximum likelihood estimation
Model chi-square test, 348-349
Model x^2, 366-369
Monte Carlo evaluation procedure, 12-13, 119, 339
Multicollinearity, 342, 386-387
Multi-item scale, 20
Multilevel modeling, 393
Multinominal logistic regression, 338, 393
Multiple linear regression, *v.* logistic regression, 325-326
Multiple logistic regression, 361-394
advantages/limitations & alternatives to, 393
binary logistic regression, alternatives, 393
classification tables, 370-372
Cook's distance, 390-391
Hosmer-Lemeshow goodness of fit test, 369-370

influence values, 390
interaction effects, impact of on full model, 379-384
Internet resources for, 366
likelihood ratio tests, 372-373
linearity of the logit, 384-385
methods of entry in, 362-364. *See also* Methods of entry, in logistic regression
model x^2, 366-369
multicollinearity, 386-387
odds ratio, confidence levels interpretation, 373-375
output, computer-generated, 364-391. *See also* Output, computer-generated
research examples, 394-395
research question, 361-362
residuals, 388-389
results, presentation of, 391-392
R^2 values, 370
Wald statistic, 372
Multivariate analysis of variance. *See* MANOVA
Multivariate outliers, assess, 37

Nagelkerke R^2, 352
Natural order, 313
Negative skew, 22-25
Neurological Sciences, 280
Neurology, 164
Neuropsychological Rehabilitation, 395
New England Journal of Medicine, 5
Nominal level of measurement, 17-18
Nondirectional alternative hypothesis, 77
Nonparametric longitudinal data, 401
Nonparametric receiver operating characteristic (ROC) curve, 401
Nonparametric statistics:
alternatives, to higher level techniques, 400-402
characteristics of, 3-4
development of, 2-3
for groups, 266
health care research and, 4-6
identified procedures for, 397-400
misperceptions about, 5-6
parametric tests, characteristics, 1-2
tests, summary of (tab.), 398
tests characteristics, 3
types of tests, 6
Nonparametric tests:
choosing parametric or, 12-16
situations suggesting use of (box), 14
when to use, 15-16
Normality:
of distribution, assessing, 21-35. *See also* Distribution, normality of
statistical tests of, 31-33
Normalized residuals, 358
Normal probability plot, 28-31
Null hypothesis:
alpha and, 11
in binomial tests, 48
chi-square tests and, 62, 165, 203
Cochran's *Q* test and, 125-126
Cramér's *V* coefficient, 277
Fisher's exact test, 153-154
Friedman test and, 136
kappa coefficient, 282-283
Kendall's tau coefficient, 312
Kolmogorov-Smirnov one-sample test and, 77-78
Kolmogorov-Smirnov two-sample test and, 84
Kruskal-Wallis one-way ANOVA by rank, 236, 237 (fig.)
Mantel-Haenszel chi-square test for trends, 220
McNemar test and, 93-94
Median test, 226-227
phi coefficient, 270-271
point biserial correlation, 293-294
sign test and, 102
simple bivariate regression, 336, 337 (tab.)
Spearman rank-order correlation coefficient, 302
statistical hypothesis testing and, 8-9
two-way ANOVA by ranks, 253-254
Wilcoxon-Mann-Whitney *U* test, 178-179
Wilcoxon signed-rank test and, 112
Nursing Older People, 251
Nursing Research, 197, 300
Nuisance factor, 123
Nutrition, Metabolism, and Cardiovascular Disease, 225

Observations:
- binomial testing and, 56
- interobserver agreement, 281
- parametric tests and (box), 2

Obstetrics and Gynecology, 83

Odds ratio, 218
- calculating, 332-333
- confidence interval, obtain for, 333-335
- interpret confidence interval, 335, 356-357, 373-375
- logistic regression and, 326
- *See also* Logistic regression; Relative risk

OLS regression, 324, 325-326. *See also* Logistic regression

OR. *See* Odds ratio

Ordinal level of measurement, 18-19, 393

Ordinary least squares (OLS), 324

Outcomes:
- hypothesis testing (box), 9
- McNemar test, using website, 99-100

Outliers, 35-38
- logistic regression and, 342
- multivariate, 37
- univariate, assess with boxplot, 36-37
- what to do about, 37-38

Output, computer-generated:
- binomial tests, 57-59
- chi-square test, for two independent samples, 168-171
- classification tables, 370-372
- Cochran's *Q* test, 129-130
- Cook's distance, 390-391
- Fisher's exact test, 158-161
- Friedman test, 140-143
- impact, of interaction effects on full model, 379-384
- influence values, 390
- Kendall's tau coefficient, 316-317
- Kolmogorov-Smirnov one-sample test, 80-82
- Kolmogorov-Smirnov two-sample test, 86-88
- Kruskal-Wallis one-way ANOVA by rank, 242
- likelihood ratio tests, 372-373
- linearity of the logit, 384-385
- for McNemar test, 96-99
- Median test, 230-233
- model χ^2, 366-369
- multicollinearity, 386-387
- odds ratio, confidence level, 373-375
- residuals, 388-389
- R^2 values, 370
- sign test, 106
- Spearman rank-order correlation coefficient, 307-309
- standardized logistic regression beta coefficients, 376-379
- two-way ANOVA by ranks, 258-262
- Wald statistics, 372
- Wilcoxon-Mann-Whitney *U* test, 188-190
- Wilcoxon signed-rank test, 114-117

Output, computer-generated:
- multiple logistic regression, 364-391
- point biserial correlation, 296-299

Overfitting, 340

Pairwise comparisons, 246-247

Palliative & Supportive Care, 110

Parametric test:
- choosing nonparametric or, 12-16
- nonparametric alternatives (tab.), 399

Parametric tests, characteristics, 1-2

PASS 12 (software), 11, 43, 60, 339

Pearson correlation coefficient, 173

Pearson correlation (*r*), 222-224, 272, 309, 311

Pearson product-moment correlation coefficient, 20, 44, 172, 175, 278, 311, 398. *See also* Pearson correlation (*r*)

Pearson residuals, 358-359

Pearson skewness coefficient, 25

Pediatrics, 197, 319, 395

Percentage agreement, 281

Phi coefficient, 269-276
- advantages/limitations & alternatives to, 275
- chi-square test, for two independent samples and, 172-173
- computer commands, 272
- critical assumptions, 272
- examples of research, 275-276
- Internet resources for generating, 274-275
- null/alternative hypotheses, 270-272
- output, computer-generated, 272-274

overview, 271-272
research question, 270
results, presentation of, 275
SPSS for Windows, 272-274
Physical Therapy, 197
Platykurtic, 25
Platykurtic distributions, 38-39
PLoS Medicine, 218, 225
PLoS ONE, 164, 177
Point biserial correlation, 293-301
advantages/limitations & alternatives to, 300
critical assumptions of, 295-296
examples from research, 300-301
Internet resources for generating, 299
null/alternative hypotheses, 293-294
output, computer-generated, 296-299
overview, 294-295
p value, 298
research question for, 293
results, presentation of, 300
SPSS for windows, 296-299
t statistic, 298
Poisson distributions, 76
Polytomous logistic regression, 338
Positive skew, 22-25
Post hoc comparisons:
Friedman test and, 143-144
Kruskal-Wallis one-way ANOVA by rank, 247-249
Power efficiently, of statistical tests, 13-14, 110, 148
Predictor variables, entering in blocks, 363
Preintervention fatigue (fig.), 27, 32, 33
Pretest-posttest measures of single sample:
McNemar test, 92-101. *See also* McNemar test
sign test. *See also* Sign test, 101-110
Wilcoxon signed-ranks test, 111-120. *See also* Wilcoxon signed-ranks test
Probability. *See* Relative risk
Probability plots, 28-31
normal (fig.), 32
Protective effect, 373, 374
Psuedo-R^2, 350-352, 370
PsychInfo database, 178, 236, 253, 301
Psycho-Oncology, 311
Pub Med, 164
Puri-Sen approach, to transformation, 262
P value, point biserial correlation and, 298-299

Quade test, 149
Quantpsy.org. website, 65-67, 217
Question(s). *See* Research question

Randomized block design, 123
Rank differences, post hoc comparisons Friedman test and, 143-144
Rank ordering, of scores, 4
Rank-transformed tests, 252-253
Ratio:
likelihood, 56
odds. *See* Odds ratio
Ratio levels of measurement, 20-21
ReCal, 290
Regression:
diagnostics, 357
logistic, 61
Relative risk:
calculating, 329-333
confidence level for, obtain, 331-332
defining, 329-330
See also Logistic regression; Odds ratio
Research alternative, stating, 8
Research examples:
binomial test, 60-61
chi-square test, 75-76
chi-square test, for *K* independent samples, 218
chi-square test, for two independent samples, 177
Cochran's *Q* test, 134-135
Cramér's *V* coefficient, 280
Fisher's exact test, 163-164
hypothetical, 7-8
kappa coefficient, 292
Kendall's tau coefficient, 319
Komogorov-Smirnov one-sample test, 83
Komogorov-Smirnov two-sample test, 88
Kruskal-Wallis one-way ANOVA by rank, 251
Mantel-Haenszel chi-square test for trends, 225
McNemar, 101
Median test, 235

multiple logistic regression, 394-395
phi coefficient, 275-276
point biserial correlation, 300-301
sign test, 110
Spearman rank-order correlation coefficient, 311
Wilcoxon signed-ranks test, 120
Research in Nursing and Health, 87
Research question:
binomial test, 48
chi-square test, 61
chi-square test, for *K* independent samples, 202-203
chi-square test, for two independent samples, 164-165
Cochran's *Q* test, 124-125
Cramér's *V* coefficient, 276
Fisher's exact test, 153
Friedman test, 135
kappa coefficient, 282
Kendall's tau coefficient, 312
Kolmogorov-Smirnov one-sample test, 77
Kolmogorov-Smirnov two-sample test, 83-84
Kruskal-Wallis one-way ANOVA by rank, 236
Mantel-Haenszel chi-square test for trends, 219
Median test, 226
Multiple logistic regression, 361-362
phi coefficient, 270
point biserial correlation, 293
simple bivariate regression, 336
Spearman rank-order correlation coefficient, 301
two-way ANOVA by ranks, 253
Wilcoxon-Mann-Whitney *U* test, 177-178
Wilcoxon signed-rank test, 111-112
Research report, report testing assumptions/violations in, 44
Residuals:
cell influences, examine, 211
output for, 388-389
standardized/studentized, 358-359
Respiratory Care, 177
Results, presentation of:
binomial test, 59
chi-square test, 73-74
chi-square test, for *K* independent samples, 217
chi-square test, for two independent samples, 175
Cochran's *Q* test, 133-134
Cramér's *V* coefficient, 279-280
Fisher's exact test, 162
Friedman test, 146-147
kappa coefficient, 290-291
Kendall's tau coefficient, 318
Kolmogorov-Smirnov one-sample- test, 82
Kolmogorov-Smirnov two-sample- test, 88
Kruskal-Wallis one-way ANOVA by rank, 249-250
Mantel-Haenszel chi-square test for trends, 224
McNemar test, 100
Median test, 234
multiple logistic regression, 391-392
phi coefficient, 275
point biserial correlation, 300
sign test, 108-110
simple bivariate regression, 360
Wilcoxon-Mann-Whitney *U* test, 195-196
Wilcoxon signed-ranks test, 119
Reverse natural order, 313
Revised Trauma Score (RTS), 61
R^2 values, 370
Risk. *See* Relative risk

SamplePower3.0.1 (software), 11, 43, 60
Sample size:
binomial tests, 60
estimate requirements, 11
minimum, 42-43
parametric tests and, 2
Scale(s). *See* Levels of measurement
Score(s), rank ordering of, 4
Scot's Pi, 290
Self-Estimated Functional Inability Because of Pain (SEFIP), 101
Sensitivity, 353, 371
Shapiro-Wilks statistics, 31-33, 35
Significant level, 8
Sign test, 101-110
advantages/limitations & alternatives to, 110
critical assumptions of, 104
examples from research, 110

hand-calculating value of, 103-104
null/alternative hypotheses, 102
output, computer-generated, 106
overview of, 102-103
presentation of results, 108-110
research question for, 101-102
SPSS for Windows, commands, 104-105
using Internet to determine outcome of, 106-108
Simple bivariate regression, 335-361
advantages/limitations & alternatives to, 360-361
critical assumptions, 336-343
Internet resources, to generate, 344-348
interpreting logistic regression analysis, 343-359. *See also* Interpreting logistic regression analysis
null/alternative hypotheses, 336, 337 (tab.)
research question for, 336
results, presentation, 360
SPSS for Windows, 343-349
Size measure, effective, Wilcoxon-Mann-Whitney *U* test and, 194-195
Skewness, 22-26
Smoothing, kernel density estimation methods, 400
Software determined entry, logistic regression, 363-364
Spearman rank-order correlation coefficient, 301-311
advantages/limitations & alternatives to, 311
computer commands for, 307
critical assumptions of, 306
determining relationship strength, 309
examples from research, 311
Internet resources for generating, 309
null/alternative hypotheses for, 302
output, computer-generated, 307-309
overview, 302-306
research question for, 301
results, presentation of, 309-311
SPPS for Windows and, 307-309
Spearman rho coefficient, 222-224, 225, 398
Specificity, 353
SPSS® for Windows (software), 11, 43, 54
binomial tests in Windows, 54-56, 57-59
boxplots, univariate outliers and, 36-37
chi-square test, commands, 69-72
Chi-square test, for two independent samples, 168-171
chi-square test for *K* independent samples, 206-213
classification tables, 352-353
Cochran's *Q* test and, 129-133
coefficient of determination and, 350-351
Cramér's *V* coefficient, 278-279
distributions of dependent variable by subgroup, 33-35
Fisher's exact test, 158-161
frequencies and histograms, 27-28
Friedman test and, 139-143
interpreting logistic regression analysis, 343-349
kappa coefficient, 287-290
Kendall's tau coefficient, 316-317
Kolmogorov-Smirnov one-sample test, 79-82
Kolmogorov-Smirnov two-sample test and, 85-88
Kruskal-Wallis one-way ANOVA by rank, 241-249
Levene's test, 39-42
likelihood ratio test, 355-356
Mantel-Haenszel chi-square test for trends, 222-224
McNemar test and, 96-99
Median test, 230-233
Multiple logistic regression, 364-391. *See also* Output, computer-generated
odds ratio/confidence level, interpret, 356-357
output for binomial test (fig.), 58
pairwise comparisons, 247
phi coefficient, 272-274
platykurtic/leptokurtic distributions, 38-39
point biserial correlation, 296-299
post hoc differences, comparing in, 144-145
sign test and, 104-106
Spearman rank-order correlation coefficient, 307-309
standardized/studentized residuals, 358-359
T2 data, calculating for, 228-229
tests of normality and, 31-33

two-way ANOVA by ranks, 255-262
using, 21-22
Wald statistics, 354-355
Wilcoxon-Mann-Whitney *U* test, 186-193
Wilcoxon signed-rank test and, 114-117
Standardized logistic regression beta coefficients, 376-379
Standardized residuals, 358-359
Statistical hypothetical testing:
hypothesis, possible outcomes (box), 9
steps in (box), 8
Statistical test, determine power of, 13-14
Statistics calculators, 50
Statpages.org, website, 133
Stepwise backward, 364
Stepwise forward, 363
Stroke (Framingham Study), 75
Structural equation modeling, 393
Studentized residuals, 358-359
Subgroups:
distribution, dependent variables and, 33-35
equal number of subjects within, 43-44
Subtables, analyze partitioned, chi-square test for *K* independent samples, 213

Tetrachoric correlation, 275
Transformation
Box-Tidwell, 384-385
logistic, 327
Transforming data, 38-39
Conover-Iman rank transformation, 261-262
Puri-Sen approach, 262
Transfusion Medicine, 301
Trends. *See* Mantel-Haenszel chi-square test for trends
T statistic, calculating, point biserial correlation and, 298
T test, 119
Two independent samples. *See* Chi-square test, for two independent samples
Two-way ANOVA, 44
Two-way ANOVA by ranks, 251-265
advantages/limitations & alternatives to, 265
computer commands, 255-258
Conover-Iman rank transformation, 261-262
critical assumptions of, 255
data transformations, 252
Internet resources for, 262-264
null/alternative hypotheses, 253-254
output, computer-generated, 258-262
overview, 254-255
Puri-Sen approach, 262
rank-transformed tests, 252-253
research question, 253
results, presentation, 264
Wald-type/weighted *F* statistics, 252
Type I error, 10, 12-13, 353
Type II error, 10, 353

Uniform distribution, 77
Univariate outliers, 36-37
Up-and-Go Scale, 77
User-specific entry, in logistic regression, 362-363

Variables:
determining strength of association between two, 172-174
dichotomous, 47
distribution and, 235
dummy-coded, 363
grouping, 185-186
Hosmer's seven-step process for selecting meaningful independent (tab.), 341
level of measurement of, in tests, 14
logistic regression analysis, 343-344
predictor, entering in bocks, 363
ratio-level, 20-21
simple bivariate regression and, 338
Variance, homogeneity of, 39-42
Vassarstats.net, 99-100, 156, 163, 174-175, 213, 249

Wald interval, 53, 54
Wald statistic, 354-355, 372
Wald-type, 252
Websites:
ams.med.uni-goettingen.de, 401
cardiff.ac.uk, 194
CRAN.R-project.org, 401
danielSoper.com, 50, 174-175, 213
danielsoper.com, 156
determine outcome of McNemar test using, 99-100

EpiTools, 221
justusrandolph.net, 290
medcalc.org, 133
medicine.cf.ac.uk, 194
ncbi.nlm.nih.gov, 10
obg.cuhk.edu, 290
quantpsy.org, 65-67, 217
socr.ucla.edu, 108, 118-119, 146, 194
statpages.org, 133
vassarstats.net, 99-100, 156, 163, 174-175, 213, 249, 344
wessa.net, 317
xlstat.com, 133

Weighted *F* statistics, 252
Weighted kappa, 292
Wilcoxon-Mann-Whitney (WMW) test, 44, 101
Wilcoxon-Mann-Whitney *U* test, 177-197
advantages/limitations & alternatives to, 196-197
assessing shape of distributions, 187
calculating for intensity of fatigue data, 180-183
computer commands, 186-187
confidence interval, 95%, differences in medians and, 190-193
confidence interval for median of differences, 183-185
critical assumptions of, 185-186
examples from research, 197
Internet generated (fig.), 193
Internet resources for generating, 194
null/alternative hypotheses, 178-179
output, computer-generated, 188-190
overview, 179-180
presentation of results, 195-196
research question, 177-178
size measure, obtain effective, 194-195
SPSS for windows and, 186-193

Wilcoxon-Mann-Whitney (WMW) test, 13
Wilcoxon signed-rank tests, 101, 111-120
advantages/limitations & alternatives to, 119
critical assumptions of, 113-114
examples, research, 120
Friedman test and, 149
hand-calculating value of, 113
Hodges'-Lehmann confidence interval for, 117
null/alternative hypotheses, 112
outcome, Internet resources to determine, 118-119
output, computer-generated, 114-117
overview of, 112-113
presentation of results, 119
research question for, 111-112
SPSS for Windows, commands, 114

WMW test, 13

Xlstat.com, 133

Yates correction, 170-171

Z approximation, binomial distribution and, 51-52
Z statistic, 354-355